ABRAHAM E. NIZEL, D.M.D., M.S.

Professor Emeritus in Nutrition and Preventive Dentistry
Tufts University, School of Dental Medicine

ATHENA S. PAPAS, D.M.D., PH.D.

Assistant Professor in General Dentistry
Co-Director Division of Geriatric Dentistry
Director of Oral Health Management Clinic
Tufts University, School of Dental Medicine

Nutrition
in
Clinical
Dentistry

THIRD EDITION

1989

W. B. SAUNDERS COMPANY

Harcourt Brace Jovanovich, Inc.

Philadelphia   London   Toronto
Montreal   Sydney   Tokyo

W. B. SAUNDERS COMPANY
Harcourt Brace Jovanovich, Inc.

The Curtis Center
Independence Square West
Philadelphia, PA 19106

Library of Congress Cataloging in Publication Data

Nizel, Abraham E.

Nutrition in clinical dentistry/Abraham E. Nizel, Athena S.
Papas.—3rd ed.   p.   cm.

Includes bibliographies and index.

1. Nutrition and dental health.   I. Papas, Athena S.
II. Title. [DNLM: 1. Dentistry.   2. Nutrition.
WU140 N735n]

RK281.N58 1989   617.6'01   DNLM/DLC   88–31853 CIP

ISBN 0–7216–2423–5

Listed here are the latest editions of this book together with the language of the
translation and the publisher.

Japanese *(1st Edition)*—Gakuken Shoin Ltd., Tokyo, Japan

Editor: John Dyson
Designer: Terri Siegel
Production Manager: Pete Faber
Manuscript Editor: Judith Gandy
Illustration Coordinator: Lisa Lambert
Indexer: George Vilk

Nutrition in Preventive Dentistry: Science and Practice   ISBN   0–7216–2423–5

Last digit is the print number: 9   8   7   6   5   4   3   2   1

Preface

In this third edition of "Nutrition in Clinical Dentistry," we have continued the format of the previous editions of "Nutrition in Clinical Dentistry" and "Nutrition in Preventive Dentistry: Science and Practice." Essentially, we have covered (1) relevant advances in the science of food and nutrition and (2) the application of this knowledge to nutrition counseling of patients who want to prevent or control dental-oral problems such as dental caries, dental erosions, stomatitis, glossitis, periodontal disease, and other nutrition-related oral health problems. The procedures used in nutrition counseling evolved from experience gained in private dental practice and from feedback from predoctoral students in the Preventive Dentistry Counseling Clinic at Tufts University School of Dental Medicine.

Dr. Athena S. Papas, the co-author of this book, matriculated at the Massachusetts Institute of Technology in the Oral Science section of the Department of Nutrition and Food Science when I was Visiting Associate Professor in the same department. In addition to enjoying the benefits from the guidance and teachings of Professors Robert S. Harris and Nevin S. Scrimshaw, both she and I had the good fortune to be associated with Drs. Sanford Miller and Juan Navia, two scholars and superb researchers in nutrition and dental-oral health.

After Dr. Papas received her Ph.D. in nutrition from MIT, she continued her graduate studies at Harvard University School of Dental Medicine, from which she received a doctorate in dental medicine. She is now assistant professor in general dentistry at Tufts University School of Dental Medicine where she engages in research, teaching, and clinical supervision.

From the foregoing, it is evident that our paths have crossed many times in the past and fortuitously we are now co-authors of this third edition of "Nutrition in Clinical Dentistry."

This book is written for both the student and the practitioner of dentistry or dental hygiene who want updated knowledge of the science and practice of nutrition and the effects of nutrients, foods, and diet on both oral and general health. Nutritionists who want to serve as consultants for dentists will find this book helpful because it explains the nature and mechanisms involved in common dental-oral health problems such as dental caries and periodontal disease.

We are grateful to our typists Donna Russell and Donald J. Hamm, and to the competent editors and production staff members of the W.B. Saunders Company for their expertise and guidance in helping to make this book a reality.

We especially express our appreciation to our respective mates, Jeanette Nizel and Arthur Papas, for their encouragement, patience, and cooperation, which helped make what at times seemed impossible not only possible but fulfilling.

ABRAHAM E. NIZEL

Contents

11

12

13

14

15

16

17

18

19

20

Appendix 1

1

Energy Values of Foods and Nutrients; Obesity; Rules for Achieving Desirable Weight

Because energy is of prime importance in the life processes, the study of nutrition is concerned with the basic question of how the human body metabolizes or transforms the elements of food into energy.

In fact, our need for energy has such a high priority that a nutrient such as protein—whose primary function is to build tissue—can be used to provide energy when adequate amounts of carbohydrates and fats—the usual nutrient energy sources—are not eaten. Thus one of the fundamental requirements for life is to obtain adequate sources of food for energy.

The energy from food is made available to the body in four basic forms: chemical, for synthesis of new compounds; mechanical, for muscle contraction; electrical, for brain and nerve activity; and thermal, for regulation of body temperature. These various forms of energy are converted from one to another. Humans are inefficient energy users because they can convert only 25% of chemical energy from the food they eat into mechanical energy (walking, typing, and so forth). Most of the energy is dissipated as heat.

ENERGY VALUE OF FOODS AND NUTRIENTS

Because heat is produced by the transformation of food energy to body energy, calories are used as units of energy measurement. In nutrition, we measure energy in kilocalories (kcal, formerly Calories, or large calories), which provide 1000 times the heat of the gram (g), or small calorie, used in chemistry. Thus the nutritional kilocalorie is defined as the amount of heat required to raise the temperature of 1 kilogram (kg) (2.2 lb) of water 1°C (from 14.5 to 15.5°C). When the International System (SI) is used, the unit of energy is the joule (J); 1 kcal = 4.18 kilojoule (kJ).

The energy value of a food depends on the relative amounts of carbohydrate, fat, protein, and alcohol it contains. To determine the heat produced by the combustion of a food, a weighed amount is placed in a device called a bomb calorimeter, which is charged with oxygen and submerged in 1 kg of water. When the food is ignited, its combustion produces heat, causing the temperature of the water to rise. The temperature increase multiplied by the volume of water gives the amount of heat liberated, or the number of calories present in the food sample.

Because the heat of combustion of a food is not the same as the available energy from an absorbed food, Atwater, who initiated calorimetry in the United States, corrected the caloric values of the average heats of combustion of the pure nutrients, which he expressed in kilocalories per gram: carbohydrate, 4.1; fats, 9.45; protein, 5.65; and alcohol, 7.1. More oxygen is required to burn fats and alcohol, because they contain relatively large amounts of carbon and hydrogen; therefore they release much more heat than do carbohydrates and proteins. The Atwater corrected caloric values are

carbohydrates	4 kcal/g or	17 kJ/g
proteins	4 kcal/g or	17 kJ/g
fats	9 kcal/g or	38 kJ/g
alcohol	7 kcal/g or	30 kJ/g

The kcal and cal values of commonly used foods can be found under the heading Food Energy in Appendix 1.

ENERGY NEEDS OF THE BODY

The overall energy needs of the body are calculated to be the sum of three factors: (1) basal metabolism, (2) energy for physical activity, and (3) a small amount of additional energy expended during digestion and absorption of carbohydrates, proteins, and fats in the gastrointestinal tract, called the specific dynamic action, or SDA, of food. Thus the energy requirement = basal metabolism + physical activity + SDA.[1] Specific dynamic action is explained in greater detail later in this chapter.

Basal Metabolism and Basal Metabolic Rate

Basal metabolism is the minimum amount of energy needed to regulate and maintain the involuntary essential life processes, such as breathing, beating of the heart, circulation of the blood, cellular activity, keeping muscles in good tone, and maintaining body temperature. This is the amount of energy expended by the body when lying quietly in a comfortable environmental temperature, relaxed but awake, and 12 to 15 hours after the last meal. Energy expenditure measured under the same conditions but at different intervals after eating is called resting metabolism.

The basal metabolic rate (BMR) is defined as the number of kilocalories expended by the organism per square meter of body surface per hour (kcal/m^2/hour). It is determined by body size, age, sex, and secretions of endocrine glands.

Basal metabolic expenditure varies in accordance with the body surface area. Because of the difficulty of actually measuring the body surface area, it has been computed by a mathematical equation. The nomogram in Figure 1–1 shows body surface area according to the height, weight, sex, and age of an individual,[2] together with the corresponding number of calories per day necessary for basal metabolism.

The BMR is higher in young people. It increases for some months after

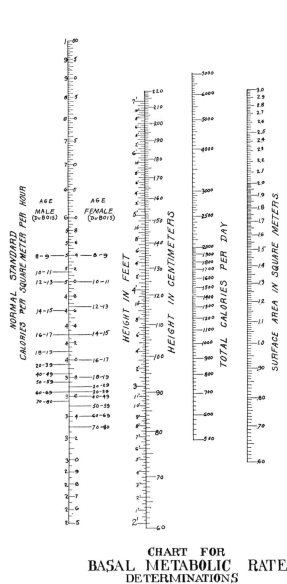

NORMAL STANDARD
CALORIES PER SQUARE METER PER HOUR

AGE MALE (DuBOIS)

AGE FEMALE (DuBOIS)

HEIGHT IN FEET

HEIGHT IN CENTIMETERS

TOTAL CALORIES PER DAY

SURFACE AREA IN SQUARE METERS

WEIGHT IN POUNDS

WEIGHT IN KILOGRAMS

CHART FOR
BASAL METABOLIC RATE
DETERMINATIONS

TOTAL BASAL CALORIES PER DAY

W.M.BOOTHBY   R.B.SANDIFORD
FEBRUARY 1921.

FIGURE 1–1. *This nomogram can be used to derive the basal metabolic expenditure (Scale V. Total Calories per Day) of normal adults whose height and weight are known. Use only a ruler with a true straight edge. Locate the person's normal weight on Scale I and his height on Scale II. The ruler joining these two points intersects Scale III at the person's Surface Area in Square Meters. Locate the age and sex of the person on Scale IV. A ruler joining this point with the person's Surface Area on Scale III crosses Scale V at the basal energy requirement. To convert Calories (kcal) to kJ, multiply by 4.184. (Nomogram of Boothby, W. M., et al. Am. J. Physiol. 116:468, 1936.)*

3

birth, then decreases (at first rapidly but later more gradually) through adolescence. In adults there is a still slower decline in BMR with increasing age.

The basal metabolism of healthy men requires about 1600 to 1800 kcal (6500 to 7500 kJ) daily; basal expenditure of women is about 1200 to 1450 kcal (5000 to 6000 kJ). Basal energy expenditure increases with increased lean body mass, which is higher in males than in females and which probably contributes to the higher BMR for men.

Thyroxine, the iodine-containing hormone secreted by the thyroid gland, regulates the rate of cellular oxidation and thus the rate of metabolism of cells. Chemically, the iodine in the thyroxine combines readily with blood protein to form protein-bound iodine (PBI), which is used as a measure of thyroid activity. The normal range for PBI is 4 to 8 micrograms (µg) per 100 milliliters (ml) of serum. A person with hyperthyroid disease has an elevated BMR and an elevated PBI.

Other factors that can increase the BMR are muscular development, body temperature, and pregnancy and lactation.

Individuals with large muscular development have a BMR from 5 to 6% greater than that of persons of the same height and weight but with less muscle mass.

As body temperature rises, there is an increase in the rate of chemical reactions in the body. A patient with a fever of 40°C may demonstrate an increase in oxygen consumption of 30 to 35%. Conversely, hypothermia decreases oxygen demands.

An additional increment for BMR must be allowed for pregnancy and lactation, because each of these activities requires additional energy. A pregnant woman needs 10 to 20% more kilocalories than one who is not pregnant. For example, a nursing mother who produces 850 ml of milk a day requires about 100 additional calories.

Major surgery, injury, infection, and burns increase body metabolism and therefore increase basal metabolism, as do other stress situations, such as pain, fear, and anxiety. Analgesics and tranquilizers are helpful in the management of these types of stress and act to reduce the BMR to normal levels.

The major endocrine medical problem that depresses the BMR is hypothyroidism.

Energy Expenditure Factors

In addition to the BMR, the two major items, already mentioned, that affect energy requirements are physical activity, and the digestive system's expenditure of heat energy in digestion and absorption, the SDA of food.

PHYSICAL ACTIVITY

Muscular activity affects both energy expenditure and heat production. Energy expenditure increases with muscular activity.

Some of the approximate percentage increases of energy expenditure above the basal or resting metabolic rate influenced by the degree of physical activity are as follows: for sedentary or maintenance activity, add a factor of 50% of the resting metabolic rate; for light activity, 60%; for moderate activity, 70%; and for strenuous activity, 100% or more.

Maintenance activity: sitting most of the day; about 2 hours of moving about slowly or standing.

Light activity: typing, teaching, shopwork, laboratory work; some walking.

Moderate activity: walking, housework, gardening, carpentry, cycling, tennis.

Strenuous activity (laborers and athletes): pick-and-shovel work, swimming, basketball, football, running, and so forth.

In general, for moderately active persons the daily energy need is increased about 300 kcal more than for light activity. For the laborer and athlete who engage in strenuous activity, the energy expenditure is increased 600 to 900 kcal.

ENVIRONMENTAL TEMPERATURE

Environmental temperature is an important factor in heat production. When the body is exposed to a low environmental temperature, it automatically produces more heat to maintain normal body temperature.

One of the body's first responses to cold is constriction of the peripheral blood vessels and reduction of blood flow to the skin, which helps to reduce heat loss. Next comes a sensation of tight muscles followed by shivering, which is the body's instinctive method for increasing heat production. In fact, vigorous shivering can raise the heat output to four times the basal level. On the other hand, a person who is obese is naturally protected against the cold and may not shiver or produce any extra heat in conditions that produce a marked response in a lean person.

SPECIFIC DYNAMIC ACTION (SDA) OF FOOD

Specific dynamic action (SDA) is the term used to describe the expenditure of calories during the digestion and absorption of food. Studies have shown that the heat increment, or thermogenic response, necessary to digest and absorb fat is 2%; for carbohydrate it is 6%; and for protein-rich foods it is about 12%. In general, the specific dynamic effect of diet is calculated to contribute approximately 10% of the consumed calories. Thus for a hypothetical person whose energy needs for the day (basal metabolism and physical activity) amount to 2000 kcal, one would add 200 more kcal for heat expended in specific dynamic action of the food.

Nutrient Needs for Active Persons and Athletes

Generally, a diet consisting of a minimum of 3 servings of milk and 2 servings each of meat or fish, plus 4 servings each of fruits and vegetables and of enriched or whole-grain breads or cereals provides the basic needs for a nutritionally balanced diet. The requirements of active individuals and athletes for types of food are similar to those of sedentary persons, except that the former need more servings of each to satisfy their energy needs.

For most athletes, a diet containing about 50 to 55% complex carbohydrates (starches), 30 to 35% fat, and 10 to 15% protein is recommended.[3, 4] However, for athletes participating in high-energy, demanding sports such as long-distance running, long-distance bicycling, and swimming, an increased carbohydrate intake prior to the event is desirable.[5] An adequate intake of water before, during, and after strenuous exercise, particularly in warm or hot weather, is critical for avoidance of such problems as cramps, exhaustion, or even stroke.[6]

The effect of exercise on food intake appears to be influenced not only by such factors as the duration and intensity of the activity but also by an individual's age, sex, and amount of body fat.

There is still little scientific evidence to support intake of vitamins and minerals above the Recommended Dietary Allowances for athletes or other physically active individuals already consuming a nutritionally balanced diet with an adequate energy content.[7]

OVERWEIGHT AND OBESITY

When food energy intake equals bodily energy expenditure, the body weight remains constant. This energy balance is the goal as long as the relationship of weight to height is desirable (Table 1–1). When food intake exceeds energy expenditure, the additional food is stored primarily as fat, resulting in overweight or obesity. *An intake of 3500 kcal more than the energy requirement accounts for approximately one pound of additional body fat.* On the other hand, when the energy expenditure exceeds food intake by 3500 kcal, one pound of body fat will be lost. Overweight refers to excessive amounts of muscle or bone and water as well as to body fat. Obesity, on the other hand, is concerned only with an abnormally increased amount of body fat. An individual who weighs *more than 10%* above the theoretical normal for his or her height is classified as *overweight,* whereas a person who weighs *20% or more* above normal is *obese.*

TABLE 1–1. Suggested Desirable Weights and Ranges for Adult Males and Females

Height*		Weight†						
		Men				Women		
in	cm	lb		kg		lb		kg	
58	147		—		—	102	(92–119)	46	(42–54)
60	152		—		—	107	(96–125)	49	(44–57)
62	158	123	(112–141)	56	(51–64)	113	(102–131)	51	(46–59)
64	163	130	(118–148)	59	(54–67)	120	(108–138)	55	(49–63)
66	168	136	(124–156)	62	(56–71)	128	(114–146)	58	(52–66)
68	173	145	(132–166)	66	(60–75)	136	(122–154)	62	(55–70)
70	178	154	(140–174)	70	(64–79)	144	(130–163)	65	(59–74)
72	183	162	(148–184)	74	(67–84)	152	(138–173)	69	(63–79)
74	188	171	(156–194)	78	(71–88)		—		—
76	193	181	(164–204)	82	(74–93)		—		—

From Bray, G. A.: DHEW Publication No. (NIH) 75-708. U.S. Department of Health, Education and Welfare, Washington, D.C., 1975, p. 107.
*Without shoes.
†Without clothes. Average weight ranges in parentheses.

Overweight and obesity, probably the most common nutritional disorders in the United States today, can contribute significantly to the development of a number of health problems, including coronary heart diseases (cardiac failure, angina, atherosclerosis), high blood pressure, diabetes, gall bladder disease, gout, and some forms of arthritis.

According to a Consensus Development Conference of the National Institutes of Health (1985), obesity afflicts 33 million Americans.[8] If a person merely adheres to a weight-reduction diet without additional exercise, there is an adaptive decline in BMR with the result that it becomes more difficult to lose weight.[9] Exercise may be effective in counteracting this decreased BMR.[10] Until recently, the role of exercise had been thought to be unimportant because it was assumed that exercise increases appetite.[11] The effect of exercise on food intake appears to be influenced by age, sex, and amount of body fat as well as by the duration and intensity of the physical activity.[12]

Etiology

A number of causes contribute to obesity, including genetic factors, eating patterns early in infancy, compulsive eating habits during adolescent and adult years, psychological factors, and lack of physical activity.

GENETIC FACTORS

Obesity runs in families. If the mother and father are both obese, there is a greater than 80% chance that the child, too, will be obese. If one parent is obese, the risk may be about 40%. If neither parent is obese, the risk is less than 10%.[13]

EATING PATTERNS EARLY IN INFANCY

From evidence derived from experiments with rodents, it is becoming apparent that one of the causes of obesity and overeating in adolescents and adults can be traced to eating patterns established during the neonatal, infant, and childhood periods.[14] It appears that the number of fat cells (adipocytes) can be increased when newborns are fed excessively. This increased number of fat cells is permanent. Therefore in adult life the adipocytes are available, so that even if an obese adult loses weight, he or she always has a more than normal number of fat cells to store fat and thus may easily become obese again.

An interesting observation is that excessive body fat rarely occurs in breast-fed infants because they do not take in excessive milk. On the other hand, the mother may force a formula-fed child to ingest more than it wants or needs, with a resultant tendency toward creating lasting obesity.

Unfortunately, current methods for measuring adipocyte number and size cannot be applied with precision to children under 2 years of age. If there were techniques available to detect and measure lipid-containing adipose cells, some problems associated with adipose tissue in obese individuals could be solved. At any rate, it is desirable to prevent obesity throughout childhood.[15]

EATING HABITS OF OBESE ADULTS

Obese persons ingest an excess number of calories because they nibble continuously, particularly if food is available and palatable. They do not seem to know when they are full. They do not refuse food, regardless of their physiological needs.

PSYCHOLOGICAL FACTORS

Unhappiness and other psychological stress factors can contribute to over-eating. Some people find comfort and relief of tension in eating or drinking.

PHYSICAL ACTIVITY

In addition to dietary management, regular physical activity is considered a vital aid for weight control. There is considerable evidence that a combination of increased physical activity and an energy-restricted diet is more effective in weight control than either diet or exercise alone.[16]

Diagnosis

A method for diagnosing overweight or obesity (in addition to the obvious ones of general appearance and weight mentioned above) is measurement of skinfold thickness, which assesses subcutaneous fatty tissue. Two areas representative of total-body fatness for this measurement are the skinfold of the triceps area on the back of the arm and the skinfold on the side of the chest. A fold of skin in either of these areas is pinched and its thickness is measured with calipers. A skinfold thickness of more than 23 millimeters (mm) (about 1 in) for males and 30 mm (about 1½ in) for females indicates obesity.

PREVENTION AND CONTROL OF OBESITY

A weight-loss program will fail unless it is accompanied by a maintenance program. This is the reason that "quickie," fad weight-loss diets (high-protein, low-carbohydrate diets, for example), therapeutic fasting, and medications for appetite suppression have failed over the long term to control obesity. On the other hand, peer pressure group therapy programs such as Weight Watchers, which provide both short-term weight reduction and long-term low-weight maintenance diets, have had some success.

The use of behavior modification for weight reduction programs appears to have enjoyed some success.[17, 18] In these programs, the reasons for a person's eating patterns are determined. On the basis of this information, selected behaviors are modified by a reeducation process in which one small habit at a time is changed. Control of environmental cues is the key to shaping and maintaining the desired behavior patterns. A diary is kept that includes an hour-by-hour detailed history of exactly what, when, where, and with whom food is eaten. In addition, information is acquired about the subject's emotional state and habits such as reading or watching television while eating. From these data, a rational program of acceptable change by the patient, supported by a reward system, is developed. The subject is asked not to attempt changes in life style that cannot be maintained.

An energy-restricted diet that is nutritionally adequate but will produce a 1- to 2-lb weight loss per week can be planned. The number of calories that an adult patient must consume to achieve this weight loss can be calculated by a rule-of-thumb formula:

Ideal weight × 20 to 25 kcal for a sedentary individual

or × 30 kcal for a moderately active individual

or × 35 kcal for a strenuously active individual

For example, a woman whose ideal weight should be 55 kg (55 × 2.2 = 121 lb) and is moderately active should eat 55 × 30 kcal, or 1650 kcal per day. If she is obese, she is probably eating much more—let us assume 2150 kcal. She must reduce her calorie intake by 500 kcal each day. At the end of a week, she will have lost 1 lb, because loss of that amount requires a reduced weekly intake of 3500 kcal.

The decreased caloric intake should be accompanied by increased calorie expenditure from regular daily exercise or physical labor. Aerobic exercise (breathing hard to sustain one's activity) such as walking, jogging, bicycling, or swimming is recommended. These exercises allow submaximal exertion levels to be maintained long enough to increase the body's capacity to process oxygen. They produce a discernible level of fatigue.

TABLE 1–2. Minutes of Exercise Required to Burn Calories in Certain Foods

Food	Walking	Bicycling	Swimming	Running	Reclining
Apple, large	19	12	9	5	78
Beer, 8-oz glass	22	14	10	6	88
Cake, 2-layer, $\frac{1}{12}$	68	43	32	18	274
Carbonated beverage, 8-oz glass	20	13	9	5	82
Carrot, raw	8	5	4	2	32
Cookie	10	6	5	3	39
Egg, boiled	15	9	7	4	59
Halibut steak, $\frac{1}{4}$ lb	39	25	18	11	158
Malted milk shake	97	61	45	26	386
Pie, apple, $\frac{1}{6}$	73	46	34	19	290
Pizza, cheese, $\frac{1}{8}$	35	22	16	9	138
Sandwich, tuna fish salad	53	34	25	14	214
Steak, T-bone	45	29	21	12	181
Strawberry shortcake	77	49	36	21	308

Source: Dr. Frank Konishi, Southern Illinois University.

A few general dietary rules for losing weight include the following:

1. *Have a calorie chart of foods available to select nutritious low-calorie types.* Also, be aware that the addition of fats, sugars, or special sauces or gravies can change a low-calorie food to a high-calorie one. For example, a baked potato has less than 100 calories, but with added butter or mashed with milk and butter, it can contribute 150 calories. A hash-browned potato can contribute as much as 500 calories.

2. *Reduce fat consumption.* Use low-fat or skim milk instead of whole milk. Avoid the marbled meats, which are high in saturated fats; use poultry instead of beef or pork. Also use margarine and vegetable oils instead of butter and shortening. Avoid fatty hamburgers, frankfurters, sausages, and cold cuts.

3. *Cut sugar intake and sugared foods such as sweet beverages, cakes, and confections.* Sugar is an empty-calorie food, which means that it provides calories but no vitamins, minerals, or other nutrients that accompany foods such as fruits, vegetables, cereals, and bread. Substitute fruits for sweets and add fibrous foods to give some bulk and a feeling of satiety (sufficiency or satisfaction).

4. *Eat smaller portions.* Eat thinly sliced breads and smaller portions of pasta, desserts, and meats. Use 4 to 6 oz of meat instead of 8 to 12. Leave food on your plate. Refuse second helpings.

5. *Cut down on alcoholic drinks.* Alcohol provides 7 kcal per gram (only 2 kcal/g less than fat and 3 kcal/g more than bread). Two cocktails can amount to 300 kcal or more.

Other factors for successful weight reduction include (1) having a positive attitude and a keen desire to lose weight in order to look and feel better, (2)

TABLE 1–3. Menu Plan

Breakfast

½ c of orange or grapefruit juice or one serving of a high–vitamin C fruit from Fruit list*
One egg or 1 oz hard cheese or 2 oz fish or ¼ c cottage, pot, or farmer's cheese
One serving from Bread for women, two servings for men
Beverage (if desired) from Beverage list

Lunch

4 oz fish (canned or fresh) or 4 oz lean meat or 4 oz poultry or ⅔ c cottage or pot cheese or 2 oz hard cheese or 2 oz farmer's cheese or two eggs
One or two servings from Vegetable A
One serving from Bread for women, two servings for men
Beverage if desired

Dinner

6 oz (women) or 8 oz (men) of fish, lean meat, or poultry
One serving from Vegetable B
One or two servings from Vegetable A
Beverage if desired

Snacks Required Daily

Two servings from Milk
Three servings from Fruit for women, five servings for men (if you've had fruit or juice for breakfast, the snack allowance is two servings from Fruit for women, four for men)

*Food list appears in Table 1–4.

TABLE 1–4. Lists of Foods in Four Food Groups

MILK

Each of the following represents one serving
  Buttermilk (from skim milk), 8 oz c
  Skim milk, evaporated, ½ c
  Nonfat dry milk solids, ⅓ c
  Skim milk, fresh, 1 c

BREAD

(includes cereals, some vegetables, and other carbohydrate sources)
Each of the following represents one serving

Bread, 1 slice	Rice or grits (cooked), ½ c
Frankfurter or hamburger roll, ½	Spaghetti, macaroni, ½ c
Matzo (6-in square), 1	Cooked noodles (not egg), ½ c
Melba toast, 4 pieces	Baked beans (no pork), ⅓ c
Bran flakes, ½ c	Lima beans, ⅓ c
Cooked cereal, ½ c	Corn, ⅓ c
Dry cereal (unsweetened), ¾ c	Popcorn (popped), 1 c
Grapefruit flakes, ¼ c	Potato, mashed, ½ c
Wheat germ, 2 T	white, ½ medium
Graham crackers, 2	sweet, ¼ c
Oyster crackers, 20	Angel cake, 1½ in cube
Saltines, 5	Sponge cake, 1½ in cube
Soda crackers, 3	Gelatin dessert, ½ c

VEGETABLES (Selection A)

Each of the following represents one serving (measured before cooking)

Asparagus, 4 spears	Mushrooms, 10 small
Broccoli, ½ stalk	Pepper, green, 1 medium
Brussels sprouts, 4 medium	Radishes, 10 small
Cabbage, ¾ c	Sauerkraut, ⅔ c
Celery, 8 stalks	Spinach, ½ c
Chicory, 3½ oz	Squash, summer, ½ c
Cucumber, 1 medium	String beans (young), ½ c
Endive, 3½ oz	Tomatoes, ½ medium
Escarole, 2½ oz	Watercress, 3½ oz
Lettuce, 3½ oz	

VEGETABLES (Selection B)

Each of the following represents one serving (measured after cooking)

Artichoke, ⅓ large bud	Pumpkin, ⅓ c
Beets, ½ c	Rutabaga, ⅓ c
Carrots, ½ c	Squash, winter, ¼ c
Onions, ½ c	Turnips, ⅔ c
Parsnips, ¼ c	
Peas, green, ⅓ c	

FRUIT

Each of the following represents one serving
Check the labels of canned fruit to make sure no sugar has been added

Apple, 2-in diameter, 1	Honeydew melon, medium, ¼
Applesauce, unsweetened, ½ c	Mango, small, ½
Apple juice or cider, ⅓ c	Orange, small,* 1
Apricots, medium, 2	Orange juice,* ½ c
Banana, small, ½	Peach, medium, 1
Blackberries, blueberries, raspberries, ½ c	Pear, small, 1
Cantaloupe, ¼	Pineapple,* ½ c
Cherries, large, 10	Pineapple juice,* ⅓ c
Cranberries, sugarless, 1 c	Plums, medium, 2
Cranberry juice, sweetened, ¼ c	Prunes, medium, 2
Dates, medium, 2	Strawberries, fresh, 1 c
Fruit cocktail, peaches or pears, ½ c	Tangerine, large,* 1
Grapefruit, small,* ½ c	Watermelon, 1 c
Grapefruit juice,* ½ c	Prune juice, ⅓ c
Grapes, medium, 12	Tomato juice,* 1 c
Grape juice, ¼ c	

BEVERAGES

No-calorie carbonated drinks, club soda, coffee (black), tea (black), water

*Denotes high in vitamin C.

learning the basic facts about good nutrition from recognized authorities, (3) modifying one's behavior and developing self-control with respect to amounts and types of foods consumed, and (4) walking at least 1½ miles each day, engaging in other types of physical exercise, or both.

The number of minutes of various physical activities required to burn calories in certain foods is listed in Table 1–2.

A number of diets that are adequate, varied, and well balanced will provide 1000 to 1200 calories per day. The menu plan and food lists shown in Tables 1–3 and 1–4 have proved effective not only in producing an initial significant weight loss but also in maintaining the recommended energy intake without the subject feeling hungry.

REFERENCES

1. Hegsted, D. M. Energy requirements. In Present Knowledge in Nutrition: Nutrition Reviews, 5th ed., p. 2. Washington, D.C., Nutrition Foundation, 1984.
2. Boothby, W. M., et al. Studies of the energy of metabolism of normal individuals. A standard for basal metabolism with a nonogram for clinical application. Am. J. Physiol. 116:468, 1936.
3. Wilmore, J. H.; Freund, B. J. Nutritional enhancement of athletic performance. Nutr. Abstr. Rev./ Rev. Clin. Nutr. 54:1, 1984.
4. American Dietetic Association. Nutrition and physical fitness. J. Am. Diet. Assoc. 76:437, 1980.
5. Williams, M. H. Nutritional Aspects of Human Physical and Athletic Performance, 2nd ed. Springfield, Ill., Charles C Thomas, 1985.
6. Murphy, R. J. Heat illness in the athlete. Am. J. Sports Med. 12:258, 1984.
7. Conoslazio, C. F. In Johnson, R. E., ed. Nutrition and Performance. New York, Pergamon Press, 1983.
8. National Institutes of Health. Consensus Development Conference. Health Implications of Obesity. Bethesda, Md., Feb. 11–13, 1985.
9. Weinsier, R. J.; Wadden, T. A.; Ritenbaugh, C., et al. Recommended therapeutic guidelines for professional weight control program. Am. J. Clin. Nutr. 40:865, 1984.
10. Thompson, J. K.; Jarvie, G. L.; Lahey, B. B., et al. Exercise and obesity: etiology, physiology, and intervention. Psychol. Bull. 91:55, 1982.
11. Katch, F. J.; McArdle, W. D. Nutrition, Weight Control and Exercise, 2nd ed. Philadelphia, Lea & Febiger, 1983.
12. Williams, M. H. Nutrition for Fitness and Sports. Dubuque, Iowa, Wm. C. Brown, 1983.
13. Mayer, J. Genetic factors in human obesity. Ann. N.Y. Acad. Sci. 131:412, 1985.
14. Winick, M., et al. Nutrition and cell growth. In Winick, M., ed. Current Concepts in Nutrition, vol. 1. Nutrition and Development, p. 49. New York, John Wiley & Sons, 1972.
15. Hirsch, J.; Knittle, J. L. Cellularity of obsese and nonobese human adipose tissue. Fed. Proc. 29:1516, 1970.
16. Bjorntop, P. In White, P. L.; Mondeika, T., eds. Diet and Exercise: Synergism in Health Mainte- nance, pp. 91–98. Chicago, Ill., American Medical Association, 1982.
17. Levitz, L. S.; Stunkard, A. J. A therapeutic coalition for obesity behavior modification and patient self-help. Am. J. Psychiatry 131:4, 1974.
18. Stuart, R. B. Behavior control of overeating. Behav. Res. Ther. 5:357, 1967.

2

Carbohydrates in Nutrition; Sweeteners; Diabetes Mellitus; Lactose Intolerance

Carbohydrates are organic compounds of the elements carbon, hydrogen, and oxygen. The carbohydrate molecule is composed of a hydrated (chemically combined with water) carbon atom, CH_2O. Carbohydrates are the principal sources of energy in the diet, but they can also act as starting materials for the synthesis of fatty acids and amino acids. In addition, carbohydrates play a role in the structure of other biologically important materials, such as glycolipids, glycoproteins, nucleic acids, acids, and heparin.

In 1980 in the United States, carbohydrate-rich foods contributed about 46% of the energy content of the diet,[1] whereas in many other populations throughout the world, as much as 80% of energy intake is derived from carbohydrates.[2] The carbohydrate portion of the American diet consists on the average of 47% starch and 53% sugar. This intake of sugar contributes to dental caries, among other problems, particularly in areas where drinking water is not fluoridated. In addition, Bibby and colleagues[3] have recently suggested that starch in foods may be a more important contribution to the cariogenicity of sugar-containing foods than has generally been believed, owing to the fact that starch-rich foods such as breads and cereals can promote the retention of sugar in close proximity to the dental plaque on the tooth surface. The degradation of the sucrose to lactic acid by the *Streptococcus mutans* bacteria in dental plaque creates the initial demineralization of the tooth enamel (see Chap. 3).

CHEMISTRY AND CLASSIFICATION

The carbohydrates that are of special interest and importance in nutrition are monosaccharides, disaccharides, and polysaccharides.

The monosaccharides are the simplest carbohydrates and are classified according to the number of carbon atoms in the chain; the most common are the pentoses ($C_5H_{10}O_5$) and the hexoses ($C_6H_{12}O_6$). A disaccharide is a carbohydrate consisting of two monosaccharides. However, disaccharides are classified as oligosaccharides, because by definition an oligosaccharide is a carbohydrate that on hydrolysis yields from two to ten monosaccharides.

Monosaccharides

The five- and six-carbon monosaccharides, called pentoses and hexoses, respectively, are important in nutrition.

PENTOSES (FIVE-CARBON SUGARS)

Two pentoses are of vital importance: ribose and deoxyribose. These pentoses, which are synthesized by the body, are components of nucleic acids (substances found in the cells of all living tissues concerned with cellular biosynthesis) and nucleotides (obtained from hydrolysis of nucleic acid), which act as coenzymes in energy production. (Hydrolysis is the splitting of a compound by adding water and is catalyzed in the body by enzymes.) The pentose sugars most commonly present in human foods are L-arabinose and D-xylose, which are widely distributed in nuts, fruits, and root vegetables.

HEXOSES (SIX-CARBON SUGARS)

Three hexoses—glucose, fructose, and galactose—are of major nutritional importance. A fourth hexose, mannose, is of more interest to sugar chemists than to nutritionists.

Glucose (also called dextrose, grape sugar, and corn sugar) is the form of carbohydrate that the body tissues can best use; it is oxidized in the cells for energy and is the principal monosaccharide existing in a free state in blood and body fluids. It is the main and perhaps the only fuel for the brain. Chemically, glucose is an aldohexose. It is a white crystalline solid that is soluble in water and is about half as sweet as sucrose (table sugar). It can be synthesized from other carbohydrates, such as starch and sucrose, and to a lesser degree from proteins, which provide the carbon and oxygen fragments. Because of the asymmetrical carbon atoms in the molecule, solutions of glucose can rotate polarized light to the right (i.e., dextrorotatory) hence, the alternative name dextrose, which is often used in industry. Dextrose is produced commercially by the hydrolysis of starch. The major food sources of glucose are honey, fruits, and corn syrup.

Fructose (levulose or fruit sugar) is structurally closely related to glucose. It is the sweetest of all the sugars and is found along with glucose in honey, fruits, and corn syrup. It is a constituent of common table sugar. Fructose is also called levulose and fruit sugar.

Galactose (and glucose) is derived from the hydrolysis of lactose, the sugar found in milk, and is a constituent of many plant polysaccharides. During lactation, the human body converts glucose to galactose in the mammary tissue for the synthesis of lactose in breast milk.

Mannose is classified as an aldohexose. It is found in various plant sources.

Disaccharides and Trisaccharides

Sucrose, lactose, and maltose consist of a linkage of two monosaccharide units and for that reason are called disaccharides. In the formation of a disaccharide, a hydrogen atom (H) is split away from one of the monosaccharide units and a hydroxyl group (OH) is split from the other to yield a molecule of water (H_2O). In general, these saccharides have a sweet taste, are water soluble, and are crystalline solids.

Sucrose (cane sugar, beet sugar, and maple sugar), the familiar table sugar in common use, is available as a refined carbohydrate in such forms as granulated, powdered, brown, and "raw" sugar. Granulated and powdered sugars are white, highly refined, or purified, sugars. Brown and raw sugars are somewhat less pure owing to the presence of some molasses. Sucrose is a disaccharide that is readily hydrolyzed into glucose and fructose by boiling with acids or by the action of a certain enzyme (invertase) forming "invert sugar," the commercial name for a product that is a mixture of glucose and fructose. Invert sugar is slightly sweeter than sucrose. Sucrose is extensively used as a sweetener in food preservation, in food processing, and in pill- or tablet-making for pharmaceutical preparations.

Lactose, or milk sugar, unique to mammals and found in mammary glands, makes up almost 40% of the solids in fresh whole milk. Lactose is said to improve the absorption of calcium and other minerals in the body. On hydrolysis with acids or an enzyme (galactase), lactose yields glucose and galactose.

Maltose is formed from the enzymatic breakdown of starch in the process of malting barley. Maltose is a component of numerous infant formulas in which partial hydroxylates of starches have been included. When maltose is hydrolyzed, it produces two molecules of glucose. It contributes a very characteristic and pleasant malt flavor to beer and ale.

Raffinose is a trisaccharide of glucose, fructose, and galactose; it is found in molasses.

Polysaccharides

Polysaccharides are complex carbohydrates made up of many (more than 10) monosaccharides linked together. Unlike the sugars, they are tasteless. Their molecular weight ranges from 20,000 to 1,000,000. Some (starch, glycogen, dextran, and insulin) are used for storing energy; others (cellulose, pectin, agar, and carrageen, for example) have structural functions.

Starch is nutritionally the most important carbohydrate, providing about 50% of the total carbohydrate intake. It is a major source of energy and provides texture and consistency to many food preparations.

Starch ($C_6H_{10}O_5$) (the value of x is between 500 and 1000) is not a single chemical substance but a natural product that occurs as a reserve food in most green plants. It consists of a mixture of amylose and amylopectin. Plants make starch granules from sugars and store them in stems, fruits, seeds, roots, and tubers. When the plant needs energy, it reconverts the starch into sugar. Starch grains freshly obtained from plants are insoluble in water. However, heat promotes a solution that may gel on cooling.

Starch is digestible by humans because it has chemical linkages for which we have an enzyme. On the other hand, cellulose is not digestible because it has linkages for which we do not have a digesting enzyme. The digestion of starch takes place in two steps and involves the action of two enzymes: first, a liquefying enzyme that converts starch to dextrins or oligosaccharides; and second, an enzyme that converts the oligosaccharides into maltose and finally into glucose.

Rice, wheat, sorghum, corn (maize), millet, and rye contain about 70% starch and are outstanding sources of carbohydrate. Potatoes and legumes, such as peas and nuts, are rich in starch, but they also contribute other essential nutrients such as proteins, vitamins, minerals, and fatty acids. Cooking renders the starch vegetables more digestible.

Dextrins are intermediate products formed during the hydrolysis of starch. They are dextrorotatory, soluble in water, and precipitable by alcohol.

Glycogen is the animal equivalent of starch and provides a food storage system for all forms of animal life. Glycogen is found in highest concentration in the liver, where it serves as an important regulator of blood glucose concentration: it is also stored in muscles, where it serves as an energy source for muscle contraction.

Dextrans are polysaccharides that form the substrate for dental plaque and serve as the energy source for potentially dental caries–producing bacteria such as *Streptococcus mutans.*

Cellulose provides the fibrous framework for the plant. It is a good source for fiber, currently advocated for greater inclusion in our diets. Because it is not digestible by humans, it provides roughage and bulk and thus aids in the production of soft stools, in peristalsis, and in the elimination of water.

Pectin is a polysaccharide found in small quantities in many fruits, young green plants, and root vegetables. In the presence of sugars and a warm, slightly acid solution, pectin turns into jelly. This property is responsible for the setting of jams and fruit preserves.

Agar is used as a food additive to improve the texture and consistency of such foods as ice cream.

Alginic acid has the useful property of forming jellies without the need for heat and is therefore used in quick-mix gelatin preparations.

Lignin is a woody substance closely bound to cellulose in plants. It provides fiber in the diet.

MUCOPOLYSACCHARIDES

Mucopolysaccharides are a group of polysaccharides that contain hexosamine. Hyaluronic acid and chondroitin sulfate are mucopolysaccharides that are found in connective tissue. Heparin, an acidic mucopolysaccharide, is the anticoagulant that helps to prevent thrombosis by interfering with the formation of fibrin clots.

DIGESTION AND ABSORPTION

If the body is to use the complex carbohydrates for energy, they must be split into monosaccharides and then absorbed. This splitting, or hydrolysis, is part of the process of digestion and is accomplished by the action of enzymes. The acidity of the gastric contents can also aid in the hydrolysis of simple sugars.

A minimal amount of digestion of starch begins in the mouth under the influence of salivary amylase (ptyalin), which works best in a neutral pH and is inactivated by the acid in the stomach.

In the small intestine, the amylose and amylopectin of food starches and the animal starch glycogen are broken down into disaccharides. The disaccharide sucrose is further hydrolyzed by the enzyme sucrase into one molecule of glucose and one of fructose; maltose is hydrolyzed by maltase into two molecules of glucose; and lactose is hydrolyzed by lactase into one molecule of galactose and one of glucose. The end products of carbohydrate digestion—glucose, fructose, and galactose—are absorbed in phosphorylated form from the intestine and pass into the portal blood. Glucose enters the blood directly. Fructose and galactose are partly converted into glucose as they pass through the intestinal wall. (Lactose intolerance, discussed in detail later in this chapter, is a digestive problem for some people.)

METABOLISM AND UTILIZATION

The primary purpose of glucose in metabolism is to furnish energy. Once glucose is in the blood stream, the individual cells take it up. In order for glucose to be used, it must combine with phosphorus as it passes into the cells. Cells oxidize the glucose to pyruvic acid, a process known as glycolysis. Ultimately the pyruvic acid is oxidized to CO_2 and water, with the production of usable energy in the form of adenosinetriphosphate (ATP).

Glucose is used to maintain blood glucose concentrations. After a high-carbohydrate meal, glucose may be stored in the liver as glycogen. This glycogen can be converted to glucose by a liver enzyme and released to the blood at a rate that will maintain a desirable level of 100 to 120 mg of glucose per 100 ml of blood. This process is called glycogenolysis. In the case of starvation and depletion of stored glucose, the liver can make glycogen from amino acids from some of the body's own protein, and/or from fatty acids and glycerol. This is called gluconeogenesis.

Whenever a meal provides more glucose than the cells can use for energy and the glycogen reserve needs of the liver and muscle are filled, the excess is deposited in adipose cells as fat. This process is called lipogenesis.

FUNCTIONS

Provide Energy

After carbohydrate becomes available to the body in the form of glucose, its major function is to provide energy for the organism to live and work. Nervous tissue depends uniquely and exclusively on a continuous supply of glucose for its energy. Other tissues can use fats and even protein. Thus a diabetic who accidentally takes excess insulin can develop hypoglycemia from a lack of glucose and may show clinical manifestations of nervous changes such as disorientation and confusion.

Facilitate the Oxidation of Fats

Fat requires carbohydrate for oxidation. If not enough carbohydrate is available, the fat will not be completely oxidized to carbon dioxide and water.

Instead, there will be an accumulation of ketone bodies (acetoacetic acid, beta-hydroxybutyric acid, and acetone) with resulting acidosis. These acids combine with sodium to form sodium salts, which are excreted, creating a severe sodium imbalance that can lead to coma. This may occur in diabetic patients whose tissues cannot oxidize carbohydrates or in persons eating many foods rich in fat, or it may occur during acute starvation.

Spare Proteins

If insufficient carbohydrates are consumed, protein will be used as an energy source. Consequently, protein will not be available for its primary function, tissue-building and cell replacement.

Contribute to Body Structure

Glucose can be converted to pentoses, such as ribose and deoxyriboses, which are important in the formation of nucleic acid in cells; to galactose, which contributes to the lipids of the cell membrane; or to mucopolysaccharides, which are involved in collagen formation.

Affect Food Consumption

Palatability and sweetness affect food consumption. Sweetness varies with the type of sugar used. If sucrose (table sugar) is considered a standard and is given the value of 100, fructose would be rated 110 to 175; glucose, 75; galactose, 35 to 70; and lactose, 15 to 30.

Excessive sugar intake can decrease the desire for food. Concentrated sugar solutions attract water. Thus when a large amount of sugar is eaten, the sugar solution in the stomach is increased, which draws water from the tissues to dilute the stomach contents, this causing the stomach to feel full.

Provide Energy for Oral and Intestinal Bacteria

A detailed discussion of the role of carbohydrates in the metabolism of oral bacteria, particularly those related to dental caries production, can be found in Chap. 3.

In the intestine, carbohydrates such as lactose, which are absorbed slowly and tend to remain in the intestine for a relatively long period, stimulate the growth of lactic acid bacteria. Starch, which is also absorbed slowly from the intestine, stimulates the growth of bacteria that synthesize some B-complex vitamins, such as biotin.

Provide Protein, Vitamins, and Minerals

Whole-grain products, fruits, vegetables, and legumes, which have high carbohydrate contents, also provide protein (e.g., legumes), B-complex vitamins, iron, some of the essential amino acids (e.g., whole-grain cereals), vitamin C (e.g., citrus fruits, tomatoes, and potatoes), and vitamin A (e.g., deep green and yellow vegetables).

Furnish Fiber for Normal Peristalsis

Dietary fiber has recently become a subject of increased interest as a result of Burkitt's claim that diverticular diseases, cancer of the colon and rectum, polyps, and ulcerative colitis might be due to a lack of dietary fiber.[4] He noted that these diseases were more prevalent in Britain and the United States than in Asia and Africa. He attributed this to the constipating characteristics of the soft consistency, low-fiber diets eaten by people in industralized countries. He reasoned that a low-fiber diet would make for slow passage of stools through the intestinal tract, allowing an increased potential for bacterial production and for absorption of toxins. It must be emphasized that these epidemiological observations simply hypothesize a correlation between low-fiber diets and the incidence of intestinal problems. They definitely do not prove a direct cause-and-effect relationship.

By definition, dietary fiber includes cellulose, hemicellulose, lignin, pectin, gums, and related compounds of plant origin. There is no adequate method for analyzing the amount of dietary fiber, so a crude-fiber analysis must be used to roughly approximate the amount of dietary fiber. Actually, crude fiber consists of only cellulose and lignin.

The following are some of the hypothetical positive health reasons for increasing dietary fiber. A high-residue, low-sugar diet supplemented by unprocessed bran, which makes it a high-fiber diet, provides bulk and is said to relieve the symptoms of abdominal pain usually experienced by patients with diverticulosis.[5] The water-absorptive properties of the fiber softens and increases the volume of the feces, causing distention of the colon and fast propulsion and elimination of its contents. Fiber may also increase the numbers of bacteria by enhancing their growth while they are in the bowel. It is speculated that the total cholesterol level in the body may be reduced, because bile salts and acids are bound to fiber and excreted. This implies that fiber will reduce hyperlipidemia and will therefore lower the incidence of ischemic heart disease.[6]

In Finland, it has been found that one of the major reasons for the low cancer rate is the high fiber intake from unrefined grain as a result of the frequent consumption of coarse rye bread.[7, 8] However, foods high in bran are high in phytates, which can theoretically interfere with absorption of calcium, iron, zinc, and other trace elements essential for good health. This may constitute a reason for not ingesting dietary fiber in large amounts.

On the basis of present knowledge, dietary fiber in itself has not been proved to have any effect on coronary heart disease, but it does seem to play a role in the prevention of constipation and diverticular disease.

DIETARY REQUIREMENTS AND FOOD SOURCES

There is no specific recommended dietary allowance for carbohydrates because they can be made in the body from some amino acids and the glycerol portion of fats. However, it is desirable to include some preformed carbohydrate in the diet to avoid ketosis, excessive breakdown of body protein, loss of cations (especially sodium), and involuntary dehydration. At least 100 g/day is required to provide energy for the nervous system and to offset the ketosis associated with high-fat diets and fasting.

Over the past 40 years, the nature and amount of carbohydrates in the American diet have changed. As a result of more prosperity, the amount of carbohydrates (particularly flour and cereal products) has decreased as the amount of meat and dairy products has increased. There has been an increase in sugars and a concomitant decrease in starches. In 1972 sugar contributed 53% of the carbohydrates in our food supply compared with 32% from 1909 to 1913 and 50% from 1957 to 1959. Primarily, the increase is due to greater use of sugar in processed foods and soft drinks.

Food science facts about carbohydrates include the following: The nature of carbohydrate is influenced by the ripening process of some plant foods. For example, in bananas starch is changed to sugar as the fruit ripens. On the other hand, the sugar in corn changes to starch as the seed matures. Drying grapes or plums to produce raisins and prunes, respectively, concentrates the sucrose content. Modified food starches are used as thickeners, fillers, moisture absorbents, and carriers for fats, oils, and flavors in such food preparations as salad dressing, fruit pie fillings, and canned soups.

Important food sources of carbohydrate are cereals, bread, vegetables (root tuber, seed, and leafy types), fruits (fresh and dried), sugar, and corn syrup. Cereals and breads consist mainly of starch. Vegetables have varying amounts of glucose and fructose. Root tuber and seed types of vegetables (e.g., potatoes, beets, beans, squash) have high starch and sucrose contents, whereas leafy vegetables consist of appreciable amounts of cellulose and hemicellulose. Fruits consist mainly of glucose and fructose with some sucrose, cellulose, hemicellulose, dextrins, and pectin. Sugar, honey, and corn syrups consist of combinations of mono- and disaccharides and contain the highest percentage of carbohydrate on a dry-weight basis.

SWEETENERS

Sugars

To most people, "sugar" is the refined granulated product used for table-top purposes, which they believe is pure sucrose obtained from sugar cane or beets. Actually, the sugar manufacturer produces three types of sugar mixtures for commercial use: (1) blended sugar (50% sucrose and 50% glucose), (2) pure invert sugar (50% glucose and 50% fructose), and (3) common invert sugar (50% sucrose, 25% glucose, and 25% fructose). "Sugars" in the plural is used to refer to all sugar. This includes the naturally occurring sugar of milk, fruit, syrup, honey, and refined cane and beet sugar.

PATTERNS OF SUGAR USE[9]

Higher Sugar Than Starch Intake. From 1900 to 1970, world sugar production rose from 8 million to about 70 million tons per year. For the world's population, consumption of white sugar has increased from 21 to 51 g (84 to 204 kcal) per person per day and has been constant for the past 30 years.[10] In the United States, the per capita consumption and production of caloric sweetening products such as sugar and corn syrup have increased so much that they now exceed our consumption of polymeric carbohydrates (starches) such as corn, wheat, rice, and their products. Around 1910, which is the base period for United States sugar statistics, our diet consisted of 68% starch and 32% sugar. Now it consists of 47% starch and 53% sugar.

Per Capita Consumption of Caloric Sweeteners. From 1965 to the present, with the exception of 1974 and 1975, when the high price of sugar tended to interrupt the trend, there was substantial growth in per capital consumption of caloric sweeteners in the United States, with corn sweeteners absorbing substantially all of the growth. In 1977 the annual per capita consumption of caloric sweeteners was 127 lb (95 lb from cane and beet sugar and 32 lb from corn sweeteners). This means that the average intake of caloric sweeteners per person per week was more than 2.4 lb.

Presweetening of Foods by Processors.[11] Although the percentage of change in consumption of types of carbohydrate, namely, that we are eating more sugars than starches now compared with 60 years ago, has been noteworthy, the most striking change in our consumption of sweets is in the origin of the sugars. More than 70% of our sugar calories comes from food products and beverages presweetened by the food processor. Only about 25% of the sugar consumed in this country was packaged and bought for household use.

A number of chemical and physical properties of sugar are important in food technology. It provides body to beverages, texture to cake, lubrication to the mixing process for cookie and cake batter, and characteristic flavor and aroma as a result of caramelization and bulking properties. Originally, sugar was primarily used as a food preservative.

Sugar is the major food additive in the United States today. Product ingredient labels reveal that sugar is used in many prepared food products—not only in sweet baked goods, desserts, and soft drinks but also in sauces, almost all fruit drinks, salad dressings, canned and dehydrated soups, frozen TV dinners, cured meats, some canned and frozen vegetables, most canned and frozen fruits, fruit yogurt, and breakfast cereals. The content of tomato ketchup is 29% sugar; of cream substitute, 65%; of salad dressing, 30%; and of ready-sweetened cereal, 57%. Some of these so-called food products contain more sugar than the 51% in a chocolate bar, which is classified as candy. Perhaps food products containing more than 50% sugar, such as presweetened cereals, might be considered to be like candy from a dental caries–producing standpoint.

Types and Processing of Sugar. Raw sugar crystals are the product of processing of sugar cane (crushing, juice extraction, chemical treatment, boiling, and crystallization). Raw sugar has a light-brown color because a thin film of molasses clings to the crystals. It is banned in this country because of its contamination with impurities (e.g., insect parts and bacteria).

Turbinado sugar is the intermediate product in the refining of raw sugar to granulated sugar. By a series of further processes, including washing, filtering, boiling, centrifuging, and drying, raw sugar is converted into white, granulated, refined sugar, which is less likely than raw sugar to be bacterially infested. Brown sugar consists of fine sugar crystals covered with molasses. In the United States, most of it is made by spraying refined white sugar with molasses syrup.

Confectioner's sugar is a white, very finely textured sugar resulting from the powdering of granulated sugar.

Invert sugar is a mixture of equal weights of dextrose and levulose that results from splitting sucrose by hydrolysis (heating it in the presence of water and acid) or by treating it with invertase enzymes. This sugar has moisture retention properties and prolongs the freshness of baked goods and confectioneries. It is used in the form of invert syrups in beverages, preserves, and icings. During the inversion process, 5.26 lb of water is taken up by every 100 lb of sugar, increasing the weight of the sugar to 105.26 lb (a positive economic factor for the food processor).

Corn syrup is a viscous liquid that contains maltose, dextrin, dextrose, and other polysaccharides. It is the product of incomplete hydrolysis of starch. The fructose found in the high-fructose corn syrup is derived by inversion from sucrose or by isomerization from dextrose.

Blackstrap molasses is the final product—a brownish black, thick, sticky liquid mass—in sugar manufacturing. It contains sugar, water, some minerals (calicum, iron, and so forth), and biotin (a B-complex vitamin) but is considered a poor source for these nutrients. Honey is essentially an invert sugar. It is formed by an enzyme, honey invertase, from nectar gathered by bees. Maple sugar and syrup are derived from the sap of maple trees and consist largely of sucrose.

All of these sugars consist largely of calories and contain very little else of nutritional value. There may be minor differences between various sugars in terms of minimal nutrients or sweetening power per calorie, but these differences are indeed minor in the face of the overriding feature of empty calories.

Starch hydrolysates are dextrin-based sucrose substitutes that have been developed by using starches from cereals or potatoes. The final products are syrups containing dextrins, maltose, and glucose.

Sugar Alcohols

Sorbitol (D-glucitol) is a sugar alcohol that is made commercially from glucose by hydrogenation. It is about 60% as sweet as sucrose and is used as a sweetening agent in diabetic foods and so-called sugarless gums and candies. (Because sorbitol is a sugar, the appropriateness of the term "sugarless" is questionable. The more accurate terms would be "without refined sugar.") In the body, 70 to 90% of the ingested sorbitol is absorbed and metabolized to glucose. However, sorbitol has a very small effect on raising the blood sugar level because its rate of absorption from the gut is very slow. An excessive intake of sorbitol can cause diarrhea because of osmotic transfer of water into the bowel. One gram of sorbitol yields 4 calories.

Mannitol and dulcitol are obtained by the hydrogenation of mannose and galactose, respectively, and have a variety of industrial uses as food improvers and sweetening agents. Like sorbitol, mannitol is commonly used in sugarless chewing gums and candies as a sweetener. Compared with sucrose, both of these polyols break down to organic acids in the mouth at a much slower rate. Thus the salivary buffering system has an opportunity to more effectively neutralize some of the acids that normally demineralize the enamel surface.

Xylitol is a naturally occurring pentose alcohol that can be derived from various types of cellulose products, such as wood, straw, cane pulp, or seed hulls. Its sweetness is similar to that of sucrose, and it produces a cooling sensation in the mouth. Like sorbitol, when taken in excess, it can produce diarrhea. One gram of xylitol yields 4 calories.

In dental plaque, microbial fermentation of most polyols proceeds at a slower rate than the fermentation of sucrose and results in the production of little or no acid: xylitol is neither fermented nor utilized by *Streptococcus mutans,* an acid-producing organism closely associated with dental caries formation.

When xylitol was used as a sugar substitute in animal and human studies, there appeared to be some initial promise that this polyol might have useful anticaries properties. However, in toxicity studies in mice, it was found that those that were fed 20% xylitol in the diet developed malignant neoplasms of the urinary bladder.[12] Therefore, the clinical caries trial that was to be conducted under contract to the National Institute of Dental Research was suspended. To satisfy the standards of safety laid down by the U.S. Food and Drug Administration (FDA), more toxicity studies by several independent investigators are required.

Flavonoid Sweeteners[13]

Three flavonoid sweeteners that are derived from citrus fruits are neohesperidin, naringin, and hesperidin. These have a pleasant sweetness that is slow in onset but lingers for a long time. Neohesperidin is 1900 times sweeter than sucrose, and naringin and hesperidin are about 300 times sweeter.

These sweeteners work best when long-lasting sweetness is desirable—in chewing gum, toothpastes, and mouthwashes. A small amount of this sweetener can make sour grapefruit juice acceptable.

Monellin[14]

Monellin is a sweet-tasting protein that is found in the fruit, initially called "serendipity berries," of a tropical shrub. Monellin evokes an intense sweet sensation that lingers. Monellin is approximately 3000 times sweeter than sucrose.

Saccharin[15]

Saccharin, discovered in 1879, is a non-nutritive artificial sweetener approximately 350 times sweeter than sugar. About 70% of saccharin used is in food and beverages as a flavoring agent. It is also used in cosmetics (e.g., lipsticks), in pharmaceuticals (e.g., dentrifices and mouthwashes), and in animal feed and industrial processes.

Sodium saccharin is used more extensively than saccharin because of its ready solubility. Saccharin is compatible with most food and drug ingredients, is stable in most processed foods, and is unchanged in the heat processing of such products as jams and canned fruits.

A clause in the Food Additive Amendments of 1958 prohibits the marketing of any food additive that has been shown to be a carcinogen. Because of the greatly increased use of saccharin, the FDA requested the National Academy of Sciences to reevaluate its safety. In long-term feeding studies, saccharin was fed to rats and mice at levels up to 7.5% of the diet. Results from 11 of the tests showed no conclusive evidence of potential hazard. In three other studies, the test animals were exposed to the saccharin in utero and for the remainder of the long-term test period. These studies showed an increased incidence of tumors in the bladders of male rats compared with controls. Other factors besides a direct cause-and-effect relationship between pure saccharin and tumors have been considered. One possibility is the carcinogenic potential of a coal tar–derivative impurity (orthotoluene sulfonamide) contained in saccharin.

Four of five epidemiological studies on saccharin showed no relationship between saccharin ingestion and bladder tumors in humans. The fifth study (Canadian) alleges a possible low-level association of bladder tumor occurrence in human males after long-term consumption of saccharin.

Two recent studies have shown that there is no saccharin-induced epidemic of bladder cancer in this country.[16, 17] The evidence is that little, if any, current bladder cancer is due to the consumption of artificial sweeteners at the doses and in the manner in which they were commonly consumed in the past. However, a plea is made for prudence in the use of saccharin. "Any use by nondiabetic children or pregnant women, heavy use by young women of childbearing age, and excessive use by anyone are ill-advised and should be actively discouraged by the medical community."[18]

The National Academy of Sciences has accepted the premise that the use of non-nutritive sweeteners in drugs and dentifrices presents insignificant risks and involves possible benefits. Most toothpastes and many drugs contain saccharin to improve palatability, thereby encouraging proper use of these products.

Aspartame[19]

James Schlatter, a chemist at G.D. Searle Co., noticed an extremely sweet taste accidentally when he touched a tiny bit of some amino acids (aspartic acid and phenylalanine) and licked it from his finger. This combination of amino acids, known as aspartame, yields 4 kcal/g, as does sucrose. But because aspartame is 180 times as sweet as sucrose, the amounts used in a 12-oz soft drink, for example, add up to a few tenths of one calorie.

Aspartame (Nutrasweet or Equal) lacks the bitter or metallic aftertaste of saccharin. Its biggest drawback is that it is about 20 times more expensive than saccharin. Some soda makers are combining saccharin and aspartame to reduce the cost.

Aspartame is unstable at high temperature, so that it cannot be used in baking products or to sweeten food that will be cooked.

One-half of the aspartame molecule is phenylalanine. Therefore, the ingestion of aspartame could be harmful to people with an inherited metabolic abnormality called phenylketonuria (PKU), because brain damage can result if they eat foods with phenylalanine.

It has been shown that even a person who carries one gene for PKU can consume twice the Acceptable Daily Intake (ADI) of aspartame without experiencing any adverse effects. In fact, a 4-oz hamburger has about 12 times more phenylalanine than an 8-oz can of aspartame-sweetened soda. The Acceptable Daily Allowance (ADA) for aspartame is 50 mg/kg (22.7 mg/lb) of body weight. To consume this much, a 150-lb adult would have to drink seventeen 8-oz cans of soda sweetened with aspartame; a 40-lb child, 4 to 5 cans. The problem is that quantities of aspartame-sweetened products, particularly for children, can take the place of more nutritious foods. This means that for children some limitation should be placed on the amount of intake of foods sweetened with aspartame.

Aspartame has been adjudged safe by the FDA even after considering all the concerns with possible alteration of normal brain function. Convincing scientific proof in this matter has not yet been presented.

DIABETES MELLITUS[20]

Diabetes mellitus is a complicated metabolic disorder in which the body cannot control its levels of sugar. The beta cells in the islets of Langerhans in the pancreas are unable to produce the hormone insulin in sufficient quantities to metabolize glucose. Consequently, glucose reaches a high level in blood and cells, causing tissue damage.

Incidence

There are more than 2 million known or undiagnosed diabetics in the United States. From 70 to 90% fall into the adult-onset group, whereas about 5 to 10% are the youth-onset type. The rate of diabetes in the elderly probably exceeds 10%.

Adult-onset diabetes is more frequent than youth-onset diabetes. About 75% of adult-onset diabetics are obese, whereas only a small percentage of youth-onset diabetics are obese. Adult-onset diabetes is usually mild to moderately severe because there is only partial failure of pancreatic beta cell function. On the other hand, youth-onset diabetes is usually severe because there is little or no endogenous insulin available.

Many controlled diabetics now live as long with diabetes as they would be expected to live without it. Yet on the average, life expectancy is still only about half of normal in youth-onset patients and roughly two-thirds of normal in adult-onset patients.

Role of Insulin

The hyperglycemia of diabetes may be caused by a failure to produce enough insulin, so that the peripheral tissues can remove the needed glucose from the blood at a reasonable rate. It may also result from excessive gluconeogenesis (the formation of glucose from molecules of protein or fat, described earlier in this chapter.

Normally, insulin signals the fat cells to take up excess glucose, convert it into fat, and store it. In muscle, insulin stimulates the transformation of glucose into glycogen. This hormone also helps amino acids in the blood stream enter the muscle cells to be synthesized as new protein. Fat traveling in the blood as chylomicrons is transported into the adipose (fat) cells with the aid of insulin.

The consequences of hyperglycemia are

- Glycosuria (excessive glucose in the urine). The glucose concentration in the blood exceeds the capacity of the renal tubules to reabsorb it from the glomerular filtrate. The renal threshold is usually about 180 mg/100 ml.
- Polyuria (increased volume of urine). The glucose increases the concentration of the glomerular filtrate and prevents the reabsorption of water into the kidney, which can cause dehydration and sodium depletion.
- Hyperketonemia (increased number of ketone bodies in the blood). Because of the body's inability to use the glucose in the circulation, fat is mobilized and partly metabolized. Acetoacetic acid is a normal intermediate in the breakdown of fats. Under normal circumstances, the body has no difficulty in completely oxidizing it, but when fat combustion is disproportionate, acetoacetic acid and its derivatives, beta-hydroxybutyric acid and acetone, begin to accumulate and appear in excessive amounts in the blood, producing ketosis.
- Ketonuria (presence of ketoacids in the urine). The amount of ketone bodies is greater than the capacity of the peripheral tissues to metabolize them.
- Increased urinary nitrogen and wasting of muscles.

Diabetes may be secondary to pancreatitis, hemochromatosis, or carcinoma of the pancreas. It may be a result of abnormal concentrations of insulin antagonists in the circulation such as growth, adrenocortical, or thyroid hormones, and epinephrine; or it may be caused by liver disease (cirrhosis, hepatitis) associated with impaired glucose tolerance.

Clinical Signs and Symptoms

Frequently there are no symptoms or abnormal physical signs except glycosuria, which is the first inkling that further examination and testing are required to rule out diabetes.

On the other hand, patients may have complaints of weakness, polydipsia (excessive thirst), polyuria (excessive excretion of urine), nocturia (excessive urination at night), and loss of weight. They may also have failing vision, peripheral vascular disease, neuropathy (diseases of the nervous sytem), infections, or an acetone (sickly sweet) breath odor, the expected complications of diabetes.

ORAL MANIFESTATIONS

The oral symptoms most commonly associated with diabetes are xerostomia (dry mouth), gingival swelling and bleeding, and advanced periodontal pocket formation.

A number of abnormal oral conditions have been associated with diabetes, namely, diffuse erythema of the oral mucosa, a burning sensation in the roof of the mouth, dryness of the mouth, and various stages of periodontal disease from a persistent marginal gingivitis to an advanced periodontosis.

Opinions differ regarding the exact relationship of diabetes to development of periodontal disease. For example, there have been investigations reporting a significant increase in the severity of periodontal disease in the diabetic compared with the nondiabetic individual.[21] In a clinical study of 50 diabetic children under control with insulin and diet compared with a matched group of normal children, greater incidence of gingival inflammation was found in the diabetic group. There was very little difference in the rate of calculus formation and periodontal disease. The decayed, missing, and filled surfaces (DMFS) rates were higher in the normal children.[22] On the other hand, Hove and Stallard noted in their clinical study that periodontal disease increased in both diabetics and nondiabetics as they increased in age and that the amount of periodontal destruction was directly correlated with the amount of accumulated plaque and calculus. They concluded that the severity of diabetes appeared to have little effect on periodontal disease.[23] However, there is general agreement that diabetics are much more susceptible to infection and inflammation in the mouth and in other parts of the body (especially the feet and the eyes).

In addition to the oral changes, diabetes affects other organs and systems: the nerves, eyes, kidneys, and blood vessels. Excess blood sugar in these areas can cause serious complications, such as hardening of the arteries, stroke, blindness, kidney disease, and serious nerve disorders.

OTHER COMPLICATIONS

There is a clear, undisputed association between diabetes and disease of the small blood vessels. Diabetes may predispose patients to coronary artery atherosclerosis. Diabetics have about twice the normal incidence of stroke resulting in death and are predisposed to arterial disease, particularly in the legs.

Diabetes is a major cause of disturbance to the nervous system called neuropathy, which may be manifested as loss of ankle reflexes and other reflexes. Pain is a common symptom. A burning sensation and a dull or sharp pain in the feet and legs are often elicited in the history. Neuropathy may also appear as dizziness, diarrhea, stomach trouble, and bladder dysfunction. Diabetic neuropathy is the second leading cause of blindness in the United States, particularly in patients who have had diabetes for more than 20 years. It is also the primary cause of new cases of blindness in the middle-aged population.

Diabetic nephropathy results in the slow loss of kidney function. Kidney disease is a serious, often fatal, consequence of diabetes. The incidence and severity of renal damage are less in insulin-dependent diabetics than in non-insulin-dependent patients, most of whom die of heart attacks.

Currently available treatments for diabetes do not achieve the degree of metabolic control needed to prevent the complications discussed and to extend the shorter life span of many diabetics. Research continues.

Dietary Management of Diabetes[24]

Dietary objectives and management for adult-onset diabetes in an obese patient are different from those for the youth-onset diabetic.

In obese diabetic patients, restricting calories and increasing exercise usually reduce hyperglycemia. This regimen usually alleviates the "overstrain" of the beta cells of the pancreas and leads to their improved function. Thus diet not only controls but actually reduces the severity of the diabetes. Glucose tolerance can conceivably return to normal when weight is reduced and the ideal weight is achieved and maintained. Although diabetologists still advise restriction or complete elimination of sugar, it is the consensus that the primary goal is reduction of calorie intake by the obese diabetic. As long as the weight is properly controlled, the amounts of dietary starch or the timing of feeding periods for this type of diabetes is not critical.

On the other hand, the dietary regimen for the lean diabetic is quite strict. Here, calories should not be restricted below normal levels. Because these patients take insulin, they must eat five or six times a day to correspond with the time-action pattern of the insulin so that they do not develop hypoglycemia. In contrast with obese patients, there must be no delay in mealtime and no unusual exercise. If any stress, such as stenuous exercise or a surgical procedure, occurs, insulin and diet are adjusted to the situation.

In both types of diabetes there is decreased emphasis on the priority of carbohydrate restriction. In the long run, insulin requirements are related to the fuel supply rather than to the amount of dietary carbohydrate itself. It is now evident that diets generous in starch are well tolerated, provided that the levels of calorie consumption are appropriate. Furthermore, if carbohydrate levels are sharply restricted, it is difficult to construct a diet that is not high in fat and cholesterol.

A typical diabetic diet contains the number of calories necessary to achieve or adhere to the ideal weight. Refined sugars are either totally eliminated or sharply limited. Natural sugars from fruit, vegetables, and milk are allowed at the 10 to 15% level. Fat is limited to between 25 and 35% (foods with unsaturated fat are used more than those with saturated fat). Protein provides 12 to 24% of the diet, and the remaining calories, usually 30 to 40%, are derived from starches. Emphasis is placed on starches high in fiber.

Hypoglycemia (Low Blood Sugar)[25]

It has been suggestd that the cause of hypoglycemia is excessive carbohydrate intake, especially that of sugar. There are two types of hypoglycemia, fasting and reactive. The more common is the reactive type, which is a reaction to the ingestion of food, including sugar.

Reactive hypoglycemia may produce symptoms such as lightheadedness, palpitations, and sweating that may trigger a ripple effect of fatigue and depression. These ripple effects are more frequent in individuals who have situations of personal stress such as marital, job, sex, or aging problems.

A low-carbohydrate, high-protein diet can afford variable relief, but more important, attention should be given to dealing with the emotional problems through counseling. Also, the possibility of an underlying chemical diabetes should be investigated.

LACTOSE INTOLERANCE

Lactose intolerance is a digestive problem for some people. They may experience gastrointestinal discomfort such as abdominal cramps, flatulence, watery stools, or all of these when they drink milk or ingest milk products. However, the aforementioned symptoms per se are not diagnostic of lactose intolerance. A hydrogen breath-analysis test, which gives a quantitative determination of the relative completeness of lactose digestion, must be done to confirm the diagnosis of primary adult lactose deficiency, recently called lactose nonpersistence.[26] Milk intolerance generally refers to some intestinal discomfort within a few hours after an individual ingests one or two glasses of milk.[27] In the United States, less than 12% of the whites but more than 70% of the blacks experience lactose nonpersistence.[26, 28]

Because dairy products contribute 75% of the calcium intake, the total elimination of lactose-containing foods from the diet is both unwise and not necessary.[29] The person may consume one-half glass of milk two or three times a day rather than a full 12-oz glass of milk once a day. Tolerance can be improved by consuming milk with a meal especially if it is accompanied by bananas, corn flakes, or hard-boiled eggs, because they reduce the rate of lactose fermentation. Whole milk is tolerated better than skim milk, and chocolate milk is tolerated better than unflavored milk.[30] Unpasteurized yogurt is tolerated better than milk because it has intrinsic lactase activity that substitutes for the individual's endogenous lactase.[31] As a result of the availability of commercial food-grade lactases at pharmacies, milk and milk products can be incubated with food-grade lactase for 24 hours, which will reduce the lactose content in the milk by 40 to 90%. Thus better tolerance is achieved by persons with lactose nonpersistence. Findings of preliminary studies in which exogeneous beta-galactosidases are added to milk at mealtime show that this method is convenient and improves lactose absorption while decreasing caloric hydrogen production.[32]

REFERENCES

1. Committee on Dietary Allowances, Food and Nutrition Board, National Academy of Sciences-National Research Council. Recommended Dietary Allowances, 9th rev. ed. Washington, D.C., National Academy Press, 1980.
2. Anderson, T. A. Recent trends in carbohydrate consumption. Annu. Rev. Nutr. 2:113, 1982.
3. Bibby, B. G.; Mundorff, S. A.; Zero, D. T., et al. Oral food clearance and the pH of plaque and saliva. J. Am. Dent. Assoc. 112:333, 1986.
4. Burkitt, D. P. Some diseases characteristic of modern Western civilization. Br. Med. J. 1:274, 1973.
5. Painter, M. S., et al. Unprocessed bran in treatment of diverticular disease of the colon. Br. Med. J. 2:137, 1972.
6. Trowell, H. C. Ischemic heart disease and dietary fiber. Am. J. Clin. Nutr. 25:926, 1972.
7. Reddy, B. S. Dietary fiber and atherosclerosis. In Vahouny, G. V.; Kritchevsky, D., eds. Dietary Fiber in Health and Disease, p. 265. New York, Plenum Publishing Corp., 1982.
8. Englyst, H. N.; Bingham, S. A.; Wiggins, H. S., et al. Nonstarch polysaccharide consumption in four Scandinavian populations. Nutr. Cancer 4:50, 1982.
9. Cantor, S.M. Patterns of use of sugar. In Shaw, J. H.; Roussos, G. G., eds. Proceedings, Sweeteners and Dental Caries, p. 111. Spec. Suppl. Feeding, Weight and Obesity Abstracts. Washington, D.C., Information Retrieval, Inc., 1978.

10. Dahlquist, A. Carbohydrates. In Present Knowledge in Nutrition:Nutrition Reviews, 5th ed. Washington, D.C., Nutrition Foundation, 1984.
11. Shannon, I. L. Brand-Name Guide to Sugar, p. 171. Chicago, Nelson-Hall, 1978.
12. Shaw, J. H. The metabolism of polyols and their potential for greater use as sweetening agents in foods and confections. In Shaw, J. H.; Roussos, G. G., eds. Proceedings, Sweeteners and Dental Caries, p. 171. Spec. Suppl. Feeding, Weight and Obesity Abstracts. Washington, D.C., Information Retrieval, Inc., 1978.
13. Horowitz, R. M.; Gentili, B. Citrus-based dihydrochalone. In Shaw, J. H.; Roussos, G. G., eds. Proceedings, Sweeteners and Dental Caries, p. 291. Spec. Suppl. Feeding, Weight and Obesity Abstracts. Washington, D.C., Information Retrieval, Inc., 1978.
14. Cagan, R. C., et al. Monellin, a sweet tasting protein. In Shaw, J. H.; Roussos, G. G., eds. Proceedings, Sweeteners and Dental Caries, p. 311. Spec. Suppl. Feeding, Weight and Obesity Abstracts. Washington, D.C., Information Retrieval, Inc., 1978.
15. Zienty, F. B. Present status and uncertainties concerning saccharin. In Shaw, J. H.; Roussos, G. G., eds. Proceedings, Sweeteners and Dental Caries, p. 253. Spec. Suppl. Feeding, Weight and Obesity Abstracts. Washington, D.C., Information Retrieval, Inc., 1978.
16. Hoover, R., et al. Progress report to the Food and Drug Administration from the National Cancer Institute concerning the National Bladder Cancer Study. Bethesda, Md., National Cancer Institute, 1979.
17. Morrison, A. S.; Buring, J. E. Artificial sweeteners and cancer of the lower urinary tract. N. Engl. J. Med. 302:537, 1980.
18. Hoover, R. Saccharin—bitter aftertaste? N. Engl. J. Med. 302:573, 1980.
19. Bost, R. G.; Ripper, A. Aspartame, a commercially feasible aspartic acid based sweetener. In Shaw, J. H.; Roussos, G. G., eds. Proceedings, Sweeteners and Dental Caries, p. 269. Spec. Suppl. Feeding, Weight and Obesity Abstracts. Washington, D.C., Information Retrieval, Inc., 1978.
20. West, K. M. Diabetes mellitus. In Schneider, H. A., et al., eds. Nutritional Support of Medical Practice, p. 278. Hagerstown, Md., Harper & Row, 1977.
21. Cohen, D., et al. Diabetes mellitus and oral periodontal disease: two year longitudinal observations. Part I. J. Periodont. 42:709, 1970.
22. Benick, S., et al. Dental disease in children with diabetes mellitus. J. Peridont. 46:241, 1975.
23. Hove, K.; Stallard, K. Diabetes and the periodontal patient. J. Periodont. 41:713, 1970.
24. Sussman, K.; Metz, R. Diabetes Mellitus, vol. IV, Diagnosis and Treatment. New York, American Diabetes Association, 1975.
25. Danowski, T. S. The Hypoglycemia Syndromes, 1st ed. Pittsburgh, Pa., Harper Press, 1978.
26. World Health Organization. Workshop on Lactose Malabsorption. Moscow, June 10–11, 1985.
27. Hourigan, J. A. Nutritional implications of lactose. Aust. J. Dairy Technol. 39:114, 1984.
28. Bayless, T. M.; Rothfield, M.; Massa, C., et al. Intolerance of recommended amounts of milk and lactose by lactose-intolerant adults. Am. J. Clin. Nutr. 26:465, 1973.
29. Marston, R. M.; Roper, N. R. The nutrient content of the food supply. Natl. Food Rev. 29:5, 1985.
30. Newcomer, A. D.; Mcgill, D. B. Clinical importance of lactose deficiency (editorial). N. Engl. J. Med. 310:42, 1984.
31. Kolars, J. C.; Levitt, M. D.; Aouji, M., et al. Yoghurt—an autodigesting source of lactose. N. Engl. J. Med. 310:1, 1984.
32. Solomons, N. W.; Guerrero, A. M.; Torun, B. Dietary manipulation of postprandial colonic lactose fermentation: II. Addition of exogenous microbial beta-galactosidases at mealtime. Am. J. Clin. Nutr. 41:209, 1985.

3

The Role of Carbohydrates in the Production of Dental Caries

THE NATURE OF DENTAL CARIES

Dental caries (from the Latin word *carius*, meaning rottenness) is more commonly known as tooth decay. It is a pathological process involving the localized demineralization of the inorganic mineral portions of the tooth followed by proteolysis (breakdown of proteins into simpler compunds), resulting in a carious lesion, or cavity.

The chemicoparasitic theory for the initiation and development of dental caries proposed by Miller in 1890 is accepted as the mechanism for the carious process by most dental scientists and clinicians.[1] Miller showed that carbohydrate foods, such as bread or potatoes or sugar, when mixed with saliva and incubated at 37°C were degraded to lactic acid. Further, he noted that only the dental plaque bacteria adherent to the tooth surface were responsible for the tooth destruction, not the bacteria of the oral environment. From these observations, he concluded that dental decay is a two-stage process comprising (1) a chemical phase consisting of demineralization of the inorganic structure by acid from bacterial fermentations of carbohydrate foods and (2) a bacterial, or "parasitic," phase consisting of dissolution of the "albuminous substances" by the "peptonizing" and digestive action of the bacteria.

MAJOR FACTORS IN THE DENTAL CARIES PROCESS

Five dental and oral environmental factors, namely, (1) the tooth chemistry, (2) the amount of salivary flow, (3) the types of dental plaque bacteria, (4) the type of fermentable carbohydrate eaten, and (5) the frequency of daily food intake, especially the between-meal snacks, are the causative agents concerned with the initiation and extension of dental caries. The dental decay process begins with the initiation of the lesion at the interface between the enamel or cemental surface and the base of the dental plaque. The enzymes of the dental plaque bacteria act upon the fermentable carbohydrates and break them down relatively rapidly to one or more of the following organic acids—lactic, pyruvic, acetic, propionic, formic—which can begin to demineralize the enamel or cemen-

31

tum rather quickly. Stephan showed that within 2 to 4 minutes of rinsing with a glucose or sucrose solution, the plaque pH fell from about 6.5 to about 5 (the pH for enamel decalcification is 5.5 or below) and gradually returned to the original pH within 40 minutes.[2] According to the Stephan curve (Fig. 3–1), during a period of 20 to 30 minutes, tooth enamel undergoes some decalcification because the plaque pH is 5.5 or below for that period.

Tooth Structure

The internal structure of the enamel is affected by systemic nutrients (e.g., protein, calcium, phosphorus, fluoride) in the circulatory system during tooth formation, development, and calcification. When the tooth is newly erupted and

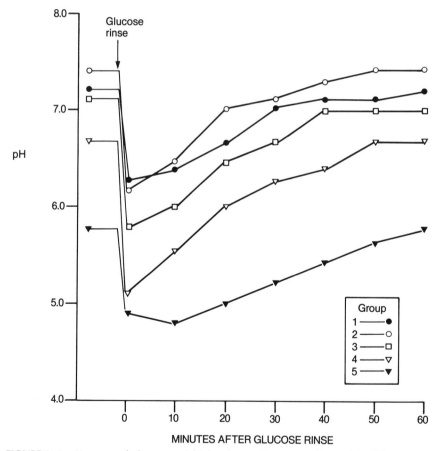

FIGURE 3–1. pH curves of plaques on labial surfaces of lower anterior teeth in different caries activity groups. Groups: 1 = caries-free; 2 = previous caries but caries-inactive during period of study; 3 = slight caries activity; 4 = marked caries activity; 5 = extreme caries activity. (From Stephan, R. M. Extra-oral hydrogen ion concentrations associated with dental caries activity. J. Dent. Res. 23:261, 1944.)

during its early maturation or mineralization, stage, the outer surface of the enamel is acted on by ionic exchange by local oral environmental factors (trace elements, e.g., fluorides or other minerals in drinking water; mouth rinse; toothpaste; saliva). Although enamel cannot regenerate like bone and other vital tissues, it has been shown by radioactive isotope techniques not to be completely inert. Enamel contains some fluid and is to a certain extent permeable, allowing minor modifications of its chemical composition and structure. Because the crystals are small, considerable activity in the intercrystalline spaces provides a large surface area available for reaction. The uptake of the ions takes place primarily in the hydration shell around the crystals, but some exchange is believed to occur on the crystal surfaces as well.

The 45° angulated incline planes of the cusps meet to form the deep occlusal pits and fissures of the posterior teeth, which are highly susceptible to dental caries because both dental plaque bacteria and food particles are readily trapped and retained in these crevices. Other caries-susceptible tooth enamel surface areas are the buccal pits and grooves of the lower molars, and the lingual cingulum of the upper incisors.

Teeth that are crowded or overlap are common sites for the development of dental caries because the thorough removal of dental plaque and food from between the teeth is often overlooked or may be difficult.

Saliva

An inadequate salivary flow rate can interfere with proper oral clearance of cariogenic food substrates. (The average flow rate of unstimulated whole saliva in adults is about 0.3 ml/min.) An inadequate volume of saliva would decrease the amount of natural buffers in the oral environment that normally neutralize most of the organic acids formed from the sugar fermentation.

As normally secreted, saliva contains very little glucose and no sucrose. However, ingestion of sugar-rich confections may produce a salivary sugar concentration that remains above 1 mg/ml, producing a pH low enough to produce tooth demineralization.[3] If a patient has a slow oral clearance of food or if he or she ingests a food with a high sugar content, sugar would be available to the oral microorganisms long enough to make acid production and subsequent caries development probable.

Dental Plaque Bacteria

Dental plaque is a sticky, jellylike mass that may cover the enamel on all its surfaces. It is composed of a great number of oral bacteria (see Roles of Specific Types of Plaque Bacteria, later in this chapter) plus salivary degradation products and products of microbial metabolism. Although food debris is often mixed with dental plaque, only those nutrients that are soluble, readily diffusible through the dental plaque, and quickly metabolized by the bacterial enzymes have a direct role in the caries process; the debris itself does not. According to Fosdick,[4] dental plaque acts as a permeable membrane and obeys the laws of diffusion. In the case of carbohydrates, the more soluble the mono- and disaccharides and the more concentrated the sugars, the better the diffusion through the dental plaque.

Fermentable Carbohydrate

The concentration of sugar in a food can be a key factor in the dental caries process. The reason is that the molar concentration, or particles per liter (a 1-molar [1-M] solution of sugar contains 342.3 g of sugar in a liter of water, or 0.3 g/1 ml), of the available sugar determines the rate of diffusion through the plaque. Fosdick stated that a concentration of 0.8 M must be present for sugar to pass through 1 mm of dental plaque and ferment to a harmful level (pH 5.2) within a 5-minute interval.[4] On the other hand, solutions of sugar on the order of 0.3 M, about that of fruit juices, were found to be too weak to penetrate 1 mm of plaque during a 30-minute interval. This may explain why the normal usage of fruit juices is not considered cariogenic.

The total sugar content per serving of a food is not a major consideration in determining its cariogenic potential. Small amounts of highly concentrated caloric sweeteners are just as cariogenic as large amounts. For example, one medium apple has a sugar content of 17 g and 1 oz of a sugar-frosted cereal has a sugar content of 16 g, but the sugar concentration of the apple (because of its water content) is only 11%, whereas that of the frosted cereal is 57%. Also, the speed of oral clearance of the apple is much greater than that of the presweetened cereal. Thus even though the sugar content per serving is about the same, the cariogenic potential of the presweetened cereal is much greater than that of the raw fruit owing to its higher sugar concentration and slower clearance from the oral cavity.

The role of starches and sugars in dental caries will be discussed in greater detail later in this chapter.

Time for Caries Lesion to Develop and Frequency of Between-Meal Snacks

It takes 18 months plus or minus 6 months from the incipient attacking forces of the organic acids on the tooth enamel surface until a carious lesion can clinically be detected.[5] In some persons with xerostomia resulting from either Sjögren's syndrome or radiation therapy to the head and neck, caries can be detected clinically within 3 months.

Caries prevalence is directly related to the frequency of between-meal snacking. This is true in individuals who frequently omit breakfast and overeat at other meals or between meals to make up for it. One-fourth to one-third of the total caloric intake of adolescents comes from between-meal snacks, a major factor in their high dental caries susceptibility.

The Cariogenic Potential of Foods as Measured by the Enamel-Demineralizing pH of Plaque

A food is classified as a potential cariogenic food if, when it comes into contact with the plaque bacteria, the plaque pH falls below 5.5, the tooth

TABLE 3–1. Some Foods that Cause the pH of Human Interproximal Plaque to Fall Below 5.5

Apples, dried	Gelatin, flavored dessert
Apples, fresh	Grapes
Apple drink	Milk, whole
Apricots, dried	Milk, 2% fat
Bananas	Milk, chocolate
Beans, baked	Oatmeal, instant cooked
Beans, green, canned	Oats, rolled
Bread, white	Oranges
Bread, whole wheat	Orange juice
Caramel	Pasta
Carrots, cooked	Peanut butter
Cereals, non-presweetened	Peas, canned
Cereals, presweetened	Potato, amylase
Chocolate, milk	Potato, boiled
Cola beverage	Potato, chips
Cookies, vanilla sugar	Raisins
Corn flakes	Rice, instant cooked
Cornstarch	Sponge cake, cream-filled
Crackers, soda	Tomato, fresh
Cream cheese	Wheat, flakes
Doughnuts, plain	

From Schactele, C. F. Changing perspectives on the role of diet in dental caries formation. Nutrition News™, vol. 45, no. 4, 1982, courtesy of National Dairy Council®, Rosemont, Ill.

demineralization pH. Table 3–1 lists some of the foods that according to Schactele fall into this category.[6] Foods that are classified as nonacidogenic include cheeses, namely, blue cheese, Cheddar, Gouda, Monterey Jack, mozzarella, and Swiss, because after contact with them, plaque pH usually registers pH 6 or higher. The common characteristics of the noncariogenic foods are that they (1) not only create a plaque pH of 6 or higher but (2) are relatively high in protein content, (3) have a moderate fat content to facilitate oral clearance, (4) contain a minimal concentration of fermentable carbohydrate, (5) exert a strong buffering action, (6) have a high mineral content, including calcium and phosphorous, and (7) include cheeses such as those noted above that are firm enough to stimulate salivary flow.

The conclusions from this research are that both noncariogenic snack foods such as those described and the development of products capable of neutralizing plaque acids might contribute significantly to the prevention of dental caries.

RELATIONSHIP OF SUGAR ALCOHOLS, STARCHES, AND SUGARS TO DENTAL CARIES

Sugar Alcohols

Sugar alcohols have little or no effect on plaque pH. Thus it is generally agreed that sorbitol-containing chewing gums may not contribute significantly to tooth decay, but there is some reasonable doubt that sugar alcohols are completely inactive in producing caries.

In answer to the question Should the dentist recommend the use of chewing gum, one could say that the dentist might recommend the alternative use of confections containing sugar alcohols instead. But in general, it is best to dissuade the patient from the use of mints or chewing gum.

Starch-Rich Foods

Two studies, reported in 1981 and 1982, have shown that starch-rich foods that tend to be retained on and around the teeth for a prolonged period of time are ultimately degraded to organic acids and thus contribute to the demineralization phase of the dental caries process.[7,8] In a third study, it has been reported that starch and sucrose act in synergism to produce acids in the presence of *Streptococcus sanguis*.[9] Bibby and co-workers reported that starch-rich foods, although containing less sugar than some other foods, were retained in the mouth for a longer time and therefore depressed the pH of the plaque longer, a potentially cariogenic factor.[10] They found an inverse relationship between the pH of plaque and the content of total carbohydrates in the saliva. In short, the impression is that the retention of food in the mouth (prolonged with starch-rich foods) may be as critical a factor in the production of dental caries as the amount of acidity the food produces in the plaque. *Thus the contribution of starch in sugar-containing foods may be a more important factor to caries production than has commonly been thought.*

Sugar-Rich Foods

Clinical evidence to support the profound effect of readily fermentable carbohydrates on dental caries has been reviewed by Newbrun,[11] Sreebny,[12] and Bowen.[13, 14] Although sucrose, the sugar most frequently used as sweetener, is usually regarded as the most cariogenic of the sugars, the fact is that there is little difference in cariogenic action between sucrose and glucose or fructose.

The physical form in which sugar is ingested influences its cariogenicity. Gustafson and colleagues[15] reported that subjects who chewed sticky toffee developed more caries than subjects who ingested a comparable amount of sugar in a nonsticky form.

The following are descriptions of three well-controlled clinical trials: the Vipeholm study, the Hopewood House study, and the Turku study. They have contributed the most convincing evidence of a direct cause-and-effect relationship between increased sugar consumption and increased dental caries.

VIPEHOLM STUDY

The classic clinical study that first demonstrated the importance of between-meal eating of sweets in producing dental caries was the Vipeholm study.[15] This was a 5-year nutritional study of 436 mental patients with a mean age of 32 who were confined more or less permanently in an institution in Vipeholm, Sweden. Diets were carefully supervised as to preparation, and nurses were able to ensure cooperation of the patients in following the experimental prescriptions.

The first year constituted an adjustment period during which a baseline caries index was established, and the patients consumed a diet rich in vitamins and other protective foods four times a day with no candy or chocolate and no between-meal snacks. The next 4 years consisted of the carbohydrate study period during which subgroups were fed the same basal diet, but the subgroups differed from one another in that some groups had increased amounts of sugar at mealtime and others had increased amounts of sugar between meals. There were nine groups who could essentially be categorized as eating one of the following four diets:

1. Basal diet
2. Basal diet and additional sugar in solution at meals
3. Basal diet and additional sugar in bread consumed at meals
4. Basal diet and additional sugar in the form of sweets between meals (It has been pointed out that caramels, toffees, and chocolates were not given at meals in spite of the fact that it is so recorded on the graph in Fig. 3–2.)

Those who were on the basal diet (the control group throughout the study) had low caries activity (Fig. 3–2). In those groups who had as much as 300 g of sucrose added to the meal in liquid form, as a beverage, or in food preparation, the caries activity was only slightly increased. It is worth noting that the same slight caries activity increase was seen in the group given bread containing only 50 g of refined sugar with meals.

In all groups other than those given the basal diet, there was a significant increase in dental caries. Even if there was a small amount of sugar added, as with those who ate candy between meals, there was a marked increased in caries activity, indicating that the quantity of sugar was not the most important factor. Furthermore, when the sweets were withdrawn from between meal periods, the caries activity decreased to the level of the initial preparatory period.

The important conclusions from this experiment were that the risk of increasing caries activity was least (1) if sugar with only a slight tendency to be retained in the mouth (such as sucrose solution) was ingested at meals or (2) if sugar-rich bread, which has a strong tendency to be retained, was consumed at meals. When sugar with a strong tendency to be retained was frequently eaten betweeen meals, the risk of increased caries activity was greatest.

Lundqvist measured the time sugar could be detected in the saliva of the participants of the Vipeholm study.[16] In Figures 3–2 and 3–3, it can be seen that in those groups ingesting sugar at meals—whether it was the control group, the sucrose group, or the bread group—only four peaks of sugar in the saliva were noted, corresponding to the four meals. Of special interest is that the sucrose groups, who ate twice as much sugar as the control group (but at meals), had an identical salivary glucose level.

In short, dental caries activity increased in connection with consumption of sugar in sticky form between meals but decreased when the consumption was interrupted. Furthermore, when sugar was consumed in solutions at meals, in amounts twice the average consumption, no increase in dental caries was observed. (It is important to note that there was no group consuming sugar in solution between meals.)

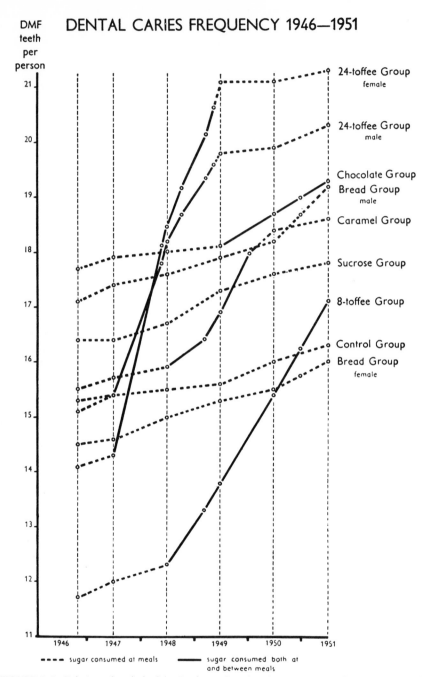

FIGURE 3–2. *Relation of carbohydrate intake to dental caries. (From Gustafsson, B., et al. The Vipeholm dental caries study: the effect of different levels of carbohydrates intake on caries activity in 436 individuals observed for five years. Acta Odont. Scand. 11:232, 1954.)*

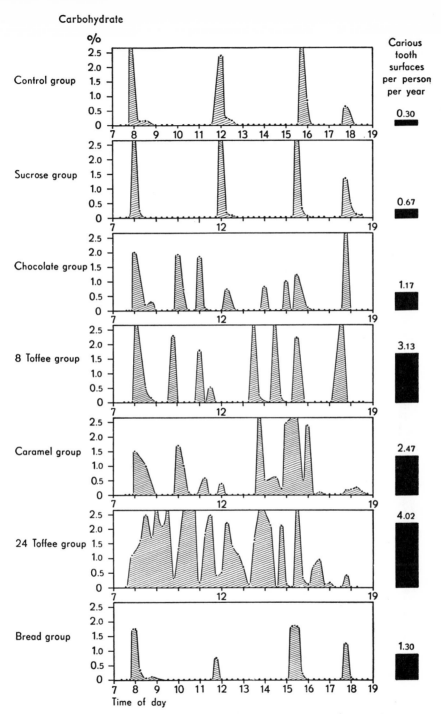

FIGURE 3–3. *Sugar clearance in day-series in different study groups. One individual series in agreement with each group's average value is chosen. The caries activity is expressed as an average value for each group within which clearance determination has been performed. (From Lundqvist, C. Odont. Rev. 3[Suppl. 1]:5, 1952.)*

Gustafsson's and Lundqvist's studies proved several points:

1. Sugar exerts its caries-promoting effect locally on the tooth surfaces.

2. Starch-rich foods such as bread with minimal sugar are not as cariogenic as sugar-rich foods (e.g., cookies).

3. The amount of sugar is not of paramount importance.

4. The form and composition of the sweets may be critical (prolonged retention is more cariogenic than short-term or nonretention).

5. The frequency of sugar consumption is a prime factor in caries activity.

Confirmation of Vipeholm Study Conclusions. The preceding conclusions, particularly those distinguishing between the influence of at-meal and between meal timing of sugar intake on caries incidence, were confirmed by the results of Mack,[17] King and co-workers,[18] Jay,[19] and Potgieter and colleagues.[20] There are more confirmatory data on the marked cariogenicity of the between-meal snack habit. Weiss and Trithart, in their clinical study of several hundred 5-year-old children, found that the children experienced a caries increase linearly related to the number of between-meal snacks they ate.[21] Specifically, those who ate one snack had a caries score of 4.8; two snacks, 5.7; three snacks, 8.5; and four or more snacks, 9.8 (Fig. 3–4). It appears that the most important difference between cariogenic and noncariogenic diets is not the amount of sugar ingested but the frequency of intake.

In 18 other clinical caries diet studies reviewed by Bibby, he noted the investigators' reasons for the high caries incidence they observed in their subjects.[22] Some of the reasons were "More desserts," "More frequent eating," "More candies, cookies, and sodas," and so forth (Table 3–2). In general, the principal conclusions of the investigators were that the high candy consumption and frequency of eating were mentioned most often as causes of caries, followed closely by the use of flour-containing foods.

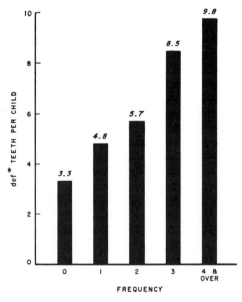

FIGURE 3–4. Effects of between-meal eating on caries activity in children. (From Weiss, R. L.; Trithart, A. H. Am. J. Public Health 50:1097, 1960.)

TABLE 3–2. Summary of Reports on Diets of Subjects with High and Low Caries Incidence

Authors	Date	Location	Caries Group High	Caries Group Low	Age	Authors' Reasons for High Caries
Pepin & Miller	1934	Michigan	90	80	School	More desserts
Bibby	1935	Various	19 racial groups		Various	More frequent eating, not nutrition
Collett	1936	Norway	40	11	School	More sweets and soft bread
Read and Knowles	1937	England	12	12	3–14	Between-meal eating, more sweets and fermentable carbohydrates
Staz	1943	S. Africa	41	20	5–12	More frequent sweets
Hyde et al.	1945	New England	275 in 5 groups		Military	More meals and snacks
Bazant et al.	1954	Czechoslovakia	—	—	School	Sugar and white flour
Potgieter et al.	1956	Connecticut	864 in 3 groups		11–14	Poor diet, somewhat more between-meal eating, candy and soft drinks
Kridakara et al.	1956	Thailand	2300 in 2 groups		4–18	More sugar and wheat flour
Eppenberger	1958	Switzerland	249 in 2 groups		14–15	Higher sugar and white bread
Oravecz	1959	Hungary	3859 in groups		3–6	Early weaning, high sweets, between-meal eating
Zita et al.	1959	Indiana	200 in 4 groups		5–13	More between-meal sugar
Weiss and Trithart	1960	Tennessee	1375 in 5 groups		5	More frequent candies, cookies, and sodas
Bradford and Crabb	1961	England	72	157	4–11	More frequent carbohydrates
Fukui et al.	1962	Japan	808 in 4 groups		School	More cakes and candy after supper
MacGregor	1963	Ghana	383 in 3 groups		6–12	More sweets
Niwa	1969	Japan	155 subgrouped		2–3	More frequent eating
Palmer	1971	England	366	355	7–10	Cariogenic food and liquid at bedtime
Samuelson et al.	1971	Sweden	1401 subgrouped		4, 8, and 13	More frequent sweets, buns, and cakes
Martinson	1972	Sweden	156	167	14	Frequency of eating toffee, gum, and sweetmeats

HOPEWOOD HOUSE STUDY

There is strong supportive evidence for the positive relationship of dietary sugar to prevalence of dental caries in the 1957 to 1961 study done at Hopewood House, a home for children in Bowral, Australia.[23] Eighty-two residents of the institution, aged 10 to 15 years at the beginning of the study, were observed for 5 years. These children were fed a balanced lactovegetarian diet without sweets. When compared with a control group of children who had continuously eaten an unsupervised, high-sugar diet, the Hopewood House 15-year-olds had half the caries, even though there was rapid caries development in these children after they left Hopewood House (Table 3–3). This result can be interpreted either as a reflection of the residual caries-protective effect of a balanced diet during the pre-eruptive development of permanent teeth or as an effect of sweets consumption after the teeth erupt, which in a comparatively short period can overwhelm the earlier low caries incidence.

TURKU STUDY

Probably the most unequivocal evidence of the importance of readily fermentable sugars in the causation of caries comes from a clinical trial in Turku, Finland.[24] This was a 2-year feeding study dealing with measuring and evaluating the dental and general health effects of the exclusive use of one type of sweetener—sucrose or fructose or xylitol—on a total of 125 subjects whose mean age was 27.6 years.

Each group ate a variety of foods sweetened with only one of the three sugars being tested. One of the most important results was the remarkable reduction in the incidence of dental caries in the xylitol group (Fig. 3–5). Although fructose was less cariogenic than sucrose, it caused a substantial number of caries, an important consideration because of the increased use by food and beverage processors of corn syrup, which is high in fructose. In fact, soft drinks, which have a high sugar content and a low pH, really contain the acidified conversion products of sucrose, namely, fructose and glucose.

OTHER CLINICAL STUDIES

A number of dental clinics have included nutritional guidance in their dental care programs. Each has been able to effectively reduce the caries increments in their patients by prescribing diets that emphasize reduction of

**TABLE 3–3. Number of DMF Teeth of Hopewood Child
(Lactovegetarian Diet, Almost Complete Absence of Refined
Carbohydrate) Compared with Those of State School Child
(Usual Diet, High in Refined Carbohydrates)**

	Age (Years)					
Residence of Child	10	11	12	13	14	15
Hopewood House	0.85	1.00	1.81	3.50	6.20	6.46
State school	5.28	6.98	9.32	10.70	12.78	13.91

From Harris, R. M. J. Dent. Res. 42:1387, 1963.

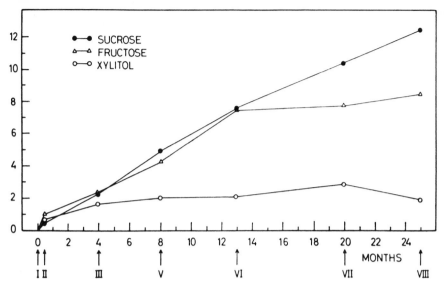

FIGURE 3–5. Turku sugar studies. Development of caries activity index, comprising all clinical and radiographic quantitative and qualitative changes during the 2-year feeding study. (Scheinin, A.; Mäkinen, K. K. Acta Odont. Scand. 33[Suppl. 70], 1975.)

sugar intake. For example, 30 or 40 years ago, several investigators, Jay,[25] Becks,[26] and Templeman[27] used a restricted, refined carbohydrate intake regimen and increased the daily intake of foods of high nutrient density (milk, eggs, meats, vegetables). Using the *Lactobacillus acidophilus* test, now an outmoded caries-monitoring device, an individualized diet of low cariogenic potential seemed to be achieved. Becks claimed rather dramatic results in reducing caries increments as a result of his dietary counseling.

In 1942 Howe and co-workers compared dental caries increments in 189 children who had been under nutritional supervision (emphasis on increased intake of protective foods and decreased intake of sugar-sweetened foods) with those of 225 children of the same ages who had no special supervision.[28] The overall reductions in dental caries for all age groups in those children who received general and dental health nutrition guidance was 50% (Fig. 3–6). It should be pointed out that this study was done before the period of availability of any type of systemic or topical fluoride regimen.

The Comparative Cariogenicity of Starch and Sugar in Humans

Other clinical studies confirm the concept that diets high in sugar produce more caries than diets high in starch, without or with minimal sugar. Several dental clinicians have independently noted that a group of individuals who cannot metabolize fructose because of a genetic error also have practically no dental decay. This disease is known as hereditary fructose intolerance.[29, 30] Whenever such patients eat any food containing fructose, they become nauseated. Because sucrose is broken down, absorbed, and utilized as both glucose and

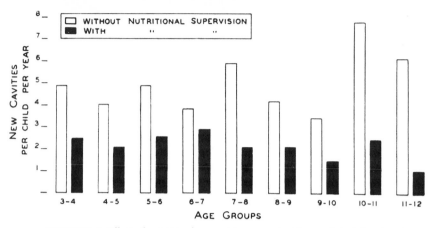

FIGURE 3–6. Effect of nutritional supervision upon incidence of dental caries.

fructose, these patients must abstain from using sugar. The carbohydrates they can eat freely are starches such as wheat, rice, potatoes, and other root vegetables, because the final breakdown product of carbohydrate is glucose (dextrin to maltose to two molecules of glucose).

A survey of patients with hereditary fructose intolerance revealed that 15 of 27 individuals were caries-free and the others for whom a DMFT score could be ascertained had a low caries rate (Table 3–4). Newbrun stated that in one study, normal siblings of children with hereditary fructose intolerances show the usual high caries prevalence because they can ingest and tolerate sugars.[31]

Guatemalan children on a dietary regimen that included candy, cake, and other sweets had more caries and more polysaccharide storing bacteria in their dental plaque than children who ate a high-starch diet and practically no sugars.[32]

The control group in the Vipeholm study was fed a starchy diet that was almost sugar-free and they developed virtually no new caries. Also, in the previously mentioned Turku clinical trial, the groups using xylitol as a sweetener consumed significant amounts of starch, and these subjects did not develop any new decay.

Nursing Bottle Caries

Nursing bottle caries is a type of caries characterized by rapid onset and extensive destruction of most of the deciduous teeth in infants who hold nursing bottles and pacifiers in their mouths over long periods of time, e.g., falling asleep with the nipple of the bottle or pacifier in the mouth (Fig. 3–7). In this situation there is direct contact of the teeth with water, juice, or milk sweetened with sugar, syrup, or honey. Some pedodontists have even seen this type of rampant caries in children who drink unsweetened milk from their nursing bottles. Usually, the nursing bottles are used as pacifiers at bedtime for children who are much beyond the bottle-feeding age.

TABLE 3–4. Dental Caries Experience of Patients with Hereditary Fructose Intolerance

Patient	Age	Sex	DMFT	Comment	Reference
RKC	7	M	0	Dark stain in groove of 2nd primary molar	
DFC	15	M	5	Deep developmental grooves, prophylactic fillings?	Cornblath et al.[1]
JC	9	F	0		
MJD	26	F	0		
JAC	18	F	4		
KE	39	F	2	Teeth surprisingly intact	
EP	33	M	1	No active caries	Froesch et al.[2]
P	>33	M	1	No active caries	
	39	M	2	Very good dental health	Hubschmann and Cobet[3]
IG	18	F	?	Excellent dental health	
FS	54	F	?	Good dental health	
OS	63	M	?	Teeth in good condition	Linden and Nisell[4]
BB	50	M	?	Excellent dental health	
EB	57	M	?	Good dental health	
AEH	41	M	0	No caries, calculus present	
LR	32	F	0	No caries, calculus present	Newbrun[5]
JB	6	M	0		
AB	10	M	0		
EB	14	F	9		
AC	20	M	11		
EC	24	F	0		
MH	34	F	14		
PE	38	M	1		Marthaler and Froesch[6]
MP	38	M	6		
EA	10	M	0	No caries	Levin et al.[7]
OW	54	M	0	No restorations, no caries	Auerswald and Kupetz[8]
F	83	F	0	No caries	Brauman et al.[9]
EA	42	F	0	No caries, calculus present	Newbrun[10]
A	7	F	0	Caries-free	
V	13	F	0	Caries-free	
M	15	F	0	Caries-free	
U	11	M	2	Interprox. lesions	Hess and Graf[11]

From Newbrun, E. Cariology. Baltimore, Williams & Wilkins, 1978.

1. Cornblath, M.; Rosenthal, I. M.; Reisner, S. H., et al. Hereditary fructose intolerance. N. Engl. J. Med. 269:1271, 1963.
2. Froesch, E. R.; Wolf, H. P.; Baitsch, H. Hereditary fructose intolerance. Am. J. Med. 34:151, 1963.
3. Hubschmann, K.; Cobet, G. Contribution to hereditary fructose intolerance. Dtsch. Med. Wochenschr. 89:938, 1964.
4. Linden, L.; Nisell, J. Hereditary intolerance to fructose. Svensk. Läkartidn. 61:3185, 1964.
5. Newbrun, E. Dextransucrase from *Streptococcus sanguis*. Further characterization. Caries Res. 5:124, 1971.
6. Marthaler, T. M.; Froesch, E. R. Hereditary fructose intolerance—dental status of 8 patients. Br. Dent. J. 123:597, 1967.
7. Levin, B.; Snodgrass, G. J. A. I.; Oberholzer, V. G., et al. Fructosaemia observations on seven cases. Am. J. Med. 45:826, 1968.
8. Auerswald, W.; Kupetz, G. W. Beitrag zur Klinik der hereditären Fruktose-Intoleranz. Dsch. Gesundheitsw. 24:875, 1969.
9. Brauman, J.; Kentos, P.; Frisque, P., et al. Intolerance hereditaire au fructose chez une femme de 83 ans. Acta. Clin. Belg. 26:65, 1971.
10. Newbrun, E. Polysaccharide synthesis in plaque. In Stiles, H. M.; Loesche, W. W.; O'Brien, T. C., eds. Microbial Aspects of Dental Caries. Spec. Suppl. Microbiol. Abstr. 3:649, 1976.
11. Hess, J.; Graf, H. Zahnplaque-pH bei Patienten mit hereditären Fruktose-Intoleranz. Schweiz. Monatsschr. Zahnheilk. 85:141, 1975.

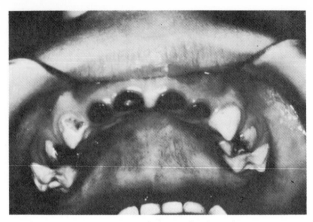

FIGURE 3–7. *Rampant caries owing to use of nursing bottle with sugar-sweetened beverages as a pacifier.*

The child usually lies with the nursing bottle in the mouth. The tongue extends slightly out of the mouth and covers the lower anterior teeth. As the child falls asleep, active sucking stops, so that the movements of the jaw that normally stimulate the anticaries factors, salivary flow and salivary buffering, no longer take place. In short, the problem is compounded by low salivary flow during sleep.

This is a perfect oral environment for the enhancement of the carious process, particularly when a sugary beverage pools around the teeth. The beverage spreads over the upper teeth and the lower posterior teeth, but not over the lower incisors, which are covered and protected by the tongue. The unprotected teeth undergo rampant caries (Fig. 3–7).

Winter and colleagues noted the dietary habits of 200 children with rampant caries and came to the conclusion that there was a direct cause-and-effect relationship between the sugar-sweetened contents of the nursing bottle and the extensive carious damage to the teeth.[33]

EVIDENCE FOR THE RELATIONSHIP OF CARIES TO BACTERIA AND CARBOHYDRATES

To arrive at a scientific explanation for and to postulate the mechanisms producing carious lesions, we must consider the evidence concerning the effects of both bacteria and carbohydrates on dental caries.

Roles of Specific Types of Plaque Bacteria

There is an association between predominance of specific bacteria, caries activity, and bacterial tooth sites (*Streptococcus sanguis* and *Streptococcus mutans* in fissures and smooth surfaces of the crown and *Actinomyces viscosus* on the root surfaces).[34, 35] *S. mutans* characteristically clumps together in the form of a sticky plaque that adheres readily to all tooth surfaces and crevices.

This plaque is a jellylike mass composed of a large number of bacteria plus other cellular matter (bacterial extracellular polysaccharides, white cells, salivary mucin, and epithelial cell remnants).[36]

Although *S. sanguis* and *A. viscosus* have been shown to be involved in the development of caries, the two major bacteria are *S. mutans* (first initiates the carious process) and *Lactobacillus acidophilus* (extends the process). However, there appears to be some slight controversy as to the precise role of each of these bacteria in caries development. The decay-producing potential of these organisms results in part from the fact that they both readily ferment sugars to acid. *S. mutans* also has the ability to synthesize and store complex carbohydrates (fructans, or levans, and glucans, or dextrans) for future fermentation. These polysaccharides provide the streptococci with the sticky coating that allows them to clump together as a tenacious mat on the tooth surfaces.

It is clear that sucrose is of central importance in the plaque formation process. However, according to Brown, all dietary carbohydrates, not sucrose alone, contribute to plaque formation and to the development of caries. Sucrose and other dietary carbohydrates are most important in the caries process as fermentable energy sources for the bacteria.[37]

Effects of Carbohydrate Metabolism on Bacterial Metabolism

Both sucrose and glucose are degraded to lactic acid as a result of the enzymatic activity of streptococci and lactobacilli. At the same time that acid is formed, the polysaccharides glycogen, glucan (dextran), and fructan (levan) are formed and stored in the dental plaque by various polysaccharide-storing streptococci. When the bacteria need more of the simple sugars for energy and metabolism, the dextran, levan, and glycogen stored in the dental plaque may be broken down.

Highly concentrated, readily fermentable mono- and disaccharides diffuse into the plaque quickly, where they are used by the microorganisms for energy. However, large, insoluble, nondiffusible starch molecules have little direct effect on the plaque and therefore on the dental caries process. The rate of development of the carious process involving starch is very much slower than the reactions with sugar.

Effect of Low-Carbohydrate Diet on Numbers of Bacteria

A low-carbohydrate diet will reduce the number of *Lactobacillus, S. salivarius,* and *S. mutans.* However, when there is a decrease in *S. mutans* because of a low carbohydrate intake, there is usually an increase in the numbers of *S. sanguis.*

Numbers of polysaccharide-storing streptococci are directly influenced by the amount of dietary carbohydrate. For example, van Houte[38] noted that when he severely limited his own daily carbohydrate to 10 g over a 2-week period, there was a significant reduction in the number of polysaccharide-storing microorganisms in the dental plaque. When he resumed a normal, carbohydrate-containing diet, the proportions of polysaccharide-storing organisms increased to the original counts. It is interesting to note that even though the numbers of specific bacteria changed, the types of bacteria did not change during the different dietary regimens.

Physical-Chemical Properties of Starch and Sugar

The physical and chemical properties of starch, a polysaccharide, are much different from those of the simple sugars, sucrose, glucose, fructose, maltose, and lactose.

The polysaccharide, being of high molecular weight, is a macromolecule (very large molecule) and thus does not readily diffuse through plaque, is relatively insoluble, and does not ferment readily. It therefore is not immediately available as an energy source for oral microorganisms. On the other hand, the simple sugars, which are low molecular weight micromolecules (small), diffuse readily through plaque, are easily soluble, and are readily fermentable. These simple sugars are readily available as an energy source for microorganisms.[39]

The differences in physical and chemical properties provide further evidence that starch is less cariogenic than sugar. Starch must be hydrolyzed into smaller units before it can enter the plaque. In reality, very little starch is enzymatically broken down in the mouth. When this does occur, it takes time, allowing the buffering capacity of the saliva to exert its neutralizing effects on acid formation much more effectively than on the rapidly fermented sugars.

Cariogenicity of Soft Drinks

Research on the relative cariogenicity of liquid sweets or soft drinks shows that sugary drinks are just as likely to promote cavities as solid sweets. Stephan's findings in 1938[40] and 1944[41] showed that after rinsing with a glucose solution, the pH of the dental plaque remains acidic for about 30 minutes. This was confirmed in 1971 and 1983 by Muhlemann[42] and Imfeld,[43] respectively.

Ismail and co-workers assessed the relative cariogenicity of soft drinks in a representative sample of the American population, using a case control, epidemiological approach.[44] The soft drinks included in the study were consumed between 1971 and 1974, the period during which NHANES I data were collected. NHANES I was a comprehensive survey of a national sample of 20,749 Americans aged 1 to 74, whose health and nutritional status were measured. The interviewers collected 1-day food intakes on the basis of 24-hour dietary recall.

The soft drink group included about 29 carbonated and noncarbonated sucrose-sweetened beverages, mostly colas and fruit-flavored drinks. The data showed that the frequencies of consumption of the sugar-sweetened soft drinks at and between meals were directly correlated with high DMFT (Decayed, Missing, and Filled Teeth) scores in age groups 12 to 14, 15 to 17, 21 to 23, and 24 to 26. No association was found between high DMFT scores and the consumption of soft drinks in age groups 9 to 11, 18 to 26, and 27 to 29. Since the time covered in this study, sweeteners other than sucrose, such as high-fructose corn syrups, saccharin, and aspartame, have been used. The impact of these other sweeteners on the cariogenic potential of soft drinks is not yet known.

Clearly, this study shows that caries formation is related to frequency of ingestion of sugar-sweetened drinks. Thus the results of this study indicate that equal weight should probably be given to reduction of high-sugar snacks in both solid and liquid form.

SUMMARY

Dental caries occur when demineralization agents such as an acid-producing plaque acting on tooth enamel overwhelm the buffering capacity and remineralization ability of the oral and dental environment.

The major food factors that provide the media for proliferation of cariogenic bacteria *(S. mutans)* are carbohydrates—both monosaccharides and disaccharides—sugar alcohols, and starchy foods containing even small amounts of sugar. Each food characteristic, namely, composition, texture, solubility, potential for retention, and ability to stimulate salivary flow, should be considered when determining the relative cariogenic potential of a food.

The frequency of ingestion and the physical form of the sugars are important influences in caries development. The more often retentive sugars are eaten, the greater the risk of developing caries. However, when sugar-containing solutions such as soft drinks are consumed frequently, they also produce caries.

Clearly, the amount, composition, and physical form of readily fermentable carbohydrate-rich foods and especially the meal pattern and frequency of consumption of these foods in the daily diet influence the incidence of caries.

Therefore one major method for preventing and controlling dental caries is to decrease the formation and enzymatic activity of bacterial plaque. This can be done by reducing the supply of readily fermentable carbohydrates.

REFERENCES

1. Miller, W. D. The microorganisms of the human mouth. Philadelphia, S. S. White Dental Mfg. Co., 1980. Cited in Noto, W. A., ed. Oral Microbiology, 2nd ed., p. 251. St. Louis, Mo. C. V. Mosby Co., 1973.
2. Stephan, R. M. Changes in hydrogren ion concentration on tooth surfaces and in carious lesions. J. Am. Dent. Assoc. 27:718, 1940.
3. Kleinberg. I. Prevention and dental caries. J. Prevent. Dent. 5:9, 1978.
4. Fosdick, L. S. Biochemical aspects of dental caries. Dent. Clin. North Am. July:369, 1964.
5. Parfitt, G. J. The speed of development of the carious cavity. Br. Dent. J. 100:204, 1956.
6. Schactele, C. F. Changing perspectives on the role of diet in dental caries formation. Nutr. News 45(4):13, 1982.
7. Mormann, J. E.; Muhlemann, H. R. Oral starch degradation and its influence on acid production in human dental plaque. Caries Res. 15:166, 1981.
8. Jensen, M. E.; Schactele, C. F. The acidogenic potential of reference foods and snacks at interproximal sites in the human dentition. J. Dent. Res. 62:889, 1982.
9. Buehrer, E. A.; Miller, C. H. Sucrose and starch synergism in *Streptococcus sanguis* acid production. Proc. J. Int. Dent. Res., Abstract no. 137, 1984.
10. Bibby, B. G.; Mundorff, S. A.; Zero, D. T., et al. Oral food clearance and the pH of plaque and saliva. J. Am. Dent. Assoc. 112:333, 1986.
11. Newbrun, E. Sugar and dental caries: a review of human studies. Science 217:418, 1982.
12. Sreenbny, L. M. The sugar-caries axis. Int. Dent. J. 32:1, 1982.
13. Bowen, W. H. Role of carbohydrates in dental caries. In Shaw, J. H.; Roussos, G. G., eds. Proceedings, Sweeteners and Dental Caries, pp. 147–152. Spec. Suppl. Feeding, Weight and Obesity Abstracts. Washington, D. C., Information Retrieval, Inc., 1978.
14. Colman, G.; Bowen, W. H.; Cole, M. F. The effects of sucrose, fructose, and a mixture of glucose and fructose on the incidence of dental caries in monkeys. Br. Dent. J. 142:217, 1977.

15. Gustafson, B. E.; Quensel, C. E.; Swenander, L., et al. The Vipeholm dental caries study: effect of different levels of carbohydrate intake on dental caries activity in 436 individuals observed for 5 years. Acta Odont. Scand. 11:232, 1954.
16. Lundqvist, C. Oral sugar clearance. Its influence on dental caries activity. Odont. Rev. 3(Suppl. 1):5, 1952.
17. Mack, P. B. A study of institutionalized children with particular reference to the caloric value as well as other factors of the diet. Soc. Res. Child Dev. 13:62, 1949.
18. King, J. D.; Mellanby, M.; Stones, H. H., et al. The effect of sugar supplements on dental caries in children. Med. Res. Council, Spec. Rep. Serv. No. 288. London, 1955.
19. Jay, P. The reduction of oral lactobacilli counts by the periodic restriction of carbohydrate. Am. J. Orthop. 33:162, 1947.
20. Potgieter, M.; Morse, E. H.; Erlenback, F. M., et al. The food habits and dental status of some Connecticut children. J. Dent. Res. 35:638, 1956.
21. Weiss, R. L.; Trithart, A. H. Between-meal eating habits and dental caries experience in preschool children. Am. J. Public Health 50:1097, 1960.
22. Bibby, B. G. The cariogenicity of snack foods and confections. J. Am. Dent. Assoc. 90:126, 1975.
23. Harris, R. M. Biology of the children of Hopewood House. J. Dent. Res. 42:1387, 1963.
24. Scheinin, A., et al. Turku sugar studies. V. Final report on the effect of sucrose, fructose and xylitol diets on caries incidence in man. Acta Odont. Scand. 34:179, 1976.
25. Jay, P. The role of sugar in the etiology of caries. J. Am. Dent. Assoc. 27:293, 1940.
26. Becks, H. Carbohydrate restriction in the prevention of dental caries using the L.A. count as one index. J. Calif. Dent. Assoc. 26:53, 1950.
27. Templeman, A. J. The dietary control of dental caries. Aust. Dent. J. 9:163, 1964.
28. Howe, R. P.; White, R. L.; Elliott, M. D. The influence of nutritional supervision on dental caries. J. Am. Dent. Assoc. 29:38, 1942.
29. Marthaler, T. M.; Froesch, E. R. Hereditary fructose intolerance. Dental status of eight patients. Br. Dent. J. 123:597, 1967.
30. Cornblath, M., et al. Hereditary fructose intolerance. N. Engl. J. Med. 269:1271, 1963.
31. Newbrun, E. Cariology, pp. 79–81. Baltimore, Williams & Wilkins Co., 1978.
32. Loesche, W. J.; Henry, C. A. Intracellular microbial polysaccharide production and dental caries in a Guatemalan Indian village. Arch. Oral Biol. 12:189, 1967.
33. Winter, G. B., et al. Role of the comforter as an etiologic factor in rampant caries of the deciduous dentition. Arch. Dis. Child 41:207, 1966.
34. Gibbons, R. J. Bacteriology of dental caries. J. Dent. Res. 43:1021, 1964.
35. Rosen, S. Laboratory animals and their contribution to oral microbiology. In Nolte, U. A., ed. Oral Microbiology, 2nd ed. St. Louis, Mo., C. V. Mosby Co., 1973.
36. Gibbons, R. J.; Van Houte, J. Dental caries. Annu. Rev. Med. 26:121, 1975.
37. Brown, A. T. The role of dietary carbohydrates in plaque formation and oral disease. Nutr. Rev. 33:353, 1975.
38. Van Houte, J. Relationship between carbohydrate intake and polysaccharide storing microorganisms in dental plaque. Arch. Oral Biol. 9:91, 1964.
39. Newbrun, E. Sucrose, the arch criminal of dental caries. Odontol. Revy 18:373, 1967.
40. Stephan, R. M. Hydrogen ion concentration of the dental plaque. J. Dent. Res. 17:251, 1938.
41. Stephan, R. M. Intra-oral hydrogen ion concentrations associated with dental caries activity. J. Dent. Res. 23:257, 1944.
42. Muhlemann, H. R. Intra-oral radio telemetry. Int. Dent. J. 21:456, 1971.
43. Imfeld, N. Identification of low caries risk dietary components. Monographs in Oral Science, vol. 11, pp. 101–189. New York, S. Karger, 1983.
44. Ismail, A. I.; Burt, B. A.; Eklund, S. A. The cariogenicity of soft drinks in the United States. J. Am. Dent. Assoc. 109:241, 1984.

4

Lipid Nutrition in Health and Disease

Lipids are a group of compounds that are not of uniform composition but are related by their relative insolubility in water and their solubility in organic solvents such as ether, alcohol, and chloroform. The term lipids is an all-inclusive one for fats and fat-like substances. It embraces (1) the true fats (e.g., butter, margarine, vegetable oils, and body depot fat); (2) substances whose molecular structure includes fatty acids or fatty acid derivatives, such as cholesterol (a sterol); and (3) compounds present in minor amounts associated with lipids in nature, such as ergosterol (a fat-soluble vitamin) or a steroid sex hormone.

Nutritionists further subdivide the true fats into visible and invisible types. Visible fats are foods such as butter, lard, margarine, vegetable shortening, and salad oils. Invisible fats are those that are hidden in food, such as the marbleized fat in roast beef, the butterfat in milk, or the oil in avocados. A few other invisible fats are those in ice cream, peanut butter, potato chips, and many highly processed food products. Visible fats that remain solid at room temperature are called fats, whereas those that are liquid are called oils.

DIETARY INTAKE AND FOOD SOURCES

An increase in annual per capita domestic consumption of food fat from 126 lb in 1969 to about 135 lb in 1979 was noted by the U.S. Department of Agriculture. The increase was of both visible and invisible fat.[1] According to the Recommended Dietary Allowances, the total fat intake, particularly in diets below 2000 kcal, should be reduced to 35% of the total dietary energy.[2] However, the American Heart Association and the Committee on Diet, Nutrition, and Cancer of the National Research Council recommend that a prudent diet should contain only 30 to 35% of calories as fat in order to reduce the incidence of coronary heart disease[3] and cancer.[4]

In the food supply, 90% of the fat comes from (1) salad and cooking oils, butter, and margarine; (2) meat, poultry, and fish; and (3) milk, cheese, and yogurt. In 1982 fats and oils provided 44% of the fat available in the food supply; meat, poultry and fish, 34%; and dairy foods, 12%.[5] Individuals who want to reduce fat intake without adversely affecting the total nutrient intake in their diet should decrease their intake of mayonnaise and salad dressing and be prudent with the amounts of butter, margarine, and vegetable oils they ingest. The last three foods are the most desirable in the fat group of foods because they provide fat-soluble vitamins A and E and also some essential fatty acids.

51

Because fats lack water and are reduced (have added hydrogen at some bonds), they are highly concentrated stores of potential energy, and when metabolized by tissue cells, they can combine with more oxygen and release more energy than either carbohydrate or protein. On a gram-for-gram basis, dietary fat provides 9 calories, a little more than twice the number of calories of carbohydrates or proteins. Affluence, social customs, and psychological and physiological factors influence the amount and type of fat consumed. The higher the income, the more fat is eaten and the more vegetable fats and oils (e.g., corn oil), rather than animal fats such as lard, are used in cooking. For good health, fat is an essential component of the diet, but an intemperate intake at the expense of other nutrients can contribute excess calories and thus can lead to such serious health problems as diabetes, obesity, and atherosclerosis.

TRUE FATS (TRIACYL GLYCEROLS)

Chemically, lipids contain carbon, hydrogen, and oxygen, as do carbohydrates, but lipids contain greater proportions of carbon and hydrogen and much less of oxygen. Complex lipids may contain additional elements, such as phosphorus and nitrogen.

A pure fat is composed of molecules of glycerol to which one, two, or three fatty acids are linked to form monoglycerides, diglycerides, or triglycerides, respectively. Natural fats, as in meat, grain, and nuts, are made up mostly of triglycerides. Animal fats consist primarily of triglycerides but also contain cholesterol. Processed fats, such as shortenings, contain up to 20% mono- and diglycerides.

FATTY ACIDS

Saturated and Unsaturated Fatty Acids

The basic structural unit of lipids is the fatty acid (carbon atoms arranged in a straight chain, with the acid part on one end). Fatty acids that are common in food fats and oils fall, according to their degree of saturation, into three broad classes: (1) fully saturated, (2) monounsaturated, and (3) polyunsaturated. Fatty acids also vary in chain length according to the number of carbon atoms. Short-chain fatty acids have 2 to 4 carbon atoms; those with medium chains have 6 to 10 carbon atoms; and those with long chains have 12 to 26 carbon atoms.

Fully saturated fatty acids consist of carbon atoms connected to hydrogen atoms by a single bond and cannot take up any more hydrogen. They are stable compounds. The common ones are stearic acid (18 carbons), found in beef and lard, and palmitic acid (16 carbons), found in animal fat and palm oil. Others are myristic acid (14 carbons) and lauric acid (12 carbons). The latter is found in milk and coconut oils. These fatty acids can increase the serum cholesterol level. Unsaturated fatty acids contain one or more free bonds and may take up more hydrogen atoms; in other words, they are not "saturated" with hydrogen atoms. Monounsaturated fatty acids are those with one reactive unsaturated linkage or one double bond and no hydrogen atom. Palmitoleic acid and oleic acid are the most common ones found in nature. Oleic acid is found in olive oil, shortenings, lard, peanut oil, lamb, and poultry fat. These fatty acids have no effect on serum cholesterol.

Polyunsaturated fatty acids have two, three, or four double bonds per molecule. An example is linoleic acid, the essential fatty acid found in soybean, cotton, cottonseed, and other vegetable oils. These fatty acids lower the cholesterol levels in the serum.

Essential Fatty Acids (EFA)

Certain unsaturated fatty acids have been identified as essential because the body cannot synthesize them, and if missing from the diet, they will produce a deficiency state.

Linoleic acid and arachidonic acid are essential fatty acids. Arachidonic acid has been found to be indispensable for rodents. However, arachidonic acid can be formed in humans from linoleic acid, and therefore only linoleic acid is actually essential for humans.

EFA and their derivatives (1) maintain the function and integrity of cell membranes, (2) are used to esterify cholesterol in plasma, and (3) are required for the metabolism of cholesterol and other lipids. It has been shown that a diet high in EFA reduces high levels of serum cholesterol.

Linoleic acid derivatives have been shown to be precursors for a group of hormonelike compounds called prostaglandins, which are among the most potent biologically active substances yet discovered. Prostaglandins cause contraction of smooth muscle and dilation of certain vascular beds. They have been suggested for use in preventing conception, inducing labor at term, terminating pregnancy, preventing or alleviating gastric ulcers, controlling inflammation, lowering blood pressure, and relieving asthma and nasal congestion.

When there is a linoleic acid deficiency, signs and symptoms of scaly skin, sparse hair growth, poor wound healing, and thrombocytopenia (decrease in blood platelets) may appear. Infants fed skim milk formulas for extended periods of time without fatty acid supplementation can become deficient in fatty acids. EFA deficiency has been noted in hospitalized patients who have not been fed by mouth but instead have been kept on a fat-free diet by being fed intravenously for several weeks.

Good sources of linoleic acid are corn, cottonseed, peanut, soybean, and safflower oils. It is recommended that 1 to 2% of the total calories consumed should be EFA.

LINOLEIC AND LINOLENIC ACIDS

There may be a relationship between the polyunsaturated fatty acids linoleic and linolenic acids with prostaglandin production, blood platelet–vessel wall interactions, and clot-forming tendencies. Among other physiological roles such as helping regulate the body's use of cholesterol, prostaglandins influence smooth muscle contraction, reproduction, venous functions, and cardiopulmonary processes, including the accumulation of blood platelets. It has been claimed that the balance between two prostaglandins, thromboxane and prostacyclin controls activities related to the arrest of blood flow and to clot formation.[6, 7] It is premature, however, to suggest that an increase in dietary polyunsaturated fatty acids would be desirable for stopping bleeding.[8]

SOME OTHER LIPIDS

Phospholipids. A class of compound lipids called phospholipids consists of esters of fatty acids and glycerol combined with phosphoric acid and a nitrogenous base. These phospholipids are subdivided into three groups—phosphatides, sphingomyelins, and plasmalogens.

The phosphatides form part of the cell walls and mitochondria (filamentous or granular components of cytoplasm). One of these phosphatides, lecithin, is composed of glycerol, fatty acid, and choline and has a role in the transport and use of fat and fatty acids. The major food sources of lecithin are egg yolks and meat. Commercial preparations are made from soybeans. Lecithin is used as an emulsifying agent in mayonnaise and salad dressings. Contrary to the claims of food faddists, there is no good evidence that extra lecithin intake will lower serum cholesterol levels or that it is helpful in the treatment of coronary disease. It will not aid in the removal of fat deposits in obese subjects. Cephalin, another phosphatide, is found in egg yolks and in brain. It is present in thromboplastin, which is needed in the blood-clotting process.

Sphingomyelin normally is a component of a fatlike sheath substance, the insulation around nerve fibers. These nerve fibers are spoken of as being myelinated or medulated. In Niemann-Pick disease, a lipid-storage disorder of childhood, an excess of sphingomyelin accumulates in all organs and tissues of the body.

Plasmalogens may be related to the specialized function of platelets in blood coagulation.

Cholesterol. Another group of lipids consists of sterols, which are complex alcohols of high molecular weight capable of forming esters with fatty acids. Cholesterol is one of these and occurs either in stored form or as free cholesterol. The esters (compounds formed from an alcohol and an acid by removal of water) are the storage form of cholesterol and are found in the plasma, constituting two-thirds of the total plasma cholesterol. Most of the cholesterol that accumulates in the walls of atherosclerotic arteries is esterified (converted into an ester). Free cholesterol is found in plasma lipoproteins and does not provide energy; rather, it is a structural component of cell membranes and is essential for normal cell function. It is a precursor to steroid sex hormones, bile acids, adrenocortical hormones (one of the steroids produced by the adrenal cortex), and vitamin D. It has an important role in the transport of fatty acids.

Cholesterol is a fat-soluble substance that is synthesized only by the animal organism. It is regulated primarily by the liver. It is estimated that the body synthesizes approximately 1.5 to 2 g of cholesterol per day.

Only animal foods (Table 4–1), including meat, glandular organs (liver, kidney), eggs, whole milk, cheese, and fats, are sources of dietary cholesterol; plant foods are not. We absorb 50% of dietary cholesterol, so the ideal intake should be in the range of 100 to 300 mg of dietary cholesterol per day, far less than the 600 to 1200 mg that the average North American eats per day. Diets

TABLE 4–1. Cholesterol Content of Common Measures of Selected Foods

Food	Amount	Cholesterol (mg)
Milk, skim, fluid or reconstituted dry	1 c	5
Cottage cheese, uncreamed	½ c	7
Lard	1 tbsp	12
Cream, light table	1 fl oz	20
Cottage cheese, creamed	½ c	24
Cream, half and half	¼ c	26
Ice cream, regular (approximately 10% fat)	½ c	27
Cheese, cheddar	1 oz	28
Milk, whole	1 c	34
Butter	1 tbsp	35
Oysters, salmon	3 oz, cooked	40
Clams, halibut, tuna	3 oz, cooked	55
Chicken, turkey, light meat	3 oz, cooked	67
Beef, pork, lobster, chicken, turkey, dark meat	3 oz, cooked	75
Lamb, veal, crab	3 oz, cooked	85
Shrimp	3 oz, cooked	130
Heart, beef	3 oz, cooked	230
Egg	1 yolk or 1 egg	250
Liver (beef, calf, pork, lamb)	3 oz, cooked	370
Kidney	3 oz, cooked	680
Brains	3 oz, raw	more than 1700

From Feeley, R. M.; Criner, P. E.; Watt, B. K. J. Am. Diet. Assoc. 61:134, 1972; Fats in Food and Diets, p. 6. USDA Information Bulletin No. 361, 1974.

high in cholesterol, saturated fats, or both raise the total plasma cholesterol level.

In addition to the saturated animal fats already mentioned that raise blood cholesterol, other cholesterol-producing fats can be found in hydrogenated shortenings, coconut oil, cocoa butter, and palm oil (in cookies, pies, and nondairy milk substitutes).

The polyunsaturated fats, which lower blood cholesterol, are liquid oils that originate from corn, cottonseed, safflower, sesame seed, soybean, sunflower, and other vegetable sources. Olive oil and peanut oil are low in polyunsaturated fats but neither raise nor lower blood cholesterol. Chicken, turkey, fish, and lean veal are low in total fat and are recommended for low-cholesterol diets.

In 1982 cholesterol in the food supply was 42% from eggs; 38% from meat, poultry, and fish; 15% from dairy foods; and 5% from fats and oils.[5]

Plasma cholesterol levels are considered normal by many physicians when they are in the range of 200 to 300 mg. However, normal is not optimal, nor does it imply any protection from heart disease. In fact, a plasma cholesterol level of 260 mg or higher carries with it five times more risk for heart disease than does the acceptable level of 220 mg or lower. Only in societies in which the level of plasma cholesterol is below 150 to 160 mg do physicians find virtually no deaths from heart disease.

Whether or not we consume dietary cholesterol, the normal human body can and will produce all the cholesterol that it requires. A biological feedback mechanism theoretically inhibits the synthesis of cholesterol when dietary cholesterol is increased; conversely, the synthesis of cholesterol is increased when dietary cholesterol is low. However, the feedback mechanism is not completely effective in compensating for the dietary intake level.

Another significant finding has been that lipoproteins are carriers of cholesterol and other fatty substances in the blood stream. Two lipoproteins have been found to be of particular interest: LDL, or low-density lipoprotein, and HDL, or high-density lipoprotein. High levels of LDL have been directly correlated with heart disease, whereas high levels of HDL appear to be protective with respect to heart disease. (This topic and others dealing with the control of serum cholesterol levels are discussed in the section concerning atherosclerosis in this chapter.)

FUNCTIONS OF LIPIDS

Lipids have many important functions in human nutrition:

- Phospholipids are an integral component of cells and contribute to their proper functioning.
- True fats are an excellent source of energy. They provide 9 calories per gram of substance compared with 4 calories per gram of carbohydrate or protein. (In short, they are twice as efficient as a source of energy.)
- Lipids provide the essential fatty acids—arachidonic for animals and linoleic for humans—that are indispensable for normal growth and skin health.
- Lipids are carriers for and facilitate the absorption of the fat-soluble vitamins, A, D, E, and K.
- Fats maintain body temperature by insulating against the cold and act as a cushioning mechanism against injury, affording protection of vital organs such as the kidneys and reproductive organs.
- Fats provide a pleasant flavor and consistency to food. They contribute physical properties to food that are important in processing and cooking.
- Fats in a meal cause a sense of fullness and satisfaction (satiety).

THE PHYSIOLOGY OF FATS

Digestion and Absorption

Fatty foods stimulate enterogastrone, a duodenal hormone that inhibits gastric motility and retards the discharge of food from the stomach. This is the reason a meal rich in fat digests slowly and provides a sense of fullness, or satiety.

The major digestive action of fat takes place in the small intestine with the aid of bile salts, which emulsify the fat (divide it into small globules). This increases the surface area and lowers the surface tension, allowing better access and penetration by enzymes (pancreatic and enteric lipases), which break up the fat into mono- and diglycerides, fatty acids, and glycerol.

Glycerol, monoglycerides, and medium-chain fatty acids are absorbed directly into the portal system from the intestine and are transported to the liver.

Long-chain fatty acids are first esterified to form neutral fat within the mucosal wall of the intestine. They then combine with cholesterol, phospholipids, and protein to form chylomicrons (particles of emulsified fat), which are the chief vehicles for the transport of lipids from the alimentary canal to the liver. The chylomicrons are absorbed from the intestine into the lymphatic system and are transported from the thoracic duct to the left subclavian vein, where they enter the venous blood and are carried to the liver. Sixty to seventy percent of dietary fat is absorbed via this lymphatic system. The remainder of the dietary fat, esterified cholesterol, and phospholipids is transported via the portal circulation.

Metabolism and Storage

Most ingested fat is oxidized to provide energy, if needed. If not needed for energy, it is stored in adipose tissue. Before oxidation takes place, fat is broken down into glycerol and fatty acids, which follow different chemical paths of oxidation, both finally becoming carbon dioxide and water. The rate at which fragments from fatty acid metabolism are oxidized, producing energy, depends primarily on the number of carbohydrate fragments also being oxidized.

In abnormal conditions such as diabetes, carbohydrate is not well utilized. Two-carbon fragments derived from fatty acid oxidation begin to accumulate and are eventually converted to compounds known as ketone bodies, which can be partly responsible for the acidosis or ketosis that may accompany diabetes, starvation, or protein-sparing fasting.

Lipid metabolism releases large amounts of adenosine triphosphate (ATP), a potential source of energy for molecular movements, synthesis of tissues, and heat.

The liver performs important functions in lipid metabolism. It synthesizes triglycerides, cholesterol, phospholipids, and lipoprotein. It also clears phospholipids, cholesterol, and lipoprotein from plasma.

A large number of hormones (e.g., insulin, growth hormone, thyroxine, and glucagon) cause fat to be mobilized, synthesized, utilized, and released from tissue stores.

Fat in excess of that needed to supply energy is stored as adipose tissue (lipogenesis), particularly under the skin, thus insulating the body and cushioning internal organs. These stores and the body weight they add can be reduced only when bodily energy needs are greater than caloric food intake.

ATHEROSCLEROSIS, CORONARY HEART DISEASE, AND CANCER

Atherosclerosis is a degenerative disease that produces a loss of elasticity and a hardening of the large and medium arteries. It is characterized by the formation of atheromata (deposits of lipids) on the inner walls of the large and medium-sized arteries, narrowing them. As it ages, the plaque becomes fibrotic or hardens with calcium deposits. It may ulcerate the lumen (cavity or channel) of the vessel, causing narrowing, roughening, and scarring of the channel through which the blood flows. Marked deformity and occlusion of the arteries may occur because the deposits have grown together or because a blood clot plugs the narrowed passageway. Atherosclerosis is responsible for ischemia (a lessened blood supply).

Atherosclerosis in the coronary arteries can cause myocardial infarction (presence of a localized area of ischemic [blood-deficient] necrosis [death of cells]), resulting in coronary heart disease, the commonest cause of cardiovascular disability and death. In the United States, coronary disease occurs most commonly in men between the ages of 50 and 60; in women it usually occurs between the ages of 60 and 70. It expresses itself clinically as angina pectoris (acute pain in the chest caused by interference with the supply of oxygen to the heart), acute myocardial infarction, arrhythmia, and congestive (abnormal accumulation of blood) heart failure. When atherosclerotic plaque cuts off the blood supply to the brain, cerebral infarction (stroke) ensues. In the leg arteries, atheroma causes claudication (resulting in lameness) and gangrene, and in the renal arteries it may produce hypertension and poor kidney function.

Most people have some degree of atherosclerosis, even children, adolescents, and young people in their twenties, but some are more susceptible than others. Evidence now suggests that hyperlipidemia (high lipid level in the blood) contributes to this disease process.

Blood Levels of Lipids in Atherosclerosis

Hyperlipidemia is an elevation of serum cholesterol or triglycerides, or both. Cholesterol, triglycerides, and phospholipids are carried in the plasma bound to specific proteins and thus are called lipoproteins. Five classes of lipoproteins have been identified according to their density: (1) chylomicrons; (2) pre-beta–cholesterol, or very low-density lipoprotein (VLDL); (3) beta-cholesterol, or low-density lipoprotein (LDL); (4) alpha-cholesterol, or high-density lipoprotein (HDL); and (5) a transient, intermediate, low-density lipoprotein (ILDL) that appears during the conversion of VLDL to LDL. Chylomicrons come from the diet and are cleared rapidly. VLDL, LDL, and HDL are manufactured by the body.

The higher the HDL levels, the lower the risk of cardiovascular disease. On the other hand, the more LDL that remains in the blood stream, the greater the likelihood of developing atherosclerosis.

As a result of research done by Goldstein and Brown,[9] the 1985 Nobel Prize winners in Medicine from the University of Texas Health Science Center in Dallas, we now know that "receptors" on the outer membranes of cells control blood LDL levels. These receptors act as gatekeepers that attach themselves to the LDL, remove it from the blood, and pull it inside the cell where it can perform its important role. However, if cholesterol begins to accumulate inside the cells, fewer LDL receptors are produced. These investigators suspect that persons who eat a great deal of food containing fat and cholesterol become unable to process cholesterol because their cells have metabolized all the LDL they can handle, and many receptors shut down. Without these receptors, cholesterol accumulates in the blood, causing atherosclerosis. As a result of this research, drugs are being developed that will stimulate cells to produce more LDL receptors so that cholesterol can be cleared from the blood at a normal rate.

When the amount of HDL increases, the risk of developing coronary heart

**TABLE 4–2. Plasma Lipid and Lipoprotein Concentrations
(Suggested Normal Limits*)**

Age	Total Cholesterol (mg/100 ml)	Triglyceride (mg/100 ml)	Pre-beta-cholesterol (mg/100 ml)	Beta-cholesterol (mg/100 ml)	Alpha-cholesterol (mg/100 ml)	
					Males	*Females*
0–19	120–230	10–140	5–25	50–170	30–65	30–70
20–20	120–240	10–140	5–25	60–170	35–70	35–75
30–39	140–270	10–150	5–35	70–190	30–65	35–80
40–49	150–310	10–160	5–35	80–190	30–65	40–85
50–59	160–330	10–190	10–40	80–210	30–65	35–85

From Fredrickson, D. S. Reprinted by permission of the New England Journal of Medicine (276; 151, 1967).
*Based on 95% fiducial limits calculated for small samples; all values rounded to nearest 5 mg. (For practical purposes, differences between the sexes have been ignored except for alpha-lipoprotein concentrations.)

disease is low. This explains why some patients with high blood cholesterol levels do not fit the general pattern. They have a higher ratio of HDL to LDL than normal. HDL transports cholesterol. As a result, excess cholesterol is carried out of the system before it can do harm. Table 4–2 gives the normal limits of the plasma lipids and lipoproteins for different age groups.

Hyperlipoproteinemia occurs when serum lipoproteins are elevated and are accompanied by an elevation of cholesterol, triglycerides, or both. According to Fredrickson, five types of hyperlipoproteinemia are significant in the diagnosis and treatment of various serum lipid disorders.[10] For further information on the method of management of each of the five types of hyperlipoproteinemia, the reader is referred to a medical nutrition text.[6]

The five major types of hyperlipoproteinemia are affected by the following dietary factors: cholesterol, fat, saturated fat, polyunsaturated fat, carbohydrate, and alcohol.

Of these five types, type II and type IV are the most common. The aim in the dietary management of type II, which is characterized by an elevated cholesterol of LDL origin, is to reduce the saturated fatty acids and cholesterol and to increase polyunsaturated fatty acids. The diet for this type should contain less than 300 mg of cholesterol daily (one egg yolk contains 250 mg), no more than 6 to 10% of total calories from saturated fats, and a polyunsaturated to saturated fatty acid ratio of about 2:1.

Type IV, or hypertriglyceridemia, is characterized by an elevation of endogenous (formed in body cells) VLDL. Triglycerides are elevated, and a slight elevation of cholesterol may be found. Since most of the patients with type IV are overweight, weight reduction is most important. Limitation of carbohydrate (especially sweets) and alcohol, moderate cholesterol restriction (usually 300 to 500 mg/day), and substitution of polyunsaturated for saturated fats are also recommended.

Methods for Reducing Blood Lipids

It is advisable to reduce the total dietary fat to about 33% of the total calories, to reduce the saturated fats by 50%, and to double the intake of polyunsaturated fats. This procedure could lower the blood cholesterol by at least 15%. In a National Diet–Heart Study the serum cholesterol level was reduced about 11% as a result of reducing cholesterol intake to about 400 mg with a polyunsaturated to saturated fat ratio of 1.5:1.

FATS AND OTHER LIPIDS

It is not advisable or even possible to eliminate saturated fats and cholesterol completely, because they are present in many essential foods.

The food patterns that can reduce the blood lipids in humans are as follows:

- The diet should furnish all other nutrients—proteins, vitamins, minerals, and carbohydrates—in adequate and balanced quantities (Fig. 4–1).
- The diet should provide adequate calories for maintenance of a desirable weight but should avoid an excess.
- The intake of fatty foods rich in saturated fats should be lowered to less than 10% of the total calories. In their place, one might select foods rich in polyunsaturated fats to compose up to 10% of total calories. A polyunsaturated to saturated fat ratio of 2:1 is desirable.
- The cholesterol-rich foods can be controlled by eating no more than three egg yolks a week, including eggs used in cooking, and by limiting intake of shellfish and organ meats. Cholesterol intake should be under 250 mg daily.
- The amount and type of fat can be controlled by using fish, chicken, turkey, and veal; by trimming visible fat from meats; by avoiding deep-fat frying and instead baking, boiling, broiling, roasting, or stewing; by restricting the use of fatty delicatessen foods such as salami and sausages; by using liquid vegetable oils and corn oil margarines instead of butter and hydrogenated fats; by using skimmed milk and skimmed milk cheeses rather than whole milk and cheeses made from whole milk.
- In addition, the intake of simple, refined carbohydrate (sugar) and table salt (below 4 g daily, one-third of what is normally consumed by the average American) should be limited.

These dietary modifications seem safe, but we do not have enough scientific data to say that they are optimal and incontrovertible.

Other Methods for Reducing Risk of Atherosclerosis

For the dietary control of atherosclerosis to be successful, it must be instituted early in life. Children at high risk for adult atherosclerosis, such as those with diabetes or familial hypercholesterolemia, should be advised to lower their fat intake under close medical supervision.

Since many factors contribute to coronary heart disease, the nutritional approach is only one of several that must be instituted to realize any benefits. Other factors that contribute to atherosclerosis are obesity, cigarette smoking, lack of exercise, high blood pressure, nervous tension, gorging at mealtime, diabetes, excessive salt intake, and an inherited tendency to heart disease.

Thus the risk of having a heart attack can be lessened for the person whose diet will not increase the serum cholesterol levels, and who maintains normal weight, exercises regularly, eliminates the stress of emotional tensions, does not smoke, and obtains medical treatment if high blood pressure or diabetes is present.

According to the "lipid hypothesis," elevated blood lipids, particularly cholesterol and LDL, can cause coronary heart disease. Moreover, dietary fat, especially saturated fatty acids and cholesterol, is suggested as the main dietary factor influencing blood lipids.[11] Some scientists support the lipid hypothesis and believe that diet modification can help prevent coronary heart disease.[12, 13] They base their conclusion on clinical studies demonstrating an effect of dietary fat and cholesterol on blood lipids and lipoproteins. On the other hand, others emphasize the complex etiology of coronary heart disease, including a genetic predisposition to the disease and the inability of intervention trials to decrease total mortality rates in subjects.[14, 15]

Examination of data from the Framingham Heart Study revealed that intake of eggs, one of the highest sources of cholesterol in the diet, was unrelated to blood cholesterol levels or to the incidence of coronary heart disease.[16, 17]

In only about 20% of persons with high bood cholesterol do cholesterol levels return to normal as a result of dietary modifications.[18] To date, clinical studies in which diet is manipulated and the course of the disease is followed have not proved or disproved the lipid hypothesis. Results of trials designed to reduce the incidence of coronary heart disease in individuals through lowering blood cholesterol levels either by diet or drugs have not shown a reduction in total mortality.[19] Also, the Multiple Risk Factor Intervention Trial in the United States, involving men with a mean blood cholesterol level of 240 mg/100 ml at entry, failed to result in a decreased total mortality, even when they ate a cholesterol-lowering diet.[20] (The risk of suffering from coronary heart disease increases when blood cholesterol exceeds 250 mg/100 ml.[21])

Nevertheless, the American Heart Association recommends that the general public consume a "prudent" diet containing 30 to 35% of calories as fat with equal amounts of saturated, monounsaturated, and polyunsaturated fatty acids and no more than 300 mg of cholesterol per day.[3]

On the other hand, the Food and Nutrition Board recommends that for patients with hyperlipidemia or proven vascular disease diet modification is indicated. However, they do not recommend that all healthy individuals reduce intake of fat and cholesterol to prevent or delay the development of atherosclerosis and coronary heart disease.[22] It should also be noted that the American Academy of Pediatrics emphasizes the need for dietary fat and cholesterol at least during the first year of life; therefore they do not recommend the use of reduced-fat milks during infancy.[23]

With respect to the relationship between total fat intake and cancer, the committee on Diet, Nutrition, and Cancer of the Assembly of Life Sciences recommends that the average current total fat intake of 40% of the diet be reduced to 30% of the diet to reduce the risk of cancer.[24] This recommendation was based on animal experiments seeming to show that a high intake of fat is associated with development of breast and colon cancers.[25]

FATS AND ORAL HEALTH

Dental Caries

There is indirect evidence that dietary fats may help prevent caries in humans. For example, those Eskimos whose diets are almost solely of animal

> Every day, select foods from each of the basic food groups in lists 1–5, and follow the recommendations for number and size of servings.

1 MEAT POULTRY FISH DRIED BEANS and PEAS NUTS · EGGS

1 serving . . .

3-4 ounces of cooked meat or fish (not including bone or fat) or 3-4 ounces of a vegetable listed here

Use 2 or more servings (a total of 6-8 ounces) daily

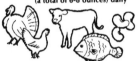

RECOMMENDED

Chicken • turkey • veal • fish • in most of your meat meals for the week.

Shellfish: clams • crab • lobster • oysters • scallops • shrimp • are low in fat but high in cholesterol. Use a 4-ounce serving in a meat meal no more than twice a week.

Beef • lamb • pork • ham • in no more than 5 meals per week.

Choose lean ground meat and lean cuts of meat • trim all visible fat before cooking • bake, broil, roast, or stew so that you can discard the fat which cooks out of the meat.

Nuts and dried beans and peas:

Kidney beans • lima beans • baked beans • lentils • chick peas (garbanzos) • split peas • are high in vegetable protein and may be used in place of meat occasionally.

Egg whites as desired.

AVOID OR USE SPARINGLY

Duck • goose

Heavily marbled and fatty meats • spare ribs • mutton • frankfurters • sausages • fatty hamburgers • bacon • luncheon meats.

Organ meats: liver • kidney • heart • sweetbreads • are very high in cholesterol. Since liver is very rich in vitamins and iron, it should not be eliminated from the diet completely. Use a 4-ounce serving in a meat meal no more than once a week.

Egg yolks: limit to 3 per week including eggs used in cooking.

Cakes, batters, sauces, and other foods containing egg yolks.

2 VEGETABLES and FRUIT

(Fresh, frozen, or canned)

1 serving . . . ¹/₂ cup
Use at least 4 servings daily

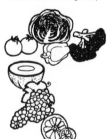

RECOMMENDED

One serving should be a source of Vitamin C:
Broccoli • cabbage (raw) • tomatoes. Berries • cantaloupe • grapefruit (or juice) • mango • melon • orange (or juice) • papaya • strawberries • tangerines.

One serving should be a source of Vitamin A—dark green leafy or yellow vegetables, or yellow fruits:
Broccoli • carrots • chard • chicory • escarole • greens (beet, collard, dandelion, mustard, turnip) • kale • peas • rutabagas • spinach • string beans • sweet potatoes and yams • watercress • winter squash • yellow corn.
Apricots • cantaloupe • mango • papaya.

Other vegetables and fruits are also very nutritious; they should be eaten in salads, main dishes, snacks, and desserts, in addition to the recommended daily allowances of high vitamin A and C vegetables and fruits. If you must limit your calories, use a serving of potatoes, yellow corn, or fresh or frozen cooked lima beans in place of a bread serving.

AVOID OR USE SPARINGLY

Olives and avocados are very high in fat calories and should be used in moderation.

FIGURE 4–1. The Five Basic Food Groups.

3 BREAD and CEREALS

(Whole grain, enriched, or restored)

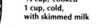

1 serving of bread . . . 1 slice

1 serving of cereal . . .
    ¹/₂ cup, cooked
    1 cup, cold,
    with skimmed milk

Use at least 4 servings daily

RECOMMENDED

Breads made with a minimum of saturated fat:
White enriched (including raisin bread) • whole wheat • English muffins • French bread • Italian bread • oatmeal bread • pumpernickel • rye bread.

Biscuits, muffins, and griddle cakes made at home, using an allowed liquid oil as shortening.

Cereal (hot and cold) • rice • melba toast • matzo • pretzels.

Pasta: macaroni • noodles (except egg noodles) • spaghetti.

AVOID OR USE SPARINGLY

Butter rolls • commercial biscuits, muffins, donuts, sweet rolls, cakes, crackers • egg bread, cheese bread • commercial mixes containing dried eggs and whole milk.

4 MILK PRODUCTS

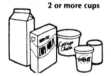

1 serving . . . 8 ounces (1 cup)

Buy only skimmed milk that has been fortified with Vitamins A and D.

Daily servings:
Children up to 12 . . .
    3 or more cups
Teenagers . . .
    4 or more cups
Adults . . .
    2 or more cups

RECOMMENDED

Milk products that are low in dairy fats:

Fortified skimmed (non-fat) milk and fortified skimmed milk powder • low-fat milk. The label on the container should show that the milk is fortified with Vitamins A and D. The word "fortified" alone is not enough.

Buttermilk made from skimmed milk • yogurt made from skimmed milk • canned evaporated skimmed milk • cocoa made with low-fat milk.

Cheeses made from skimmed or partially skimmed milk, such as cottage cheese, creamed or uncreamed (uncreamed, preferably) • farmer's, baker's, or hoop cheese • mozzarella and sapsago cheeses made with partially skimmed milk.

AVOID OR USE SPARINGLY

Whole milk and whole milk products:

Chocolate milk • canned whole milk • ice cream • all creams including sour, half and half, whipped • whole milk yogurt.

Non-dairy cream substitutes (usually contain coconut oil which is very high in saturated fat).

Cheeses made from cream or whole milk.

Butter.

5 FATS and OILS

(Polyunsaturated)

An individual allowance should include about 2-4 tablespoons daily (depending on how many calories you can afford) in the form of margarine, salad dressing, and shortening.

RECOMMENDED

Margarines, liquid oil shortenings, salad dressings and mayonnaise containing any of these polyunsaturated vegetable oils:

Corn oil • cottonseed oil • safflower oil • sesame seed oil • soybean oil • sunflower seed oil.

Margarines and other products high in polyunsaturates can usually be identified by their label which lists a recommended *liquid* vegetable oil as the *first* ingredient, and one or more partially hydrogenated vegetable oils as additional ingredients.

Diet margarines are low in calories because they are low in fat. Therefore it takes twice as much diet margarine to supply the polyunsaturates contained in a recommended margarine.

AVOID OR USE SPARINGLY

Solid fats and shortenings:

Butter • lard • salt pork fat • meat fat • completely hydrogenated margarines and vegetable shortenings • products containing coconut oil.

Peanut oil and olive oil may be used occasionally for flavor, but they are low in polyunsaturates and do not take the place of the recommended oils.

FIGURE 4–1 Continued

origin and furnish about 70 to 80% of their total calories as fat experience little if any decay. It is only when the fat content of the diet is reduced to 25% or less that decay starts to appear.[26, 27]

The mechanisms whereby fats act to reduce dental caries are probably as follows: (1) coating of the tooth surfaces with an oily substance would mean that food particles will not be so readily retained; (2) a fatty protective layer over plaque would prevent fermentable sugar substrate from being reduced to acids; (3) high concentrations of fatty acids may interfere with the growth of cariogenic bacteria; and (4) increased dietary fat will decrease the amount of dietary fermentable carbohydrate necessary for organic acid formation.

Parotid Enlargement

Chronic swelling of the parotid glands can be the result of the disturbed lipid metabolism that accompanies alcoholism. It is known that alcoholism will produce fatty infiltration in the liver, and similar infiltrations of the parotid glands have also been reported. Thus the fatty deposits in the parotid glands will result in enlargement.[28]

REFERENCES

1. USDA National Food Review. U.S. Fats, Oils Consumption Rises (report). J. Am. Oil Chem. Soc. 57:538a, 1980.
2. Committee on Dietary Allowances, Food and Nutrition Board, National Academy of Sciences-National Research Council. Recommended Dietary Allowances, 9th rev. ed. Washington, D.C., National Academy Press, 1980.
3. American Heart Association, Nutrition Committees, and Council on Atherosclerosis. Recommendations for treatment of hyperlipidemia in adults. Circulation 69:1082A, 1984.
4. Committee on Diet, Nutrition and Cancer, National Research Council. Diet, Nutrition and Cancer. Washington, D.C., National Academy Press, 1982.
5. Marston, R. M.; Welsh, S.O. Nutrient content of the U.S. food supply, 1982. Natl. Food Rev. 25:12, 1984.
6. Bazan, N. G.: Paoletti, R.; Ianconora, J. M., eds. New Trends in Nutrition, Lipid Research and Cardiovascular Disease. New York, Alan R. Liss, Inc., 1981.
7. Galli, C. Adv. Nutr. Res. 3:95, 1980.
8. Harlan, J. M.; Harker, L. A. Hemostasis, thrombosis, and thromboemboli. Med. Clin. North Am. 65:855, 1981.
9. Award-winning breakthrough on cholesterol. Tufts Univ. Diet Nutr. Lett. 3(10):1, 1985.
10. Fredrickson, D. S. Fat transport in lipoproteins—an integrated approach to mechanisms and disorders. N. Engl. J. Med. 276:151, 1967.
11. Stamler, J. In Hegyeli, R. J., ed. Nutrition and Cardiovascular Disease, pp. 245–308. New York, S. Karger, 1983.
12. Zilversmit, D. B. Diet and heart disease. Prudence, probability and proof. Arteriosclerosis 2:83, 1982.
13. Ahrens, E. H., Jr. Obesity and coronary heart disease: new dimensions. Arteriosclerosis 4:177, 1984.
14. Reiser, R. A commentary on the rationale of the diet-heart statement of the American Heart Association. Am. J. Clin. Nutr. 40:654, 1984.
15. Dawber, T. R.; Nickerson, R. J., Brand, F. N., et al. Eggs, serum cholesterol and coronary heart disease. Am. J. Clin. Nutr. 36:617, 1982.
16. Anonymous. The influence of eggs upon plasma cholesterol levels. Nutr. Rev. 41:272, 1983.
17. Glueck, C. J. Dietary fat and atherosclerosis. Am. J. Clin. Nutr. 32:2703, 1979.
18. Samuel, P.; McNamara, D. J.; Shapiro, J. The role of diet in the etiology and treatment of atherosclerosis. J. Annu. Rev. Med. 34:179, 1983.
19. Mitchell, J. R. A. What constitutes evidence on the dietary prevention of coronary heart disease? Costly beliefs or harsh facts? Int. J. Cardiol. 5:287, 1984.

20. Multiple Risk Factor Intervention Trial Research Group. Multiple Risk Factor Intervention Trial—risk factor changes and mortality results. JAMA 248:1465, 1982.
21. Reiser, R. Oversimplification of diet, coronary heart disease relationships and exaggerated diet recommendations. Am. J. Clin. Nutr. 31:865, 1978.
22. Food and Nutrition Board, National Research Council. Diet, Nutrition, and Cancer. Washington, D.C., National Academy of Sciences, 1980.
23. Committee on Nutrition, American Academy of Pediatrics. The use of whole cow's milk in infancy. Pediatrics 72:253, 1983.
24. Committee on Diet, Nutrition, and Cancer, National Research Council. Diet, Nutrition and Cancer. Washington, D.C., National Academy Press, 1983.
25. Perkins, E. G.; Visek, W. J., eds. Dietary Fats and Health, pp. 721, 791. Champaign, Ill., American Oil Chemists Society, 1983.
26. Volker, J. F.; Finn, S. B. Food and dental caries. In Finn, S.B., ed. Clinical Pedodontics, p. 518. Philadelphia, W.B. Saunders Co., 1973.
27. Dennison, C.J.; Randolph, P.M. Diet and dental caries. In Randolph, P.M.; Dennison, C.J., eds. Diet, Nutrition, and Dentistry, p. 205. St. Louis, Mo., C.V. Mosby Co., 1981.
28. Mandel, L.; Baurmash, H. Parotid enlargement due to alcoholism. J. Am. Dent. Asoc. 82:369, 1971.

5

Protein Nutrition; Its Role in Infection

The word *protein* is derived from the Greek word meaning "of the first rank." Protein is of prime importance to all of life—because it is an indispensable constituent of the cytoplasm and nuclei of all cells and serves as building blocks for cellular membranes and tissue structures. Proteins are precursors of antibodies and are also essential components of enzymes and hormones, which act as catalysts and regulators in metabolism. They can even serve as a source of energy if the intake of dietary carbohydrates and fats is inadequate.

Protein, next to water, is the most plentiful substance in the body. Half the dry weight of the body is protein. One-third of body protein is found in muscle, one-fifth in bone and cartilage, and one-tenth in the skin. The remainder is in other tissues and body fluids.

CHEMICAL NATURE, CLASSIFICATION, AND PROPERTIES OF PROTEINS

Proteins are large, complex molecules that basically contain carbon, hydrogen, oxygen, and nitrogen atoms arranged into amino acids. In addition, they often include phosphorus, sulfur, and (less frequently), iron, copper, iodine, zinc, and manganese.

Chemically, proteins consist of a number of amino acids held together by peptide linkage, which means that the carboxyl (COOH) group of one amino acid is linked with the amino (NH_2) group of another. The numbers of amino acids so linked determine the type of protein: a compound of two amino acids, a dipeptide; a compound of three amino acids, a tripeptide; a compound of an intermediate substance between a protein and a peptone, a proteose; or a compound of an intermediate product formed in the digestion of protein, a peptone. Amino acids are formed by the combination of several identical molecules in a specific pattern, which provides genetic and immunological characteristics and gives individuality to the species. It is often said that there are 20 amino acids, but if cystine and ornithine are counted, there are 22. They combine with one another and with other compounds in many different ways.[1] The human body contains an estimated 10,000 to 50,000 different kinds of protein. Of these, only about 1000 have been identified.[1]

Proteins are classified as simple, conjugated, and derived, based on solubility and other physical properties as well as on chemical composition. The *simple* proteins yield only amino acids on hydrolysis, e.g., globulins found in legumes

66

such as beans and peas. *Conjugated* proteins are compounds formed by attachment of a protein molecule such as globin to a nonprotein molecule or prosthetic group, such as heme (e.g., globin + heme = hemoglobin). *Derived* proteins are products resulting from the hydrolysis of proteins, e.g., proteose and cooked egg albumin.

DIGESTION, ABSORPTION, AND METABOLISM

Digestion and Absorption. Proteins are not only acquired exogenously (from outside the body) from the diet but are also obtained endogenously (from within the body) from shed or worn out cells and digestive enzymes. No protein digestion takes place in the mouth because there are no protein-hydrolyzing (cleavage) enzymes in the saliva.

The first step in the digestion of protein takes place in the stomach as a result of the flow of hydrochloric acid from the gastric glands and the protein-splitting enzyme pepsin. These hydrolytic substances rupture the peptide bonds, forming proteoses, peptones, and polypeptides. Rennin (chymosin), found only in the infant's stomach, is an enzyme that slows down the passage of milk and acts on casein, the protein in milk, to form a more easily digested curd. When there is a deficiency of this enzyme, milk passes too quickly through the stomach, causing milk intolerance.

The next step in protein digestion occurs in the alkaline medium of the small intestine. Enzymes of the pancreatic (trypsin) and intestinal (erepsin) juices further digest the products of protein by splitting them into small polypeptides and some amino acids. Most of these are finally hydrolyzed to amino acids when taken up by the mucosal cells lining the small intestine.

The absorption of dipeptides has been shown to play a significant role in the assimilation of dietary protein.[2] Peptide absorption is a major route of amino acid uptake.

Metabolism. The liver is the main site of catabolism (breakdown into simpler compounds, with release of energy) of most of the essential amino acids. The other amino acids are primarily degraded in muscle and kidney. The degradation of essential amino acids by the liver is regulated by body requirements.

Food protein provides the amino acids that are absorbed from the small intestine into the portal blood. Thereafter they undergo a variety of metabolic transformations. They may be synthesized into tissue proteins, structural proteins of cellular membranes, plasma proteins, enzymes, or hormones. An adequate supply of both essential and nonessential amino acids is necessary for protein synthesis. Once the essential and nonessential amino acids are present in the cell, synthesis of specific body proteins is genetically controlled by deoxyribonucleic acid (DNA) located in the cell nucleus. The genetic information for the amino acid sequence (the primary structure of the protein) is stored in DNA. This information is carried by messenger RNA (ribonucleic acid) to the cell cytoplasm, where the specific protein is produced.

Amino acids that are not utilized for protein synthesis may be partially deaminated, i.e., different amino portions are removed. Some fragments may be converted into carbohydrates and oxidized for needed energy.

Decarboxylation (removal of the carboxyl, COOH, group) of amino acids during metabolism may also result in formation of new compounds. An example is serotonin, a neurotransmitter necessary for central nervous system function.

The nitrogen-containing end products of protein metabolism that are excreted in the urine consist primarily of urea, small amounts of ammonia, uric acid, and creatinine from muscle protein. A small portion of dietary nitrogen is unabsorbed and is excreted as fecal nitrogen.

Interchange of Amino Acids and Metabolites Among Organs. Amino acid metabolism depends on a cooperative interchange among organs.

Some aromatic acids can be precursors of hormones, e.g., tryptophan for serotonin. Wurtman and Fernstrom have reported that tryptophan administration increases the free tryptophan content of the brain and consequently its serotonin production and content, resulting in a tendency to sleep.[3]

PROTEIN TURNOVER

The tissues of the body are under constant repair. The rates at which they are broken down and replaced vary greatly. For example, the mucosa (mucous membrane) lining of the small intestine is renewed every 1 or 2 days and the oral mucosa, within a week; red blood cells are replaced in about 120 days.

As much as 300 g of the 10 kg of body protein is replaced daily. This is about three times the customary protein content of the Western diet. Body tissues supply and use different amounts of body protein. Some 70 g of endogenous protein is secreted daily into the gut, and about 20 g/day of plasma proteins is released into the circulation from the liver. The muscle tissue used considerable protein because of the amount in the body as well as its rate of metabolism.

Some tissue proteins are continuously broken down and resynthesized, thereby creating a dynamic state in which nitrogen flows from one tissue to another. In fact, more protein is supplied endogenously, daily, than is ordinarily consumed in the diet. Amino acids from dietary and tissue proteins enter a metabolic pool, supplying amino acids for tissue synthesis, for the formation of carbohydrate or fat, or for the release of energy. The pool, an aggregate of both exogenous and endogenous protein metabolism, is influenced by various factors, such as the amount and quality of dietary protein, the rate of absorption of amino acids, and the endocrine balance. Exogenous metabolism varies with the quantity and quality of dietary protein and is associated with the excretion of urea. Endogenous metabolism deals with the formation and excretion of creatinine, presumably from the breakdown of muscle tissue, and is independent of amino acid intake.

Is the amino acid pool a storage depot? Amino acids consumed in excess of the amounts needed for synthesis of nitrogenous tissue constituents are not stored. They are rapidly degraded to a source of energy and are excreted as urea. No organ in the body contains a static reserve of protein similar to glycogen in muscle or fat in adipose tissue; therefore there is no value in consuming extra proteins in anticipation of stress. The time for eating the extra protein is during illness, especially when convalescing, not before.

However, when the body is deprived of protein, cellular proteins—enzymes and nonessential structures not absolutely vital for keeping the body alive—are broken down to supply amino acids to the pool. These are protein reserves called labile protein.

NITROGEN BALANCE

Nitrogen balance means that a balance exists between intake and output of nitrogen in the body. It should be pointed out that nitrogen is found not only in amino acids but also as nonprotein nitrogen such as in urea, uric acid, ammonia, creatine, creatinine, and other body tissues and fluids.

A subject is said to be in nitrogen balance when the nitrogen intake in the diet equals the nitrogen output (urine and feces, for example). A negative nitrogen balance (when output exceeds intake) results from breakdown of body protein. It can occur as a result of infection, fever, surgical trauma, blood loss, or loss of plasma because of burns.

Because meeting the body's energy requirements is the first priority in nutrition, eating foods rich in carbohydrates and fats for this purpose is most desirable from the standpoint of the body's economy. However, if a person ingests inadequate amounts of these two nutrients, dietary or body protein will be used for energy, creating a negative nitrogen balance.

Nitrogen balance also depends on the amounts and proportions of essential amino acids in the diet plus the total nitrogen intake. In an adult, nitrogen equilibrium signifies an adequate diet.

AMINO ACID REQUIREMENTS OF HUMANS

Essential and Nonessential Amino Acids

The major issue in protein nutrition is the body's requirements for specific types, amounts, and proportions of amino acids rather than protein per se.

Twenty-two different amino acids ordinarily are required for synthesis of tissue proteins, and the absence of any one could prevent body protein formation. The body can synthesize some of these, which are called nonessential only because they need not be supplied in the diet. They are as important as the essential amino acids to growth and body metabolism.

Although the nitrogen balance technique (the amount of body protein metabolized is equal to the amount taken in from food) can be criticized for its sources of error because of inherent technical difficulties,[4] it has nevertheless been a means for identifying which amino acids are essential for humans and for determining protein requirements. A joint committee of the Food and Agriculture Organization, the World Health Organization, and the United Nations University has estimated the essential amino acid requirements in infants, 2-year-old children, 10- to 12-year-old schoolboys, and adults based mainly on nitrogen balance measurements (Table 5–1).

The body must obtain the essential amino acids (those it cannot synthesize) from the diet. With dietary provision of these essential amino acids in adequate amounts and in proper proportion, a nitrogen balance can be achieved. A dietary supply of nine or ten amino acids is essential for adult humans. They are

TABLE 5–1. Estimates of Amino Acid Requirements at Different Ages (Milligrams Per Kilogram Per Day)

Amino Acid	Infants	Two-Year-Old Children	Schoolboys (10–12 Years)	Adults
Histidine	28	?	?	8–12
Isoleucine	70	31	30	10
Leucine	161	73	45	14
Lysine	103	64	60	12
Methionine + cystine	58	27	27	13
Phenylalanine + tyrosine	125	69	27	14
Threonine	87	37	35	7
Tryptophan	17	12.5	4	3.5
Valine	93	38	33	10
Total essential amino acids	714	352	261	84

From Food and Agriculture Organization/World Health Organization, 1983.

histidine, isoleucine, leucine, lysine, methionine + cystine, phenylalanine + tyrosine, threonine, tryptophan, and valine.

CONTENT AND QUALITY OF PROTEIN IN FOODS

The protein concentration of food is generally estimated by measuring its total nitrogen content. Since a total nitrogen analysis measures nitrates, nitrites, and other nitrogenous substances that are not necessarily part of the protein molecule, the assumption that the total nitrogen value measures protein alone is not completely valid. However, for most purposes, this total is sufficiently accurate. Based on the assumption that the protein of food contains 16% nitrogen, a factor of 6.25 multiplied by the number of grams of nitrogen can be used to calculate the food's protein content.

The nutritive value, or quality, of a protein food depends on its digestibility and amino acid composition. The terms used in describing the quality of protein are protein efficiency ratio (PER), biological value (BV), and net protein utilization (NPU). The PER is defined as the change in the body weight relative to the amount of protein eaten. BV is an index of protein quality that reflects the percentage of absorbed nitrogen from dietary protein actually utilized and retained by the body. NPU is an index that takes into account the relative digestibility of protein. It is simply the biological value multiplied by digestibility. Proteins are 90% or more digestible.

Animal proteins such as eggs, milk, and meats have excellent proportions of all the essential amino acids, and their net utilization by the body is accordingly high. On the other hand, plant proteins such as soybeans, wheat, corn, and rice are deficient in one or more of the essential amino acids, which greatly reduces the proportion of total amino acids available for protein synthesis. This accounts for their low NPU values.

The foods with high BV and NPU can be used in relatively small quantities to meet daily protein requirements.

COMPLETE AND INCOMPLETE PROTEINS

When a food consists of all the essential amino acids in significant amounts and in proportions fairly similar to those found in the body, it is called a complete protein. These proteins can completely supply the needs of the body for maintenance, repair, and growth. The best examples of complete proteins are those derived from animal sources such as meat, fish, eggs, milk, and cheese. As previously stated, their high biological value enables small quantities of these foods to meet the daily protein requirement. The only food from an animal source that is not a complete protein is gelatin; it has practically no tryptophan and is low in other amino acids.

Plant proteins are less complete food proteins that by themselves cannot be synthesized into body proteins because they are missing or deficient in one or more of the essential amino acids. The best examples of these foods are grains, nuts, fruits, and vegetables. The proteins of plant origin are deficient in quantity and proportion of amino acids but not necessarily totally lacking in them. The concentration of one or more of the essential amino acids in these plant foods is too low to be helpful in body growth and maintenance. According to the American Dietetic Association, and of interest to strict vegetarians who do not eat any animal foods, certain plant foods and food combinations eaten at the same meal, as described under the next section Complementary Proteins, do in fact provide all the essential amino acids.[5]

COMPLEMENTARY PROTEINS

Amino acids from incomplete proteins are better used if the missing essential amino acids are supplied by other foods so that all the essential amino acids can be eaten at the same meal. This is what is meant by complementary protein feeding.

All of the essential amino acids need to be available in the right proportions to each other at about the same time so that the body can use them for tissue synthesis. The body cannot construct proteins from food with adequate amounts of only six essential amino acids eaten at one meal and from food with adequate amounts of the rest of the esential amino acids eaten at a later meal. Amino acids cannot be stored in tissues until others come along later.

To provide good nutrition, plant proteins of lower quality must be supplemented by other foods that will supply the missing or inadequate amino acids. Even a protein of low biological value may be useful if it is supplemented by another protein that provides the missing constituent. For example, corn, which is high in methionine and low in lysine, should be eaten with beans, which are a good source of lysine but low in methionine. Bread or cereal (low in lysine and threonine) and milk (high in lysine and threonine) or macaroni with cheese are complementary proteins. It is important to reemphasize that these foods should be eaten at the same meal because amino acids are not stored for any appreciable length of time. For the synthesis of protein, all of the essential amino acids should be available in adequate amounts and in the proper ratio in the cells at about the same time. In fact, the amount of protein that is produced is limited by the one essential amino acid that is present in the smallest amount in relation to the need of the organism. This is called the limiting amino acid.

It should be emphasized that it is possible to be well nourished while consuming only proteins of plant origin as long as the diet contains plant proteins that provide the entire spectrum of essential amino acids in adequate amounts. Some good plant protein combinations are legumes and rice, or beans and wheat. Also, small quantities of eggs or dairy products along with vegetable proteins (such as those consumed by lacto-ovovegetarians or lactovegetarians) will ensure the intake of a sufficient amount of amino acids.

RECOMMENDED DIETARY ALLOWANCES AND FOOD SOURCES

The optimal amount of dietary protein in the daily diet appears to be controversial. However, on the basis of a review of nitrogen balance studies, the Food and Nutrition Board has suggested protein allowances based on the average requirement of 0.47 g of protein per kilogram of body weight.[6] After taking into consideration individual variability and correcting for efficiency of utilization, the Recommended Dietary Allowance (RDA) was set at 0.8 g/kg of body weight, or about 56 g of protein for a 70-kg (154 lb) man and 44 g of protein for a 55-kg woman.[6] The RDA for protein remains the same on a weight basis throughout adulthood. The elderly may require somewhat more dietary protein as a result of changes in the body's efficiency in using protein.

For age groups from 1 to 18, an amount of protein has been added to cover the needs for growth.

An additional 30 g of protein per day is recommended for women from the second month of pregnancy until the end of gestation. Lactation requires an additional 20 g of protein per day above the maintenance allowance.

Most people, particularly Americans, eat more protein than is required. To determine one's protein needs, divide your weight in pounds by 2.2 (2.2 lb = 1 kg) and then multiply that number by 0.8. For example, if one calculates the protein RDA for a man weighing 165 lb, the RDA is 60 g. This amount of protein can be easily acquired if one eats 3.5 oz of roasted chicken (31.5 g), two slices of whole wheat bread (2.5 g), ½ c of cottage cheese (14.0 g), and 1 c of milk (10.0 g).

Exercise or heavy work does not significantly increase one's need for protein. High-protein diets or use of high-protein drinks by athletes is an unnecessary expense. Performance is not improved by a high-protein diet.

According to the December 1977 edition of the Dietary Goals for the United States prepared by the staff of the Select Committee on Nutrition and Human Needs of the U.S. Senate, the diet of Americans contains almost twice as much protein as recommended by the Food and Nutrition Board of the National Academy of Sciences. Furthermore, there is no scientific evidence of a nutritional need for the current high level of protein intake.

About 12% of the calories in the American diet is protein. Red meats tend to be high in fat; thus the percentage of protein ounce for ounce is lower than in fish or poultry. The ratio of animal protein to vegetable protein is 2:1, 8% of the calories being derived from animal protein and less than 4% from vegetable protein. This amount of animal protein, if derived from beef, lamb, or pork, can contribute significantly to elevated plasma cholesterol levels, which explains why vegetarians have a lower incidence of coronary heart disease.

Meat, fish, poultry, soybeans, and other dried beans are the best sources of protein.

PROBLEMS ASSOCIATED WITH EXCESS OR DEFICIENCY OF PROTEIN IN THE DIET

Effects of Protein Excess

Do high-protein diets cause toxicity? Diets that include usually two or three times the RDA for protein can be tolerated by the average healthy individual, because the excess protein is used for energy, although this is an expensive way to obtain energy. However, a high-protein diet may be hazardous to a person who has a kidney problem and retains nitrogen or one who has a liver problem and cannot metabolize protein. A high intake of protein also increases the dietary phosphorus level to the point that it may significantly alter the desirable dietary ratio of calcium to phosphorus from 1:1 to 1:3 or more. This has been suggested as a possible contributing factor to the prevalence of osteoporosis in population groups having a high intake of animal products. This large intake of protein—600 g/day or about 80 to 85% of the total energy intake as protein—can cause kidney problems and excessive loss of calcium in the urine. There is also a danger that fruits and vegetables will be omitted from the diet, with the result that the diet will be inadequate in other nutrients.

High-protein, low-carbohydrate, very low-calorie diets can be effective for weight loss for obese people. After an initial loss of water, significant amounts of fat are also lost. However, these diets can be hazardous and are not recommended for people who have small amounts of weight to lose. Such diets must be supervised by a physician.

Effects of Protein Deficiency

Protein Deficiency Problems Common in Developed Countries. In developed countries, a common medical problem resulting from protein deficiency is nutritional liver disease. It is seen most often in alcoholics who have an adequate caloric intake but ingest inadequate amounts of protein. These people develop fatty liver disease, which can be moderated by a high-protein diet.

Trauma, anxiety, fear, and other causes of stress have an effect in altering protein requirements. Stress results in an increase in the catabolism of muscle protein, leading to the transport of amino acids away from muscle and peripheral tissues to the liver, where they are converted to glucose for energy purposes. This process creates a deficit in the protein content of the body. Injuries such as burns, fractured bones, or surgical operations are followed by a period of negative nitrogen balance.

Phenylketonuria is an inborn error of protein metabolism in which phenylalanine is not oxidized and accumulates in the blood, producing mental deficiency unless treated. Treatment of this condition consists of a careful restriction of dietary phenylalanine.

Hunger edema associated with starvation may result from simple protein deficiency. Secondary, or conditioned, protein deficiency may arise from kidney disease, hemorrhage, and intestinal disorders.

The Adverse Effect of Protein Undernutrition. Kwashiorkor is caused by a severe dietary protein deficiency, which is manifested clinically by anemia, edema, pot belly, depigmentation of the skin, and loss of hair or change in hair color. A prolonged dietary deficiency of both protein and calories in young children is called marasmus. In the past these two conditions were incorrectly considered to be similar, which made treatment of these patients difficult.[7]

Increased morbidity (a pathological or diseased state) from infectious diseases has been shown to be due to an inadequate immune response.[8] Humoral (blood and lymph) immunity and cell-mediated immunity are the two major components of the immune response.[9] Serum immunoglobulin A may be slightly elevated if infection is present.[10]

How the individual amino acids affect the immune response in humans is unknown.[11, 12]

Individuals with a mild to moderate deficiency of only protein (which is relatively rare; there are usually deficiencies of other nutrients as well) exhibit defects in their phagocytic (scavenger cells that can ingest bacteria) system.[13]

Under experimental conditions marginal deficiencies of protein have been shown to promote the progress of periodontal disease because the permeability of the sulcular epithelium is decreased. Therefore its barrier function is concomitantly decreased.[14]

PROTEIN NUTRITION IN ORAL HEALTH AND DISEASE

Effects of Protein Deficiency on the Jaw and Teeth

Formation, Eruption, and Alignment. An adequate protein diet during pregnancy has been shown to benefit significantly the bone and dental development of the child. Conversely, 71% of infants whose mothers had a poor protein diet during pregnancy had retarded development of bone and teeth.[15]

As for all other body structures, protein nutrition is a basic consideration in the growth and development of the oral cavity. If the diet includes too little or none of the essential amino acid during the critical period of active growth, permanent structural damage can occur. Synthesis of protein in the cell is disrupted, resulting in disturbed tissue growth and development.[16] For example, the weaning period is a critical time during which the infant's diet, predominantly liquid and soft foods, begins to include more solids, usually going from a low-protein to a high-protein diet. If solid, protein-rich food intake (meat with 20% protein compared with milk with 5% protein) is not adequate, jaw and tooth malformations are possible. Lack of growth stimulus from chewing firm foods may also be a factor.

Teeth of children who suffer from protein-calorie malnutrition tend to be crowded and rotated, possibly caused by inadequate development or retarded growth of the jaw bone. Newly forming bone tissue is extremely sensitive to protein deprivation. Teeth of normal size in an undersized jaw will produce a crowded arch.[17, 18]

In Nigerian children with kwashiorkor, protein deficiency may be one reason for the delayed eruption and hypoplasia of their deciduous teeth.[17, 18]

When borderline protein-deficient diets are fed to female rats throughout the reproductive cycle, the offspring have several dental defects.[19] The teeth are smaller and more caries-prone than normal. Third molars in the protein-deficient offspring erupt late and have altered cuspal patterns.[20]

In other experiments on feeding protein-deficient diets to rats, stringent deficiencies of the amino acids lysine[21] or tryptophan[22] produced an irregular predentin layer and a number of interglobular spaces in poorly calcified dentinal matrix.

Effect of Protein Deficiency on Dental Caries

A protein-deficient diet fed to experimental animals during the pre-eruptive tooth development period increases their caries susceptibility.[23–26] The caries may be caused either by a quality defect in the matrix of the tooth enamel or, equally important, by alterations in the salivary gland.

Experimental caries in rodents have been reduced significantly by adding casein to an otherwise cariogenic diet. Since casein is a phosphoprotein, it is possible that the phosphate in this protein compound may have exerted some significant anticariogenic effect.[27] Several animal feeding studies show that amino acids such as lysine[28] and glycine[29] help prevent caries. Both the amount and quality of protein appear to be important factors influencing dental caries development in rodents.

In humans there is no direct evidence of a correlation between dental caries experience and dietary supplements of protein. Protein deficiency after tooth eruption probably means increased ingestion of carbohydrates, frequently resulting in caries-conducive bacteria in contact with the tooth enamel surface over prolonged periods. On the other hand, nuts, eggs, meats, and some dairy products do not decrease plaque pH under experimental conditions.[30]

ROLE OF PROTEIN IN THE BIOCHEMISTRY OF PERIODONTAL TISSUES

The periodontal tissues are composed of epithelium, connective tissue, and bone. The biochemistry of these tissues is essentially the same as that of other body structures, with the exception that it is modified slightly by environmental stresses that the periodontium undergoes.[31]

The epithelium of the gingival crevice or pocket adheres to the tooth surface by physicochemical forces mediated by the proteins and glycoproteins in the gingival fluid.

The connective tissue consists of cells and fibers embedded in a ground substance composed of serum proteins, glycoproteins, and mucoproteins. The glycoproteins are associated with oligosaccharides, and the mucoproteins contain such acid mucopolysaccharides as hyaluronic acid and chrondroitin sulfate. The mucoproteins are essential for the maintenance of a regular distribution of water and electrolytes in the tissues. They also have the ability, by cross-linking, to bind collagen fibrils into fibers. Some glycoproteins are associated with cell adhesion; others belong to immunoglobulins.

The fibers that are embedded in the ground substance are made of collagen. Collagen deficiencies in connective tissue may be due to any of three factors: (1) an inability of fibroblasts to synthesize collagen (owing to a deficiency in amino acids, such as in proline and lysine); (2) a failure of soluble collagen to form insoluble fibers; and (3) a degeneration of collagen. In fact, periodontal disease may be measured by the relative amounts of soluble and insoluble collagen in tissues. The degeneration of collagen may develop as a result either of lysozomal activity of the white cells present in inflamed tissue or of a collagen-liquifying enzyme derived from *Bacteroides melaninogenicus,* an anaerobic organism associated with periodontal disease.[32]

The alveolar bone provides rigidity to the periodontium but is sensitive to changes in protein and mineral metabolism. A most important fact is that collagen is required for bone crystallization.

Periodontal disease is in part a reflection of the proteolysis of proteinaceous material found both in the ground substance as mucoproteins and in fibers as collagen. The bacterial enzymes that contribute to tissue proteolysis may be hyaluronidase, collagenase, or other proteases.

EFFECT OF PROTEIN ON PERIODONTAL DISEASE

Present knowledge concerning the biochemistry of periodontal tissues and periodontal disease indicates that dietary protein is an important factor in maintaining the health of the tooth-supporting structures. In experimental animals, it has been shown that a dietary protein deficiency negatively affects the activity of fibroblasts, osteoblasts, and cementoblasts. Histologically, atrophic and degenerative changes in the connective tissue of the gingiva and periodontal ligaments are usually seen. The mineralized tissues, bone and cementum, also show similar evidence of breakdown because the size of cancellous bone spaces are increased and there is retardation of cementum deposits. When a foreign body is introduced into the periodontal pocket in a protein-deficient animal, the resorption of the alveolar crest, the downgrowth of the epithelial attachment, and the inflammatory exudate are increased and accentuated. However, the effects of deficiency have been reversed when the animal is fed a normal diet complete in protein.[33]

Findings about the correlation between periodontal health in humans and their protein status have been inconclusive and controversial because of the number of uncontrollable variables involved in the causes of periodontal disease. One group found that a protein supplement had a favorable effect on gingival health.[34] Other researchers could find no correlation between serum protein or parotid salivary protein levels and the subject's periodontal health.[35]

In conclusion, knowledge concerning nutrition-periodontal health relationships in humans is minimal. As Stahl states, "Nutritional deficiencies apparently do not initiate periodontal disease, but may modify the severity and extent of the lesion by altering the resistance and repair potential of the affected local tissue. . . . a great deal of information is necessary to further define the role of nutritional deficiencies as potential co-destructive factors in periodontal disease."[36] On the basis of our knowledge of nutrition-infection interactions, it is plausible that subclinical deficiencies in several nutrients (protein, vitamin A, and so forth) may unfavorably influence one's immunity to chronic and acute periodontal infections. This statement should be proved or disproved by well-designed and properly controlled experiments.

REFERENCES

1. Rosenfeld, A. The great protein hunt. Science 81:64, 1981.
2. Adibi, S. A.; Soleimanpour, M. R. Functional characterization of dipeptide transport system in human jejunum. J. Clin. Invest. 53:1368, 1974.
3. Wurtman, R. J.; Fernstrom, J. D. Effects of the diet on brain neuro transmitters. Nutr. Rev. 32:193, 1974.
4. Munro, H. N.; Young, V. R. In Howard I. A. H.; Baird, D. M., eds. Recent Advances in Clinical Nutrition, pp. 33–41. London, Libby, 1981.
5. American Dietetic Association. Position paper on vegetarian approach to eating. J. Am. Diet. Assoc. 77:61, 1980.
6. Committee on Dietary Allowances, Food and Nutrition Board, National Academy of Sciences-National Research Council. Recommended Dietary Allowances, 9th rev. ed. Washington, D.C., National Academy Press, 1980.
7. Landman, J. P.; Jackson, A. A. The role of protein deficiency in the aetiology of kwashiokor. West Indian Med. J. 29:229, 1980.
8. Chandra, R. X. Cell-mediated immunity in nutritional imbalance. Fed. Proc. 39:3086, 1980.
9. Good, R. H.; Fernandes, G.; West, A. Nutrition and immunity. In Present Knowledge in Nutrition: Nutrition Reviews, 5th ed., pp. 693–710. Washington, D.C., Nutrition Foundation, 1984.
10. Chandra, R. K. Nutrition, immunity and infection: present knowledge and future directions. Lancet 1:688, 1983.
11. Beisel, W. R.; Edelman, R.; Nauss, K., et al. Single-nutrient effects on immunologic functions. Report of workshop sponsored by the Dept. of Food and Nutrition and its nutrition advisory group of the American Medical Assoc. JAMA 245:53, 1981.
12. Beisel, W. R. Single nutrients and immunity. Am. J. Clin. Nutr. 35(Suppl.):417, 1982.
13. Vitale, J. J. In Vitale, J. J.; Broitman, S. A., eds. Advances in Human Clinical Nutrition, pp. 81–97. Boston, John Wright-PSG Inc., 1982.
14. Navia, J. Research advances and needs in nutrition in oral health and disease. In Pollack, R. L.; Kravitz, E., eds. Nutrition in Oral Health and Disease, p. 448. Philadelphia, Lea & Febiger, 1985.
15. Stuart, H. C. Findings on examinations of newborn infants and infants during the neonatal period which appear to have a relationship to the diets of their mothers during pregnancy. Fed. Proc. 4:271, 1945.
16. Winick, M.; Noble, A. Quantitative changes in DNA, RNA and protein during prenatal and postnatal growth in the rat. Dev. Biol. 12:451, 1965.
17. Trowell, H. C.; Davies, J. N. P.; Deard, R. F. A. Kwashiorkor. London, E. Arnold & Co., 1954.
18. Enwonwu, C. O. Prevalence of enamel hypoplasia in well-fed and malnourished Nigerians. 48th General Meeting of International Association for Dental Research, Abstract no. 51, 1969.
19. Shaw, J. H.; Griffith, D. Dental abnormalities in rats attributable to protein deficiency during reproduction. J. Nutr. 80:123, 1963.
20. Shaw, J. H. Influence of marginal and complete protein deficiency for varying periods during reproduction on growth, third molar eruption and dental caries in rats. J. Dent. Res. 48:310, 1969.
21. Irving, J. T. Action of the hypophysis and of dietary protein on the calcifying tissues. Nature 178:1231, 1956.
22. Bavetta, L. A.; Bernick, S.; Geiger, E., et al. The effect of tryptophan deficiency on the jaws of rats. J. Dent. Res. 33:309, 1954.
23. Navia, J., et al. Effect of undernutrition during the perinatal period on caries development in the rat. J. Dent. Res. 49:1091, 1970.
24. Shaw, J. Protein deficiency and tooth and salivary gland development. Nutr. Rev. 12:34, 1974.
25. Menaker, L.; Navia, J. Effect of undernutrition during the perinatal period on caries development in the rat. J. Dent. Res. 52:680, 688, 692, 1973.
26. Menaker, L.; Navia, J. Effect of undernutrition during the perinatal period on caries development in the rat. V. Changes in whole saliva volume and protein content. J. Dent. Res. 53:592, 1974.

27. Nizel, A. E. Amino acids, proteins and dental caries. In Harris, R. S., ed. Dietary Chemicals vs. Dental Caries, p. 23. Advances in Chemistry Series, no. 94. Washington, D.C., American Chemical Society, 1970.
28. McClure, F. J.; Folk, J. E. Lysine and cariogenicity of two experimental rat diets. Science 122:557, 1955.
29. Harris, R. S., et al. Effects of dietary supplement of glycine on dental caries development in rats. Proc. Int. Dent. Res. 451:151, 1967.
30. Schachtele, C. F.; Harlander, S. K. Will the diets of the future be less cariogenic? Can. Dent. Assoc. J. 50:213, 1984.
31. Schultz-Haudt, S. D. The biochemistry of periodontal tissues. Alabama J. Med. Sci. 5:289, 1968.
32. Beerstecher, E. The periodontium. In Lazzari, E. P., ed. Dental Biochemistry, p. 92. Philadelphia, Lea & Febiger, 1968.
33. Miller, S. A.; Nizel, A. E. Proteins in nutrition. In Nizel, A. E., ed. The Science of Nutrition and Its Application in Clinical Denistry, 2nd ed., p. 45. Philadelphia, W.B. Saunders Co., 1966.
34. Cheraskin, E., et al. An ecologic analysis of gingival state: effect of prophylaxis and protein supplementation. J. Periodont. 39:316, 1968.
35. Shannon, I. L., et al. Uric acid and total serum in parotid fluid in relation to periodontal status. J. Dent. Res. 45:1539, 1966.
36. Stahl, S. S. Nutritional influences on periodontal disease. World Rev. Nutr. Diet. 13:277, 1971.

6

Water and Electrolytes; Hypertension

WATER

Water is a vital nutrient crucial to every bodily function and second only to oxygen in importance to the body. One can live only a few days without water.

Water provides a suitable medium for chemical reactions in the body. It serves as a solvent and as a vehicle to transport inorganic nutrients. It contributes to the structure of tissues such as whole blood, muscle, and bone. Evaporation of water from the skin and exhalation of water in air from the lungs contribute to temperature regulation. Water transports heat from one part of the body to another and thus stabilizes body temperature. The body uses water to keep the kidneys functioning normally. Most of the body's waste products are excreted through the kidneys. Enzymes (substances that initiate and accelerate a chemical reaction), hormones (glandular secretions that act as messengers to body organs by stimulating certain life processes and retarding others), and coenzymes (a portion of an enzyme that is required for the activation of a protein molecule to form a whole enzyme) are dissolved in watery body fluids. Water serves as a lubricant in digestion and other body processes, and the water in saliva facilitates chewing and swallowing. Water plays an active role in the hydrolysis of nutrients (conversion of sucrose into fructose and glucose, for example). Water helps maintain electrolyte balance, which will be discussed later in this chapter.

The body's major source of water is drinking water and beverages. Under normal conditions, this should be about six to eight glasses per day for an adult. Water is also ingested in solid foods such as raw fruits and vegetables (90 to 95% water), cooked meat, eggs, and even bread.

Water requirements are based on body size and are determined per kilogram of body weight (Table 6–1). Based on recommended energy intake, the daily intake of water should be 1 ml/kcal for adults (or 2 liters or 2 quarts for a person ingesting the usual 2000 kcal/day) and 1.5 ml/kcal for infants. Special attention must be given to the water needs of infants given high-protein formulas; comatose patients; patients with fever, polyuria, vomiting, or diarrhea; persons taking diuretics or consuming high-protein diets; and all persons in hot environments. Free access to water as well as salt is essential whenever sweat losses are significantly increased.

TABLE 6–1. Water Requirement*

	Age (Years)	Water (ml per kg Body Weight)
Infants	Birth–1	120–100
Children	0–10	60–80
Adolescents	11–18	41–55
Adults	19–51	20–30

Adapted from Bell, G. H. Textbook of Physiology and Biochemistry, 6th ed., p. 166. Baltimore, Williams & Wilkins Co., 1965; and Waring, W.; Jeansonne, I. Practical Manual of Pediatrics, p. 217. St. Louis, Mo., C. V. Mosby Co., 1975.
*The daily maintenance required is based on body surface area, at 1500 to 2000 ml/m² of surface area per 24 hours.

Body Fluids

The body fluids are intimately involved in the basic cellular processes. These fluids consist of water, protein, and solutions of electrolytes (minerals that when dissolved dissociate into positive and negative ions and thus can conduct electricity) and nonelectrolytes. Sodium, potassium, and chloride are the major electrolytes. Others are magnesium, calcium, phosphate, sulfate, and carbonate. Nonelectrolytes such as glucose and urea are present in body fluids in very small quantities in comparison with the electrolytes.

In a healthy person, the volume and composition of the body fluids are carefully regulated and homeostasis (tendency to uniformity or stability) is maintained. However, during illness or after trauma or surgery, alteration in body fluid composition can occur, producing dehydration, with consequent shock and even death if the fluids and electrolytes are not replaced.

In humans, most of the body weight (65%) is water, and as little as a 10% water loss can cause metabolic disorders. The exact percentage of water normally present depends on the amount of fat in the body—the more fat, the less water. The water content of an obese person is nearly 50% of the total weight, whereas a lean person's body is about 70% water. Thus in an average 70-kg (150-lb) man with an average amount of fat the body water weighs about 45 kg (100 lb). Total body water is related to body surface area and metabolic activity, so that at birth the body water may be about 78% of the body weight, whereas during adulthood it decreases to about 65%.

Intracellular (within cells) fluid contains 60% of the body water and the other 40% is in the extracellular blood plasma and interstitial fluid. The intracellular fluid consists of water and solutes (substances dissolved in it) and is the site of metabolic processes. Two types of extracellular fluids provide the environment surrounding the cells—interstitial (between a small space or gap in a tissue) fluid and blood plasma.

The intracellular and extracellular fluids differ from each other sharply in the type and amounts of electrolytes and protein they contain. The ionic solutes of the intracellular fluid are potassium and magnesium cations (positively charged ions) plus mostly protein and phosphate with small amounts of carbonate and sulfate anions (negatively charged ions). In the extracellular fluid, sodium is the major cation, and chloride and bicarbonate are the principal anions. The small amount of protein in the extracellular fluids is essentially in the blood plasma. Other components of the extracellular fluids are the same for both the blood plasma and the interstitial fluid.

Importantly, during health the cell fluid and its surrounding extracellular fluids are stable because they are in osmotic equilibrium. However, during illness, losses or gains in sodium or potassium, the major active solutes, will alter osmotic pressure and thus cause an abnormal shift of water into or out of the cells, resulting in impaired cellular function.

Water Balance

Water balance is achieved when there is an osmotic equilibrium between the different body fluid compartments and when the water intake equals the water output.

The extracellular fluid is separated from the intracellular fluid by membranes that are permeable to water. Water will move from the extracellular fluid to the intracellular fluid when the latter has a higher solute concentration (more electrolytes in solution). The reverse process occurs when the solute concentration of the extracellular fluid is higher—water then moves to it. This is the body's mechanism for regulating a balance between water intake and water output.

The pressure exerted by a solute on a semipermeable membrane is called osmotic pressure. Dehydration, for example, causes changes in plasma osmotic pressure that stimulate receptors in the hypothalamus, which in turn have neural connections with the posterior pituitary. As a result of this stimulation, antidiuretic hormone (aldosterone) is released, causing the renal (kidney) tubules to reabsorb water and decrease urine volume. Conversely, ingestion of fluids in excess of the requirement decreases plasma osmotic pressure, suppresses aldosterone (an electrolyte-regulating hormone of the adrenal cortex) release, and increases urine volume to reestablish fluid equilibrium.

Under normal conditions, the water intake is satisfied by drinking liquids or from fluids derived from ingesting solid foods. Water is also obtained from the metabolism of carbohydrates, proteins, and fats in the body (Table 6–2). The latter is called metabolic water.

For the most part, water is excreted in the urine and the feces. There is also an insensible (not perceptible) loss of water resulting from evaporation from the skin and from expired air. With elevated temperature or vigorous exercise, water is also lost by sweat.

TABLE 6–2. Normal Routes of Intake and Output of Water

Intake		Output	
Preformed water	1200 ml	Urine	1500 ml
Water in food	1000 ml	Stool	100 ml
Metabolic water	300 ml	Insensible water	900 ml
Total	2500 ml	Total	2500 ml

SODIUM

Sodium serves a number of important functions in the body and is considered an essential nutrient.[1] It not only maintains extracellular fluid volumes and cellular osmotic pressures, it also aids in (1) the transmission of nerve impulses; (2) permeability of cell membrane; and (3) muscular contraction.[2]

Common table salt and foods of plant and animal origin (Table 6–3) supply sodium in the diet.

Sodium needs can vary from person to person, depending on age, environmental temperature, humidity, and the amount of physical activity. The need for sodium increases as a result of its significant loss during periods of excess sweating, diarrhea, or both. A minimum dietary intake of 200 mg/day (0.5 g sodium chloride, or salt, which is 39% sodium) is necessary to maintain physio-

TABLE 6–3. Sodium Content of Selected Foods

Food	Description	mg/100 g Edible Portion
Rich Sources		
Bread	All types	265–674
Sausages	Cold cuts and luncheon meats	740–1234
Fish	Fresh, unsalted	54–177
Cheese	Cream	250
Cheese	Cheddar	700
Butter	Salted	987
Margarine	Salted	987
Prunes	Dehydrated	329–940
Eggs	Whole, fresh	122
Eggs	Whole, dried	427
Milk	Whole, dried	405
Moderate Sources		
Vegetables	Carrots, beets, corn, peas, spinach	
	Raw	2–71
	Canned	2–46
Ham	Cooked	65
Bacon	Cooked	65
Oatmeal	Rolled or ground	1–218
Meats	Beef, pork, lamb (cooked)	60–70
Milk	Whole, pasteurized	50
Ice cream	All types	33–63
Breakfast cereals	Corn, oats, rice, wheat (dry)	2–1267
Chocolate	Candy, sweet	33
Coffee	Dry, powder	72
Poor Sources		
Butter	Unsalted	10
Fruit	Apples, pears, bananas	
	Fresh	1
	Dried	1–5
Nuts	Roasted, unsalted	1–5
Fruit juices	Orange, pineapple, grapefruit (fresh)	1–5
Marmalades, jams, preserves	All types	14

Data from Nutrition and Your Health. Dietary Guidelines for Americans. USDA Handbook no. 8. Washington, D.C., U.S. Department of Agriculture and U.S. Department of Health and Human Services, 1985.

logical balance in adults.[3] The Food and Nutrition Board considers 1100 to 3300 mg of sodium (2.8 to 8.4 g of salt) a "safe and adequate" daily dietary intake for healthy adults.[1] As much as 3 to 4 g of salt/day may be necessary to maintain normal daily physiological activity. Sodium balance is maintained by renal and hormonal mechanisms in the kidneys and adrenal glands. One teaspoon of table salt contains approximately 2000 mg of sodium. Of the total salt intake, about one-third is added during cooking or as a condiment at the table.[4] The other two-thirds is added to commercially processed food or occurs naturally.

Salt and other sodium-containing compounds are used as flavoring agents or for technological reasons. Sodium chloride is used to raise the boiling point of water. It can also be used to lower the freezing point of water when making ice cream, for example. Salt is used as a preservative and can dehydrate some vegetables. The preparation of kosher meat by the removal of blood is accomplished by sprinkling salt over the raw meat and allowing it to stand for an hour or so. Salt preserves a number of perishable foods by suppressing the growth of undesirable bacteria, helps cure meats (e.g., kosher beef frankfurters and corned beef), ferments foods (e.g., turns cabbage into sauerkraut), controls the texture of foods (e.g., cheese), and regulates yeast fermentation in bakery products.

The average daily consumption of sodium, including both the sodium found naturally in food plus the discretionary sodium intake (salt added when food is cooked or eaten) is about 4453 mg for males and 3064 mg for females.[5]

A decrease in both sodium intake and excess body weight is probably necessary for most hypertensive patients to lower blood pressure to the normo-tensive (normal blood pressure) range.

The best way to decrease sodium intake is to limit the use of discretionary sodium. If sodium intake needs to be further limited, one must carefully read the sodium information on food labels. Food processors label their products as follows: *sodium free* means less than 5 mg per serving; *very low sodium* means 35 mg or less per serving; *low sodium* means 140 mg or less per serving; *reduced sodium* means a 75% reduction in sodium content. The labels *unsalted, no salt added,* and *without salt* mean that salt was not used in preparation of the food so labeled.[6]

POTASSIUM[7]

Potassium is the principal cation in intracellular fluid, and is present in very small amounts in the extracellular fluid. The potassium content of the body is derived solely from dietary intake—meat, milk, and many fruits (Table 6–4).

Intracellular potassium is essential in many cellular enzymatic functions, such as glycogen synthesis, glucose degradation, and amino acid uptake. The chief function of extracellular potassium is to control cardiac function and muscle and nerve irritability.

The minimum amount of potassium that the body needs to function is approximately 300 mEq (milliequivalents) per day, whereas the maximum is 400 mEq/day. The ordinary American diet supplies from 50 to 100 mEq of potassium or 3.7 to 7.4 g of potassium chloride per day.

TABLE 6–4. Potassium Content of Selected Foods

Food	Description	mg/100 g Edible Portion
Bacon	Cooked	390
Bread	All types	67–454
Breakfast cereals	Corn, oats, rice, wheat (dry)	99–947
Butter	Salted	23
Butter	Unsalted	10
Cheese	Cream	74
Cheese	Cheddar	82
Chocolate	Candy, sweet	269
Coffee	Dry, powder	3256
Eggs	Whole, fresh	129
Eggs	Whole, dried	463
Fish	Fresh, unsalted	160–525
Fruit	Apples, pears, bananas	
	Fresh	110–370
	Dried	144–1477
Fruit juices	Orange, pineapple, grapefruit	
	(fresh)	162–940
Ham	Cooked	390
Ice cream	All types	95–181
Margarine	Salted	23
Marmalades, jams, preserves	All types	33–88
Meats	Beef, pork, lamb (cooked)	370–390
Milk	Whole, pasteurized	144
Milk	Whole, dried	1330
Nuts	Roasted, unsalted	464–773
Oatmeal	Rolled or ground	61–352
Prunes	Dehydrated	760–2170
Sausages	Cold cuts and luncheon meats	140–269
Vegetables	Carrots, beets, corn, peas, spinach	
	Raw	280–470
	Canned	96–250

Data from Nutrition and Your Health. Dietary Guidelines for Americans. USDA Handbook no. 8. Washington, D.C., U.S. Department of Agriculture and U.S. Department of Health and Human Services, 1985.

Healthy adults need about 2500 mg of potassium per day. The estimated safe range is 1875 to 5625 mg.

Potassium Deficiency

Under normal dietary circumstances, a deficiency is unlikely to occur because potassium is so widely distributed in foods.

A deficiency can occur from a prolonged potassium-free diet or from excessive losses resulting from diarrhea; diabetic acidosis; or use of drugs such as diuretics, steroids, and purgatives.

Potassium depletion is manifested by muscle weakness, paralysis, reduced or absent reflexes, and mental confusion. The cardiovascular signs are electrocardiogram changes, poor pulse, and weak heart sounds.[8]

Potassium supplementation must be administered with care when potassium deficiency occurs.

Potassium Excess

Excess potassium will result from sudden increases in intake of about 18 g of potassium by an adult; this can cause fatal cardiac arrest.

The consequences of potassium excess are muscle weakness and cardiac dysfunction.

CHLORIDE

Chloride occurs in combination with sodium or potassium cations. The highest concentrations of chloride are found in the secretions of the gastrointestinal tract and in the cerebrospinal fluid. It is found in relatively low concentrations in muscle and nerve tissues. It is the predominant anion in extracellular fluid and is almost entirely absent within the cells. It is the anion component of hydrogen chloride (HCl) in gastric juice; HCl is important in initiating the digestion of protein.

The principal function of chloride is to regulate the osmotic pressure and water balance in the body. The chloride anion also acts as a coenzyme (facilitates action of enzymes) in the digestive process. A third function is to help maintain the acid-base balance of the blood. Chloride enhances the ability of the blood to carry large amounts of carbon dioxide to the lungs for exhalation. Chloride also aids in the conservation of potassium.

Chloride Deficiency

Starvation, fever, diarrhea, excessive vomiting, and excessive sweating can cause a decrease in plasma chloride. As with potassium, a marked loss of chloride can result in hypokalemic alkalosis. With a decrease in the chloride concentration in the extracellular fluid, there is an accompanying increase in the bicarbonate concentration, leading to a state of alkalosis (accumulation of base). Chloride and potassium supplementation is needed to correct a deficiency of potassium in the blood.

Abnormalities of chloride metabolism are generally accompanied by abnormalities in sodium metabolism.

Food Sources

Most dietary chloride is derived from sodium chloride (common table salt) and dairy and meat products; a lesser amount is derived from fruits and vegetables. The chloride content of foods is roughly proportional to the sodium content and inversely proportional to the potassium content. The daily chloride intake is about 2 to 3 g.

ACID-BASE BALANCE[3]

Only when the blood is maintained within a narrow range of neutrality between pH 7.35 and 7.45 is health for the human possible. This precise equilibrium is maintained by the lungs and kidneys, to prevent shifts in electrolyte patterns. First, the rate of excretion of carbonic acid (a weak acid) through the lung acts as a very fine adjustment. Second, the kidney is able to excrete urine with either an acid or an alkaline reaction. Thus acidosis (accumulation of acid) or alkalosis (accumulation of base) can result if either the lung or the kidney is diseased. Compared with the renal and respiratory aspects of acid-base balance, the dietary aspects, discussed briefly here, are minor.

Foods are grouped as alkali-producing, acid-producing, or neutral. This is determined by the properties of the minerals each food contains. For example, fruits (with the exception of cranberries, prunes, and plums), vegetables (except corn and lentils), milk, and nuts contain alkali-forming minerals—namely, sodium, potassium, calcium, and magnesium. When these foods are metabolized, or "burned," in the body, they yield an alkaline ash and are thus referred to as alkaline foods. Some confusion may exist, however, because although fruits and vegetables are alkali-producing foods from a physiological point of view, they may taste acidic and are often thought to be "acid" foods. Intake of large quantities of fruits and vegetables does not cause acidosis. On the other hand, foods such as meat, cereals, and eggs, which contain acid-forming elements (phosphorus, sulfur, and chlorine) will yield acid end products.

For the average, healthy individual, there is no evidence regarding the practical importance of balancing acid and alkaline foods. The human body has a wide range of adaptability.

However, lactic acid and acetoacetic acid, which are produced in the body in excessive amounts under certain disease conditions, can give rise to acidosis. Large quantities of lactic acid may accumulate in the blood after strenuous muscular exercise. However, the rapid breathing that occurs during recovery from exercise helps to restore the acid-base balance by expelling carbonic acid. In diabetes that has been treated inadequately, or in other conditions in which fat metabolism predominates, acetoacetic acid and beta-hydroxybutyric acid accumulate in the blood. Because these two acids are stronger than carbonic acid, they displace the bicarbonate in the blood. As a result there may be a serious fall in the alkalinity of the blood, and the dangerous condition of acidosis may develop.

Effects of Water and Electrolyte Imbalances on Oral Health

Like the other soft tissues in the body, the mucosa of the oral cavity has a high water content (70 to 80%). Therefore any systemic factors that produce either general dehydration or edema of tissues will similarly cause shrinkage or swelling of the oral tissues. As mentioned previously, patients who ingest high-salt diets and retain the sodium will accumulate body water. Conversely, patients on a low-carbohydrate, high-fat diet or a high-protein diet for rapid loss of weight will tend to lose large amounts of water from the excessive oxidation of body fat.

Patients wearing full upper dentures who lose large amounts of body water will experience denture looseness and the accompanying discomforts. On the other hand, denture wearers who retain water will tend to have pressure-induced sore spots on the underlying swollen mucosa.

Dehydration can cause a decrease in salivary flow, which tends to promote xerostomia (dry mouth). A common clinical oral problem associated with xerostomia is the lack of lubrication of mucosal surfaces. The roof of the mouth and tongue develop a burning sensation and the corners of the mouth become macerated and infected owing to a tendency to moisten them by licking. Also, xerostomia promotes increased dental plaque formation and the consequences of gingival irritation and more rapid dental caries production.

HYPERTENSION

Hypertension affects about 60 million adults in the United States today. If uncontrolled, this condition can lead to stroke, heart failure, and kidney failure.[10]

Hypertension is defined as a pattern of consistently elevated arterial blood pressure; the systolic (phase when the heart is actually contracting) pressure is consistently greater than normal (Table 6–5) for the age group, and the diastolic (resting phase between the heart contractions) pressure is also greater than normal. Although elevation of both systolic and diastolic pressures is considered important, most clinicians make a distinction between them. For example, the systolic pressure is often elevated by hardening of the arteries as part of the aging process, and in practice true systolic hypertension is considered to exist after allowing for a factor of 100 plus age. Elevation of systolic pressure alone can be caused by other diseases, such as an overactive thyroid. On the other hand, diastolic elevations are most closely related to what is customarily considered hypertension. Mild hypertension may be said to be present when the diastolic pressure is 90 to 105, moderate hypertension when the diastolic is 105 to 120, and severe hypertension when the diastolic pressure exceeds 120.

Hypertension is associated with damage to the heart (coronary heart disease), the brain (stroke), and the kidney (renal failure). The higher the blood pressure, the more serious is atherosclerotic disease.

Mild pressure elevations in young persons are more serious than in older persons. Among adults more men than women have hypertension, although after menopause the incidence of elevated blood pressure in women rises. Approximately one of every six adults has hypertension. The incidence of hypertension among the black population in the United States is almost twice as high as in the white.

TABLE 6–5. Upper Limits of Normal Blood Pressure by Age Group

Age Group (Years)	Blood Pressure (mm Hg)
Infants	90/60
3–6	110/70
7–10	120/80
11–17	130/80
18–44	140/90
45–64	150/95
65 and older	160/95

From Batterman, B. Hypertension. Part 1: detection and evaluation. Cardiovasc. Nurs. 11:38, 1975.

Causes of Hypertension

Hypertension may be caused either by unknown factors (essential hypertension) or by known factors (secondary hypertension). The disease has a number of causes.[11] Some contributing factors associated with the etiology of hypertension are genetic, environmental, and nutritional ones. Factors increasing the risk, in addition to race and age mentioned above, include family history of hypertension, obesity, smoking, psychological stress, diabetes, elevated cholesterol levels, and excessive sodium intake.[12]

Epidemiological surveys show that among some of the Indians in Brazil who ingest comparatively little salt, hypertension is rare. However, when such people move to more industrialized areas where they tend to use more salt, hypertension becomes more common. In Northern Japan, where salt intake is high, hypertension is more prevalent.[13]

Clinical observations that restrictions on the use of dietary sodium intake can decrease blood pressure in patients with hypertension support the concept that dietary sodium intake can be a major factor in hypertension.[14]

The association of cardiovascular disease with excessive weight appears to be due, not to the weight per se, but to the higher incidence of hypertension, diabetes, and elevated cholesterol levels in obese persons. Conversely, it has been demonstrated that weight loss can serve as an effective treatment for high blood pressure and is sometimes all that is needed in mild cases.

Stress can be responsible for at least a temporary rise in blood pressure. Techniques of relaxation, meditation, and biofeedback have been reported to relieve mild hypertension.

PATHOLOGICAL CHANGES IN THE ARTERIES

Specific pathological changes observed in the arteries when hypertension is present include increased collagen in the arterial walls, increased elastic fibrils and acid mucopolysaccharides in the arterial walls, increased sodium and calcium in the arterial walls, and a proliferation of smooth muscle cells in the arterial walls. All of these lead to an increased arterial thickness and a narrowing of the lumen, which results in increased blood pressure.

Treatment

In the treatment of essential hypertension, the intake of electrolytes is carefully regulated. Originally, the major treatment for hypertension was a rigid dietary sodium restriction accomplished by the use of a Kempner (rice-fruit) semistarvation diet. Now a sodium intake limit of 200 to 250 mg is recommended.[15] A number of oral diuretics (agents that increase formation and output of urine) are also prescribed. Sodium restriction by avoiding certain foods, suggested in Table 6–6, plus a diuretic medication produces saluresis (salt loss) and diuresis (water loss), resulting in a reduction of extracellular fluid volume, plasma volume, and total exchangeable sodium with the desirable fall in blood pressure. An associated decrease in cardiac output then occurs. However, after

TABLE 6–6. Foods to Avoid on Sodium-Restricted Diets

Salt

Obviously salty foods such as salted crackers, potato chips, pretzels, salted nuts, pickles, olives, sauerkraut

Smoked, cured, or pickled meats and fish such as ham, bacon, frankfurters, bologna, salami, other cold cuts, salted fish and pork, corned beef

Seasonings such as catsup, prepared mustard, Worcestershire sauce, celery salt, onion salt, garlic salt, soy sauce, barbecue sauce, monosodium glutamate

Bouillon cubes, concentrated canned or frozen soups, dried soup mixes

Baking soda, seltzers, or antacids

Most commercial salad dressings

From Mikkola, M. L. In Howard R. B.; Herbold, S. H. Nutrition in Clinical Care, p. 337. New York, McGraw-Hill Book Co., 1976.

a few weeks on this therapy, the cardiac output returns to normal while the blood pressure remains low.

Side effects of these diuretics include a low serum potassium (hypokalemia), high serum uric acid, and high blood sugar. Hypokalemia can be treated with dietary sources of potassium such as bananas, broccoli, cantaloupe, grapefruit juice, orange juice, potatoes, and perhaps a potassium elixir.

Other antihypertensive medications are often used in combination with diuretics to achieve a maximum reduction in blood pressure with a minimum of side effects. These agents reduce the peripheral vascular resistance and thus produce a decrease in blood pressure. Restriction of high-calorie foods, which results in weight loss, will reduce blood pressure in obese hypertensive patients as well as in hypertensive patients of normal weight.[16, 17]

In conclusion, the U.S. Food and Drug Administration (FDA) in "A Word About Low-Sodium Diets" gives the following advice:

- Use the saltshaker sparingly. Don't use it until you've tasted your food.
- Read food labels. Look for the amount of sodium in a product. See where salt or sodium is on the ingredient list.
- Look for low-salt, low-sodium, or sodium-reduced products. These days the low-sodium list runs literally from soup to nuts.
- Try cooking with less salt. Use spices and other seasonings.
- Remember: a teaspoon of salt contains almost 2000 mg of sodium.
- Give yourself a little time to get adjusted to a diet lower in sodium. Most people make the adjustment and enjoy it.

For more information, write to U.S. Department of Health and Human Services, Public Health Service, Food and Drug Administration, 5600 Fishers Lane, Rockville, MD 20857 for *Sodium*, HFE-88, HHS Publication no. (FDA) 84–2179 and to Frances Stern Nutrition Center, N.E. Medical Center Hospital, 188 Harrison Avenue, Boston, MA 02111 for *Ideas for Adding Flavor to Sodium Restricted Diets.*

REFERENCES

1. Committee on Dietary Allowances, Food and Nutrition Board, National Academy of Sciences-National Research Council. Recommended Dietary Allowances, 9th rev. ed. Washington, D.C., National Academy Press, 1980.

2. Fregly, M. J. Estimates of sodium and potassium intake. Ann. Intern. Med. 98:792, 1983.
3. Sebranek, J. G.; Olson, D. G.; Whiting, R. C., et al. Physiological role of dietary sodium in human health and implications of sodium reduction in muscle foods. Food Technol. 37:51, 1983.
4. Fregly, M. J. Sodium and potassium. In Present Knowledge in Nutrition: Nutrition Reviews, 5th ed., pp. 439–458. Washington, D.C., Nutrition Foundation, 1984.
5. Carroll, M. D.; Abraham, S.; Dresser, C. M. Dietary Intake Source Data, United States, 1976–80. Vital and Health Statistics Series 2, no. 231. Public Health Series Publication no. 83–1681. Washington, D.C., GPO, March 1983.
6. Food and Drug Administration, Department of Health and Human Services. Food Labelling; Declaration of Sodium Content of Foods and Label Claims for Foods on the Basis of Sodium Content: Final Rule. Fed. Regist. 49:15510, April 18, 1984.
7. Meneely, G. R.; Battarbee, H. D. Sodium and potassium. Nutr. Rev. 34:259, 1976.
8. Krehl, W. A. The potassium depletion syndrome. Nutr. Today 1:20, 1966.
9. Goldberger, E. A Primer of Water, Electrolyte and Acid-Base Syndromes, 5th ed. Philadelphia, Lea & Febiger, 1975.
10. Van Italie, T. B. Symposium on current perspectives in hypertension. Hypertension 4(Suppl. III):177, 1982.
11. Shank, F. R.; Park, Y. K.; Harland, B. F., et al. Perspective of Food and Drug Administration on dietary sodium. J. Am. Diet. Assoc. 80:29, 1982.
12. Callaway, C. W. Nutritional factors and blood pressure control: an assessment. Ann. Intern. Med. 98:884, 1983.
13. Food and Nutrition Board, National Research Council. Toward Healthful Diets. Washington, D.C., National Academy Press, 1980.
14. Tobian, L. Interrelationship of sodium, volume, C.N.S. and hypertension. In Hegeli, R. J., ed. Nutrition and Cardiovascular Disease, pp. 208–229. New York, S. Karger, 1983.
15. Dustan, H. R. Diuretic and diet treatment of hypertension. Arch. Intern. Med. 133:1007, 1974.
16. Maxwell, M. H.; Kushiro, T.; Dornfeld, L. P., et al. BP changes in obese hypertensive subjects during rapid weight loss. Comparison of restricted v unchanged salt intake. Arch. Intern. Med. 144:1581, 1984.
17. Imai, Y.; Sato, K.; Abe, K., et al. Effect of weight loss on blood pressure and drug consumption in normal weight patients. Hypertension 8:223, 1986.

7

The B Complex Vitamins

Frederick G. Hopkins, a biochemist at Cambridge University, England, and a Nobel Prize winner, reported in 1906 that there was an unknown something in food essential for life and health. In 1912, he had experimental data that supported this statement.[1]

Casimir Funk, a Polish chemist, obtained an antiberiberi substance from rice polishings. He believed that the active factor that he found was a protein, i.e., an "amino." Since he considered this amino to be the vital element in the food, he called it a "vitamine."[2] It was found that very few of these "vitamines" were truly protein so the final *e* was dropped.

A vitamin is defined as an organic substance that occurs in foods in small amounts and is necessary for the normal metabolic functioning of the body. Vitamins may be water soluble or fat soluble. In this chapter, the water-soluble B complex vitamins are discussed.

As new vitamins were discovered, successive letters of the alphabet were assigned to them.[3] However, in some cases a letter was used because it was the first letter of a word describing the principal characteristic of the vitamin. For example, vitamin K, which is concerned with the coagulation of blood, was derived from the Scandinavian word *koagulation.*

In addition to letters, numerical subscripts were added to identify separate factors in a vitamin group. This produced some confusion, so that the present, more acceptable procedure is the use of a chemical name for some of the B complex vitamins (for example, thiamin instead of vitamin B_1).

Vitamins usually act as coenzymes (organic molecules necessary for activation of an apoenzyme). When vitamins enter the body, they are combined with an associated apoenzyme (the protein part of an enzyme) to form a holoenzyme, commonly referred to simply as an enzyme (an organic compound produced by living tissue to accelerate metabolic reactions). The vitamin is able to function only when combined with its apoenzyme within the cell. Because the quantity of protein that will combine with the vitamin is limited, any excess vitamin ingested beyond that which can combine with apoenzyme cannot function as a vitamin. In short, amounts of vitamins many times the recommended dietary allowances may not only be worthless but may, in fact, be harmful.[4] Reviews on toxicity of megadoses of vitamins have been published.[5–7]

Vitamins do not contribute directly to the structure of the body, nor do they supply energy. Instead they regulate metabolism by releasing energy from fats and carbohydrates. Vitamins can be involved in amino acid metabolism and also assist in forming blood, bones, and tissues. As noted above, they act as catalysts that hasten biological changes or enable them to take place.

CLASSIFICATION OF THE B COMPLEX VITAMINS

In 1915 the beriberi factor was named water-soluble vitamin B by McCollum and Davis.[8] At that time, vitamin B was thought to be a single substance. However, later research showed that it actually consisted of a number of different chemical substances with a few similar properties. Therefore these substances were grouped together and called B complex vitamins. All B complex vitamins have three common properties: they are natural constituents of yeast and liver, they are water soluble, and they promote the growth of bacteria.

Eleven different vitamins have been discovered and categorized as belonging to the B complex group. On a functional basis, this general grouping might be subdivided into (1) those vitamins that primarily release energy from carbohydrates and fats, namely thiamin, niacin, riboflavin, pantothenic acid, and biotin; (2) those that catalyze formation of red blood cells, namely folic acid and vitamin B_{12}; (3) the vitamin that is important in protein and amino acid metabolism, vitamin B_6; and (4) the vitaminlike compounds (discussed briefly later in this chapter).

THE ENERGY-RELEASING B VITAMINS

Thiamin (Vitamin B₁)

Discovery and History. Beriberi, a thiamin deficiency disease, was known in the Orient as early as 2600 B.C. (The word *beriberi* means *I cannot* in Singhalese, signifying that the person who has the disease is too sick to function.) Investigation into the cause of the disease in the late nineteenth century led to the discovery of the B vitamins.

More than a hundred years ago, Dr. K. Takaki, a Japanese physician, began to suspect that there was something lacking in the polished rice diet of Japanese sailors that caused them to succumb to beriberi.[9] He drew this conclusion from a feeding experiment in which the rice diet usually eaten by his country's sailors was replaced by a British diet of whole-grain barley, milk, meat, and vegetables. One group was given the usual Japanese diet and another was fed the British diet. The Japanese sailors who ate the British diet did not develop beriberi, whereas those who ate the usual Japanese rice diet succumbed to the disease.

At about this same time a Dutch physician, Dr. Christian Eijkman, made the chance observation that chickens fed milled white rice contracted beriberi, whereas those living on unhusked brown rice did not.[9] When the ailing chickens were placed on a diet of brown rice, they were cured almost overnight. This experiment demonstrated the cause and cure of beriberi. A few years later it was discovered by U.S. Army doctors in the Philippines that feeding a brown rice diet rather than white polished rice to soldiers imprisoned in army hospitals prevented beriberi.

The first pure preparation of thiamin from rice polishings was made by Jansen.[10] Ten years later, Williams and Cline synthesized thiamin and determined its chemical structure.[11]

Chemistry and Properties. Thiamin is broken down by heat in neutral or alkaline solutions. This ready solubility and the ease with which it is destroyed are important, because overcooking may result in significant losses of this vitamin. However, destruction of thiamin can be retarded in acid media; e.g., it is resistant to heat up to 120°C in an acid solution.

Absorption and Metabolism. Thiamin is easily absorbed from the small intestine. It is combined with phosphate within the mucosal cells of the intestine and transported via the portal vein into the general circulation. Alcohol and barbiturates decrease thiamin absorption.

As with most water-soluble vitamins, the body is unable to store thiamin in any great quantity. Some thiamin may be found in liver, heart, brain, and muscle tissue. Diuretics containing mercury increase urinary loss of this vitamin. There is no benefit to be derived from taking large doses, because the excess will be rapidly excreted in the urine.

Function. Thiamin, as thiamin pyrophosphate, is an important coenzyme in energy metabolism. It acts as a coenzyme in the production of ribose, the sugar needed by all cells for the formation of ribonucleic acid (RNA), which helps produce protein and deoxyribonucleic acid (DNA), the basic substance of genes. Thiamin is needed for the metabolism of carbohydrates, proteins, and fats.

Thiamin has a specific role in neurophysiology that is independent of its coenzyme function. It has been isolated from stimulated nerve fibers, suggesting that it is in some way related to the transmission of neural impulses. In fact, the neuritis of alcoholism is similar to the polyneuritis of beriberi, and sometimes therapeutic doses of B complex vitamins, especially thiamin, are prescribed.

Clinical Diagnosis of Deficiency. Deficiency of this vitamin in the United States may be prevalent in people with restricted dietary habits, in food faddists, and in alcoholics. It will also occur among people in those countries in which polished rice is used as the main source of calories. Also, thiaminase, an antivitamin present in uncooked shellfish and some types of freshwater fish, when ingested, can produce a thiamin deficiency.

Severe thiamin deficiency is called beriberi. It affects principally the cardiovascular, muscular, and nervous systems.

Beriberi can be separated into three forms: (1) wet, (2) dry, and (3) infantile. In wet beriberi, edema (accumulation of fluid in tissue spaces) of the legs, cardiac disturbances such as enlarged heart, systolic murmurs, and dyspnea (difficulty in breathing) may develop. The pulse is rapid and irregular, and the neck veins are distended. In dry beriberi, edema does not occur. Rather, a condition consisting of paresthesia (prickling or burning) and numbness of the feet and cramps in the legs is present.[12] Infantile beriberi, caused by inadequate thiamin in the breast milk, is characterized by dyspnea, cyanosis, and cardiac failure.

In the alcoholic, a severe thiamin deficiency may lead to Wernicke's syndrome, which is characterized by confusion, paralysis of eye muscles, and loss of memory. Peculiar gait and foot and wrist drop are seen in advanced cases. The administration of excess thiamin during treatment can be justified whether deficiencies are present or not because when thiamin is given in large amounts, passive absorption can overcome deficiencies.[13]

The possible oral manifestations of a deficiency of this vitamin are increased sensitivity of the oral mucosa, burning tongue, and loss or diminution of taste. However, these symptoms may be related to other nutritional deficiencies as well.

Diagnostic Laboratory Findings. The concentration of pyruvate in the blood is increased, so that the ratio of lactic acid to pyruvic acid becomes abnormal. The measurement of transketolase (an enzyme) activity in erythrocytes is a useful test in the diagnosis of thiamin deficiency.

Recommended Dietary Allowance. The thiamin requirement is related to caloric intake, particularly from carbohydrates. When the caloric intake is increased as a result of greater metabolic requirements (e.g., spurt growth, pregnancy, or lactation), thiamin requirements are correspondingly increased. The recommended daily dietary allowance for thiamin is 0.5 mg/1000 kcal,[14] which means that the average adult using about 2000 kcal a day should ingest about 1 mg of thiamin per day. However, when kilocalorie intake is less than 2000 (as may occur in older people), the thiamin intake should not fall below 1 mg daily. Because stores of thiamin in the body are negligible, this amount is not excessive, particularly if one experiences a disease with associated fever or increased metabolism.

Food Sources. The main dietary sources of thiamin are cereals, meats, and legumes. The richest sources are brewer's yeast, lean pork, liver, beef, dried peas and beans, nuts, and whole wheat and enriched cereals and breads. Other foods such as milk, eggs, fruit, and leafy vegetables contribute worthwhile amounts to the diet. The American food supply provides 2.07 mg/day per capita.[15]

Thiamin can be lost by milling cereals, overheating milk, and canning meat. Because it is water soluble, the vitamin can be lost in cooking, and its loss is accelerated by the addition of baking soda (used to improve the appearance of vegetables). The amount of thiamin lost will depend on the amount of water used and the length of the cooking period; as much as one-third of the original thiamin content may be lost through overcooking. Meat can lose a significant amount of thiamin if it is roasted too long. Freshly frozen vegetables are as rich in thiamin as the original product. Canned vegetables, however, suffer a loss of this vitamin because of its solubility and the heating during the canning process.

The presence of thiamin in foods and enriched staples is so widespread that with a varied, balanced, and adequate diet, one's needs will be met.

Therapy. A good diet and administration of 5 to 10 mg of thiamin hydrochloride three times a day will help the usual cases of nutritional polyneuropathy (a disease involving several nerves). There is no reliable evidence that thiamin supplementation is useful in any other disorder of the nervous system. Alcoholics or others who may develop beriberi should also have some multivitamin B complex tablet supplement in a therapeutic dose (which is two or three times the supportive dose), brewer's yeast, liver extract, or wheat germ.

Niacin

Niacin should be used as the generic description for derivatives exhibiting qualitatively the biological activity of nicotinamide.

Discovery and History. Pellagra was described more than 200 years ago by Casal, a court physician to King Philip V of Spain, soon after the introduction of corn (maize) into Europe. An Italian physician, Frappoli, named the disease *pelle agra* (*rough skin* in Italian). The disease reached epidemic proportions in the southern part of the United States in the early 1900s; more than 10,000

Americans died. In 1915 Dr. Joseph Goldberger of the U.S. Public Health Service became convinced that a faulty diet rather than a bacterial infection was the cause after he was able to eliminate the disease in a Mississippi orphanage by adding milk, meat, and eggs to the children's diet of corn, pork, hominy, and molasses.[16] He confirmed that this disease was caused by a nutritional deficiency as a result of an experiment on 12 convicts on a prison farm. Goldberger divided the volunteer group into six control and six experimental subjects. All were housed in wards of the same type; the only difference between the two groups was in their diet. The six in the experimental group were fed the typical pellagrin (one suffering from pellagra) diet consisting of cornmeal, cornstarch, sweet potatoes, rice, syrup, and pork fat. This was known as the 3-M ration— maize, molasses, and meat (pork fat). The six in the control group were fed the regular prison fare. After six months on their respective diets, the experimental group developed pellagra, whereas the control group did not. More convincing proof that the disease was indeed the result of dietary deficiency was the fact that it was possible to cure the sick of their illness by improving their diet with meat, eggs, vegetables, and fruits. Attempts to transmit the disease from a pellagrin to a healthy person by inoculation failed. This was indeed proof that pellagra did not result from a bacterial infection.

In 1938 Elvehjem and his group demonstrated that with nicotinic acid they could cure black tongue in dogs, a condition similar to one seen in humans with pellagra.[17] Shortly thereafter, niacin was shown to be effective in the prevention and treatment of pellagra.

Why infants who live on milk do not develop pellagra in spite of the fact that milk is very low in niacin remained unanswered until it was discovered that tryptophan, an amino acid found in milk, is a precursor (forerunner) of niacin and that humans can manufacture their own niacin if their diets contain tryptophan.[18] We now know that approximately 60 mg of dietary tryptophan furnishes 1 mg of niacin. Accordingly, estimated human requirements of niacin must take into account the tryptophan content of the diet.

Chemistry and Properties. Niacin is a slightly water-soluble, light- and heat-stable, weak organic acid. Although chemically related to nicotine, it possesses very different physiological properties. Niacin is one of the most stable vitamins, but because it is water soluble, it may be lost in cooking water.

Metabolism. Niacin is absorbed in the upper part of the small intestine. It is stored only sparingly in the kidney, heart, brain, and liver and is excreted in the urine.

As mentioned above, niacin is synthesized from tryptophan with the aid of other B vitamins, namely, pyridoxine, riboflavin, and thiamin.

Functions. Niacin forms the active portion of the coenzymes that play an essential role in supplying organ tissues, making its presence necessary for the health of all cells. Niacin's biochemical role is carried out by two coenzymes— nicotinamide adenine dinucleotide and nicotinamide adenine dinucleotide phosphate, known collectively as the pyridine nucleotides. These coenzymes act as catalysts in accepting and releasing hydrogen in cellular respiration, carbohydrate metabolism, and fat synthesis. A deficiency of this vitamin will disturb tissue respiration and glycolysis (the process by which sugar is broken down to produce energy) and the formation of fat. The energy released during the oxidation of food substrate is captured as high-energy adenosine triphosphate

(ATP). Therefore, niacin is vital in the normal function of the central nervous system, in maintaining the integrity of the skin and mucous membranes, and especially in supplying the needed coenzyme for the energy cycles.

Clinical Diagnosis of Deficiency. Pellagra is a niacin deficiency disease caused by a primary inadequate dietary intake or by a secondary conditioning (systemic) factor such as alcoholism, gastrointestinal disease, hyperthyroidism, or infection that inhibits absorption and use of nutrients.

Pellagra is characterized as the disease causing the 4 Ds—dermatitis, diarrhea, depression, and if not corrected, death.

Early symptoms of pellagra are similar to those produced in other B complex deficiency states: weakness, persistent fatigability, irritability, headache, and depression. Soreness and inflammation of the tongue (glossitis) and mouth (stomatitis) aggravated by highly seasoned foods is also a frequent complaint.

The dermatitis tends to be most severe in areas of exposure to chronic irritation, sun, or heat. The most likely to be affected are the face, neck, backs of the hands, wrists, elbows, knees, and perineal folds. The lesions are usually symmetrical. The margins of the lesions are usually sharply demarcated from normal skin, one of the more important features that differentiate it from other types of dermatitis. At first there is redness and thickening of the skin, followed eventually by a variegated dermatitis with brown, scaly areas alternating with areas of depigmented, shiny, shrunken skin.

The tongue is sore, swollen, scarlet in color, and smooth. Secondary infection with fungi or bacteria (e.g., fusiform bacilli and spirochetes) characteristic of acute necrotizing ulcerative gingivitis (Vincent's infection) is common. Eating and swallowing are so painful that food is often refused, which may contribute to worsening of the disease.

Diarrhea is due to inflammation of the mucosal lining of the esophagus, stomach, and colon.

Depression, confusion, hallucinations, and delirium can result from degeneration of nerve and brain cells.

The clinical diagnosis of pellagra rests largely on the identification of the skin and oral changes (cheilosis, a fissured condition of the lips, and angular stomatitis, inflamed corners of the mouth) plus complaints of gastrointestinal upsets.

Because of vitamin B complex interrelationships, in pellagra there may be deficiencies of riboflavin, thiamin, and pyridoxine in addition to the deficiency of niacin.

Diagnostic Laboratory Findings. Urinary excretion of niacin metabolite falls to low levels. Excretion of 0.5 mg of N'-methylniacinamide per gram of creatinine suggests a niacin deficiency.

Recommended Dietary Allowance. The daily requirement for niacin is influenced by the amount of tryptophan present in the diet. Recall that the body can manufacture niacin from the amino acid tryptophan. An average of 60 mg of tryptophan is equivalent to 1 mg of niacin in the diet. Thus, one niacin equivalent is defined as 1 mg of niacin or 60 mg of dietary tryptophan.

The recommended daily dietary allowance for niacin is 13 niacin equivalents when one eats a diet of 2000 kcal or less. The recommended amounts for different age groups are specified in Appendix 2. With high caloric intakes, the allowance increases at the rate of 6.6 niacin equivalents per 1000 kcal. Most diets in the United States supply 16 to 33 niacin equivalents per day.

For pregnant and lactating females over the age of 18, the recommended daily allowance is 15 and 18 niacin equivalents, respectively.

Food Sources. Niacin is found in appreciable amounts in liver, yeast, meat, legumes, peanuts, and whole cereals. In some cereals, such as corn, most of the niacin is unavailable unless it is hydrolyzed. Treatment of cereals with alkali, which some population groups have traditionally done in making tortillas, releases much of the bound niacin. Cooking does not appear to increase availability.

Foods that are good sources of tryptophan, such as animal protein (except gelatin) and vegetable protein, are good sources of niacin, because as stated earlier, the body has the capacity to convert tryptophan into niacin.

Because niacin is relatively heat stable and resistant to oxidation, there are usually no large losses of this vitamin during cooking or processing. Niacin that is lost in cooking will be found in the cooking water.

Therapy. In treatment of mild niacin deficiency, administration of 50 mg of nicotinamide orally three times a day is recommended.

For the treatment of pellagra, 300 to 500 mg of nicotinamide daily in divided doses, as well as supplements of other nutrients that are frequently deficient, is prescribed.[19] If pellagra is complicated by deficiency of other B complex vitamins, which is often the case, it is advisable to give an additional multivitamin capsule containing 5 mg thiamin, 5 mg riboflavin, 5 mg vitamin B_6, and 10 mg pantothenic acid. Brewer's yeast, 10 to 30 g/day, is an alternative to the multivitamin capsule.

Milk, eggs, strained cereals, and pureed vegetables are usually well tolerated by sore mouths. These foods are high in tryptophan, which is a precursor to niacin.

Toxicity and Pharmacological Effects. Nicotinic acid, not nicotinamide, can cause a transitory dilation of blood vessels, resulting in a tingling and flushing of the skin.

Pharmacological doses of niacin (3 g or more) have been used to prevent recurrent nonfatal myocardial infarctions. However, because of the excess incidence of arrhythmias, gastrointestinal problems, and abnormal chemistry, the use of niacin for this purpose is not recommended. Massive doses of niacin have also been used in treatment of schizophrenia without convincingly positive effects.

Massive doses of this vitamin can cause liver toxicity and peptic ulcers.

Riboflavin (Vitamin B_2)[20]

Discovery and History. Chemical research on riboflavin was begun in 1879 by an English food chemist, Winter Blyth, who observed some pale yellow material in the whey of milk, which he called lactoflavin. However, the importance of this vitamin in nutrition was not discovered until 1926, when it was shown that the heat-stable portion of vitamin B complex had growth-promoting properties when fed to rodents.

A yellow enzyme essential for cell respiration was isolated from yeast by Warburg and Christian in 1932. But it was Kuhn and his co-workers who reported in 1935 on the synthesis of riboflavin and the relation of its activity to green fluorescence. The latter group established that lactoflavin and the vitamin are the same. This was the first evidence that a vitamin functions as a coenzyme.[9]

Chemistry. Riboflavin is an orange-yellow crystalline substance slightly soluble in water. It is stable to heat in neutral or acid solutions but may be destroyed by heating in an alkaline solution or by exposing to light. Under ultraviolet light, it exhibits a characteristic green fluorescence. This aids in its identification in tissue sections.

Absorption and Metabolism. Riboflavin must be phosphorylated (combined with phosphate) in the intestinal tract before it can be absorbed. Absorption of the vitamin is best when eaten with a meal. Very little of the vitamin is stored, and it must be supplied daily. Excess riboflavin is excreted in the urine.

Drugs such as tetracycline and diuretics increase urinary excretion. Sulfonamides depress bacterial synthesis of the vitamin. However, the extent to which bacteria serve as a source for this vitamin is probably not very great.

Function. Most of the riboflavin in the body is found in two coenzymes, flavin mononucleotide and flavin adenine dinucleotide. These coenzymes are attached to enzymes called flavoproteins, which act as hydrogen carriers. Hydrogen is passed along from one substance to another until it unites with oxygen to form water. Energy in the form of ATP is produced in this process. Thus riboflavin is an electron-transfer vitamin participating in the exchange of oxygen and hydrogen between plasma and tissue cells. In addition to taking part in the formation of ATP, riboflavin assists in the metabolism of carbohydrates, proteins, and fats.

Clinical Diagnosis of Deficiency. The basis for a riboflavin deficiency is an inadequate dietary intake, most often seen in alcoholics and the economically deprived. Also, a severe gastrointestinal disease that causes vomiting and hypermotility of the gastrointestinal tract can produce this deficiency, as can polyuria resulting from uncontrolled diabetes.

Clinically, riboflavin deficiency may be found in conjunction with a lack of other B vitamins such as pyridoxine, niacin, and folic acid. The reason for the multiplicity of vitamin deficits is that dietary deficiencies tend to be multiple because the food sources are similar.

Besides cracks in the corners of the mouth (angular stomatitis) and inflammation of the tongue (glossitis), there are characteristic eye and skin changes. The eye changes include an increase in blood vessels and inflammation of the conjunctivae. The cornea is invaded by capillaries, producing opaque areas and even ulceration. Dermatitis characterized by a greasy and scaly reddened lesion develops in the skin around the nasolabial folds and may extend to a butterfly shape on the cheeks. There may also be lesions at the corners (canthi) of the eyes and lobes of the ears.[21]

The diagnosis of a riboflavin deficiency depends not only on the mouth, eye, and skin signs and changes just described but also on nutritional history and laboratory tests. The positive response to therapeutic levels of riboflavin is the key to confirming the diagnosis of riboflavin deficiency.

Diagnostic Laboratory Findings. Excretion in the urine of less than 27 mg of riboflavin per gram of creatinine indicates a deficiency.

The concentration of riboflavin in red blood cells of less than 14 mg/100 ml is considered to indicate a potential deficiency.

Recommended Dietary Allowances. The body size, metabolic rate, and growth rate influence the amount of riboflavin that should be ingested. The recommended daily dietary allowance is about 1.5 mg for adults. The recommended amounts for different age groups are given in Appendix 2.

The need for riboflavin, like that for protein, is increased during growth, pregnancy, and lactation. It does not seem to be related to caloric consumption.

Food Sources. The best food sources of riboflavin are milk, liver, heart, and kidney. Lean meat, cheese, eggs, and leafy green vegetables are also good sources. The whole-grain and enriched cereals and breads contribute important amounts of riboflavin to the diet. However, riboflavin differs from other components of the vitamin B complex in that milk rather than cereal is its major source in the diet.

Very little riboflavin is lost in cooking because of its stability. However, bottled milk exposed to sunlight will lose a significant amount. For this reason, milk packaged in opaque paper cartons is better.

Therapy. In the treatment of riboflavin deficiency, a good diet of liver, meat, eggs, and enriched cereal plus a special emphasis on a quart of milk daily is a first consideration. One quart of milk furnishes 2 mg of the riboflavin. Also, a therapeutic multivitamin capsule containing at least 5 mg of riboflavin should be taken two or three times a day.

Pantothenic Acid[22]

History. The discovery of pantothenic acid stemmed from investigation of yeast growth factor and a liver filtrate factor. It was named pantothenic acid by R. J. Williams in 1938 because of its distribution in many foods. It cured a dermatitis around the eyes and beaks of chickens. When black rats ate diets deficient in this vitamin, their hair turned gray.

Chemistry and Properties. Free pantothenic acid is a yellow oily liquid that has never been crystallized. It is easily destroyed by heat. The calcium salt (calcium pantothenate) crystallizes readily, and this is the form in which it is generally available. It is soluble in water and is more stable to heat than pantothenic acid.

Function. Pantothenic acid is of great biological importance because of its incorporation with coenzyme A, which assists in acetylation reactions (the introduction of an acetyl group into an organic molecule). It is involved in the release of energy from the catabolism of carbohydrates, proteins, and fats. It initiates the Krebs cycle and releases ATP. It is the starting substance for the biosynthesis of long-chain fatty acids. Pantothenic acid is concerned with the biosynthesis (creation of a compound by physiological processes in a living organism) of cholesterol and other sterols as well as porphyrin, a component of hemoglobin.

Clinical Diagnosis of Deficiency. In humans a deficiency can be induced experimentally. The symptoms are fatigue, sleep disturbances, headaches, malaise, nausea, and abdominal stress. Burning, prickling sensations (paresthesia) of the hands and feet, cramping of the leg muscles, and impaired coordination are additional findings.

Diagnostic Laboratory Findings. Urinary excretion of less than 1 mg/day is considered abnormally low in adults.

Recommended Dietary Allowance. A daily intake of 3 to 4 mg is probably adequate for children; adults should receive 4 to 7 mg daily.

Food Sources. Pantothenic acid is widely distributed, occurring abundantly in yeast and in animal tissues such as liver and eggs, whole-grain cereals, and legumes. Other fair sources are milk, fruits, and vegetables such as broccoli, cauliflower, and potatoes. It is usually present when the diet is adequate in other B vitamins. Pantothenic acid is probably also synthesized by intestinal bacteria.

Therapy. No definite therapeutic regimen for dealing with pantothenic acid deficiency has been presented. A balanced, adequate diet in the United States usually supplies 10 to 15 mg of pantothenic acid, which more than meets the recommended daily allowance. Multivitamin B complex preparations usually contain pantothenic acid.

Biotin[23]

Chemistry. When biotin was discovered, it was considered part of the "bios" factor needed for yeast growth. Raw egg white contains avidin, which strongly binds biotin. However, when egg white is cooked, avidin loses its ability to bind biotin.

Function. Biotin is a very active biological substance. As little as 0.005 microgram (μg; one-millionth of a gram) stimulates the growth of yeast and bacteria.

Biotin functions as a coenzyme for reactions involving the addition of carbon dioxide in the formation of purines. The latter are essential constituents of DNA, a basic substance of genes that controls the development of the organism, and of RNA, which takes part in protein synthesis.

Clinical Diagnosis of Deficiency. Researchers[24] produced a biotin deficiency by feeding four volunteers a diet adequate in all of the B complex vitamins except biotin. This diet was composed largely of dried egg white, which is high in avidin. Other known components of the B complex were added in synthetic form. After 10 weeks of this diet, the subjects developed inflammation of the skin and the tongue (dermatitis and glossitis), loss of appetite and sleep, nausea, muscular pains, increased skin sensitivity (hyperesthesia), and burning and prickling sensations (paresthesia). All of these signs and symptoms were relieved by the injection of a concentrated preparation (0.15 to 0.3 mg) of biotin daily.

Human biotin deficiency has been encountered in infants treated with sulfa drugs and in adults whose diet consisted mainly of raw egg whites. Biotin deficiency has been reported in patients maintained for long periods of time on intravenous feeding. Characteristic symptoms were loss of hair (alopecia) and skin disease (dermatosis).[25, 26] The predominant sign, dermatitis, responded to biotin treatment.

Consumption of an occasional raw egg, as in eggnog, will not precipitate deficiency symptoms. It is only when large amounts (20 or more eggs per day) are consumed that a problem occurs.

Recommended Dietary Allowance. A daily intake of 100 to 200 μg of biotin is considered adequate.

Food Sources. The richest sources of biotin are liver, kidney, milk, egg yolk, and yeast. It occurs primarily in combined forms. Because it is found in most foods and is also synthesized by intestinal bacteria, deficiency states are recognized only when diets have included large amounts of raw egg white.

VITAMIN B₆

History. Vitamin B_6 is not a single vitamin but rather a group of metabolically and functionally interrelated pyridines: namely, pyridoxine, pyridoxamine (the amine of pyridoxine), and pyridoxal.[27] Each of these substances is widely distributed in foods and is present in both free and bound forms.

This vitamin factor was discovered in 1934, when it was demonstrated that there was another factor besides riboflavin in the heat-stable fraction of the vitamin B complex.[28] The researcher also showed that this vitamin could cure scaly dermatitis in rats, which is the reason it is called the antiacrodynia (antiscaling) factor. Pyridoxal and pyridoxamine occur mainly in animal products, whereas pyridoxine is found mostly in plant products.[29] Pyridoxine has often been used as the collective term for all three, but in the current nomenclature the term *vitamin B_6* is used as the generic descriptor for all three.

Chemistry. Pyridoxine is a water-soluble, white crystalline compound that is stable to heat and strong acids. In contrast, dilute solutions of pyridoxamine and pyridoxal are quite labile to heat and air and are readily destroyed by them.

Function. The principal vitamin activity resides in the enzymatically active coenzyme form, pyridoxal-5-phosphate, which serves as a cofactor for numerous enzyme systems concerned with protein and amino acid metabolism. This vitamin plays no role in energy production. Instead, it is involved primarily with reactions involving both the synthesis and the breakdown of amino acids. Therefore, it is critical to protein synthesis.

Vitamin B_6 aids in the conversion of tryptophan to niacin. This ability serves as the basis for determining whether a deficiency of vitamin B_6 is present. A deficient individual or animal will excrete large amounts of xanthurenic acid, an abnormal metabolite that develops when large amounts of tryptophan are administered.

Vitamin B_6 has many other unrelated functions. It aids in the metabolism of polyunsaturated fatty acids. It is involved in some way in hemoglobin synthesis and red blood cell regeneration, and it aids in the normal functioning of nervous tissue. It is part of an enzyme, glycogen phosphorylase, that is responsible for the conversion of glycogen to glucose. More than 50% of the body's total vitamin B_6 is attached to this enzyme.

Estrogens (such as those used in contraceptive pills) and corticosteroids have an effect on vitamin B_6 metabolism.[30]

Clinical Diagnosis of Deficiency. Infants and children who have been fed a canned milk formula deficient in pyridoxine have developed severe irritability and convulsions. The symptoms have been relieved by administration of the vitamin. It is possible that other infants and children who develop this deficiency disease, which is very rare, have an inborn error of metabolism for this vitamin.

A frank deficiency of vitamin B_6 in humans is rare because of its widespread distribution in natural foodstuffs. An experimental deficiency was produced in humans by feeding a vitamin B_6–deficient diet together with a vitamin antagonist (substance that nullified action of the vitamin). Experimental subjects developed cheilosis (fissured condition of the lips and angles of the mouth), glossitis and stomatitis (inflammation of the tongue and mouth), and an itching and burning dermatitis with redness in the nasolabial (pertaining to the nose and lips) folds. Subjective symptoms accompanying these signs were loss of appetite, nausea, drowsiness, and peripheral neuropathy. These signs and symptoms resemble those seen in deficiencies of riboflavin, niacin, and thiamin, which attests to the close metabolic relationship of the B complex vitamins.

Patients with hypochromic anemia not readily responsive to iron therapy have improved dramatically with regimens of pyridoxine. Pyridoxal phosphate plays a role in hemoglobin synthesis as a cofactor in the formation of a precursor to porphyrin, an essential part of the hemoglobin molecule.

Diagnostic Laboratory Findings. Vitamin B_6 deficiency produces increased urinary excretion of xanthurenic acid after administration of a test dose of tryptophan. Normal subjects excrete less than 30 to 50 mg of xanthurenic acid in a 24-hour period.

Recommended Dietary Allowance. For the infant up to 1 year of age, 0.3 to 0.6 mg daily is recommended. There is a correlation between the vitamin B_6 needs and the protein content of breast milk or cow's milk (0.015 mg/g of protein). In children the recommended daily dietary allowance is 0.9 to 1.6 mg, which is available in a normal diet. It is important to meet this allowance in order to avoid a detrimental effect on physical and mental growth and development. In adolescents the recommended allowance is 1.8 to 2.0 mg daily.

If the daily intake of protein is 100 g or more (common in the United States today), an intake of vitamin B_6 of 2.0 mg/day is recommended. During pregnancy and lactation, an intake of 2.5 mg/day is desirable.

Food Sources. The best sources of vitamin B_6 are the same as for other members of the B complex: liver, muscle meats, yeast, legumes, whole-grain cereals, wheat germ, and wheat bran. Milling of whole grains causes more than half the vitamin B_6 content of the wheat to be lost. Because addition of vitamin B_6 to processed grain products is not yet legally required, there is little in flour, white bread, precooked rice, noodles, macaroni, and spaghetti.

Therapy. When primary deficiency of this vitamin is suspected in an adult, a daily dosage of 10 mg is given. In iron-resistant hypochromic anemia, doses up to 100 mg/day have been given. Certain medications, such as isoniazid and penicillamine, produce a need for a supplement of vitamin B_6.

Toxicity. Pyridoxine toxicity has been described when used in excess by the alcoholic to overcome a vitamin B_6 deficiency. A sensory nervous system dysfunction has been noted in women taking 2 to 6 g of vitamin B_6 per day.[31]

VITAMINLIKE COMPOUNDS[3]

Although choline, *myo*-inositol, coenzyme Q (ubiquinone), lipoic acid, *p*-aminobenzoic acid, and the bioflavonoids are often erroneously considered to be vitamins, according to our present knowledge they are not.

Each of these vitaminlike substances fails to meet one or more of the following criteria for a vitamin: (1) they do not have an essential biological role; (2) the animal body can synthesize adequate amounts; and (3) they are present in the diet in larger amounts than the vitamins that exert a catalytic function.

FUNCTION OF B COMPLEX VITAMINS IN CARBOHYDRATE METABOLISM

The interrelationship among the B complex vitamins is so close that a deficient intake of one impairs the use of the others. No single vitamin of the B complex is more important than another because the normal chain of metabolism can be broken by the lack of any one.

For example, in addition to minerals, thiamin, riboflavin, niacin, and pantothenic acid are required in the metabolism of carbohydrates. Each of these vitamins plays a key role in the metabolism of glucose.

Biotin is important in the conversion of acetic acid to long-chain fatty acids. It is also important in the production of energy from glucose and in the synthesis of glycogen.

Thus the complete metabolism of carbohydrates depends on the presence of adequate amounts of each of the five energy-releasing vitamins (niacin, thiamin, riboflavin, pantothenic acid, and biotin), which fall under the general classification of B complex vitamins. The B complex vitamins also play a role in the metabolism of protein and fat.

DISORDERS CAUSED BY VITAMIN B COMPLEX DEFICIENCY

The same type of close interrelationship between each of the B vitamins in the complex that contributes to the metabolism of carbohydrates, proteins, and fats also exists in the deficiency diseases that they produce. Although the signs and symptoms of a deficiency of a particular member of the B complex group may predominate, deficiency of a single vitamin seldom occurs. However, when each B complex vitamin was discovered, some characteristic clinical deficiency disorders were ascribed to it because some signs and symptoms stood out. Therefore, when each of the vitamins was discussed here, a brief description of the general dysfunction associated with its lack has been given.

Oral Signs of Vitamin B Complex Deficiencies

The oral tissues are composed of cells that grow rapidly and are replaced frequently. Therefore an adequate supply of nutrients, particularly the B complex vitamins, must be available for these tissues to maintain their integrity. When oral tissues are denied adequate nourishment, they succumb readily to infection.

The inflammatory changes seen in the mucosa of the lips, particularly at the corners of the mouth or lip junctions (referred to as labial commissures) may be a manifestation of a deficiency of one or more of the following nutrients: riboflavin, niacin, pyridoxine, folic acid, vitamin B_{12}, protein, and iron. Usually, patients develop lip lesions that begin with a pallor of the mucosa at the lip junctions. Redness, softening, and fissuring of the corners of the mouth occur. A secondary staphylococcal infection may follow, producing a yellow crust. After proper cleansing and nutritional therapy, particularly the intake of vitamin B complex in therapeutic doses, the crusty corners of the mouth will heal.[32]

Painful ulcerations of the tongue, especially at the sides, are seen with B complex deficiencies. Usually, these changes can be reversed by therapeutic doses of vitamin B complex supplements.

In most cases of acute nutritional deficiencies seen in alcoholics, there is an atrophy of both types of papillae (small projections) so that the dorsum (top surface) of the tongue is smooth, shiny, and red. If in addition to improving the quality and quantity of the food intake, a multivitamin preparation of the B complex vitamins in therapeutic doses is taken daily, the tongue will return to its normal color and texture in a few weeks.[33]

A generalized inflammation of the buccal and palatal mucosa of the mouth characteristic of stomatitis with red, swollen, and tender areas can be mitigated (lessened in severity), in part, by the intake of therapeutic doses of B complex supplements if other possible contributing factors such as allergies or irritants are eliminated.

THE HEMATOPOIETIC (BLOOD CELL–FORMING) B VITAMINS: FOLACIN AND VITAMIN B_{12}

Many nutrients are involved in the formation and maintenance of blood. However, the major ones that deal with blood formation (hematopoiesis) are folic acid and vitamin B_{12}. (Iron, the key nutrient in the formation of hemoglobin, and other nutrients— e.g., protein, pyridoxine, ascorbic acid, vitamin E, vitamin K, calcium, copper, and cobalt—that are also concerned with hematology are discussed elsewhere in this text.)

Anemia is defined as a below normal reduction in (1) number of red cells (erythrocytes) per cubic millimeter (mm^3) of blood, (2) quantity of hemoglobin, or (3) volume of packed red cells per 100 ml of blood. These abnormalities occur when blood loss is greater than blood production. A diagnosis with respect to the type of anemia is made in part on the basis of the relative maturity of the red cells. For this reason it is important to understand the genesis (origin) and development of the red cells.

Genesis of Red Blood Cells

The early red cell precursor is a megaloblast or a proerythroblast that arises from the primordial (simplest and most undeveloped) cells located in the bone marrow. The basophil (blue-staining) erythroblast (immature red cell) is the next stage in the genesis of red blood cells and is the stage when synthesis of hemoglobin begins. As the cell matures from erythroblast to normoblast (late stage in the development of red cells), the nucleus shrinks, and the quantities of hemoglobin increase. When the bone marrow produces red blood cells at a very rapid rate, reticulum (a small network) remains in the cytoplasm, giving rise to immature reticulocytes (young non-nucleated cells). When the reticulum completely disappears, the cytoplasm is filled with hemoglobin and the cell is considered to be a mature erythrocyte.

If the maturation of the red blood cells in the bone marrow is impaired by lack of folate or vitamin B_{12}, the cells that enter the blood stream are large and irregular in size and shape. If there is insufficient iron for the formation of hemoglobin, the red blood cells are pale and small.

The laboratory indicator of a folate or vitamin B_{12} deficiency is an increased mean corpuscular volume (MCV). This volume is derived from a ratio of PCV to RBC (packed cell volume or volume of blood cells to the number of red blood cells), which normally is 87 ± 5 cubic micrometers (μm^3). A value of 96 or more means that the red cells are larger than normal, which indicates the prevalence of the immature megaloblast cells associated with a deficiency of folate or vitamin B_{12}.

When the number of reticulocytes in the peripheral blood makes up more than 1% of the total blood cell count, this indicates that the bone marrow is more active than normal. This happens when a patient is responding to vitamin B_{12} therapy and confirms a diagnosis of vitamin B_{12} deficiency.

Folacin (Folic Acid)

The term folacin is the generic descriptor for folic acid, pteroylmonoglutamic acid, and related compounds exhibiting the biological activity of folic acid.

Discovery and History. The story of the discovery of folic acid begins during the 1930s and 1940s with the classic studies of Dr. Lucy Wills, who described an antianemic factor for the treatment of tropical macrocytic anemia in pregnant women. This factor was present in green leaves and thus was labeled folic acid. It was effective in the treatment of megaloblastic anemia of pregnancy and of tropical sprue.[34]

Quite unrelated to the discovery of the "Wills factor" were the findings by a group of researchers in 1941 that dietary anemia in chicks could be cured by a *Lactobacillus casei* growth factor preparation derived from the leaves of spinach.[35] The word *folic* is derived from the Latin word *folium,* meaning leaf. Therefore, the preparation was called folic acid. Folic acid (folate or folacin) was finally synthesized in 1946 by a team of industrial chemists.

Because it was known that synthetic folic acid could cure dietary anemia in chicks and monkeys, it was tried on humans with pernicious anemia, and it brought about a remission. However, it was not a satisfactory curative agent because it worsened the nerve lesions that accompany this anemia. Thus Wills's observation that two different accessory food factors are necessary for successful treatment of megaloblastic anemia was confirmed.

Chemistry. Folic acid is a yellow crystalline substance, sparingly soluble in water, that is destroyed when heated in neutral or alkaline media. The conjugated forms of the vitamin, known as a "folate," are converted to folic acid in the tissues.

Function. Tetrahydrofolic acid (the active form of this vitamin) acts as a coenzyme for the synthesis of purines and pyrimidines and is thus concerned with the formation of thymidylate, the base for DNA or nucleic acid. Folic acid coenzymes are also responsible for the formation of body protein from glycine and serine. A folic acid deficiency, then, would be characterized by impaired production of DNA, increase in size of the cell nucleus, and increase in cellular stroma (framework), thus preventing complete cell maturation.

Folic acid is essential for the manufacture and maturation of blood cells. The bone marrow is the organ that manufactures blood cells, but it cannot complete the process in the absence of folic acid. In short, folic acid is necessary for the normal functioning of the hematopoietic system.

Cells in the immune system are replaced relatively rapidly. Therefore they need to produce DNA continuously. These cells are especially susceptible to a folic acid deficiency.

Folate from food is absorbed by the gastrointestinal tract and is stored primarily in the liver. It supports the growth of such microorganisms in the body as *Lactobacillus casei* and *Streptococcus faecalis.*

Folic Acid Deficiency.[36] Folic acid deficiency is probably the most common vitamin deficiency in humans. It has been estimated that in the United States, 45% of adults who have little or no income are deficient in folic acid. Alcoholics also show this type of deficiency readily.

The commonest causes of a folic acid deficiency are disorders of malabsorption associated with infectious disease (tropical diseases) or certain metabolic and endocrine disorders. Megaloblastic anemia of pregnancy results from excessive vomiting of the mother and the increased requirement of the fetus for folic acid to aid in growth. The anemia caused by sprue and celiac disease is successfully treated with folic acid.

CLINICAL DIAGNOSIS OF DEFICIENCY. Folic acid deficiency often occurs in chronic alcoholics and malnourished elderly persons. The use of antiepileptic drugs can reduce serum folate, but megaloblastic anemia is rarely a complication of anticonvulsant therapy. Administration of folic acid antagonists (e.g., methotrexate) in the treatment of leukemia (increased numbers of abnormal white cells in the blood-forming tissues) may produce the picture of folic acid deficiency. Oral contraceptives can also impair folate metabolism.[37]

Clinically, the patient has tissue anemia characterized by weakness, fainting attacks, severe paleness of skin, and congestive heart failure. This is very often seen in the alcoholic with cirrhosis of the liver. There are no central nervous system abnormalities, which is a key factor in distinguishing between folic acid deficiency and vitamin B_{12} deficiency. It should be stressed that a folacin supplement will cure the anemia caused by vitamin B_{12} deficiency but will not alleviate the neurological symptoms that accompany this anemia.

The principal oral symptom is a burning sensation in the tongue and oral mucosa. The tongue is red, sore, and swollen. Angular cheilosis and gingivitis are also present.

Because the junctional epithelium in the gingiva is made up of rapidly multiplying cells, and because a deficient intake of folic acid might impair this type of cellular metabolism, it could be theorized that a folic acid inadequacy may condition the gingiva to react unfavorably to irritation from plaque accumulation. On this premise, two researchers, Vogel and Deasy, conducted a pilot study of the effect of a folic acid supplement on experimentally produced gingivitis.[38] They noted a significantly greater degree of gingival inflammation in a control group compared with a group receiving a supplement of 2 mg of folic acid twice daily over a 14-day period. These researchers suggested that folic acid supplements may increase gingival resistance to local inflammatory agents.

DIAGNOSTIC LABORATORY FINDINGS. The normal serum folate level ranges from 6 to 10 nanograms (ng; one-billionth of a gram) per milliliter. Folate deficiency is possible if the serum level is below 6 ng/ml. Normal values for red cell folacin are 160 to 650 ng/ml. Therefore a level of less than 160 ng/ml in red cells is indicative of a deficiency. A folic acid absorption test consisting of determining the plasma concentrations of folic acid at intervals after a dose of folic acid is given by mouth has been suggested for determining if a deficiency is present.

The laboratory findings in folic acid deficiency show the presence of free acid in the stomach. This is in contrast to a pure vitamin B_{12} deficiency, in which no free acid is found. The patient with a folic acid deficiency will readily excrete radioactive cobalt. On the other hand, a patient with vitamin B_{12} deficiency retains the radiolabeled vitamin B_{12}.

Recommended Dietary Allowance. The requirement for folate in food is approximately 0.4 mg daily for an adolescent and a nonpregnant, nonlactating adult.

During pregnancy an allowance of 0.8 mg/day is recommended; during lactation the requirement is 0.5 mg.

Consumption of alcohol will increase the body's folic acid requirements.

Food Sources. Folate is found in liver, kidney, yeasts, dark green leafy vegetables (e.g., spinach), asparagus, broccoli, soybeans, nuts, and orange juice. A balanced diet contains approximately 0.15 to 0.2 mg of folate. The intestinal bacteria may be a source of folic acid.

Therapy. Folic acid is required in the treatment of nutritional megaloblastic anemias, the megaloblastic anemias of pregnancy and infancy, and in some cases, the anemia produced by malabsorption syndrome. Folic acid is available in 1-mg tablets. A dose of 1 mg three times a week is more than adequate. It has been found in some instances that as little as 0.025 to 0.1 mg may be adequate. If the patient's reticulocyte count goes up significantly with this regimen, the diagnosis of folic acid deficiency can be made. In patients who have a history of megaloblastic anemias during pregnancy, recurrence of the problem can be prevented by taking 5 mg of folic acid daily during subsequent pregnancies.

Folic acid should not be used in the treatment of pernicious anemia, because it may make the neurological features of the disease worse. The use of folic acid to treat megaloblastic anemia resulting from the use of anticonvulsant drugs may aggravate the epileptic condition.

A prescription is required for more than 0.1 mg of folic acid per day, for although an amount in excess of this may prevent anemia, it may at the same time allow neurological manifestations of pernicious anemia to continue or even worsen.

Vitamin B$_{12}$ (Cobalamin)[39]

Discovery and History. Pernicious anemia leading inevitably to a patient's death in 2 to 5 years was first described by Thomas Addison of London in 1849. A constitutional or genetic predisposition to the disease was suggested. More recently, it has been shown to be the result of autoimmune reactions. The disease was considered fatal until 1926, when two researchers showed that a remission could be achieved by the ingestion of large amounts of whole liver.[40] In 1929 W. B. Castle demonstrated that ingesting a combination of beef muscle and gastric juice was also effective in the treatment of pernicious anemia.[41] Castle called the gastric juice intrinsic factor and the beef muscle extrinsic factor. These two factors had to be given at the same time to produce an effective result. Castle concluded that the disease was not dietary in origin but was caused by a failure of the stomach to secrete the intrinsic factor for the absorption of the dietary extrinsic factor.

The need for giving intrinsic factor to overcome pernicious anemia could be circumvented either by giving large amounts of liver by mouth or by injecting protein-free extracts of liver. In 1948 Shorb reported that the liver extracts used to overcome anemia also had growth-promoting properties for a *Lactobacillus* species.[42] Using this microorganism, Rickes and associates were able to isolate the red crystalline cyanocobalamin (vitamin B$_{12}$).[43] Originally, about one ton of fresh liver was needed for the isolation of 20 mg of the red crystals of vitamin B$_{12}$. It differed from folic acid in that it corrected both the anemias and the nervous system disorders, whereas folic acid could improve only the anemia. Vitamin B$_{12}$ binds to the intrinsic factor in the stomach and then the complex passes to the ileum where the vitamin is released from the complex, enters the circulation, and is transported as transcobalamin II. Evidently, vitamin B$_{12}$ is the extrinsic factor in food that is aided in its absorption into mucosal cells of the small intestine by intrinsic factor, secreted by cells of the gastric mucosa. Thus to be effective in a patient who cannot manufacture gastric juice (e.g., after a total stomach removal) vitamin B$_{12}$ must be given by injection rather than by mouth.

Chemistry. Vitamin B$_{12}$ is called cyanocobalamin because it consists of a cyanide ion and a cobalt ion, contained in a porphyrinlike ring linked to a nucleotide.

Vitamin B$_{12}$ is not a single substance but consists of several closely related compounds having similar activity; besides cyanocobalamin there are hydroxycobalamin (which is even more effective therapeutically than cyanocobalamin) and nitrocobalamin.

Vitamin B$_{12}$ is now produced as a by-product in the manufacture of streptomycin. Microbes are the primary source of vitamin B$_{12}$.

Function. Like folic acid, vitamin B$_{12}$ is a coenzyme involved in the synthesis of nucleoproteins by participating in the metabolism of purines and pyrimidines. Vitamin B$_{12}$ is necessary for the synthesis of thymidylate, the nucleotide of thymine, which is the characteristic base of DNA. In general, vitamin B$_{12}$ affects cells that are dividing rapidly, such as those dealing with the formation of blood, and in its absence there is a block in DNA synthesis that results in megaloblastic hematopoiesis. The macrocytic anemias are due to both reduced rates of blood formation and increased rates of destruction of the cells that are formed.

Vitamin B_{12} plays a biochemical role in the maintenance of myelin (the sheath around nerve fibers).

Vitamin B_{12} Deficiency. Vitamin B_{12} is unique in that it has a highly specialized absorption mechanism. A deficiency of vitamin B_{12} is usually not due to a dietary inadequacy. Rather it is caused by a failure to absorb the vitamin from the intestinal tract as a result of the absence of the intrinsic factor, a glycoprotein secreted by some of the cells of the stomach. This glycoprotein seems to bind vitamin B_{12} during its transit to the small intestine and attaches to a highly specific binding site in the intestinal mucosa. Calcium seems to be required in this process. In the intestinal cell membrane, vitamin B_{12} is released from the intrinsic factor and absorbed into the blood. The failure to produce the intrinsic factor in pernicious anemia arises from an autoimmune reaction that destroys the secreting glands in the stomach. This reaction may be a genetically determined defect.

Other contributing factors that may cause interference with the assimilation of vitamin B_{12} are the severely shrunken gastric mucosa found in elderly persons, tapeworms (from eating raw or insufficiently cooked fish), and such malabsorption disorders as sprue, intestinal inflammation, and strictures.

Resection of the stomach or the ileum (part of the small intestine) can result in a deficiency of this vitamin.

CLINICAL DIAGNOSIS OF DEFICIENCY. Dietary deficiency of vitamin B_{12} is rare, occurring almost exclusively in vegetarians who do not include any foods of animal origin in the diet. Vitamin B_{12} deficiency usually occurs because of a defect in absorption rather than an inadequate dietary intake. Pernicious anemia is a disease in which intrinsic factor is not produced and consequently vitamin B_{12} is not absorbed. Pernicious anemia is the most important condition resulting from vitamin B_{12} deficiency.

A deficiency can be detected by the presence of megaloblasts in bone marrow biopsy specimens. When megaloblasts are present in the bone marrow, the red cells in the peripheral circulation are usually macrocytic.

Histologically, there are nests of megaloblasts. These cells are different from normal erythroblasts in that they are larger, with a delicate, finely reticulated nuclear chromatin and a basophilic cytoplasm. Normoblasts are few, and maturing red cells are absent. The red cells formed by the megaloblasts are characteristically macrocytic.

There are atrophic changes in the alimentary tract, and in the central nervous system, there is myelin degeneration of the spinal cord.

Clinically, pernicious anemia is insidious in onset and characteristically fluctuates, with remissions and relapses. The usual complaints are weakness, numbness, and tingling in the extremities. Patients may have difficulty in walking and in coordination of movements; vibratory sense may be absent. These neurological signs are a major distinguishing characteristic of pernicious anemia. Generally, the patient may have a lemon-yellow complexion as a result of jaundice caused by red cell destruction, early graying of the hair, fast heartbeat, ankle swelling, hyperactive reflexes, and peripheral neuritis. This is called combined system disease (central nervous system damage associated with blood disturbances).

The patient also has a bright red, smooth, sore, and burning tongue resulting from an atrophic glossitis.

DIAGNOSTIC LABORATORY FINDINGS. The major laboratory findings that contribute to a diagnosis of pernicious anemia are (1) low gastric acidity, even after administration of histamine; (2) some megaloblastic red cells; (3) oval-shaped red cells; (4) greatly segmented neutrophils that have six or seven lobes instead of the usual three; (5) mean corpuscular volume (MCV) elevated above 96 μm^3; and (6) a positive Schilling test.

The Schilling radioactive B_{12} absorption and excretion test is conducted as follows:

The principle of the test is that a large injection of B_{12} will saturate all the transcobalamin in the blood at the same time the labeled dose is absorbed so that it will enter the blood stream unbound and will be excreted in the urine.

A measured amount of radioactive vitamin B_{12} is given orally, followed by a 1-mg dose of the nonradioactive vitamin. The percentage of radioactivity is determined in the urine excreted over a 24-hour period. Normal people excrete 10 to 40% of the B_{12} given, whereas patients with pernicious anemia retain most of the vitamin B_{12}, excreting less than 1%. To prove that the absorption failure is due to lack of intrinsic factor, the test is repeated with labeled B_{12} accompanied by normal gastric juice or a concentrate of intrinsic factor, which should restore absorption to normal.

Recommended Dietary Allowance. If absorption is normal, a dietary intake of 0.003 mg (3 μg) of vitamin B_{12} per day is adequate for adolescents and normal adults. A diet containing 0.015 mg/day will replenish body stores, and in the United States the average diet contains this much B_{12}. Actually, the amount of vitamin B_{12} stored in the normal liver is enough to meet the daily requirements for more than 2 years.

The recommended dietary allowance for pregnant and lactating women is 0.004 mg (4 μg) per day.

Food Sources. Vitamin B_{12} is unique among vitamins because it is not found in any plant. It occurs primarily in animal foods, and liver is the richest source. Meat, eggs, milk, cheese, and fish are also good sources of this vitamin.

Therapy. A deficiency caused by inadequate ingestion of the vitamin (i.e., strict vegetarian patients) can be effectively treated by oral ingestion of 0.001 to 0.003 mg (1 to 3 μg) of the vitamin daily.

In malabsorption disorders that manifest as combined system disease, 0.05 to 0.1 mg of vitamin B_{12} may be administered by injection daily for 2 weeks at the outset and twice a week thereafter until the laboratory findings return to normal. Administration of vitamin B_{12} is followed by a marked increase in reticulocytes (red cells at a certain stage of development) that reaches a maximum in 5 to 8 days. Then 0.1 mg is injected once a month for the patient's lifetime.

REFERENCES

1. Hopkins, F. G. Deficiency diseases and discovery of vitamins. Cited in Lowenberg, M. E.; Todhunter, E. N., et al. Food and People, 3rd ed., p. 156. New York, John Wiley & Sons, 1979.
2. Funk, C. Cited in Lowenberg, M. E.; Todhunter, E. N., et al. Food and People, 3rd ed., p. 156. New York, John Wiley & Sons, 1979.
3. Anderson C. E. Vitamins. In Schneider, H. A.; Anderson, C. E.; Coursin, D. B., eds. Nutritional Support of Medical Practice, p. 24. Hagerstown, Md., Harper & Row, 1977.

4. Herbert, V. The vitamin craze. Arch. Intern. Med. 140:173, 1980.
5. DiPalma, J. F.; Ritchie, D. N. Vitamin toxicity. Annu. Rev. Pharmacol. Toxicol. 17:133, 1977.
6. Committee on Safety, Toxicity and Misuse of Vitamins and Trace Minerals. National Nutrition Consortium on Vitamin-Mineral Safety, Toxicity and Misuse. Chicago, American Dietetic Association, 1978.
7. Herbert, V. Megavitamin therapy. N.Y. State J. Med. 79:278, 1975.
8. McCollum, E. V.; Davis, M. J. Cited in Lowenberg, M. E.; Todhunter, E. N., et al. Food and People, 3rd ed., pp. 156–157. New York, John Wiley & Sons, 1979.
9. Robinson, C. H.; Chenoweth, W. L., et al. Normal and Therapeutic Nutrition, 17th ed., pp. 178, 182. New York, Macmillan Publishing Co., 1986.
10. Jansen, B. C. P. Vitamin B_1. Cited in Lowenberg, M. E.; Todhunter, E. N., et al. Food and People, 3rd ed., p. 157. New York, John Wiley & Sons, 1979.
11. Williams, R. R.; Cline, J. K. Thiamin. In Present Knowledge in Nutrition: Nutrition Reviews, 5th ed., p. 273. Washington, D.C., Nutrition Foundation, 1984.
12. Isebacher, K. J.; Adams, R. D.; Braunwald, E., et al. eds. Harrison's Principles of Internal Medicine, 9th ed., pp. 426, 1040. New York, McGraw-Hill Book Co., 1980.
13. Hoyumpa, A. M., Jr. Alcohol and thiamine metabolism. Alcoholism (N.Y.) 7 (Winter) 11, 1983.
14. Committee on Dietary Allowances, Food and Nutrition Board, National Academy of Sciences-National Research Council. Recommended Dietary Allowances, 9th rev. ed., pp. 82–87. Washington, D.C., National Academy Press, 1980.
15. Marston, R. M.; Welsh, S. O. Nutrient content of the U.S. food supply, 1982. Natl. Food Rev. 25:12, 1984.
16. Goldberger, J. Cited in Lowenberg, M. E.; Todhunter, E. N., et al. Food and People, 3rd ed., p. 155. New York, John Wiley & Sons, 1979.
17. Elvehjem, C. A. Nicotinic acid. Cited in Lowenberg, M. E.; Todhunter, E. N., et al. Food and People, 3rd ed., p. 155. New York, John Wiley & Sons, 1979.
18. Carter, E. G. A.; Carpenter, K. J. The bioavailability for humans of bound niacin from wheat brans. Am. J. Clin. Nutr. 36:855, 1982.
19. Sandstead, H. H. Clinical manifestations of certain deficiency diseases. In Goodhart, R. S.; Shills, M. E., eds. Modern Nutrition in Health and Disease, 6th ed., pp. 685–696. Philadelphia, Lea & Febiger, 1980.
20. Rivlin, R. S. Riboflavin. In Present Knowledge in Nutrition: Nutrition Reviews, 5th ed., p. 285. Washington, D.C., Nutrition Foundation, 1984.
21. Goldsmith, G. A. In Rivlin, R. S., ed. Riboflavin, pp. 221–224. New York, Plenum Publishing Corp., 1975.
22. Anderson, C. E. Pantothenic acid. In Schneider, H. A.; Anderson, C. E.; Coursin, D. B., eds. Nutritional Support of Medical Practice, p. 29. Hagerstown, Md., Harper & Row, 1977.
23. Woodward, J. D. Biotin. Sci. Am. 204:139, 1961.
24. Syndenstricker, V. P., et al. Observations of the "egg-white injury" in man and its cure with biotin concentrate. JAMA 118:1199, 1942. Cited in Robinson, C. H.; Lawler, M. R.; Chenoweth, W. L., et al. Normal and Therapeutic Nutrition, 17th ed., p. 191. New York, Macmillan Publishing Co., 1986.
25. McClain, C. J., et al. Biotin deficiency in the adult during home parenteral nutrition. JAMA 247:3116, 1982.
26. Innis, S. M.; Allardyce, D. B. Possible biotin deficiency in adults receiving long term total parenteral nutrition. Am. J. Clin. Nutr. 37:185, 1983.
27. Henderson, L. M. Vitamin B_6. In Present Knowledge in Nutrition: Nutrition Reviews, 5th ed., p. 303. Washington, D.C., Nutrition Foundation, 1984.
28. Anderson, C. E. Pyridoxine (vitamin B_6). In Schneider, H. A.; Anderson, C. E.; Coursin, D. B., eds. Nutritional Support of Medical Practice, p. 35. Hagerstown, Md., Harper & Row, 1977.
29. Gregory, J. F.; Kirk, J. R. The bioavailability of vitamin B_6 in foods. Nutr. Rev. 39:1, 1981.
30. Gershoff, S. Vitamin B_6. In Present Knowledge in Nutrition: Nutrition Reviews, 4th ed., p. 149. Washington, D.C., Nutrition Foundation, 1976.
31. Schaumberg, H.; Kaplan, J., et al. Sensory neuropathy from pyridoxine abuse. A new megavitamin syndrome. N. Engl. J. Med. 309:445, 1983.
32. Dreizen, S. Oral indications of the deficiency states. Postgrad. Med. 49:97, 1971.
33. Nizel, A. E. Oral problems. In Schneider, H. A.; Anderson, C. E.; Coursin, D. B., eds. Nutritional Support of Medical Practice, pp. 432–440. Hagerstown, Md., Harper & Row, 1977.
34. Herbert, V., et al. Folic acid and vitamin B_{12}. In Goodhart, R. S.; Shills, M. E., eds. Modern Nutrition in Health and Disease, 6th ed., pp. 229–259. Philadelphia, Lea & Febiger, 1980.
35. Mitchell, H. K.; Snell, E. E.; Williams, R. J. The concentration of "folic acid." J. Am. Chem. Soc. 63:2284, 1941.
36. Herbert, V. The five possible causes of nutrient deficiency: illustrated by deficiencies of vitamin B_{12} and folic acid. Am. J. Clin. Nutr. 26:77, 1973.
37. Lindenbaum, J., et al. Oral contraceptive hormones, folate metabolism and the cervical epithelium. Am. J. Clin. Nutr. 28:346, 1975.

38. Vogel, R. I., Deasy, M. H. The effect of folic acid on experimentally produced gingivitis. J. Prevent. Dent. 5:30, 1978.
39. Herbert, V. Vitamin B_{12}. In Present Knowledge in Nutrition: Nutrition Reviews, 5th ed., pp. 347–364. Washington, D.C., Nutrition Foundation, 1984.
40. Minot, G. R.; Murphy, W. P. Treatment of pernicious anemia by a special diet. JAMA 87:470, 1926.
41. Castle, W. B. Vitamin B_{12}. Cited in Lowenberg, M. E.; Todhunter, E. N., et al. Food and People, 3rd ed., p. 157. New York, John Wiley & Sons, 1979.
42. Lau, K. S. Cobalamins in man. Pathology 13:189, 1981.
43. Rickes, E. L.; Brink, N. G.; Koniusgy, F. R., et al. Crystalline vitamin B_{12}. Science 107:396, 1948.

8

Vitamin C (Ascorbic Acid)

DISCOVERY

The first accurate and scientific discussion of the cause and cure of scurvy was made in 1753 by a Scottish surgeon, James Lind, in his first edition of "A Treatise on the Scurvy." He described scurvy as the disabling disease that affected the 110 men who sailed from France to Newfoundland in 1536 under the command of the French explorer Jacques Cartier. Cartier overcame this health problem by using a remedy suggested by Indians; this consisted of feeding his men a broth made from boiling the needles from evergreen trees (which have now been shown to contain 50 mg of vitamin C per 100 g).

A few years later Lind wrote a second edition of his treatise in which he described a controlled feeding experiment that he conducted on the ship *Salisbury* on 12 sailors who were sick with scurvy. He described their signs and symptoms as hemorrhagic spots in the skin; anemia; putrid, bleeding gums; general lassitude; and weakness in the knees. He further noted that their diet was limited to watery gruel sweetened with sugar, mutton broth, biscuits with sugar, barley, raisins, and wine. After dividing the 12 men into 6 groups of 2 each, he added to the basic diet of each pair one of the following diet supplements: (1) cider, (2) vinegar, (3) vitriol (sulfuric acid, alcohol, extract of ginger, and cinnamon), (4) sea water, (5) a mixture of garlic, mustard, and herbs, or (6) two oranges and one lemon. The two men who recovered in about 6 days were the ones who ate the oranges and lemon in addition to their regular fare. The pair given the cider supplement also gradually improved, but none of the other four diet supplements was adequate to overcome the scurvy.

A year after Lind's death in 1895, the British Navy recognized his scientific finding and ordered that every sailor be given a daily ration of lemon juice. The feeding of this dietary supplement proved to be the means of preventing scurvy in the British Navy. Since lemons in those days were called limes and were always included in their diet, the British sailors were nicknamed limeys.[1]

The first significant scientific advance in the study of scurvy is attributed to two researchers who in 1907 were able to induce scurvy in guinea pigs. With this experimental model, they were able to study the effects of diet supplements of fresh fruits, vegetables, and their juices when added to a scorbutic (scurvy-producing) diet of grain. Their observations are credited with a breakthrough in the isolation, identification, and eventual synthesis of the antiscorbutic food factor.

In 1932 C. G. King isolated vitamin C from lemons and identified it as the antiscorbutic (scurvy-preventing) vitamin, and at the same time Szent-Gyorgyi was making the same discovery using sweet red peppers.

Because this vitamin was the third to be discovered, it was called vitamin C. It is also called ascorbic acid (a shortened form of antiscorbutic) because it is an acid with antiscorbutic properties.

CHEMISTRY

L-Ascorbic acid can be synthesized by oxidation of glucose and has a chemical configuration similar to it. The difference is that glucose ($C_6H_{12}O_6$) has six carbon atoms firmly joined to each other by single bonds, but ascorbic acid ($C_6H_8O_6$) has six carbon atoms that are joined together by single bonds (except that between the second and third carbons there is a double bond) and four fewer hydrogen atoms. L-Ascorbic acid is readily oxidized to L-dehydroascorbic acid. The latter is only slightly less effective than L-ascorbic acid as an antiscorbutic nutrient. However, if L-dehydroascorbic acid is exposed to light or an alkaline solution, it will lose its potency. Ascorbic acid is water soluble and has strong reducing properties.

Humans, other primates, and the guinea pig, unlike other animal species, cannot synthesize ascorbic acid in their tissues.[2] Therefore, they require a daily dietary source of this vitamin in order not to develop scurvy.

STORAGE

There is no extensive storage of vitamin C, but certain tissues, such as the adrenal cortex, contain relatively large amounts of ascorbic acid. Leukocytes take up the vitamin when tissue demands have been met, and white blood cell levels have been used to evaluate vitamin C status in humans.

FUNCTION[3]

No role in biological oxidation systems in which vitamin C serves as a specific coenzyme has been described. However, vitamin C has a role in the formation of collagen (a protein matrix of connective tissue), particularly in the course of wound healing. It also contributes to the integrity of cells associated with fibroblasts, osteoblasts, and odontoblasts, which are cells that are respectively involved in the development of connective tissue, bones, and teeth.

Vitamin C appears to play a key role in the synthesis of collagen.[4, 5] This vitamin is necessary in the hydroxylation (the addition of OH to other radicals to form hydroxides) of such amino acids as proline and lysine to form hydroxyproline and hydroxylysine, the essential precursors for collagen biosynthesis. Without ascorbic acid for collagen synthesis, connective tissue formation and maintenance would be impaired and so would wound healing and scar tissue formation. Theoretically, in the absence of ascorbic acid, the body could not properly form the collagen fibers that lie between the fibroblasts. The intercellular cement, i.e., collagen, is said to hold the tissue cells together in discrete organized systems.

Because collagen is the matrix (groundwork) in which calcium is deposited to form bones, a deficiency in vitamin C would impair their formation and could even cause bones to fracture easily. Collagen is also necessary for the formation of healthy teeth, skin, and tendons.

Even though all the details about how vitamin C participates in ensuring normal collagen formation are not entirely clear,[6] we do know that without vitamin C, blood vessel walls would be fragile and would allow diffuse tissue bleeding. Clinically, this condition is seen in tender, bleeding gums; easy bruising; and pinpoint hemorrhages of peripheral skin and joints. A possible consequence of capillary fragility and permeability is infection.

Vitamin C enhances iron absorption and plays a number of roles that relate to hematology. It is important in preventing the megaloblastic anemia of infancy and perhaps other types of macrocytic (abnormally large red blood cell) anemia.

Vitamin C is involved in phagocytosis (the engulfing of bacteria) and acts as a detoxifying (reduction of poisons) agent. In adequate amounts, it can increase the resistance of traumatized and injured tissues to infection. Inadequate intake of ascorbic acid increases susceptibility to infection; in turn, infection, burns, and injuries decrease the amount of ascorbic acid in tissues and body fluids, increasing the need for a larger intake of this vitamin.

The participation of vitamin C in the synthesis of hormones by the adrenal glands may account for its high concentration in adrenal tissues. Although it had been thought that vitamin C supplementation might exert an antistress action, this has not been shown to take place in humans.

Vitamin C plays a part in the metabolism of the amino acid tyrosine.

Collagen Biosynthesis[6]

Collagen is the main organic component of the extracellular matrices of many tissues, including dentin, bone, and the gingiva. Collagen has a unique molecular structure. In tissues, collagen molecules are aggregated together to form ropelike fibers that serve to connect the cells and other components to one another.

Collagen, like all proteins, is composed of a polypeptide arrangement of amino acids. It has a unique amino acid composition in which about two-thirds of the amino acid residues are made up of glycine, proline, hydroxyproline, and hydroxylysine. Quantitatively, these four amino acids make up 67% of the collagen molecule. The remaining 33% consists of alanine, valine, aspartic acid, glutamic acid, and arginine plus about eight other amino acids.

The synthesis of collagen starts, like the synthesis of the proteins, by the formation of a polypeptide chain. The polypeptide chain is built from amino acids that are linked together in a very orderly pattern, which provides the essential specificity to the protein molecule.

The collagen-forming cell is the fibroblast, which is the location for the formation of a proline-rich polypeptide chain. After proline and lysine are incorporated into a polypeptide, they are hydroxylated by ascorbic acid into hydroxyproline and hydroxylysine. These two amino acids are uniquely characteristic of collagen and are necessary precursors for the formation of collagen. Thus a polypeptide chain consisting mainly (two-thirds of the protein molecule) of glycine, proline, hydroxyproline, and a small amount of hydroxylysine is formed. These polypeptide chains form a coiled helix. Three of these helices combine to form tropocollagen, which is the basic building block for the formation of collagen. The combination of tropocollagen units in a staggered arrangement forms a collagen fibril. These fibrils are then combined to form the fiber that is the functional unit of collagen. The process of fiber formation is called fibrogenesis.

Under the electron microscope, collagen has a characteristic 640-angstrom (10^{-7} mm) periodicity (recurs at regular intervals) with a number of interband periods.

Mucopolysaccharides, the ground substance, have not been shown to be involved in the formation of the collagen fibril. However, even though they are not active in fibrogenesis, they play an important secondary regulatory role: they help to arrange the collagen fibrils in ordered fashion. This arrangement is important for the structural stability of connective tissue.

Wound Healing

The first biochemical step in the healing of a wound is the accumulation of ground substance or mucopolysaccharides. In normal animals, this accumulation rises rapidly during the first 3 or 4 days and then begins to decline (Fig. 8–1). With the decline of ground substance formation, fiber formation begins. In

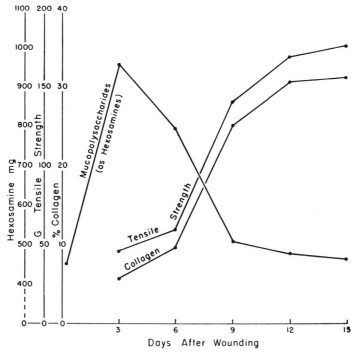

FIGURE 8–1. Normal pattern of wound healing. (Dunphy, J. E.; Udupa, K. N. N. Engl. J. Med. 253:847, 1955.)

contrast to normal wound healing, the animal with scurvy experiences a continued increase in mucopolysaccharide accumulation beyond the fourth day (Fig. 8–2). This ground substance surrounds the fibril and prevents fiber synthesis. However, if vitamin C is added to the diet, the formation of ground substance will decline, and the fibril formation will correspondingly increase.

The amount of hydroxyproline present in the wound parallels the presence of collagen fibrils, which start to appear at day 4 and reach a peak around day 11. This hydroxyproline is part of tropocollagen.

Thus, a scorbutic wound differs from a normal wound in that there is a marked decrease if not a total absence of collagen fibrils, and a large amount of amorphous (shapeless) material within the intercellular space. Histologically, in a scorbutic wound the fine network (known as the endoplasmic reticulum within the cytoplasm of the fibroblast) is altered, and there may be lipid deposits within the fibroblasts.

Scorbutic wounds generally appear to be composed of thick, chaotically arranged precollagenous fibers, which suggests that there is simply an accumulation of mucopolysaccharides around a precollagen core. The accumulation of mucopolysaccharides interferes with subsequent maturation of the collagen.

The maintenance of a wound, or its tensile (capable of being drawn out into threads) strength, is proportional to the collagen content, which, in turn, is related to an adequate plasma ascorbic acid level and the intake of foods rich in this vitamin.

SYSTEMIC SIGNS OF VITAMIN C DEFICIENCY

In Adults. The onset of scurvy in humans is slow. It is rare for frank scurvy to occur, because a diet completely deficient in ascorbic acid is very unusual.

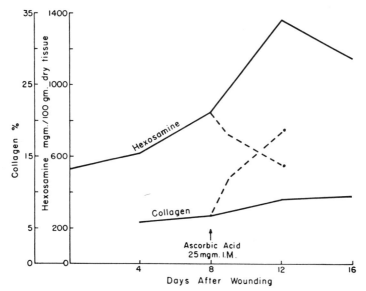

FIGURE 8–2. Wound-healing pattern in scorbutic animals. (Dunphy, J. E.; Udupa, K. N.; Edwards, L. C. Ann. Surg. 144:307, 1956.)

However, less acute signs and symptoms may occur in the malnourished, especially elderly persons whose diets consist mainly of "tea and toast," alcoholics, and food faddists.

Hodges et al.[7] studied the effects of a vitamin C–deficient diet on five male prisoners. They were given a liquid, vitamin C–deficient diet for 84 to 97 days. Decreases in ascorbic acid urinary concentration, plasma concentration, and tissue and leukocyte concentration occurred before the first symptoms of fatigue. Rough skin and pink or hemorrhagic skin follicles appeared on the buttocks, thighs, legs, and arms. The men also had hemorrhages from blood vessels in the eyes. The skin changes were noted as early as day 29 of the vitamin C–deficient diet. Swollen and bleeding gums did not occur until several weeks later, contrary to the common belief that these oral changes are one of the first signs of scurvy. Other signs and symptoms were pains in the joints, changes in the salivary and tear glands, tender mouth, dry and itching skin, and excessive loss of hair. Giving vitamin C overcame all the symptoms after a 3- to 10-week period.

In Infants. Unless the mother's diet is deficient, scurvy rarely develops in breast-fed children. The disorder is most often seen in infants whose diets are not supplemented with fruit juice or a vitamin C preparation and who are fed almost exclusively on heat-treated cow's milk, which is naturally low in ascorbic acid. These infants may also be anemic. In young children, the symptoms of latent scurvy are failure to grow properly, weakness, restlessness, irritability, and swollen joints. There is an aversion to moving the extremities because of pain caused by hemorrhage in the joints. Small hemorrhages and bone changes (beading, or fracture of ribs at the junctions with cartilage, and x-ray "scurvy lines" on tibia or femur) are seen. If the teeth have erupted, the gums are likely to be swollen, tender, and hemorrhagic.[8]

ORAL SIGNS OF VITAMIN C DEFICIENCY

Gingival and Periodontal Tissues

The characteristic oral sign of scurvy is an enlargement of the marginal gingivae that envelopes and almost completely conceals the teeth (Fig. 8–3). The gingivae are bluish red, are soft, and hemorrhage spontaneously or with slight provocation. In areas without teeth there are no mucosal changes. The inflamed gums can become secondarily infected by organisms that will result in an acute necrotizing ulcerative gingivitis (Vincent's infection, which in lay terms is referred to as trench mouth because this was a common problem in soldiers). Clinically one sees characteristic "punched-out," membranous interdental papillae and fetid breath. There is lack of periodontal support, which may make the teeth loose to the point of exfoliation (falling out). On x-ray there is evidence of interruption of the lamina dura, suggesting disturbance of periodontal collagen.

Histologically (i.e., under the microscope), the gingivae show a chronic, inflammatory cellular infiltration, with engorged capillaries and a noteworthy lack of fibroblasts and collagen fibrils. In experimentally vitamin C–deficient animals, there is microscopic evidence of destruction of the periodontal fibers,

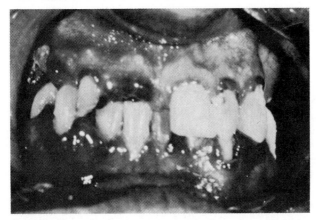

FIGURE 8–3. *Gingival enlargement as a result of ascorbic acid deficiency.*

disturbance in alveolar bone formation, increased osteoclastic resorption, and engorged capillaries.

Gingivitis with hemorrhagic, enlarged bluish-red gingivae is a classic sign of scurvy, but gingivitis is not caused by lack of vitamin C per se. Nor do all vitamin C–deficient individuals necessarily have gingivitis. If gingivitis is present in a vitamin C–deficient individual, it is caused by local irritants plus the conditioning effect of the deficiency upon the gingival response to local irritation.[9]

Several investigators found no correlation between ascorbic acid plasma levels and gingivitis.[10–13] The opposite viewpoint has been expressed by others, who have suggested that gingivitis is a manifestation of a latent or subclinical vitamin C deficiency and can be improved by supplementation with this vitamin.[14–19] This difference of opinion is understandable because of the difficulty of isolating and measuring a single variable in a complex disorder such as periodontal disease with its many causes.

A review of the current information on nutrition and periodontal disease cites research on the role of ascorbic acid in the etiology of gingivitis in humans.[17] In biopsies taken from clinically healthy gingival areas from 11 subjects, the amount of ascorbic acid in the gingival sulcular epithelium, the gingival connective tissue, and the peripheral white blood cells was measured. An inverse correlation was found between the concentration of ascorbic acid in the epithelium of the sulcus and epithelial permeability. But there was no significant correlation between the ascorbic acid levels in the white blood cells and either the gingival concentrations of the vitamin or epithelial permeability.

In another study by Mallek,[18] in which some subjects were given a vitamin C supplement daily and others received a placebo, both groups showed an inverse correlation between tissue levels of ascorbic acid and epithelial permeability. On the other hand, there was no correlation between ascorbic acid levels in white blood cells and permeability or tissue concentration of the vitamin. In the supplemented group, the vitamin C level in the gingival connective tissue increased almost threefold, and the vitamin C level of the sulcular epithelium was almost doubled. Mallek concluded that supplementation of the diet with vitamin C can result in increased collagen synthesis and decreased permeability of sulcular epithelium to bacterial infection.

Teeth

The effects of vitamin C deficiency have been demonstrated histologically on the guinea pig incisor tooth, which grows 2 mm each week. Odontoblasts atrophy, thereby producing a haphazard irregularity in the usual orderly palisade arrangement, which results in an irregular dentin or no dentin at all. The pulp is engorged and dilated from the increased blood. A few of the odontoblasts form some isolated dentin, which becomes entrapped in the pulp. In fact, the rate of dentin formation is so closely related to vitamin C levels in the diet that it could be used as a bioassay criterion (test of potency).

LABORATORY FINDINGS

During depletion, blood and urinary ascorbic acid levels fall more rapidly to zero than does ascorbic acid concentration in blood cells and fixed tissues. The normal plasma ascorbic acid level is approximately 0.6 to 1.5 mg/100 ml; the red cells contain twice this much, and the white cells, 20 to 40 times as much.

Ascorbic acid must be supplied to the body regularly from the diet because very little is stored in the body. The urinary excretion level is an index of vitamin C nutrition, and only when the level of ascorbic acid has declined significantly in the white cells can a diagnosis of scurvy be made. The concentration of ascorbic acid in the white cell–platelet layer of blood decreases to 2 mg/100 g or less when scurvy develops.

An oral-loading ascorbic acid test can be used to confirm the diagnosis of scurvy. The normal serum level of ascorbic acid is 0.8 mg/100 ml. If scurvy is present, an oral test dose of 5 mg of ascorbic acid per kilogram of body weight (250 mg for a 70-kg [154-lb] man) will not give a serum ascorbic acid level of more than 0.25 mg/100 ml. If the test is positive, large doses of ascorbic acid (200 mg or more per day) are given, so that a total dosage of 6 to 7 g is achieved to bring the plasma ascorbic acid to the normal 0.8 mg/100 ml.

A load test that is simple to use in infants is administration of 200 mg ascorbic acid intramuscularly, with serum concentration determined before and 4 hours after the dose. In scurvy, the 4-hour value is usually less than 0.012 mg/100 ml, indicating depleted tissue stores.

RECOMMENDED DIETARY ALLOWANCE

About 15 mg of ascorbic acid a day is a bare minimum to prevent scurvy, but 30 mg/day is desirable to replenish the quantity of ascorbic acid metabolized daily in an adult human. At an intake of 60 mg/day, 80 to 90% of vitamin C is absorbed and will maintain an adequate body pool of 1500 mg, which is the recommended dietary allowance (RDA) for males and females from ages 15 to 60. The RDA calls for 60 mg/day.

Although it is not precisely known, the infant's need for ascorbic acid seems to be met satisfactorily by the amount provided by the breast milk of the adequately fed mother. For children up to 11 years of age, 45 to 50 mg/day is recommended. Pregnant women should receive 80 mg/day, with an increase to 100 mg/day during lactation to ensure that milk contains enough vitamin C for their breast-fed baby. Babies fed commercial formulas receive their necessary 35 mg of vitamin C, because the formulas are fortified with the vitamin. When the baby switches to regular milk, it is necessary to include vitamin C–rich fruits and juices. Youngsters from the age of 1 to 10 need about 45 mg/day, which can be achieved by consuming one orange or its equivalent in other citrus fruits per day.[19]

A variety of factors can influence vitamin C requirements. Cigarette smokers have been shown to require as much as 50% more vitamin C than nonsmokers.[20] Women taking birth control pills and elderly persons may have lower blood levels of ascorbic acid than desirable. Also, it has been shown that work in hot climates may increase vitamin C requirements. Although vitamin C appears to be involved in the synthesis of the stress hormones epinephrine and norepinephrine, there is no evidence that engaging either in physically stressful exercises or psychological stress creates a higher requirement for vitamin C.

FOOD SOURCES

Green peppers, red peppers, parsley, and turnip greens are the best plant sources of ascorbic acid (100 to 350 mg/100 g). Citrus fruits such as oranges, lemons, limes, and grapefruit and leafy vegetables such as broccoli, cabbage, and spinach are also very good sources (25 to 140 mg/100 g). Green peas, green beans, tomatoes, strawberries, cantaloupes, carrots, turnips, and potatoes are fair sources of vitamin C (10 to 25 mg/100 g). Potatoes do not have a high concentration of vitamin C; however, if they are properly prepared and eaten in large quantities, they can contribute significantly toward meeting the recommended allowances of vitamin C.

The loss of ascorbic acid by oxidation in foods is hastened by the action of ascorbic acid oxidase, an enzyme that is present in raw fruits, squash, and other vegetables. This enzyme becomes active when leaves or fruits are damaged by drying, bruising, or cutting. Ascorbic acid may also be lost if vegetables are cooked in more water than is necessary and the water is then thrown away. To preserve the vitamin C content of frozen vegetables, the vegetables should be plunged into already boiling water; baking soda should never be added to the cooking water; and there should be a minimum of chopping and cutting of the vegetables before cooking.

Less well-known, expensive, but good sources of vitamin C are acerola cherries, rose hips, papayas, guavas, and black currants. They are *not* recommended in place of the more common sources mentioned previously.

Cow's milk is relatively low in ascorbic acid, as are eggs and meat (10 mg/100 g). Human milk contains three to four times as much vitamin C as cow's milk unless the mother's diet is deficient for a long period.

The chemical form of vitamin C is exactly the same substance as that extracted from oranges or rose hips, for example. The body cannot distinguish between natural and chemical sources.

TOXICITY

Ordinarily ascorbic acid is not toxic, because in most cases excessive amounts are usually readily excreted by the kidneys. However, ascorbic acid is a strong reducing substance, is an acid, and is biologically very potent. Therefore, it is important to be cautious in its use.

These are some of the undesirable effects that, in theory at least, might occur from megadoses. First, as an acid, large doses could irritate the mucosa of the intestinal tract. The second adverse effect of a large vitamin C intake has been the false-positive results found in oral glucose-tolerance tests; this is a result of the cross-reactivity of urinary ascorbic acid and glucose. Third, high dosage can promote the production of oxalates or kidney stones of urate (salt of uric acid) or cystine (an amino acid) because of acidification of the urine in chronic urinary tract infections. Fourth, the withdrawal effect on blood levels when cutting back after prolonged intake of megadoses is potentially harmful. For example, physicians have warned that a large ascorbic acid intake during pregnancy may create a vitamin C–dependent fetus whose requirements after birth may exceed the normal level.

Blood levels of the ascorbic ion reach a saturation level at an intake of 100 to 150 mg/day, and the intake of even several thousand milligrams a day does not change this level. The average adult can metabolize only about 40 mg/day. However, if a person takes large amounts of vitamin C for a few weeks and then stops the extra intake, the blood levels can drop to well below normal for several days.

THERAPY

In treating infantile scurvy, 50 to 100 mg of ascorbic acid may be added to the milk four times daily. After a week, the amount of ascorbic acid may be reduced to about 30 mg/day.

In treatment of adult scurvy, 250 mg should be administered four times daily for a week, after which the dose may be decreased to 50 to 100 mg four times daily until normal vitamin C plasma levels of 0.6 to 1.5 mg/100 ml are attained.

Patients with wound disruptions who have a concentration of ascorbic acid of less than 8 mg/100 g in the white cell–platelet layer of blood should receive 250 mg of ascorbic acid four times daily until the healing is complete.

In general, when therapeutic doses of vitamin C are taken, they should be accompanied by therapeutic doses of the B complex vitamins; in short, a multivitamin preparation of the water-soluble vitamins is usually the desirable way of raising the serum levels of vitamin C. It prevents a possible B complex inadequacy.

PREVENTIVE USES

It has been suggested by Linus Pauling,[21] the Nobel laureate, that a daily intake of 2 to 10 g of vitamin C will diminish susceptibility to colds and other infections. This amount of vitamin C is 33 to 166 times larger than the allowance recommended by the Food and Nutrition Board of the National Research Council. Pauling has postulated that vitamin C can reduce the incidence of viral colds by enhancing the synthesis of interferon (a protein produced by cells infected by a virus), which spreads to neighboring cells and changes them in such a way as to increase their resistance to infection.

The regimen that Pauling recommends is 1 or 2 g of vitamin C (1000 to 2000 mg) daily. Some persons may require less and others more, up to 5000 mg/ day (5 g/day). Pauling recommends that, at the first sign of cold, one should take one or two 500-mg tablets, and continue the treatment for several hours, taking an additional tablet or two every hour if necessary until a limit of 10 g is reached.

This theory of the effect of high concentration of ascorbic acid on colds has been subject to criticism on several counts.[22] First, there is no scientific evidence that this is fact and not fancy. The basis for Pauling's claims are subjective impressions of a few of his close friends. The present view of nutrition and medical authorities is that there is no evidence that ascorbic acid has any protective effect against or any therapeutic effect on the course of the common cold in healthy people. There is also no evidence for a general antiviral or symptomatic prophylactic effect of ascorbic acid.[23] It is also questionable whether increasing the intake of vitamin C will result in a correspondingly higher blood concentration of ascorbic acid. It appears that the maximum quantity that can be metabolized by an adult is only 40 mg/day. Thus amounts greater than this would be readily excreted in the urine.

Review by the American Medical Association of controlled studies on the usefulness of ascorbic acid in preventing or treating the common cold revealed that there was not enough evidence to support claims of clinically important efficacy.[24] The most compelling evidence was a study suggesting that 1 g of ascorbic acid taken daily may increase the proportions of individuals who remain free of illness (from 18 to 26%) and that 4 g of ascorbic acid taken daily during a cold may reduce the number of days a person is confined to the house by approximately one-half day. These findings could not be confirmed by a second study.[25] Therefore the American Medical Association does not advocate the unrestricted use of vitamin C for the prophylaxis or treatment of common colds.

The Committee on Diet, Nutrition, and Cancer of the National Research Council has provided some interim guidelines on diet and cancer that include the beneficial effects of vitamin C intake on gastric cancer. The evidence was consistent with the hypothesis that vitamin C probably protects against gastric cancer by blocking the reaction of amines with nitrite that forms nitrosamines (carcinogens). It was found in epidemiological surveys that protection against gastric cancer was found in individuals who ate relatively large amounts of fresh fruits and vegetables rich in vitamin C. It appears best to increase the vitamin C intake from food sources rather than from large doses (500 to 1000 mg) of vitamin C tablets, because benefits can be derived from the cellulose roughage and from other vitamins and minerals naturally present in the foods.[26]

REFERENCES

1. Lowenberg, M. E.; Todhunter, E. N., et al. Scurvy. In Food and People, 3rd ed., pp. 151–154. New York, John Wiley & Sons, 1979.
2. Kallner, A. B., et al. On the requirements of ascorbic acid in man: steady-state turnover and body pool in smokers. Am. J. Clin. Nutr. 34:1347, 1981.
3. Sauberlick, H. E. Ascorbic acid. In Present Knowledge in Nutrition: Nutrition Reviews, 5th ed., p. 260. Washington, D. C., Nutrition Foundation, 1984.
4. Gould, B. S. Ascorbic acid (vitamin C) and its role in wound healing and collagen formation. In Nizel, A. E., ed. The Science of Nutrition and Its Application in Clinical Dentistry, 2nd ed., pp. 169–182. Philadelphia, W. B. Saunders Co., 1966.
5. Peterkofsky, B.; Udenfriend, S. Enzymatic hydroxylation of proline in microsomal polypeptide leading to formation of collagen. Proc. Natl. Acad. Sci. USA 53:335, 1965.
6. Setting the record straight on vitamin C. Tufts Univ. Diet Nutr. Lett. 2(11):3, 1985.
7. Hodges, R. E., et al. Clinical manifestations of ascorbic acid deficiency in man. Am. J. Clin. Nutr. 24:432, 1971.
8. Pao, E. M.; Mickle, S. J. Problem nutrients in the United States. Food Technol. 35:58, 1981.
9. Glickman, I. Nutrition in the prevention and treatment of gingival and periodontal disease. J. Dent. Med. 19:179, 1964.
10. Radusch, D. F. Vitamin C therapy in periodontal disease. J. Am. Dent. Assoc. 29:1652, 1942.
11. Restarski, J. S.; Pijoar, M. Gingivitis and vitamin C. J. Am. Dent. Assoc. 31:1323, 1944.
12. Perlitsh, M.; Nielsen, A. G.; Stanmeyer, W. R. Ascorbic acid levels and gingival health in personnel wintering over in Antarctica. J. Dent. Res. 40:789, 1961.
13. Glickman, I.; Dines, M. M. Effect of increased ascorbic acid blood levels on the ascorbic acid level in treated and non-treated gingiva. J. Dent. Res. 42:1152, 1963.
14. Alfano, M. C.; Miller, S. A.; Drummond, J. F. Effects of ascorbic acid deficiency on the permeability and collagen biosynthesis of oral mucosal epithelium. Ann. N.Y. Acad. Sci. 258:253, 1975.
15. Alvares, O.; Siegel, I. Permeability of the gingival sulcular epithelium in the development of scorbutic gingivitis. J. Oral Pathol. 10:40, 1981.
16. Alvares, O.; Altman, L. C., et al. The effect of subclinical ascorbate deficiency on periodontal health in nonhuman primates. J. Periodont. Res. 16:628, 1981.
17. Vogel, R. I.; Alvarez, O. F. Nutrition and periodontal disease. In Pollack, R. L.; Kravitz, E., eds. Nutrition in Oral Health and Disease, pp. 141–142. Philadelphia, Lea & Febiger, 1985.
18. Mallek, H. An investigation of the role of ascorbic acid and iron in the etiology of gingivitis in humans. Ph.D. dissertation. Massachusetts Institute of Technology, 1978.
19. Committee on Dietary Allowances, Food and Nutrition Board, National Academy of Sciences-National Research Council. Recommended Dietary Allowances, 9th rev. ed. Washington, D.C., National Academy Press, 1980.
20. Pelletier, O. Vitamin C and cigarette smokers. Ann. N.Y. Acad. Sci. 258:156, 1975.
21. Pauling, L. Vitamin C and the Common Cold. San Francisco, W.H. Freeman and Co., 1970.
22. That man—Pauling. Nutr. Today 6:16, 1971.
23. Ascorbic acid and the common cold (editorial). Nutr. Rev. 25:228, 1967.
24. Dykes, M. H. M.; Meier, P. Ascorbic acid and the common cold: evaluation of its efficacy and toxicity. JAMA 231:1073, 1975.
25. Irwin, M. I.; Hutchins, B. K. A conspectus of research on vitamin C requirements of man. J. Nutr. 106:823, 1976.
26. Committee on Diet, Nutrition, and Cancer, National Academy of Sciences. Diet, Nutrition, and Cancer, pp. 144–147. Washington, D.C., National Academy Press, 1982.

9

The Fat-Soluble Vitamins: A, D, E, and K

VITAMIN A

Discovery

Night blindness was cured in ancient Greece either by ingesting cooked liver or by applying topically to the eyes the juice squeezed from cooked liver.[1]

The vitamin itself was not discovered until the early part of the twentieth century by experimental observations of serveral different independent researchers. In 1913 two teams of chemists McCollum and Davis and Osborne and Mendel extracted an accessory food factor from butterfat by the use of ether, thus proving that it was fat soluble. These two groups independently noted that the addition of butterfat to the diets of animals ameliorated xerophthalmia (abnormal dryness of cornea and membranes of the eyes). McCollum and Davis called it fat-soluble A.[2] C. E. Bloch, a Danish physician, noted that xerophthalmia in children could be cured by the addition of a milk product to their diet.[3]

Soon after, as a result of animal-feeding experiments, it was found that only certain types of fat had this curative ability. For example, vegetable oil had no effect, but butterfat, cod liver oil, and an ether extract of egg yolk were effective. Thus it was concluded that a specific active principle in these fats, which one researcher called fat-soluble A, was responsible for maintaining healthy eyes. This was the first time a letter was used to designate a specific vitamin. In 1920 the term *fat soluble* was dropped, and the factor was simply called vitamin A.

The relationship of vitamin A to the plant pigment carotene was first demonstrated in 1920 by another team. Not until 1957 was there final proof that carotene is the precursor of vitamin A and is converted in the body to the vitamin.[4]

Vitamin A includes retinol (vitamin A alcohol), retinal (vitamin A aldehyde), and retinoic acid (vitamin A acid).

Chemistry

Vitamin A is a pale yellow, almost colorless compound soluble in fat or fat solvents and insoluble in water. Because of its high degree of unsaturation, the vitamin A content of fats and oils can be destroyed by oxidation as the fats and oils become rancid. Protection by antioxidants such as vitamin E or storage in a cool, dark place will prevent the oxidation and rancidity.

Two general sources of vitamin A in the human diet are (1) preformed vitamin A, found in animal foods such as dairy foods and fish liver oils and (2) the precursor carotene (provitamin A), found in plant foods that have deep yellow or deep green pigment.

The vitamin A found in animal foods has two slightly different forms, vitamin A_1 and vitamin A_2. Vitamin A_1 is found chiefly in the liver and body fat of fish and in other foods of animal origin such as liver, milk, butter, and egg yolk. Vitamin A_2, which is of little importance in human nutrition, is found in fresh-water fish.

The provitamin A carotene, converted in the body to vitamin A, is found in orange-yellow and dark green fruits and vegetables. Three of these are known as alpha-, beta-, and gamma-carotenes, and the fourth is cryptoxanthin, the yellow pigment found in corn. For humans, beta-carotene is the most important because it has the highest vitamin A activity and is the most plentiful. Only after carotenes are absorbed and converted into vitamin A do they exert any vitamin activity.

For all practical purposes, in modern diets the major source of vitamin A is from carotenes found in plants. The deeper the yellow (orange yellow) or the deeper the green of the fruits and vegetables, the more the carotene. The green color of vegetables often masks the orange-yellow color of the carotenes. The green pigment chlorophyll does not have any vitamin A activity.

Absorption, Utilization, and Storage

The presence of fat, bile salts, and pancreatic juices is essential for complete absorption of natural vitamin A. Diseases such as sprue (a chronic disease marked by a sore mouth, a raw-looking tongue, and periodic diarrhea) or celiac (abdominal) disease, which interferes with fat metabolism, may induce a vitamin A deficiency. Other conditioning (systemic influencing) factors such as diarrhea or the excessive intake of mineral oil will also interfere with absorption.

During the conversion of absorbed carotene to retinol about half its biological activity is lost. Because only one-third of the carotene is available, the utilization efficiency of beta-carotene, on a weight basis, is one-sixth of that of vitamin A. Thus, to convert carotene into its vitamin A equivalent one must multiply the milligrams of carotene intake by the factor 0.167.

The liver stores the reserves of vitamin A in sufficient quantities to meet the nutritional needs of the individual for many months. Thus the signs and symptoms of vitamin A deficiency develop very slowly. However, in a patient with cirrhosis of the liver, the stores of this vitamin are markedly reduced.

Functions

Vitamin A has the following functions:

- Formation of visual purple for normal maintenance of the retina
- Control of the differentiation of epithelium in mucus-secreting structures such as the salivary glands, the nose, and the throat
- Promotion of bone remodeling

- Promotion of normal reproduction (in rats)
- Activation of the cell membrane systems such as the endoplasmic reticulum (the more centrally located cytoplasmic network) and the plasma membrane
- Promotion of the health of the oral structures—the teeth, periodontium, and oral mucous membrane

FORMATION OF VISUAL PURPLE

George Wald was awarded the Nobel Prize in medicine in 1967 for his discovery of the biochemical role of vitamin A in the visual system.[5]

The human retina contains rods and cones that are photoreceptor systems. Rods that contain the visual purple pigment rhodopsin are sensitive to light of low intensity. As light strikes the retina, rhodopsin is split into a protein component, opsin, and a prosthetic group, retinal, or vitamin A aldehyde (Fig. 9–1).

Visual purple is bleached to visual yellow during this process. This reaction causes a nervous excitation that is transmitted via the optic nerve so that images are transmitted to the brain. During this process some of the retinal is reduced to retinol. Most of this retinol is oxidized back to retinal. In the dark, this compound combines with opsin to form rhodopsin. But there is always some loss of degradation products that requires new supplies of vitamin A, transported by the blood.

Effects of Vitamin A Deficiency on Vision. In vitamin A deficiency, there may be a long lag in the ability of the visual mechanism to regenerate rhodopsin. This results in faulty adaptation of the eyes to the dark or even in night blindness. For example, when a person enters a dimly lit theater from a brightly lit street, there usually is a short period of adaptation to the dim light, but in vitamin A deficiency there may be a long period, or temporary blindness before adaptation. A similar situation occurs at night when drivers are confronted with the bright headlights of an oncoming car.

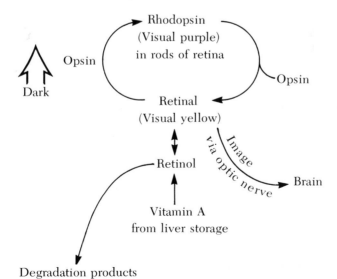

FIGURE 9–1. Function of vitamin A in the visual cycle.

It has been observed that a deficiency of vitamin A may lead to cellular changes similar to those that occur when a normal cell is transformed into a precancerous cell.[6] In fact, the Interim Dietary Guidelines for Prevention of Cancer emphasize the consumption of vegetables, especially the carotene-rich type.[7]

MAINTENANCE OF EPITHELIAL CELLS AND TISSUES

Many studies suggest that vitamin A influences genes because retinol (vitamin A alcohol) and retinoic acid (vitamin A acid) affect the differentiation and proliferation of cells.[8]

A major function of vitamin A is to maintain the health of the epithelial cells of the skin and membranes. These cells line all passages to the exterior of the body and the glands and their ducts. The epithelial cells are a first line of defense against invading bacteria and other microorganisms, but without vitamin A, they will undergo degenerative changes.

If vitamin A is present, certain cells of the epithelium that resemble a cube will form other, mucus-secreting cells. In the absence of vitamin A, the mucus-secreting cells will degenerate and produce keratin instead of mucus. Vitamin A is responsible for the production of glycoprotein, the substance from which mucus is made.

Without vitamin A, the scleral and corneal epithelia of the eye become keratinized; the normal mucosal surfaces of the conjunctiva become dry and granular; and severe secondary infection may occur (pus is exuded and the eye will hemorrhage). When keratin debris accumulates in whitish plaques, it is called Bitot's spots. The keratinization and thickening of the corneal epithelium produce xerophthalmia, which leads to impaired vision. There also may be softening of the cornea, leading to deformation and destruction; this is known as keratomalacia.

In the absence of vitamin A, the normal columnar ciliar (slender hairlike processes) epithelium of the nose, the nasopharynx, and the rest of the respiratory tract is replaced by nonciliated stratified squamous epithelium. This loss of cilia impairs the normal defensive function of the mucosa. The keratin may even act as a foreign body to produce irritation and infection. Because it maintains the defensive cilia, vitamin A was once termed the anti-infective vitamin. In fact, it was wrongly concluded that vitamin A could combat infections in nutritionally healthy individuals.

Follicular hyperkeratosis—a rough sandpaperlike skin and numerous papules caused by plugging of the hair shafts and the sebaceous gland ducts—is a characteristic response to vitamin A deficiency in humans.

PROMOTION OF BONE REMODELING

In young animals, experimentally produced vitamin A deficiency is accompanied by a cessation of bone growth. Bones fail to grow in length, and although there appears to be normal intramembranous bone formation, the remodeling sequences become abnormal and stop. The defect in bone growth is thought to result from a failure in the normal conversion of osteoblasts to osteoclasts, which causes a breakdown of bone during the process of remodeling. The bones of young vitamin A–deficient animals may become thick. Thickening of the skull or the vertebral column may compress nerve tissue, producing a nerve lesion.

An excess of vitamin A causes resorption of cartilage and old bone; in some animals, this may be so extensive that it causes spontaneous fracture.

PROMOTION OF NORMAL REPRODUCTION IN RATS

Vitamin A is essential for normal reproduction. In the absence of vitamin A, failure of spermatogenesis occurs in the male, and fetal resorption occurs in the female.

ACTIVATION OF CELL MEMBRANES

Vitamin A ensures the normal structure and function of biological membranes of cells. In severe vitamin A deficiencies, abnormalities in both RNA metabolism and protein synthesis have been reported.[9]

EFFECTS OF VITAMIN A DEFICIENCY ON ORAL STRUCTURES

In the Periodontium. In experimental animals, vitamin A deficiency produces hyperkeratosis and hyperplasia of gingival tissue. There is a tendency to periodontal pocket formation as a result of proliferation of basal cells of the gingival epithelium and a decreased cellular infiltrate of the lamina propria (the layer of connective tissue underlying the epithelium of a mucous membrane). When trauma or irritation is superimposed on this conditioned deficiency, severe pocket formation will occur as a result of decreased repair activity.

In the Teeth. In rodents a vitamin A deficiency can slow down and even completely stop the growth of the incisor teeth. Accompanying this growth retardation is a disturbance in differentiation and function of ameloblasts; therefore, enamel formation is interfered with. This interference produces hypoplastic (incompletely developed) and chalky white incisors plus a loss of the usual orange pigment. Also, disorders of the labial and lingual odontoblasts occur, producing a thick, regular labial dentin with interglobular spaces and a thin, atubular lingual dentin.

Crowding of the teeth and stunting and thickening of the tooth roots can also be seen in vitamin A–deficient animals.

In humans, the teeth are less sensitive to this deficiency. There is no absolute correlation between vitamin A deficiency and dental caries or enamel hypoplasia in humans, probably because the deficiency has to be very severe, which rarely if ever happens.

In the Salivary Glands. The atrophy of salivary glands resulting from a vitamin A deficiency will reduce salivary flow and consequently increase caries.

In the Oral Mucous Membranes. Because vitamin A deficiency is associated with epithelial metaplasia (a reversible change in which one cell type is replaced by another) and hyperkeratinization, it has been postulated that oral leukoplakia (thickened white patches on mucous membranes) might respond to large doses of vitamin A. This type of therapy has not yet received wide acceptance because its efficacy has not been clearly demonstrated.

Cleft Lip and Palate. During early development, both a deficiency and high doses of vitamin A have been reported to induce cleft lip and palate.[10]

Recommended Dietary Allowances and Food Sources

By definition, one retinol equivalent (RE) is equal to 1 microgram (μg) of retinol, or 6 μg of beta-carotene. One international unit (IU) equals 0.3 μg of retinol or 0.6 μg of beta-carotene.

The recommended allowance for the adult man is 1000 RE or 5000 IU. Because of their usually smaller body size, the allowance for women is 4000 IU, or 800 RE.[11] In 1977–78, the average intake of vitamin A nearly approached or did meet the recommended allowance for all sex and age groups.[12] However, in the 1976–80 Health and Nutrition Examination Survey, 15- to 17-year-old females ingested only about 66% of the recommended allowance for vitamin A.[13]

Food sources of preformed vitamin A (which is available only in animal products) are liver, kidney, cream, butter, and egg yolk.

The major dietary plant sources of active vitamin A are the provitamins in yellow and green vegetables and fruits, e.g., carrots, sweet potatoes, squash, apricots, spinach, collards, broccoli, cabbage, and dark leafy greens. The deeper the green or yellow color, the higher the carotene content will be.

Processing and cooking cause little loss of vitamin A because it is insoluble in water. In fact, mashing, cutting, or pureeing may increase the availability of carotenes in the plant products as a result of rupture of the cell walls.

Therapy

In the treatment of mild vitamin A deficiency (a serum vitamin A level below about 40 μg/ml) oral administration of 30,000 IU of vitamin A daily is recommended. However, this level can be toxic if taken for more than a month. (See Toxicity: Hypervitaminosis, the following section, for more discussion on this topic.)

In advanced cases of epithelial metaplasia seen in adults with xerophthalmia and skin disorders such as keratomalacia, an initial dose of 500,000 IU is suggested during the first few days of therapy. Then the dosage is gradually reduced by about one-half over the next few days and by one-fourth by the middle of the second week. By the third week, the dosage should be reduced to the 30,000 IU level.

Whether oral leukoplakia can be significantly affected by vitamin A supplementation has not been ascertained. On an experimental basis, the dosage regimen described may be a reasonable approach.

A parenteral (by injection) aqueous dispersion of vitamin A can be used initially when combined with a fatty acid such as palmitic acid, which is found in most common fats and oils; then oral administration of cod liver oil (30 ml cod liver oil provides 25,000 IU vitamin A) may be used. Aqueous preparations of vitamin A may also be used. Supportive therapy consisting of a high-protein, high-calorie diet rich in sources of vitamin A and carotene is recommended.

Toxicity: Hypervitaminosis

Because vitamin A is fat soluble, it is capable of being stored in the body; therefore the potential for toxicity exists. In adults, chronic hypervitaminosis A has occurred in individuals given 100,000 to 150,000 IU (20 to 30 times the recommended dietary allowance [RDA]) as a treatment for such dermatological conditions as acne. Others who may show signs and symptoms of vitamin A toxicity are misinformed persons who believe that if some is good, more (megadoses) is better. Anorexia, irritability, loss of weight, tenderness over the long bones, and enlarged spleen and liver are specific findings in these cases. In hypervitaminosis the concentrations of vitamin A in serum are greater than 0.1 mg/ml. Regular ingestion of more than 6700 IU of preformed vitamin A above that already in the diet should be monitored by a physician. The only effective therapy is to stop the administration of vitamin A.

Hypercarotenemia (serum carotene level above 250 μg/ml) will produce yellow-orange discoloration of the skin and oral mucosa but not jaundiced eyes. It may arise from excessive ingestion of carrots in various forms, especially as juices. When carotene ingestion is stopped, the yellow color of the oral mucosa and skin disappears.

VITAMIN D

Discovery

In 1918 Sir Edward Mellanby demonstrated that rickets in puppies was a nutritional deficiency disease that was curable by the administration of cod liver oil.[14] However, the ability of fish liver oils to cure rickets in humans had been known for centuries before. In 1922 researchers found that heated and aerated cod liver oil would not cure xerophthalmia in experimental animals (because the vitamin A in the oil had been destroyed by the heating process). However, it would cure rickets in the animals, a condition that was originally produced when they were fed diets containing abnormal calcium to phosphorus ratios.[15] Because this was the fourth vitamin to be discovered, it was called vitamin D. Two groups of investigators at about the same time independently studied the relationship of ultraviolet light to the formation of vitamin D in animals and foods.[15, 16] During the next several years, the chemistry of vitamin D was elucidated, and more recently there has been an exciting period in vitamin D research in which much new information concerning its intermediary metabolism and mechanism of action has emerged.

Chemistry

There are three types of vitamin D, but only two, vitamin D_2 and vitamin D_3, are of nutritional importance. These compounds are fat soluble and stable to cooking, processing, storage, and acids but sensitive to light.

Vitamin D_2 (ergocalciferol) is derived from the provitamin ergosterol, which is present in plants, especially in fungi and yeasts. It is a synthetic form produced by irradiating ergosterol with ultraviolet light. One milligram of vitamin D_2 is the equivalent of 40,000 IU.

Vitamin D_3 (cholecalciferol), the naturally occurring form of the vitamin in animal tissues, is produced in the skin. Its precursor (intermediate compound) 7-dehydrocholesterol is converted into D_3 when irradiated. In fact, people derive most of their vitamin D from the irradiation activity of sunlight on oils in the skin. Vitamin D_3 occurs naturally but in small amounts in egg yolk, liver, and fish such as herring, sardines, tuna, and salmon. Milk is a poor source of vitamin D unless it is fortified. Vitamin D (400 IU per quart) is added to milk to help meet the RDA for this nutrient.

Vitamins D_2 and D_3 are equally potent as dietary supplements.

Absorption, Transport, and Storage

Vitamin D is absorbed from the intestinal tract in the presence of bile salts and fats and is transported into the lymph circulation via chylomicrons (particles of emulsified fat found in the blood) in much the same way as vitamin A. Again, factors that increase or interfere with fat absorption will influence the rate at which vitamin D is absorbed. Pancreatitis, sprue, and malabsorption disorders can adversely affect vitamin D absorption. In the blood, vitamin D is carried to the liver, where it is converted to calcitrol, the most active form of vitamin D, and stored. It is also found in the skin and brain, with smaller quantities in the lungs, spleen, and bones. Large doses are retained for long periods of time, and if continued, can produce toxic effects.

Metabolism[17]

Research in 1969 by DeLuca showed that vitamin D must be converted to at least two biologically active metabolites before it can induce physiological changes. Vitamin D is initially hydroxylated in the liver and intestine to 25-hydroxyvitamin D_3 (also known as 25-hydroxycholecalciferol [25-OH-D]) and is then carried to the kidney for further hydroxylation to form 1,25-dihydroxyvitamin D_3 (also known as 1,25-dihydroxycholecalciferol or calcitrol [1,25-$(OH)_2$-D_3]). 1,25-$(OH)_2$-D_3 is the most biologically active form of vitamin D. The conversion of 25-OH-D to 1,25-$(OH)_2$-D_3 is regulated by circulating calcium, parathyroid hormone, and calcitonin.

In the small intestine, 1,25-$(OH)_2$-D_3 enters the epithelial cells of the wall and acts on nucleic acid in such a way as to produce a protein that binds calcium and thus promotes the active transport of calcium across the intestinal wall into the circulation. The increased concentration of calcium in the blood promotes bone deposition. Vitamin D thus ensures a sufficient supply of calcium to the bones.

Function

Vitamin D functions both as a vitamin and as a hormone because, in the first instance, it is present in food and, in the second instance, it is formed in the skin and acts on distant target organs, specifically the intestines and bone.

The principal action of vitamin D is to promote intestinal calcium and phosphate absorption. Both calcium and phosphorus are involved in the formation and functioning of the bones, teeth, nerves, and muscles.

Vitamin D, in conjunction with the parathyroid gland, maintains the proper levels of serum calcium and phosphorus, which promotes the calcification of bone (Fig. 9–2). In short, vitamin D is necessary for the formation of normal bone and the calcification or repair of diseased bone.

Vitamin D also stimulates renal tubular transport of calcium and phosphorus according to DeLuca.[18]

Others[19] more recently have further elucidated the functions of vitamin D and have made vitamin D available in a form that aids in the treatment of serious bone disease.

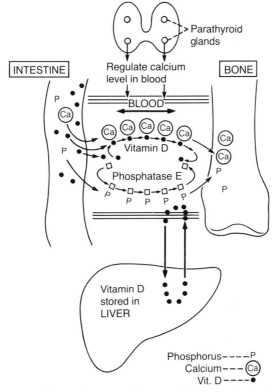

FIGURE 9–2. Diagram indicating how vitamin D may function in the body by increasing the absorption of calcium and phosphorus from the intestine, thus raising their level in the blood and promoting their deposition in bone. Reserves of vitamin D stored in the liver can be drawn on to keep up the level of this vitamin in blood and tissues during periods of low intake or extra need.

Recommended Dietary Allowance and Sources

Because sunlight provides substantial amounts of vitamin D, the dietary requirement has been difficult to assess. However, the Food and Nutrition Board recommends a daily intake of 400 IU (10 μg) from birth through 22 years of age because of the special needs of bone formation and mineralization during this period of active growth and development. Pregnant and lactating women should receive 200 IU (5 μg) more of vitamin D per day than the 300 IU (7.5 μg) recommended for the normal 19- to 22-year-old female. An allowance of 200 IU of vitamin D is recommended for adult men or women in order to maintain body calcium content throughout adult life and possibly reduce the incidence of osteoporosis in women past menopause (see Chap. 19).

Sunlight is the major nonfood source of vitamin D. The amount of vitamin D formed by the action of sunlight on the skin depends on the length and intensity of exposure to the sun and the amount of pigment in the skin. The more heavily pigmented the skin, the less able is the ultraviolet radiation to reach the deep layers of the skin where vitamin D is synthesized.

Vitamin D occurs naturally in such animal foods as fatty fish, eggs, liver, and butter but in small and insignificant amounts. Therefore, we have to rely on either fish liver oil or fortified milk as the major food sources for vitamin D. Milk and cheese products have excellent supplies of calcium and phosphorus in the ideal ratio of about 1.2:1 that vitamin D can help absorb for proper bone development. For this reason, milk and infant formulas have been selected as the only desirable vehicles for vitamin D fortification. Fortifying other foods with vitamin D is not recommended because it may contribute to overconsumption of this nutrient.

Indications for Vitamin D Supplementation

Individuals who may need vitamin D supplements are the elderly who are house-bound and have too little vitamin D in their diets and individuals who are lactose intolerant.

Mother's milk is not a particularly good source of vitamin D. Therefore vitamin D supplements are prescribed by the pediatrician for breast-fed infants.

Examples of Bone Diseases Associated with Vitamin D Deficiencies

RICKETS

Rickets is rare in the United States today because it is the general practice to add 400 IU of vitamin D to each quart of milk.

In rickets there is a lack of orderly change from cartilaginous material to calcified bone during bone development. Thus mineralization of the osteoid (young bone that has not undergone calcification) matrix does not occur. As a result, there is an overgrown and disorganized zone of cartilage, capillaries, and fibroblasts in the wide areas (at the end of long bone shafts) where bone and cartilage join.

Because of the weight of the body and the softness of the osteoid (unmineralized) bone, skeletal deformities occur. For example, there are small, round unossified areas in the membranous bones of the skull that are soft and will yield to finger pressure. The frontal and parietal bones of the skull undergo thinning and form an eminence (projection), giving the head a squared appearance. An overgrowth of cartilage at the rib-cartilage junctions causes beading of the ribs known as rickets rosary. Protrusion of the sternum and depression of the sides of the rib cage produce the condition known as pigeon breast. At the lower margin of the rib cage, the diaphragm causes a sharp depression known as Harrison's groove.

When a child with rickets begins to walk, deformities of the bone shafts of the leg develop, producing knock knees or bow legs because of the weight of the body on the soft leg bones. There also may be a spinal curvature.

A radiograph of the wrist will show characteristic changes at the epiphyses (ends of long bones, which consists of cartilage); the outline of the joint is blurred and hazy and the epiphyseal line becomes broadened. The initial laboratory diagnosis is made on the basis of a higher than normal serum alkaline phosphatase, low inorganic phosphorus level in the blood, and low or normal serum calcium.

In the treatment of rickets, vitamin D is prescribed in therapeutic doses of 1000 to 5000 IU/day, depending on the severity of the disease. Children may be given 1 ml of halibut liver oil, which has 30 to 40 times more vitamin D than cod liver oil. In addition, a food source of calcium such as four glasses (500 ml) of milk is given; if the milk is refused, a supplement of 5 g of calcium lactate should be given. The diet should include eggs and vitamin D–fortified butter or margarine. In addition, an adequate intake of a dietary supplement of iron and ascorbic acid is needed, particularly if food sources rich in these nutrients are refused. Proper hygiene and exposure to sunshine are helpful.

Vitamin D supplements should be gradually reduced to prophylactic doses of 400 IU daily after serum alkaline phosphatase decreases to normal levels.

Prevention of rickets is, of course, the desired goal, and this can be achieved by adequate exposure to sunlight and by ingestion of milk with vitamin D added. A daily maintenance dose of a vitamin preparation containing vitamins A, C, and D is advisable for infants (recommended maintenance level of vitamin D is 400 IU).

Osteomalacia

Osteomalacia, softening of the bone, is the adult counterpart of rickets. It is extremely rare in the United States.

It is most often seen in women who have experienced repeated pregnancies. It also appears to be more prevalent in women who have little exposure to the sun and who eat diets that are low in dairy products. In the United States, it is usually secondary to defective intestinal absorption or to abnormalities of renal function.

In osteomalacia, the bones become soft as a result of a failure of mineralization as they undergo remodeling. Wide zones of demineralized osteoid tissue are found at the junctions of mineralized bone and the layers of osteoblasts.

Clinically, the patient experiences pain in the ribs, spine, pelvis, and legs.

Bone tenderness to pressure is common. There is a tendency of the leg bones to bend, which leads to a waddling gait. Tetany (excessive excitability of nerves and muscles) may develop.

The biochemical test that may point toward a diagnosis of vitamin D deficiency is an elevated serum alkaline phosphatase. X-ray examination of the ribs, scapula, or femur will show translucent bands and rarefaction of bone.

The treatment for osteomalacia is 5000 to 20,000 IU of vitamin D accompanied by 5 g of calcium gluconate or calcium lactate three times a day.[20]

ENAMEL HYPOPLASIA

The first dental change seen when vitamin D deficiency occurs during tooth development and calcification is hypoplasia (incomplete development of the enamel and dentin). As a result of a lack of vitamin D, the enamel calcifies poorly and may in some areas fail to form. In the dentin, spaces that represent uncalcified dentin matrix occur. The appearance of a calciotraumatic line in the dentin is the earliest sign of an acute deficiency of vitamin D.

There have been several attempts to establish a relationship between adequate intake of vitamin D and reduced caries incidence, but this has not been clearly proved. Even though a decreased number of enamel cells occur in isolated areas of the enamel surface from vitamin D deficiency, from a chemical standpoint, the enamel is not weakened or more susceptible to caries. However, the physical roughness of the enamel surface from the characteristic pitting of teeth in rickets might dispose to the entrapment and adherence of dental plaque and sugar and thus initiate the carious process.

VITAMIN E

In the past few years, vitamin E has become one of the most misused, abused, and controversial nutrients because of many erroneous claims for its healing powers in a variety of ailments.

Discovery

In 1922 a research team discovered that female rats aborted and male rats were sterile unless lettuce, wheat germ, and dried alfalfa were added to their diet of casein, cornstarch, lard butter, and yeast.[21] A deficiency of "factor X" caused resorption of the fetus in the female and atrophy of spermatogenic tissue in the male. In 1924 another researcher came to the same conclusion, and because the then four known vitamins were called A, B, C, and D, he suggested that this "fertility vitamin" be called vitamin E.[22] In 1936 the first group isolated an alcohol having vitamin E activity from wheat germ oil and called it alpha-tocopherol from the Greek words meaning *childbirth* and *to carry*, that is, an alcohol that helps the bearing of young.[23]

Vitamin E includes the tocopherols, and also another group of compounds from plants. The most biologically active form is alpha-tocopherol.

Absorption and Metabolism

Vitamin E is absorbed best in the presence of fat. Conditions that interfere with fat absorption, such as biliary tract diseases, pancreatic insufficiency, and excessive mineral oil ingestion, reduce the amount of vitamin E absorbed.

In humans, the intestinal absorption of alpha-tocopherol is between 20 and 30%. The bulk of the vitamin enters unchanged into the lymph system and, attached to lipoproteins, is transported to the blood stream as tocopherol. It is stored largely in adipose tissue, muscle, liver, and, in somewhat smaller amounts, in heart, uterus, testes, and adrenals.

Function

Vitamin E serves as a biological antioxidant to limit free-radical chain reactions and to protect body cells from lipid peroxidation and ultimate destruction. Cellular membranes, which are high in polyunsaturated lipids, are the major sites of damage. The end result of lipid peroxidation of membranes is cell death. Thus the role of vitamin E is to make cell membranes more stable and thus spare the cell wall constituents, including those of red blood cells, from damage. Because vitamin E is an antioxidant, it prevents fats from becoming rancid. The vitamin E requirement is proportional to the amount and the degree of unsaturation of polyunsaturated fatty acids (PUFA) in the diet.[24] The less polyunsaturated fats one eats, the less vitamin E is required.

Vitamin E Deficiency

CLINICAL FINDINGS[25]

Vitamin E deficiency is rare in human beings. If it is present it is due to congenital or malabsorption disease. Some premature infants are born with an inadequate reserve of vitamin E, which is manifest as an anemia. When there is impairment of intestinal absorption of fats, red cells are susceptible to hemolysis (liberation of hemoglobin). Supplements of alpha-tocopherol can prolong the life of the red blood cells. Also, infants and children with cystic fibrosis of the pancreas have low levels of serum tocopherols and increased susceptibility of erythrocytes to hemolysis.

Infants with congenital atresia (closure) of the bile ducts have low concentrations of plasma tocopherol, abnormal erythrocyte hemolysis tests, and creatine in the urine.

Adults with either malabsorption syndromes and steatorrhea (excessive loss of fat in the feces) or xanthomatous (accumulation of lipid) biliary cirrhosis (retention of bile from obstruction of bile ducts) may develop tocopherol deficiency because they cannot absorb fat. This occurs because vitamin E is fat soluble and cannot be absorbed unless accompanied by dietary fat. Vitamin E deficiency may cause impaired neuromuscular function sometimes seen in patients with disorders that interfere with absorption or transport of the vitamin.[26]

In the only long-term study thus far reported, adult men who consumed diets low in vitamin E for 3 years showed no symptoms, even though their plasma tocopherol fell to low levels. A slight decrease in red blood cell stability was apparent, but there was no clinical sign of anemia.[27]

ORAL FINDINGS IN RATS

Vitamin E is essential for maintaining the integrity of the enamel in the rodent incisor. A deficiency of vitamin E will cause disarrangement of ameloblasts, and the rodent incisors become chalky white.

TREATMENT OF DEFICIENCY

In the treatment of vitamin E deficiency (less than 0.5 to 2.02 mg/100 ml of plasma), 30 to 100 mg daily may be prescribed. Benefits claimed for therapy with large doses of vitamin E have not been substantiated.[28] Minor symptoms of nausea and intestinal distress appeared in some human subjects ingesting more than 300 IU per day.[29] For most persons, individual doses below 300 IU are innocuous.

The only medical conditions in which vitamin E has a proven therapeutic role are genetic diseases or congenital defects causing malabsorption and thus vitamin E deficiency.

Recommended Dietary Allowance and Sources

In the ninth edition of the Food and Nutrition Board's "Recommended Dietary Allowances," the RDA values for vitamin E were unchanged from those in the eighth edition.[11] The RDA varies from 3 to 4 alpha-tocopherol equivalents in infants to 10 in men, 8 in women, 10 in pregnant women, and 11 in lactating women. If 1 IU is equal to 1 mg of *dl*-alpha-tocopheryl acetate, a range of 10 to 20 IU of vitamin E activity can be expected in balanced diets supplying 1800 to 3000 kcal, whereas some high-fat diets may contain over 25 IU.

Vitamin E has been isolated from seed oils that are present in large amounts in the germ portion of cereals (e.g., wheat germ oil). It is also found in soybean, safflower, cottonseed, corn, and peanut oils. Plants with dark green leaves, meat, milk, eggs, and fish and fish liver oils are additional sources. In the usual diet in the United States, 64% of the vitamin E is supplied by salad oils, shortening, and margarine. (Some claim that some of the vitamin E is lost during the manufacture of the last two.) A tablespoon of any of the salad oils would provide more than 15 mg of vitamin E. Other good sources of the vitamin are whole-grain breads and cereals, wheat germ, liver, nuts, and butter.

Most American diets easily meet the RDA for the vitamin because it is so widely distributed in foods. Increasing the intake of polyunsaturated fats and oils causes the requirement for vitamin E to increase. But there should be no concern, because these polyunsaturated fats and oils are naturally rich sources of vitamin E. Conversely, the less polyunsaturated fats one eats, the less vitamin E is required. If for some reason an individual consumes an excessive quantity of vegetable oil (more than 20 g/day above that already in the diet) for long periods of time, and abruptly terminates the vegetable oil intake, a deficiency of vitamin E may develop. Alpha-tocopherol is lost from tissues faster than polyunsaturated fatty acids. In such cases, supplemental vitamin E may be advisable.

The vitamin E content of the diet depends primarily on the amount and types of fat consumed (i.e., animal vs. vegetable fat) and the proportions in which they are consumed. As noted above, it has been shown that there is a relationship between the need for alpha-tocopherol and the amount of PUFA in the diet. Since the primary sources of PUFA in the U.S. food supply are soybean, cottonseed, and corn oils (which are rich in alpha- and gamma-tocopherols), increased PUFA intakes are automatically accompanied by intake of vitamin E. Satisfactory diets in the United States have ratios that average 0.4 mg vitamin E/g PUFA.[24]

Myths and Facts About Vitamin E[30]

Vitamin E supplements have been suggested as a cure for sterility and muscular dystrophy in humans. This is untrue. The claim that vitamin E supplements can slow down the aging process is also unfounded. This theory is based on the antioxidant properties of vitamin E, which should protect the lipid cell membrane from harmful oxidation. However, this has not been proved to be a scientific fact.

Vitamin E supplements are sometimes recommended to alleviate angina pectoris and other cardiac problems. Again, there is no scientific proof for this recommendation. The claims that vitamin E prevents cancer and improves athletic ability have not been proved.

Nor are there cosmetic benefits from application of vitamin E to the skin in order to remove wrinkles or heal blemishes. The only value of vitamin E on the skin is from lubrication action of the oily medium.

On the other hand, for some who suffer from a circulatory disease in the legs (intermittent claudication) that causes pain and difficulty in walking, vitamin E supplements may help.

Clearly there is still much controversy about the benefits that can be realized from the intake of vitamin E supplements.

Toxicity

Compared with high dosages of vitamins A and D, vitamin E given in similar amounts is not as toxic. However, vitamin E in large doses may increase the time required for blood coagulation. It is recommended that people given anticoagulants such as Coumadin not take high doses of vitamin E. The most common signs and symptoms of toxicity are headaches, fatigue, weakness, blurred vision, temporary nausea, flatulence, and diarrhea.

Topical application of vitamin E drops to sore breasts of nursing mothers is not advisable because the newborn may be exposed to as much as hundreds of times the recommended amount.

Daily intake of 200 to 600 mg of vitamin E is probably not harmful, but caution is indicated whenever there is consumption of daily doses above 600 mg.

VITAMIN K

Discovery

In 1931 researchers reported experiments in which chickens were protected from bleeding when they were fed fish meal that was not extracted with ether.[31] In 1935 a Danish investigator described a nutritional problem in chickens that was characterized by a type of bleeding that could be cured by a vitamin found in alfalfa and decayed fish meal.[32] Because it was considered essential for coagulation of blood, it was called the koagulation (Danish spelling) vitamin, from which the term *vitamin K* was derived. In 1939 several groups of investigators independently isolated and synthesized vitamin K.[33]

Chemistry

Vitamin K occurs in nature in two forms, K_1 and K_2; the K_1 group occurs in green plants. The K_2 group is produced by bacterial synthesis in the intestine. Vitamins K_1 and K_2 are yellowish oils, unstable in ultraviolet light, and easily destroyed by strong acids and alkalis.

Chemically, vitamin K is a derivative of 2-methyl-1,4-naphthoquinone. Vitamin K_3, a synthetic form of the vitamin, is known as menadione. There are synthetic, water-soluble vitamin K preparations that can be given orally or parenterally.

Absorption

Absorption of vitamin K requires bile and pancreatic juice, as do other fat-soluble vitamins. Vitamin K can also be synthesized by bacteria in the lower intestinal tract. It is estimated that approximately 50% of the daily requirement is derived from plant sources and the rest is from bacterial synthesis.[34] Deposition of absorbed vitamin K is greatest in the liver and spleen and is associated primarily with the mitochondria.

Function

The primary function of vitamin K is to catalyze the synthesis of a blood-clotting factor, prothrombin, by the liver. Vitamin K is also essential for the production of other clotting factors—factors VII (proconvertin), IX (Christmas factor), and X (Stuart factor). In the absence of these factors, a prothrombin deficiency develops, and blood clotting is greatly prolonged. Vitamin K has no therapeutic value for patients with hemophilia.

Prothrombin is formed by carboxylation of a precursor protein as a result of the presence of vitamin K. In the presence of thromboplastin and calcium ions, prothrombin is converted to the enzyme thrombin. This, in turn, catalyzes the conversion of the soluble fibrinogen into the insoluble fibrin, the basis of the clot. Normal human blood when shed will clot in 5 to 8 minutes at 37°C.

Diagrammatically, the fibrin clot is formed in the following manner:

1. Protein precursor $\xrightarrow{\text{vitamin K}}$ prothrombin + thromboplastin $\xrightarrow{\text{calcium}}$ thrombin in the liver.

2. Thrombin + fibrinogen $\longrightarrow$ fibrin clot.

Without vitamin K or in the presence of an antagonist to vitamin K such as coumarins (warfarin, dicumarol) or excessive salicylates (aspirin), prothrombin and other clotting factors cannot be formed, and the blood will not clot.

Deficiency

A dietary deficiency of vitamin K is unlikely because of the intestinal synthesis of the vitamin by microorganisms and because it is quite widely distributed in foods.

A deficiency of vitamin K may occur when there is a conditioning factor such as a biliary disease in which there is a deficient flow of bile into the intestine and inadequate absorption of the fat-soluble vitamin. In severe liver disease, the destruction of liver cells may cause a failure in the synthesis of prothrombin, and bleeding may result.

An intestinal disease associated with malabsorption of fat (such as celiac disease), pancreatic disease, or hypermotility of the intestine in severe ulcerative colitis may cause a vitamin K deficiency. If the normal intestinal bacteria that synthesize vitamin K are destroyed by the use of antibacterial drugs or by a surgical operation such as a cholecystectomy (removal of the gallbladder), a deficiency may result.

The most likely deficiency is the inadequate vitamin reserve of the newborn, which is now routinely prevented by injection of vitamin K. The low levels of vitamin K begin to rise after the infant is 4 to 7 days old, about the time that intestinal bacteria are established in the infant.

Dicumarol, a widely used clinical anticoagulant, appears to counteract the effect of vitamin K, producing lowered levels of the clotting factors. An important therapeutic use of vitamin K is as an antidote to the anticoagulant drug.

Vitamin K and Periodontal Disease

Vitamin K compounds have been found to be required for the growth of *Bacteroides melaninogenicus*, an organism closely associated with periodontal disease.[35] It is speculated that a suitable antimetabolite of vitamin K might interfere with the growth of this organism and, consequently, prevent the occurrence of periodontal disease.

Therapy

It is commonly recommended that infants be given a dose of 1 to 2 mg of vitamin K very shortly after birth to prevent hemorrhagic disease of the newborn.

Vitamin K therapy is indicated for patients suffering from obstructive jaundice or impaired function of the intestinal mucosa. Vitamin K may be administered to patients with a terminal disease or when it is desirable to counter the effects of dicumarol. Patients who have been on prolonged salicylate therapy for rheumatoid arthritis may also require vitamin K, because the breakdown products of the salicylates yield a compound that suppresses the formation of prothrombin in the liver. Persons on prolonged antibiotic therapy or who have poor diets may also suffer from a vitamin K deficiency brought about by a lack of intestinal bacterial synthesis of the vitamin.

The treatment of hypoprothrombinemia (prothrombin deficiency) because of vitamin K deficiency resulting from any of the previously mentioned conditions consists of the administration of 2 to 5 mg daily of a synthetic, water-soluble vitamin K tablet.

Vitamin K has been found to be the most effective preparation for the treatment of prothrombin deficiency resulting from the administration of anticoagulants. Of course, if it is possible, the use of the anticoagulant should be suspended for 1 or 2 days before oral surgery, a time that should be adequate to ensure clotting of a tooth extraction wound, and vitamin K supplements would not be needed.

It must be remembered that vitamin K has been widely abused as a blood coagulating agent. Mechanical pressure and sutures are usually all that are necessary to control blood flow in an ordinary tooth extraction wound.

Recommended Dietary Allowances and Sources

An estimated safe and adequate daily dietary intake for vitamin K has been established to be 70 to 140 µg for adults. The suggested allowances for younger age groups can be found in Appendix 3.

Usually, the bacteria in the intestine and the green leafy vegetables in the diet provide ample amounts of vitamin K. Lettuce, spinach, kale, cauliflower, and cabbage are excellent sources.

Toxicity

Excessive use of menadione in the newborn will produce hemolytic anemia, hyperbilirubinemia (excess bilirubin in the blood), and kernicterus (severe neural symptoms associated with high bilirubin levels).

REFERENCES

1. Wolf, G. Historical note on the mode of administration of vitamin A for the cure of night blindness. Am. J. Clin. Nutr. 31:290, 1978.
2. Lowenberg, M. E.; Todhunter, E. N., et al. Discovery of vitamins. In Food and People, 3rd ed., p. 157. New York, John Wiley & Sons, 1979.
3. Bloch, C. E. Clinical investigation of xerophthalmia and dystrophy in infants and young children. J. Hyg. (Camb.) 19:283, 1931.
4. Moore, T. Vitamin A. Amsterdam, Elsevier Publishing Co., 1957.
5. Wald, G. The biochemistry of vision. Annu. Rev. Biochem. 23:497, 1973.

6. Bollay, W. Vitamin A and retinoids from nutrition to pharmacotherapy in dermatology and oncology. Lancet 1:800, 1983.
7. Committee on Diet, Nutrition, and Cancer, National Academy of Sciences. Diet, Nutrition, and Cancer. Washington, D.C., National Academy Press, 1982.
8. Goodman, D. S. Vitamin A and retinoids in health and disease. N. Engl. J. Med. 310:1023, 1984.
9. Kaufman, D. G., et al. RNA metabolism in tracheal epithelium: alteration in hamsters deficient in vitamin A. Science 177:1105, 1972.
10. Navia, J. M. Research advances and needs in nutrition in oral health and disease. In Pollack, R. L.; Kravitz, E., eds. Nutrition in Oral Health and Disease, p. 451. Philadelphia, Lea & Febiger, 1985.
11. Committee on Dietary Allowances, Food and Nutrition Board, National Academy of Sciences-National Research Council. Recommended Dietary Allowances, 9th rev. ed. Washington, D.C., National Academy Press, 1980.
12. Pao, E. M.; Mickle, S. J. Problem nutrients in the United States. Food Technol. 35:58, 1981.
13. Carrol, M. D., Abraham, S.; Dresser, C. M. Dietary Intake Source Data, United States 1976–80. Vital and Health Statistics Series 2, no. 231. Public Health Series Publication no. 83–1681. Washington, D.C., GPO, March 1983.
14. Mellanby, E. A story of nutritional research. The Abraham Flexner Lectures, Vanderbilt University. Baltimore, Williams & Wilkins Co., 1950.
15. Steenbock, H.; Block, A. Fat-soluble vitamins. XVII. The induction of growth promoting and calcifying properties in a ration by exposure to ultraviolet light. J. Biol. Chem. 61:405, 1924.
16. Hess, A. F., Winstock, M. The antirachitic value of irradiated cholesterol and phytosterol. Further evidence of change in biological activity. J. Biol. Chem. 64:181, 1925.
17. DeLuca, H. F. Recent advances in the metabolism and function of vitamin D. Fed. Proc. 28:1678, 1969.
18. DeLuca, H. F. The vitamin D system in the regulation of calcium and phosphorus metabolism. Nutr. Rev. 37:161, 1979.
19. Henry, H. L.; Norman, A. W. Vitamin D metabolism and biological actions. Annu. Rev. Nutr. 4:493, 1984.
20. Goldsmith, G. C. Curative nutrition: vitamins. In Schneider, H. A.; Anderson, C. E.; Coursin, D. B., eds. Nutritional Support of Medical Practice, p. 119. Hagerstown, Md., Harper & Row, 1977.
21. Evans, H. M.; Bishop, K. S. On the existence of a hitherto unrecognized dietary factor essential for reproduction. Science 56:650, 1922.
22. Sure, B. Dietary requirement for reproduction. II. The existence of a specific vitamin for reproduction. J. Biol. Chem. 58:693, 1924.
23. Evans, H. M., et al. The isolation from wheat germ oil of an alcohol α-tocopherol having the properties of vitamin E. J. Biol. Chem. 113:319, 1936.
24. Bieri, J. G.; Evarts, R. P. Tocopherols and fatty acids in American diets. The recommended allowance for vitamin E. J. Am. Diet Assoc. 62:147, 1973.
25. Binder, H. J.; Spiro, H. M. Tocopherol deficiency in man. Am. J. Clin. Nutr. 20:594, 1967.
26. Muller, D. P. R., et al. Vitamin E and neurological function. Lancet 1:225, 1983.
27. Horwitt, M. K. Vitamin E and lipid metabolism in man. Am. J. Clin. Nutr. 8:451, 1960.
28. Supplementation of Human Diets with Vitamin E. Washington, D.C., National Academy Press, 1973.
29. Bieri, J. G. Vitamin E. In Present Knowledge in Nutrition: Nutrition Reviews, 4th ed., p. 98. Washington, D.C., Nutrition Foundation, 1976.
30. Vitamin E—exploding some myths. Tufts Univ. Diet Nutr. Lett. 3:3, 1985.
31. McFarlane, W. D., et al. The fat soluble vitamin requirement of the chick. 1. The vitamin A and vitamin D content of fish meal and meat meal. Biochem. J. 25:358, 1931.
32. Dam, H. Antihaemorrhagic vitamin of chicks; occurrence and chemical nature. Nature 135:652, 1935.
33. Dam, H. International symposium on recent advances in research on vitamins K and related quinones. Vitamins Hormones 24:295, 1966.
34. Olson, R. E. The function and metabolism of vitamin K. Annu. Rev. Nutr. 4:281, 1984.
35. McDonald, J. B.; Gibbons, R. J. The relationship of indigenous bacteria to periodontal disease. J. Dent. Res. 41:320, 1962.

10

The Macrominerals Calcium, Phosphorus, and Magnesium: Their Role in the Health of the Body and Especially the Oral Cavity

CALCIUM

Distribution

Under normal conditions, there is about 1200 g (about 2.6 lb) of calcium in an adult's body. The bones and teeth contain 99% of the body calcium in the form of hydrated tricalcium phosphate and hydroxyapatite. Young bone contains primarily amorphous (not crystallized) tricalcium phosphate, whereas mature bone contains primarily crystalline apatite. The calcium not in the bones and teeth (1%) is found in the extracellular fluid and the soft tissue, and as part of various membrane structures. The amount of the circulating calcium is independent of the dietary calcium intake. In a normal adult this amount is about 10 to 12 g.

Function

The major function of calcium is to provide rigidity and strength to the bones and teeth. Calcium salts are constantly being deposited and resorbed in dynamic tissues such as bone trabeculae (bony strands forming a meshwork of spaces filled with bone marrow) in the ends of long bones. This calcium is readily mobilized to respond to increasing body demands during the years of active growth as well as during pregnancy and lactation. On the other hand, the rate of turnover of calcium in teeth is slow. The calcium in the enamel and dentin of the teeth is stable. This calcium is not lost from a woman's teeth during pregnancy, which negates the myth that for every baby, the mother loses a tooth.

Calcium is also important in such functions as blood coagulation, muscle contraction, myocardial action, and neuromuscular irritability and is necessary for the integrity of various membranes. The specific functions of the serum calcium might be described as follows:

- Contraction and relaxation of the heart muscle depend on a proper ratio of calcium to sodium, potassium, and magnesium ions.
- Calcium, together with prothrombin and thromboplastin, is required to form the enzyme thrombin, which acts in blood coagulation. The role of calcium in this and other phases of the hemostatic (stopping of blood flow) process is shown in Figure 10–1. However, in practice, poor blood clotting is rarely if ever related to blood calcium levels.
- Low blood calcium (8 mg/100 ml) will increase the irritability of nervous tissue and may cause tetany (sustained muscular contraction) with convulsions.
- Calcium has been shown to activate enzymes such as pancreatic lipase and alkaline phosphatase. Calcium also activates rennin, which causes the curdling of milk during its digestion.
- Calcium is necessary for the release of neurotransmitters (e.g., acetylcholine, serotonin, and norepinephrine), substances from nerve endings that aid in the transmission of nerve impulses.
- Calcium regulates the transport of ions across cell membranes.

Absorption

Calcium is absorbed from the intestine by an active process that requires energy. Vitamin D and a calcium-binding protein play a role in this active absorption.[1] Calcium is also absorbed by passive ionic diffusion in another part of the small intestine. Under normal conditions, from 20 to 30% of the calcium is absorbed and the remainder is excreted in the feces, urine, and perspiration.

A number of factors can influence calcium absorption[2]:

1. Needs of the body: The relative amounts of calcium absorbed and retained depend on metabolic needs (growth, pregnancy, and lactation) and dietary habits. For example, the absorption of calcium is increased in a growing child or in a person who is healing from a bone fracture. On the other hand, an adult who has followed a diet that is deficient in calcium (300 to 400 mg daily vs. the

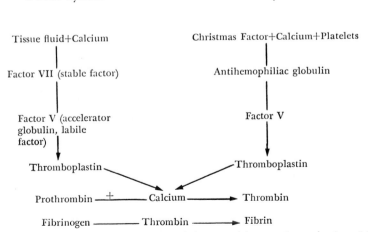

FIGURE 10–1. Diagrammatic representation of the normal hemostatic mechanism. (Modified from Robbins, S. L. Pathologic Basis of Disease, p. 55–105. Philadelphia, W.B. Saunders Co., 1974.)

recommended amount of 800 mg) can adapt to this low level.[3] It appears that as the intake of calcium is lowered, the efficiency and ability of the intestine to absorb and retain calcium are increased.

2. Gastric acidity: Gastric acidity converts the insoluble basic calcium salts into more soluble types and thus facilitates efficient absorption. Therefore it is essential that the gastric hydrochloric acid level be adequate.

3. Hormonal influences: Both the parathyroid and thyroid glands are active in influencing calcium homeostasis (see the section on regulation of calcium balance later in this chapter).

4. Vitamin D: If a person has a deficient vitamin D intake, calcium absorption is reduced and the calcium balance may be negative even when the diet has an adequate calcium level. A vitamin D metabolite (1,25-dihydroxycholecalciferol) is essential for the active transport of calcium across the intestinal mucous membrane into the circulation, thus allowing an orderly deposition of tooth and bone material. When the plasma calcium level goes down, production of the metabolite is stimulated; when the plasma calcium goes up, less metabolite is produced.

5. Calcium to phosphorus ratio: A calcium to phosphorus ratio of 1:1 or 2:1 is desirable. These are the approximate ratios found in cow and human milk, respectively, as well as in bone. Although data show that excessive dietary phosphorus increases bone resorption in animals, in a study with adults having calcium intakes from 200 to 2000 mg/day and phosphorus intakes from 800 to 2000 mg/day, changing the phosphorus intake had little effect on either calcium absorption or calcium balance.[4]

6. Lactose: The disaccharide lactose found in milk can promote calcium absorption. Lactose in the ileum can change the intestinal bacteria, which would help lower the pH and thus enhance calcium absorption.

7. Citric acid: The citric acid found abundantly in oranges, lemons, and limes also provides the low pH that is helpful in increasing calcium absorption.

8. Dietary protein and phosphorus: Some data showed that a threefold increase in protein intake caused the urinary calcium level to more than double, which changed the calcium balance from positive to negative values. The degree to which urinary calcium and calcium balance are affected by a change in protein intake depends on whether dietary phosphorus supplements are taken. Phosphorus supplements increase calcium retention.[5]

9. Oxalic and phytic acids: Increased intake of foods rich in oxalic and phytic acids may interfere with the intestinal absorption of calcium by causing formation of insoluble complexes (calcium salts) within the intestinal lumen. Oxalic acid is found in rhubarb, spinach,[6] chard, and beet greens; phytic acid is found mainly in the outer husks of cereal grain and at high levels in wholemeal flour.[7] In the average diet, the levels of these compounds consumed are not significant, provided the dietary calcium intake is sufficient.

10. Fat: Insoluble calcium salts may also be produced when there is decreased fat, bile, or bile salts caused by intestinal diseases such as sprue and celiac disease in which fat metabolism is abnormal.

11. Emotional reactions: Stress may cause hormonal changes that affect calcium metabolism.

12. Exercise: Weight-bearing exercise helps maintain calcium in bone; conversely, a sedentary lifestyle can lead to bone calcium loss.

Storage

Calcium and phosphates are stored in the trabeculae of the long bones (Fig. 10–2). However, they can be withdrawn from the trabeculae when needed because the body tends to maintain a continuous dynamic equilibrium between minerals that are stored in the bone and those found in the blood. The blood and tissue calcium acts as a pool or reserve. The diet and bone resorption contribute minerals to the pool, and bone and tooth formation in the child and lactation in the nursing mother cause the minerals to be taken from the pool.

The degree of development of the bone trabeculae, where osteoid tissue is formed, and the amount of calcium deposited are directly related to the amount of calcium available from the diet. Blood within the trabeculae transports the calcium and phosphate salts to the tissues and structures that need them.

Excretion

Of a dietary intake of 1000 mg of calcium, 700 to 800 mg is excreted in the feces. Calcium excreted in the stool is mostly unabsorbed calcium from food. When the serum calcium level or the dietary intake is low, absorption of calcium is more efficient and thus less is excreted.

During lactation a mother loses between 150 and 300 mg of calcium daily in her milk. This is replenished by calcium either from food or from bone reserves. Normally the level of calcium in the serum is unaffected by lactation, which indicates that the body through the homeostatic mechanism usually functions well with respect to calcium regulation.

After the bone and soft tissues have taken up all the calcium that they can hold, the excess is excreted in the urine. There is a relatively unimportant daily loss of 15 mg of calcium via perspiration. Calcium can also be lost via bile and digestive secretions into the intestinal tract and then excreted.

Regulation of Calcium Balance

The level of calcium in serum is regulated by parathyroid hormone, calcitonin (a hormone produced by the thyroid), and metabolically active vitamin D.

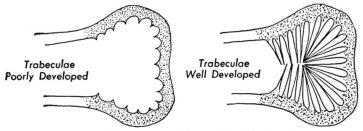

FIGURE 10–2. *Diagrammatic representations of bone trabeculae showing poor or good development according to whether the food calcium intake is low or liberal. (From Sherman, H. C. Chemistry of Food and Nutrition. New York, The Macmillan Co., 1952.)*

The calcium level is maintained at a remarkably constant concentration of 10 mg/100 ml of blood. About 60% of the serum calcium is in ion form and is physiologically active. Of the remaining serum calcium, 35% is bound to protein and 5% is in complexes with citrate, bicarbonate, and phosphate. Bone not only provides physical support to the body but also serves as a reservoir of calcium on which the body can draw in case of need to maintain the homeostasis and the constant serum concentration.

To ensure a favorable environment for bone formation and calcium balance, the proper functioning of three organ systems (bone, kidney, and intestine), at least one hormone (parathyroid hormone), and at least one vitamin (vitamin D) are essential.

ROLE OF BONE, KIDNEY, AND INTESTINE

The equilibrium between serum calcium and bone calcium depends especially on the balance of cellular activity (osteoblast, involved in bone production, vs. osteoclast, involved in bone absorption) within the skeleton. During growth, the addition of mineral to bone exceeds the amounts that are removed.

The kidney can efficiently resorb calcium. If this were not so, humans would have to ingest enormous quantities of calcium. The kidney conserves both calcium and phosphorus and is responsible for regulating the serum calcium and phosphate levels.

Like the kidney, the intestine helps to regulate the serum calcium and phosphate levels. Any gastrointestinal disturbances involving faulty absorption, such as cancer or diarrhea, can result in a negative calcium balance and bone loss. If calcium and phosphate levels in the diet are sufficient, vitamin D is not necessary for calcium absorption, but if they are not, vitamin D helps absorption.[8]

ROLE OF PARATHYROID HORMONE (PTH)

The normal level of serum calcium is maintained by the PTH. When the serum calcium falls below 7 mg/100 ml, the secretion of PTH increases. PTH stimulates the synthesis of an active metabolite of vitamin D (1,25-dihydroxycholecalciferol), which causes an increased absorption of calcium from bone. Conversely, if the serum calcium rises to above 10 mg/100 ml, the parathyroid will be inhibited and release of calcitonin (a hormone produced in the thyroid gland) will increase. Calcitonin can rapidly lower a high serum calcium level. These changes lead to decreased production of 1,25-dihydroxycholecalciferol, causing reduced intestinal absorption and bone resorption of calcium.

ROLE OF VITAMIN D

Vitamin D is necessary for normal intestinal absorption of calcium and helps maintain bone cells, thus regulating serum calcium and serum phosphate levels. Dietary calcium is made soluble and transported to the blood by either an acid mechanism or chelation. Vitamin D may be involved in the acid mechanism.

Recommended Dietary Allowance and Sources

Adults need calcium to maintain their skeletal structure, whereas children and pregnant and lactating women need this mineral both for maintenance and for growth of bones and production of milk.

High intakes of protein can increase the urinary calcium excretion. Therefore, it is necessary to consider the level of protein ingestion when estimating calcium needs.

The recommended dietary allowance of calcium for the average adult in the United States is 800 mg/day. This amount includes the "margin of sufficiency above the average physiological requirement." Based on calcium balance experiments, a mean intake of 500 mg daily for a 70 kg adult is the minimum required to offset the usual 400 mg losses.[9] Postmenopausal women and men more than 60 years of age probably need more than 800 mg/day.

The recommended allowance for infants below the age of 1 is 360 to 540 mg; from 1 to 10, 800 mg; from 11 to 18, 1200 mg (both boys and girls).

During the last few months of pregnancy and during lactation, the mother should ingest 1200 mg of calcium daily for her own maintenance needs plus the bone growth needs of the fetus and infant.

In 1984 the National Institutes of Health Consensus Development Conference on Osteoporosis recommended increasing the calcium intake to 1000 mg/day for premenopausal women and 1500 mg/day for postmenopausal women.[10] This recommendation is based on calcium balance studies. The final recommendation will be made when research is completed showing the amount of calcium needed to prevent fractures.

The majority of the studies support a beneficial effect of increasing calcium by 750 to 1000 mg/day, particularly in women who have been postmenopausal for 5 to 20 years.[11, 12] For early postmenopausal women in whom estrogen production is very low, Riis et al. found that estrogen replacement therapy was more effective in reducing bone loss than taking 2000 mg of calcium each day.[13]

In the United States, milk and milk products provide 85% of the calcium in the diet. Therefore it would be very difficult to meet the recommended levels of intake if these foods are not included in the diet.

Cheddar cheese has the highest level of calcium per 100 g (750 mg), but the usual 1-oz serving contributes only 225 mg, which is less than the 285 mg of calcium in an 8-oz (half-pint) glass of milk. In a normal diet, the best sources of calcium are hard cheeses, milk, and dark green leafy vegetables (the darker the green, the more the calcium) such as dandelion greens, mustard greens, turnip greens, collards, and kale. Although spinach, beet greens, and chard are high in calcium, it is in a relatively insoluble form and therefore not easily used by the body. Good sources of calcium are ice cream (140 mg), blackstrap molasses, broccoli, baked beans, dried legumes, and dried figs. Fair sources of calcium are cottage cheese (52 mg per 2 rounded tablespoons), string beans, parsnips, lima beans, lettuce and other salad greens, eggs, and bread. The following foods will together provide a little more than 800 mg of calcium: orange juice, 8 oz; milk, 8 oz; Cheddar cheese, 1 oz; broccoli, ⅔ c; whole wheat bread, 4 slices; ice cream, ⅙ quart.

Calcium Supplements

Calcium carbonate or oyster shell calcium is frequently recommended for persons who cannot eat dairy products. Calcium carbonate at a dose of 1500 mg provides 600 mg of elemental calcium. A daily supplement of 5 g of calcium lactate or calcium gluconate can also be given if not inadvisable because of lactose intolerance or diabetes, respectively. Children who are allergic to cow's milk will need a substitute such as a soy formula or a calcium lactate or calcium gluconate pill.

When children refuse to drink milk, it should be incorporated either in fluid or powder form in soups, gravies, casseroles, or baked goods.

Toxicity

Certain conditions, such as idiopathic hypercalcemia (excess calcium in the blood) of infancy, hypercalcinuria (excess calcium in the urine), hyperparathyroidism, and sometimes kidney stones, result in high levels of calcium in the serum and urine or calcification of soft tissues. The milk-alkali syndrome, caused by prolonged and excessive intake of milk and antacid tablets, produces hypercalcemia.

PHOSPHORUS

Phosphorus is one of the most essential elements of the body. It is available in all foods of plant and animal origin.

Distribution

Phosphorus is the second most abundant mineral in the body, after calcium. Of the more than 600 g of phosphorus in the normal human body, 80 to 90% is combined with calcium to form bones and teeth. In bones the proportion of calcium to phosphorus is about 2 to 1. Smaller amounts of phosphorus are found in red blood cells and plasma. The plasma inorganic phosphorus level in adults is 3 to 4 mg/100 ml. Soft tissues contain higher amounts of organically combined phosphorus than of calcium.

Absorption and Metabolism

In older children and older adults, the dietary phosphorus intake is on the order of 1.5 g/day compared with an average calcium intake of 0.7 g/day, resulting in a calcium to phosphorus ratio of 1:2. Between 50 and 70% of the phosphorus intake is absorbed. The same factors that influence calcium absorption also influence phosphorus absorption. Insoluble complexes with magnesium and iron will make phosphorus unavailable for absorption. Like calcium, the phosphorus balance is regulated by the metabolic and hormonal factors vitamin

D, calcitonin, and parathyroid hormone. Also like calcium, phosphorus in fluids and cells is in dynamic equilibrium and is constantly being released from and returned to bone.

The amount of phosphorus in the body is controlled by excretion in the urine rather than by absorption.

Function

Phosphorus has several functions, but the two major ones are formation of bone and tooth mineral and the production and transfer of high-energy phosphates. In addition, it plays a role in the absorption and transport of nutrients, is a component of essential metabolites (any substance produced by physical and chemical changes within the organism), and regulates the acid-base balance.

The attachment of phosphate to the matrix of bone and teeth is one of the initial steps in their mineralization. Failure of bone calcification results from a lack of phosphorus as often as from a lack of calcium. An increase in serum alkaline phosphatase is associated with poor bone calcification, as seen in rickets (vitamin D deficiency disease resulting in bone deformities, especially in children) and osteomalacia (softening of the bone in adults).

The release of energy as a result of the metabolism of carbohydrates, fats, and protein is accomplished by phosphates such as adenosine triphosphate (ATP). To provide energy needed by the body, ATP is split, by addition of water, into ADP (adenosine diphosphate) and phosphate. The energy so released is used to drive many energy-consuming metabolic reactions. For example, before glucose can be metabolized, it must be phosphorylated (a phosphate grouping is introduced into an organic compound) to glucose-6-phosphate. Therefore, phosphates have an important function for the absorption and transport of a nutrient.

Several of the B vitamins are active only in the phosphorylated form. Phospholipids are present in cell membranes. Phosphate plays an important role in cell protein synthesis. It is a part of the nucleic acids DNA and RNA, the substances that control heredity.

Phosphates are also buffers (chemicals that prevent change in the concentration of other chemicals) in blood and tissue and are thus important in the regulation of acid-base balance.

Recommended Dietary Allowances and Sources

Intakes of 800 to 1200 mg of phosphorus daily are recommended. As a rule, the diet is more than adequate in phosphorus, particularly when the calcium and protein needs are met.

Animal foods (meat, fish, poultry, eggs, and milk) rich in protein are also rich in phosphorus. Nuts, legumes, and whole-grain cereals are also good sources of phosphorus.

Excess dietary phosphorus in animals will increase bone loss and bone porosity, significantly decrease bone mineral, and cause calcification of the kidney, tendons, heart, and thoracic aorta. However, there are conflicting opinions as to whether reasonably high intakes of phosphorus are detrimental to health in humans. Spencer et al. found that absorption of calcium was unaffected by increasing phosphorus intake from 800 to 2000 mg/day at calcium intakes ranging from 200 to 2700 mg/day.[1, 14] High phosphorus intakes did not seem to affect calcium absorption when dietary calcium was in the low to normal range. Hegsted et al. showed that increasing the phosphorus intake from 1 to 2.5 g and maintaining a 0.5-g calcium intake resulted in a substantial increase in calcium retention and no change in apparent absorption of calcium when a high-protein diet was consumed.[15] The phosphorus supplement had no effect on calcium retention when a low-protein diet was fed. It appears that the statement that the dietary calcium to phosphorus ratio must be 1:1 has not been proved scientifically.

BONE AND TOOTH GROWTH AND MINERALIZATION

Chemistry and Biochemistry of Bone

The average adult human skeleton contains about 1200 g of calcium and 1500 g of phosphate plus a mixture of other minerals, such as magnesium, sodium, fluoride, and other trace minerals, as well as carbonate and citrate compounds. These minerals are present as tiny crystals in and around the collagen fibers. Because most of the crystals are extracellular, they are in contact with body fluids, thereby allowing an equilibrium between the calcium and phosphorus in the blood and bone (Fig. 10–3). Parathyroid hormone (PTH) and vitamin D help regulate this equilibrium. In general, however, most of the crystals in the mass of the skeleton are stable.

The chemical nature of bone on a weight basis is 60% inorganic material, 25% collagen, traces of mucopolysaccharides and other proteins, and 15% water (in the free form, not attached to colloids). About 5% of the total volume of bone consists of cells.

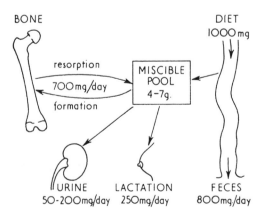

FIGURE 10–3. Calcium exchanges in the body.

Mechanism of Bone and Tooth Mineralization

There are two phases in the growth of bone: (1) the formation of calcifiable protein matrix, or collagen (produced by osteoblasts) and (2) calcification, which begins as calcium phosphate is precipitated from serum.

The initial precipitate has an amorphous (shapeless) appearance. The amorphous calcium phosphate is deposited within spaces or compartments in the collagen fibrils, a process known as seeding or nucleation. The amorphous mass is converted into hydroxyapatite (the main inorganic constituent of bone and teeth) and a fat-soluble substance, which acts to determine the growth of embryonic parts. The apatite grows in ribbons within the fibrils to form crystallites. The crystallites grow and form crystals. As the bone matures, the crystals displace the water between them (Fig. 10–4). The close relationship between the apatite crystal and the protein matrix or template at the ultrastructural level suggests that the initial event is the nucleation of the organic matrix with organic crystals. The highly ordered arrangement of the crystals in calcified vertebrate tissues strongly suggests that calcification is not a random event. The deposition, orientation, size, and shape of the crystals are controlled by several factors. The most important ones are:

1. The organic matrix
2. The degree of phosphorylation
3. The amount of ground substance

The mineralization of cementum is probably similar to that of bone. The theories for cartilage and bone calcification seem to apply equally well to dentin mineralization.

However, the calcification pattern of enamel is quite different from that of bone, cementum, and dentin. Mineralization and matrix formation occur simultaneously from the beginning of enamel development and as maturation proceeds.[16] The mineral content increases to a value of 95 to 97%, whereas the organic matrix falls to a mere trace (0.2 to 0.8%). The apatite crystals of enamel may be 200 times larger in volume than those of bone or dentin (Fig. 10–5).

In developing enamel, the major protein fraction (90%) is an aggregate of 25 small proteins, several of these being phosphoproteins. Papas et al. have isolated enamel phosphoproteins from embryonic bovine teeth.[17] These are characterized by a high content of O-phosphoserine, glutamic acid, and glycine, and their high affinity for calcium. Once the enamel is completely mineralized only small phosphopeptides (a compound of phosphorus with two or more amino acids) remain. The rest of the protein is removed.

The calcification mechanism of enamel is not as clear as that of bone, dentin, and cementum. According to Irving, the most feasible theory involves an initial

1. Osteoblasts $\rightarrow$ Ca + PO$_4$ $\rightarrow$ Amorphous mass
2. Ca + PO$_4$ + $\dfrac{\text{Amino acid}}{\text{side chains}}$ $\xrightarrow{\text{Nucleate}}$
   Ca$_{10}$ (PO$_4$)$_6$ (OH)$_2$ (Apatite)
3. Ca$_{10}$ (PO$_4$)$_6$ (OH$_2$) grows in ribbons within the fibril $\rightarrow$ Crystallites
4. Crystallites $\xrightarrow{\text{Coalesce}}$ Crystals
5. As crystal grows, it displaces the fluid

FIGURE 10–4. *Steps in mineralization of bone.*

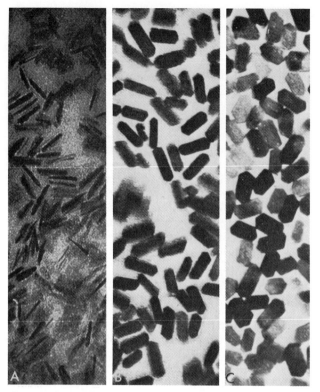

FIGURE 10–5. *Electron micrograph of three phases of enamel mineralization and maturation.* A, *Initial amorphous calcification period.* B, *Crystallite formation period.* C, *Mature crystal formation period.*

apatite nucleation on outer layer dentin crystals, followed by growth across the tissue.[18]

Collagen from hard and soft tissues has been shown to have a similar molecular structure and composition, but the organization of the fibers and physical properties are different in the two tissue types. Cross-links keep the fibers in a special three-dimensional organization, which allows crystals to form in the "hole" region.[19] When the collagen molecules are assembled in fibrils, these holes become the channels that direct the formation and growth of the mineral crystallites without disruption or distortion.

A mechanism by which cellular control could be exerted over calcification is the phosphorylation (introduction of a phosphate grouping) of specific serine (an amino acid) residues, which then would provide specifically oriented phosphate groups with which calcium ions would combine to form hydroxyapatite. Thus the cell could control not only where calcification occurred, but also the degree of calcification.[20]

There has been increasing evidence that phosphorus might link the matrix to the mineral phase. *O*-Phosphoserine (the amino acid serine combined with phosphorus) has been identified in bone, ectopic (situated other than in the normal place) calcification, dentin, and enamel. Bound phosphate in the body would react with other ions, whereas calcium would be unreactive and unable to participate in nucleation.

Osteoporosis

Osteoporosis (reduction of the quantity of bone) is the bone disease most often encountered in clinical practice and must be differentiated from osteomalacia (softening of the bone seen chiefly in adults) (Table 10–1). It is characterized by decreased bone mass per unit volume. Both diseases may be present simultaneously. Forty percent of the males and 30% of the females with hip fractures have concomitant osteomalacia as seen by bone biopsy. Osteoporosis, an atrophy of bone, is a condition in which the rate of bone resorption is greater than the rate of bone formation, resulting in decreased bone density and a reduction in the total bone mass. The quantity of bone is diminished but its composition (i.e., the ratio of mineral to organic elements) is normal. The microscopic appearance of osteoporotic bone is normal compared with that of bone in osteomalacia, where there is a failure of the matrix to mineralize and there are abnormally large amounts of osteoid (young bone that has not undergone calcification) tissue.

It is estimated that 15 to 20 million persons in the United States suffer from osteoporosis. This translates to a cost of more than 4 billion dollars annually. The rate of hip fracture increases exponentially after age 65. Thus 20% of those over age 85 will sustain at least one hip fracture, with 20 to 40% dying within a year and 75% having significant loss of function at 6 months after injury.[11]

Generalized osteoporosis is a systemic chronic bone disease that is believed to be caused by deficiencies of calcium and/or hormones (estrogens). There is some evidence that a high protein intake is associated with low calcium intake and may play a role in the pathogenesis (development) of osteoporosis. Calcium losses can be large when protein intake is high. Etiologic factors include the

TABLE 10–1. Contrast Between Osteomalacia and Osteoporosis

Osteomalacia *Abnormal Bone Calcifications*	Osteoporosis *Abnormal Organic Matrix Formation*

Due to:
Deficiency of vitamin D, Ca, and PO_4
  in adults
	Decline in anabolic hormones
	  (estrogens and pituitary)

Results in: Excessive uncalcified osteoid	Decreased ossification (bone forming activity)
Abnormal bone mineral composition	Mineral composition of bone remains normal
Clinical Manifestations: General weakness Aching	Hip and back pain (lumbago) Stooped posture Decreased height Tendency to bone fracture
Laboratory findings: Low serum Ca, PO_4 Elevated alkaline phosphatase	Normal Ca, PO_4, and alkaline phosphatase
Treatment: Dietary calcium and vitamin D	Estrogens, protein, calcium, vitamin D, and fluoride

following: (1) age; (2) endocrine abnormalities such as hypogonadism, hyperthyroidism, hyperparathyroidism, adrenal-cortical hormone excess, diabetes mellitus; (3) hereditary diseases; (4) poor nutrition: inadequate intake of foods rich in calcium; (5) use of drugs such as heparin, chemotherapeutic agents, and alcohol; (6) hematologic disorders; (7) miscellaneous: rheumatoid arthritis.

Specific factors that indicate a greater risk for osteoporosis are:

1. Heredity
2. Low bone density at skeletal maturity
3. Sedentary (lack of exercise) lifestyle
4. Smoking
5. Alcohol
6. Coffee (5 or more cups daily)
7. Low calcium intake, high fiber intake
8. Certain levels of hormones, PTH, 1,25-dihydroxycholecalciferol, calcitonin, insulin-like growth factor, estrogen, androgens, insulin, adrenal-cortical steroids, growth hormone, thyroid hormones, protein, and other factors affecting bone growth
9. Drugs, e.g., phenytoin (a type of anticonvulsant) and phenobarbital

Localized osteoporosis, it should be pointed out, is usually due to disuse or immobilization. Essentially, in both sytemic and localized osteoporosis, osteoblasts do not produce new bone and osteoclasts continue to remove bone, the result being bone atrophy.

CLINICAL DIAGNOSIS

Generalized osteoporosis occurs most commonly in older people, especially in women over age 60. They suffer a greater rate of normal bone loss, which can be as much as 35%, in contrast to the normal rate during aging of 15%. The osteoporotic individual tends to have a lower intake and a higher urinary excretion of calcium than normal persons. The clinical signs and symptoms of this disease are a loss of height because of shortening of the trunk and a collapse of the vertebrae. This is followed by a deformed rib cage. The patient may complain of bone pain, which may be due to fractures of the brittle bones and/or low back pain (lumbago). In osteoporosis the pain is intermittent, whereas in osteomalacia it is continuous.

X-rays show a loss of bone density, thinning of the bone cortex, and reduction in number and size of bone trabeculae in the spine and pelvic bones. There is greater loss of trabecular bone than cortical bone. Thirty to forty percent of the bone mineral has to be lost before the diagnosis of osteopenia (reduced bone mass) can be made. Measurement of bones in the hand is useful for comparing groups and for determining the quantity of loss over a long time.[21] Various improvements have been made in measurement techniques. Single-photon absorptiometry, which measures bone density in the forearm, has a 2 to 5% reproducibility. Dual-photon absorptiometry measures total-body calcium and bone mineral content of various regions of the body.[22] Also, computed axial tomography has been adapted to measure the mineral content in the skeleton.[23] Definitive measurements are made by bone biopsy, but even bone samples can vary.[24]

Riis et al.[13] found that 2000-mg daily calcium supplementation for 2 years had a slight effect on the loss of cortical outer layer bone, but no effect on trabecular supporting bone loss (Fig. 10–6). Calcium supplementation did not affect the rate of bone formation but estrogen did. Thus calcium supplementation alone cannot prevent postmenopausal osteoporosis.

Plasma calcium, phosphorus, and alkaline phosphatase levels are normal in osteoporosis.

THERAPY

The treatment prescribed for the generalized type of osteoporosis includes the ingestion of high-calcium diets, estrogen, fluoride, calcitonin, PTH, and the active form of vitamin D.

Estrogen and Diet. Long-term use of estrogen substantially reduces vertebral, hip, and forearm fractures but also increases the incidence of cancer of the endometrium and probably gallbladder disease. The estrogen-progesterone combination is believed to reduce this risk. Estrogen therapy is indicated in women who are thin, fair, have a family history of osteoporosis, and have early menopause. For men, methyltestosterone at a dose of 25 to 50 mg/day sublingually is prescribed. A high-calcium diet (at least a pint or more of milk) supplemented with 1 g of calcium lactate plus vitamin D is desirable.

Fluoride. Large doses (62 to 88 mg of sodium fluoride per day) of fluoride can stimulate bone formation, but side effects are common with this treatment. If a calcium supplement is not given, bone characteristic of osteomalacia is made. Even with a calcium supplement, the bone formed is abnormal chemically and crystallographically.[25]

Calcitonin. Serum calcitonin levels are normally lower in females than males, but not in osteoporosis. Calcitonin treatment can increase bone mass somewhat. A 1.5% increase has been observed in 12 to 18 months. However, the cost for this minimally effective treatment is $2,000 per year.[26]

PTH. PTH may be high, normal, or low in osteoporosis. PTH increases with age, together with calcium malabsorption, have been found to increase bone mass. Slovik et al.[27] administered a synthetic PTH fragment plus 1,25-dihydroxycholecalciferol and showed a progressive and significant increase in

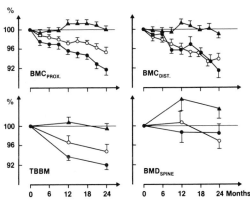

FIGURE 10–6. Bone-mass measurements in the groups treated with percutaneous estrogens (▲), calcium (○), and placebo (●). BMC$_{prox}$ and BMC$_{dist}$ denote bone mineral content in the proximal and distal forearm; TBBM, total-body bone mineral; and BMD$_{spine}$, bone mineral density in the lumbar spine. (Reprinted by permission of The New England Journal of Medicine 316; 173, 1987.)

lumbar vertebral density in the experimental group compared with the untreated control group. Large-scale studies are under way.

Localized Osteoporosis. Localized osteoporosis caused by immobility alone can be ameliorated by exercise as soon as is recommended by the physician. Extra calcium in the diet or calcium supplementation will not influence this localized problem.

PERIODONTAL DISEASE CAUSED BY DIETARY CALCIUM DEFICIENCY OR DIETARY PHOSPHORUS EXCESS

Alveolar Bone Loss

Henrikson suggested that the high incidence of periodontal disease in India might be attributed in part to a low dietary calcium intake.[28] During experiments with beagle dogs, he noted accelerated bone resorption as part of a generalized osteopenia (bone loss) related to dietary calcium deficiency and/or dietary phosphorus excess. The alveolar bone was the most susceptible to resorption, followed by the vertebrae, ribs, and finally the long bones. In a subsequent study by Krook et al., dogs that had been made osteoporotic with a low-calcium diet were placed on a diet with a tenfold increase in dietary calcium.[29] Complete remineralization occurred in all affected bones, to the greatest degree in the alveolar bone where initially there had been the greatest degree of demineralization. Lutwak et al. reported that demineralization of the alveolar bone in humans was reversed by daily dietary calcium supplements given for a year.[30] These researchers suggested that periodontal bone loss was a direct result of a calcium-deficient diet leading to secondary hyperparathyroidism and that reversal of this condition by dietary calcium supplements was due to calcitonin production.

Others have also suggested that periodontal disease is the result of alveolar bone loss caused by a nutritional deficiency of calcium or a low-calcium, high-phosphorus diet.[31-33] However, another study was unable to support this correlation.[34] It appears that the relationship between dietary calcium and periodontal health or disease has yet to be proved.[35]

One of the major problems and crucial factors in this research is that diagnoses of periodontal disease may have been questionable. Lutwak et al. did not report that they saw any decrease in the height of the alveolar crest, nor did they report apical migration of crevicular epithelium. These are the two major signs of periodontal disease. Calcium deficiency may not have been the primary cause for periodontal bone loss, because in humans and the beagle dog one can inhibit alveolar bone loss through plaque control and local treatment without any alteration of calcium in the diet. However, it is conceivable, as suggested by Glickman, that a negative bone factor such as lower dietary calcium can be a secondary conditioning factor that stimulates the periodontal disease process when excessive plaque accumulation serves as the primary cause of the periodontitis.[36]

Svanberg et al. attempted to determine whether calcium deficiency makes plaque-associated periodontal bone loss more severe in beagle dogs.[37] No difference in bone loss was observed in normal and calcium-deficient animals after 18 months.

It is clear that this postulate of a relationship between calcium deficiency and periodontal disease remains unproved.

Calcium Nutrition and Residual Alveolar Ridge Resorption

A significant amount of resorption of the alveolar ridge usually takes place after the teeth are removed. This bone shrinkage can limit the serviceability of a full denture prosthesis.

Two studies reported that the shrinkage of the edentulous alveolar ridge could be slowed.[38, 39] The latter study found that the patients who had taken a daily supplement of 750 mg of calcium and 375 IU of vitamin D experienced 36% less alveolar bone loss than those given a placebo.

PHOSPHATES AND DENTAL CARIES

In 1931 Lennox noted that the teeth of the white South Africans were extensively decayed, which, he theorized, was due to the fact that they ate foods that were grown in phosphorus-deficient soils.[40] In 1937 Osborn and Noriskin found that the African Bantus who ate unprocessed natural foods had a low incidence of caries because they did not eat such refined foods as white bread or white sugar.[41] Instead they ate bread made of an unrefined flour rich in phytates and organic phosphate.

Effect of Phosphates on Experimental Caries

In 1964 Nizel and Harris reviewed the available literature on the effect of phosphates on experimental caries in 99 different animal-feeding trials.[42] In 87 of the 99 experiments, there were decreases in caries ranging from 10% to as much as 100%. More than half of these feeding trials showed a significant caries reduction of more than 50%. Experiments comparing the cariostatic effects of phosphates and fluorides showed them to be almost equal.[43]

The different cations combined with orthophosphate were ranked from the most cariostatic to the least as follows: sodium, potassium, and calcium.[44] Ranking for the different phosphate anions combined with similar cations, from the most cariostatic to the least, was: trimeta, hexameta, tripoly, ortho, and pyro (Fig. 10–7). The conclusion drawn from these and other trials was that sodium trimetaphosphate, which reduced caries by 80 to 90%, was the most effective cariostatic inorganic phosphate.

The newly erupted period of tooth maturation seems to be the stage at which phosphates exert their major cariostatic effects. This can be interpreted to mean that the major route of anticaries action by phosphates is local topical rather than systemic.

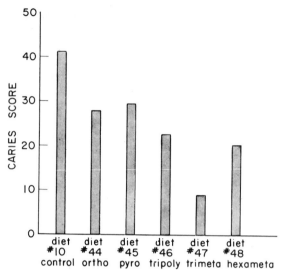

FIGURE 10–7. Cariostatic effects of several sodium phosphates fed in the diet to rats. (From Harris, R. S., et al. J. Dent. Res. 46:290, 1967.)

Clinical Trials of Phosphates Added to Cereals and Chewing Gum

The first scientifically controlled studies of the response of human caries to phosphates were conducted by Stralfors.[45] In 1956 he observed the caries-inhibiting effect of adding a 2% dicalcium phosphate suplement to bread and sugar. After 2 years with this regimen, there was a 40% decrease in caries. On the other hand, Ship and Mickelsen found no significant differences between a group given phosphate-supplemented bread and baked products and a control group.[46]

Three different independently designed and conducted clinical trials were carried out between 1957 and 1970 to test the cariostatic effectiveness of a dicalcium phosphate dihydrate additive to a sugar-based chewing gum. The first trial, conducted by Baron, showed that the group using regular gum developed significantly more caries than either the group chewing the gum with the additive or the group not chewing any gum.[47] However, the children chewing the gum with the additive had a higher caries increase than did the children not given gum.

In the second trial, conducted by Finn and Jameson,[48] there were three groups: group 1 chewed a sugar gum, group 2 chewed a sugarless gum, and group 3 chewed a sugar gum with a dicalcium phosphate additive. Each child chewed five sticks a day. At the end of 30 months there was a significant 20% reduction in DMFS (decayed, missing, and filled surfaces) in the group chewing the gum with additive compared with the group chewing the sugar gum. When only the proximal lesions were considered, there was an even greater difference and reduction in dental caries in the additive gum group compared with the sugar gum group. The conclusion was that the sugar phosphate gum was as noncariogenic as the sugarless gum.

In the third clinical trial, in which there were (1) a control group not chewing any gum, (2) a group chewing gum with dicalcium phosphate and sugar, and (3) a group chewing a sugarless gum, there were significant differences among the three groups.[49]

The results of these three clinical trials indicate that a dicalcium phosphate sugar-base chewing gum is safer for teeth than a regular sugar-base gum and is about as noncariogenic as sugarless gum.

A 30-month trial with a 1.5% sodium trimetaphosphate (TMP) additive to a sugar-base chewing gum was carried out with 5- to 16-year-old children.[50] The children were assigned to four groups: one chewing no gum, one chewing TMP sugar-base gum, one chewing a sugarless (sorbitol, mannitol, and saccharine) gum, and one chewing a TMP sugarless gum. The groups exposed to TMP had significantly fewer proximal caries than the controls (Table 10–2). The group chewing the TMP sugarless gum had significantly fewer proximal surface caries than the no gum group or the sugarless gum group. The group chewing the TMP sugar gum had about the same proximal caries as the no gum group. The results indicated that a TMP sugar-base gum was as effective as sugarless gum in not promoting tooth decay. However, there was only a marginal overall anticaries effect.

Another group of dental researchers from Indiana conducted a clinical trial that tested the anticariogenic effect of 1% sodium dihydrogen phosphate added to ready-to-eat breakfast cereals in three study groups.[51] In two of the additive groups they noted a caries reduction ranging from 20 to 40%, and in a third, the reduction was about 50% when compared with groups eating the regular presweetened cereals. They also found that the interproximal smooth surfaces were best protected against dental caries when phosphate was added to an otherwise cariogenic food. However, their experimental procedure, findings, and data analyses have been criticized.

A 3-year clinical trial in Michigan measured the relative cariostatic effectiveness of a sodium phosphate additive to cereals. The subjects were adolescents who were allowed to eat their usual variety of ready-to-eat breakfast cereals, but which were supplemented with sodium phosphate.[52] The level of supplementation was 0.2 g, which was less than half the concentration used by the Indiana group. Although no significant differences between experimental and control groups were observed, there was a definite trend toward a reduction in caries development in the experimental group. The limitation of the phosphate to only one food item made the investigators conclude that "perhaps the conditions of this study excessively restricted the phosphate anticaries effect."

TABLE 10–2. Effect of Sodium Trimetaphosphate (TMP) as a Chewing Gum Additive on Caries Increment*
(Using Analysis of Covariance)

Group	DMFS	% Difference†
1. No gum	1.63	0
2. TMP and sucrose gum	1.25	−23.3
3. Sorbitol gum	2.06	+26.4
4. TMP and sorbitol gum	0.85	−47.6

Adapted from Finn, S. B., et al. J. Am. Dent. Assoc. 96:654, 1978.
*Groups 1 and 3 are significantly different from 2 and 4. Group 1 is not different from group 3.
†Percent difference between group 1 and other groups.

In a report on a 3-year clinical study carried out in a Wisconsin boarding school, the investigators also noted no significant differences in dental caries experience between a group consuming phosphates added to presweetened or nonpresweetened ready-to-eat cereals and a control group.[53] The investigators concluded that the phosphate mixture was not potent enough to be an effective anticaries agent. Apparently a key factor in the success or failure of phosphates as anticaries agents in humans depends on the frequency of contact of the tooth surface with a food or drug product to which phosphate has been added. This group of researchers, like Rowe et al.,[52] made the important point that their findings did not negate the fact that a dietary phosphate supplement is noncariogenic, and perhaps under different experimental conditions may exert an anticaries effect. Because the need for frequent tooth surface contact seems to be critical, perhaps adding a sodium or a calcium trimetaphosphate to a number of food or drug products such as cereals, soft drinks, chewing gum, and mouthwashes may help provide more frequent tooth surface contact.

If there is some concern about the need for maintaining the 1:1 calcium to phosphorus ratio, then a calcium hydrogen trimetaphosphate supplement should be tried.

Rugg et al. studied 405 children (initially aged 11.5) by using five 3-day food diaries and 3 annual dental examinations during a 2-year period.[54] The calcium to phosphate ratio ranged from 0.56 to 1.04. They found no correlation between the calcium to phosphate ratio and caries. In fact, there was a slight relation between caries and an increased calcium to phosphate ratio. Thus Stanton's findings that caries activity is strongly related to the calcium to phosphate ratio have not been reproduced by other investigators.[54]

DIETARY AND SYSTEMIC FACTORS ASSOCIATED WITH DENTAL ENAMEL HYPOPLASIA AND HYPOCALCIFICATION

Enamel hypoplasia (incomplete development) is the end result of an interruption in ameloblast formation, which results in formation of defective enamel matrix. Hypocalcification (decreased calcification) is an imperfection in enamel resulting from inadequate mineralization.

Several systemic (affecting the whole body) stresses are associated with defective enamel formation such as venereal disease, hormonal imbalance, frank dietary calcium deficiency, frank dietary vitamin A or D deficiencies, or excess fluoride intake. However, the most likely reason for this defect is development of a high fever even for 1 or 2 days during the period of active tooth formation and calcification.

Clinically, hypoplasia is characterized by pitting, which is caused by damage to ameloblasts. A reduced amount of matrix results, but the matrix matures normally so that some places in the enamel surface are thinner than others. The pits are arranged in horizontal rows around the crown, extending into the enamel as far as the dentinoenamel junction. In severe cases the enamel on the edges of the incisors or cuspids may disappear, and the dentin on the occlusal surface of the first permanent molar is exposed.

The sign of hypocalcification is an opaque, chalky white spot on the surface of the enamel. Dietary or systemic stresses can injure the active ameloblasts, which may result in formation of a normal amount of enamel matrix but a matrix in which subsequent maturation is faulty and incomplete. Thus there is a failure to achieve full mineralization, resulting in the white spots, which may give the tooth a mottled appearance as seen in enamel fluorosis.

It is possible to estimate the age of the child at the time the disturbance occurred on the basis of the sequence of events in enamel formation. If there is interference with enamel formation during the first year of life, the permanent upper and central incisors, the lower laterals, and first permanent upper and lower molars will show pitting or white spots. The cuspids may also be involved but to a lesser degree than the incisors. If interference with calcification takes place during the third and fourth years, the first and second bicuspids and the second molars are affected.

MAGNESIUM [55]

Magnesium is one of the major cations in plant and animal tissues and is an essential constituent of bone and soft tissues. It is an essential ion in fundamental enzymatic reactions and in protein synthesis.

Distribution

The adult human body contains 20 to 35 g of magnesium, about 60% present as phosphates and carbonates in bone. The remainder is found in the cells and soft tissues, especially muscle, as well as the body fluids. Next to potassium, magnesium is the predominant metallic cation in living cells. It is the central component of chlorophyll. Magnesium is the third most abundant mineral in teeth.

Functions

Magnesium is essential for cellular respiration, functioning chiefly as an activator of numerous important coenzymes, such as cocarboxylase and coenzyme A. Thus it helps enzymes catalyze the transport of phosphate groups. For instance, it is a cofactor in the transfer of phosphate from adenosine triphosphate (ATP) to a phosphate receptor, or from a phosphorylated compound to adenosine diphosphate (ADP). This mineral is essential for the production of energy, the metabolism of carbohydrates and protein, the utilization of fat, and the mobilization of calcium from bone. Magnesium binds messenger RNA and is important in synthesis and degradation of DNA. Thus it plays a role in protein synthesis.

It ranks after potassium as the most important cation in living cells; it is thus critical for the normal metabolism and function of the living organism.

Small amounts of magnesium are present in the body fluids and take part in the transfer of water into and out of the cells; they also take part in the regulation of the acid-base balance of the body.

Absorption and Excretion

About one-third of the ingested magnesium is normally absorbed and utilized by the body. A high intake of calcium, phosphorus, and lactose will interfere with the absorption of magnesium. Unlike calcium, there is little excretion of magnesium through the intestine except that unabsorbed from the food. It is stored in bone.

Maintenance of the normal level of magnesium in the blood depends on a balance between absorption and renal excretion of sodium. There is no known hormonal regulating mechanism.

Magnesium is lost via both urine and feces. Significant amounts can be lost during prolonged episodes of vomiting or diarrhea.

Deficiency

Magnesium deficiency in humans is rare but may occur in such conditions as chronic malabsorption syndrome, acute diarrhea, chronic renal failure, and chronic alcoholism. Patients on hemodialysis should eat nutritionally wholesome foods.

The symptoms of magnesium deficiency are hyperexcitability, behavioral disturbances, weakness, depression, tremors, and convulsions.

Recommended Dietary Allowance and Sources

The recommended daily dietary allowance for normal adults is 350 mg for males and 300 mg for females.

The best food sources of magnesium are whole grains, nuts, soybeans, and green leafy vegetables. Beet greens, spinach, and all green vegetables are good sources of magnesium because it is an essential component of chlorophyll. The magnesium content of the average American diet has been estimated to be about 120 mg/1000 kcal.

Magnesium and Dental Health

Magnesium is present in both enamel and dentin, but its concentration in dentin is about twice that in enamel. If a dietary deficiency in magnesium is induced in rats, the enamel and dentin of the incisor teeth will be hypoplastic because a deficiency produces degenerative changes in ameloblasts and odonto-blasts.[56] An experimental dietary deficiency can adversely affect the periodontal structures by producing a lower rate of alveolar bone formation, widening of the periodontal ligament, and gingival hyperplasia.

An excess of dietary magnesium seems to increase dental caries development, as demonstrated by Navia, who fed rats a diet supplement of magnesium.[57]

REFERENCES

1. Spencer, H., et al. Calcium absorption and balance during high phosphorus intake in man. Fed. Proc. 34:888, 1975.
2. Allen, L. H. Calcium bioavailability and absorption: a review. Am. J. Clin. Nutr. 35:783, 1982.
3. Hegsted, D. M. In Goodhart, R. S.; Shills, M. E., eds. Modern Nutrition in Health and Disease, 5th ed., pp. 268–286. Philadelphia, Lea & Febiger, 1973.
4. Linkswiler, H. M., et al. Calcium retention of young adult males as affected by level of protein and of calcium intake. Trans. N.Y. Acad. Sci. 36:333, 1974.
5. Hegsted, M.; Schuette, S. A.; Zemel, M. B., et al. Urinary calcium and calcium balance in young men as affected by level of protein and phosphorus intake. J. Nutr. 111:353, 1981.
6. Kelsay, J. L.; Prather, E. Mineral balances of human subjects consuming spinach in low fiber diet and in a diet containing fruits and vegetables. Am. J. Clin. Nutr. 38:12, 1983.
7. Harland, B. F.; Harland, J. Fermentative reduction of phytate in rye, white and whole wheat breads. Cereal Chem. 57:276, 1980.
8. Underwood, J. L.; DeLuca, H. F. Vitamin D is not directly necessary for bone growth and mineralization. Am. J. Physiol. 246:E493, 1984.
9. Dietary phosphorus, PTH, and bone resorption. Nutr. Rev. 31:124, 1973.
10. National Institutes of Health. Consensus conference: osteoporosis. JAMA 252:799, 1984.
11. Riggs, B. L.; Melton, L. J. Involutional osteoporosis. N. Engl. J. Med. 314:1576, 1986.
12. Schafsman, G.; Van Beresteyn, E. G. H., et al. Nutritional aspects of osteoporosis. World Rev. Nutr. Diet. 49:121, 1987.
13. Riis, B.; Thomsen, K.; Christiansen, C. Does calcium supplementation prevent postmenopausal bone loss? A double-blind, controlled clinical study. N. Engl. J. Med. 316:173, 1987.
14. Spencer, H., et al. Effect of phosphorus on absorption of calcium in man. J. Nutr. 108:447, 1976.
15. Hegsted, M., et al. The effect of level of protein and phosphorus intake on calcium balance in young adult men. Fed. Proc. 38:765, 1979.
16. Sasaki, T.; Debari, K.; Garant, P. Ameloblast modulation and changes in Ca, P and S content of developing enamel matrix as revealed by SEM-EDX. J. Dent. Res. 66:778, 1987.
17. Papas, A.; Seyer, J.; Harris, R. S.; Glimcher, M. Isolation from embryonic bovine dental enamel of a polypeptide (E_3) containing as its phosphorylated sequence, Glu-O-phosphoserine-Leu. FEBS Lett. 79:276, 1977.
18. Irving, J. T. Theories of mineralization of bones and teeth. In Show, J. H., et al., eds. Textbook of Oral Biology, p. 482. Philadelphia, W. B. Saunders Co., 1978.
19. Glimcher, M. J.; Krane, S. M. In Gould, B. S.; Ramachandran, G. N., eds. A Treatise on Collagen, vol. IIb, p. 68. New York, Academic Press, 1968.
20. Glimcher, M. J. Recent studies of the mineral phase in bone and its possible linkage to the organic matrix by protein-bound phosphate bonds. Philos. Trans. R. Soc. Lond. B Biol. 304:479, 1984.
21. Wahner, H. W.; Dunn, W. L.; Riggs, B. L. Assessment of bone mineral. J. Nucl. Med. 25:1134, 1241, 1984.
22. Health and Public Policy Committee, American College of Physicians. Radiologic methods to evaluate bone mineral content. Ann. Intern. Med. 100:908, 1984.
23. Sartoris, D. J.; André, M.; Resnick, C., et al. Trabecular bone density in proximal femur: quantitative CT assessment. Work in progress. Radiology 160:707, 1986.
24. Hall, F. R.; Davis, M. A.; Baron, D. T. Bone mineral screening for osteoporosis. N. Engl. J. Med. 316:212, 1987.
25. Riggs, B. L.; Seeman, E.; Hodgson, S. T., et al. Effect of fluoride/calcium regimen on vertebral fracture occurrence in postmenopausal osteoporosis. N. Engl. J. Med. 306:446, 1982.
26. Aloia, J. F. Calcitonin in osteoporosis. Geriatric Med. Today 4:20, 1985.
27. Slovik, D. M.; Rosenthal, D., et al. Restoration of spinal bone in osteoporotic men by treatment with human parathyroid hormone (1–34) and 1,25 dihydroxyvitamin D. J. Bone and Mineral Res. 1:377, 1986.
28. Henrikson, P. Periodontal disease and calcium deficiency. Acta Odont. Scand. 26(Suppl. 50), 1968.
29. Krook, L. L., et al. Reversibility of nutritional osteoporosis: physicochemical data on bones from an experimental study in dogs. J. Nutr. 101:233, 1971.
30. Lutwak, L., et al. Calcium deficiency and human periodontal disease. Isr. J. Med. Sci. 7:504, 1971.
31. Kribbs, P. J.; Smith, D. E.; Chestnut, C. H., III. Oral findings in osteoporosis. Part II. Relationship between residual ridge and alveolar bone resorption and generalized skeletal osteoporosis. J. Prosthet. Dent. 50:719, 1983.
32. Daniell, H. W. Postmenopausal tooth loss. Contributions to edentulism by osteoporosis and cigarette smoking. Arch. Intern, Med. 143:1678, 1983.
33. Albanese, A. A. Calcium nutrition throughout the life cycle. Bibl. Nutr. Dieta 33:80, 1983.
34. Uhrbom, E.; Jacobson, L. Calcium and periodontitis: clinical effect of calcium medication. J. Clin. Periodontol. 11:230, 1984.
35. Rogoff, G. S.; Galburt, R. B.; Nizel, A. E. Role of dietary calcium and vitamin D in alveolar bone

health. In Rubin, R. P.; Weiss, G. B.; Putney, J. W., Jr., eds. Calcium in Biological Systems, pp. 591–595. New York, Plenum Publishing Corp., 1985.

36. Glickman, I. Clinical Periodontology, p. 432. Philadelphia, W. B. Saunders Co., 1972.
37. Svanberg, G., et al. Effect of nutritional hyperparathyroidism on experimental periodontitis in the dog. Scand. J. Dent. Res. 81:155, 1973.
38. Wical, K.; Swoope, C. C. Studies of residual ridge resorption. Part II. The relationship of dietary calcium and phosphorus to residual ridge resorption. J. Prosthet. Dent. 32:13, 1974.
39. Wical, K.; Brussee, P. Effects of a calcium and vitamin D supplement on alveolar ridge resorption in immediate denture patients. J. Prosthet. Dent. 41:4, 1979.
40. Lennox, J. Observations on diet and its relation to dental disease: a further consideration of calcium and phosphorus metabolism in their relation to dental caries. S. Afr. Dent. J. 5:156, 1931.
41. Osborn, T. W. B.; Noriskin, J. N. The relation between diet and caries in the South African Bantu. J. Dent. Res. 16:431, 1937.
42. Nizel, A. E.; Harris, R. S. The effects of phosphates on experimental dental caries: a literature review. J. Dent. Res. 43:1123, 1964.
43. Navia, J.; Harris, R. S. Longitudinal study of cariostatic effects of sodium trimetaphosphate and sodium fluoride when fed separately and together in diets of rats. J. Dent. Res. 48:183, 1969.
44. Harris, R. S.; Nizel, A. E. Effect of cations on the cariostatic activity of orthophosphates. J. Dent. Res. 44:416, 1965.
45. Stralfors, A. The effect of calcium phosphate on dental caries in school children. J. Dent. Res. 43:1137, 1964.
46. Ship, I. I.; Mickelson, O. O. The effects of calcium acid phosphate on dental caries in children: a controlled clinical trial. J. Dent. Res. 43:1144, 1964.
47. Baron, H. J. Modifying the cariogenicity of foods with dicalcium phosphate. In Proceedings, Workshop on Cariogenicity of Food, Beverages, Confections and Chewing Gum, p. 76. Chicago, Research Institute, American Dental Association, 1977.
48. Finn, S. B.; Jamison, H. C. The effect of dicalcium phosphate chewing gum on caries incidence in children: 30 month results. J. Am. Dent. Assoc. 74:987, 1967.
49. Richardson, A. S., et al. Anticariogenic effect of dicalcium phosphate dihydrate chewing gum: results after two years. J. Can. Dent. Assoc. 38:213, 1972.
50. Finn, S. B., et al. The effect of sodium trimetaphosphate (TMP) as a chewing gum additive on caries in increments in children. J. Am. Dent. Assoc. 96:651, 1978.
51. Stookey, G. K.; Carroll, R. A.; Muhler, J. C. The clinical effectiveness of phosphate enriched breakfast cereals on the incidence of dental caries in children: results after two years. J. Am. Dent. Assoc. 74:752, 1967.
52. Rowe, N. H., et al. The effect of ready to eat breakfast cereal upon dental caries experience in adolescent children: a three year study. J. Dent. Res. 53:33, 1974.
53. Wilson, C. J. Ready-to-eat cereals and dental caries in children: three year study. J. Dent. Res. 58:1853, 1979.
54. Rugg-Gunn, A. J., et al. Correlations of dietary intakes of calcium, phosphorus, and Ca/P ratio with caries data in children. Caries Res. 18:149, 1984.
55. Shills, M. E. Magnesium. In Present Knowledge in Nutrition: Nutrition Reviews, 5th ed., pp. 422–438. Washington, D.C., Nutrition Foundation, 1984.
56. Irving, J. T. Influences of diets low in magnesium on histological appearance of incisor teeth of rat. J. Physiol. 99:8, 1940.
57. Navia, J. Effect of minerals on dental caries. In Gould, R. F., ed. Dietary Chemicals vs. Dental Caries, p. 141. Advances in Chemistry Series 94. Washington, D. C., American Chemical Society, 1970.

11

Fluorides and Their Role in Dental Caries Prevention

OCCURRENCE AND STATUS AS AN ESSENTIAL NUTRIENT

Fluorine, a trace element, is a halogen like chlorine, bromine, and iodine. It is a very reactive gas and is not found in the free elemental form in nature. Rather it appears as the compound form, fluoride.

Fluoride is found everywhere throughout nature. The major source of ingested fluoride is water, particularly from deep artesian wells. It is found in soils rich in fluorspar (calcium fluoride), cryolite (sodium aluminum fluoride), and other minerals. It is also found in plants, foodstuffs, and body tissues. In the human, fluoride is found mainly in the calcified structures—the teeth and the skeleton.

Fluoride is a nutrient beneficial to dental health, and it is included in the 1980 Recommended Dietary Allowances, which emphasizes its importance in nutrition.[1] But the question, Does it meet the criteria for being an essential nutrient for health? has still not been satisfactorily answered. Messer and Singer have concluded from the several lines of evidence dealing with fluoride's effect on growth rate, reproduction, hematopoiesis (blood cell formation), and mineralization that evidence does not justify fluoride's inclusion in the list of essential trace elements.[2] The reason for this is that no one has been able to produce a diet totally devoid of fluoride to determine whether a fluoride supplement can support the life processes. A physiological or biochemical role that can be attributed to fluoride alone has not yet been described.

DIETARY SOURCES

Drinking Water

Although all foods contain at least traces of fluoride, waterborne fluorides are generally the most important source for humans. Modern diets are becoming increasingly important as a source of fluoride because of the increased use of fluoridated water in the preparation of processed food and beverages.

For temperate climates the optimal fluoride level in water supplies for reduction of dental caries without undesirable mottling is 1 ppm (part per million). Based on infants' and young children's normal intake of between 2 and 4 glasses of water or the equivalent per day, this level of 1 ppm would provide a total daily intake of 0.5 to 1 mg of fluoride per day. For older children, adolescents, and adults, the intake from water would be equivalent to 1.5 to 2 mg of fluoride per day because they may drink between 6 and 8 glasses of water or the equivalent (1500 ml) per day.[3]

Foods

In the United States the intake of fluoride in foods by adults averages approximately 1 mg/day in nonfluoridated communities and 2 to 3 mg/day in fluoridated communities.[4] One milligram of fluoride per liter of water equals 1 ppm fluoride. Therefore if the amount of fluoride in drinking water (6 to 8 glasses per day) were added to the amount of fluoride in food, the total daily fluoride intake would average 1.2 mg for adults living in the nonfluoridated community and 3.5 to 4.5 mg for those living in the fluoridated (1 ppm) community.[5]

The intake by children of fluoride from food and water would be proportionately less, depending on their calorie and water consumption. It is important to point out that the optimal fluoride level of 1 ppm of fluoride for drinking water was based on water intake only, even though the subjects must have ingested varying amounts of fluoride from their food. The fluoride level in food is not known to be a significant factor in producing mottled enamel (fluorosis). Only the ingestion of greater than optimal levels of fluoride in drinking water (2 ppm) caused fluorosis, as reported by Dean.[6]

In low fluoride areas, the daily diet furnishes only 0.3 mg.; in high fluoride areas, the daily intake from food is about 3.1 mg. Fruits, vegetables, and cereals contain very small amounts of fluoride (Table 11–1). The rich sources of fluoride are seafoods, especially fish with small bones such as sardines and salmon, which

TABLE 11–1. Fluoride Concentration in Fresh Foods and Beverages

Food	Range of F in ppm
Beer	0.15–0.86
Cereals	0.18–2.8
Citrus	0.07–0.17
Coca Cola	0.07
Coffee	0.2–1.6
Instant (powder)	1.7
Fish without bone or skin	1.0
Fish meal	80.0–250.0
Milk	0.04–0.55
Noncitrus fruits	0.03–0.84
Sardines	8.0–40.0
Shrimp meat	0.4
Shrimp shell	18.0–48.0
Tea	0.1–2.0
Instant (solution)	0.2
Vegetables and tubers	0.02–0.9
Wine	0.0–6.3

Adapted from Tables II and III in Hodge, H. C.; Smith, F. A. Minerals: fluorine and dental caries. In Advances in Chemistry, Series 94. Washington, D.C., American Chemical Society, 1970.

tend to take up fluoride readily. The amount of fluoride in fresh fish may be about 1.6 ppm, whereas in canned salmon, sardines, and mackerel it may be as high as 7 to 12 ppm.

On a dry weight basis, one of the richest sources of fluoride is tea; the leaves contain from 75 to 110 ppm. However, the average cup of tea may contain only 0.5 to 1.5 ppm because most of the fluoride is extracted when the tea is steeped in hot water.

Milk products taken along with sodium fluoride can reduce flouride's availability to bones and teeth by 50 to 79%.[7]

It is important to realize that the average diet in the United States is low in fluoride, and the best way to achieve optimal fluoride levels on a regular daily basis is by fluoridating the communal water supplies.

METABOLISM

To answer questions about the safety of fluoride as an additive to water supplies or foods, it is important to understand how the body metabolizes this nutrient.[8] In other words, one must understand how fluoride is absorbed, how it is distributed to the various tissues after absorption, and how the body through its excretion and storage mechanisms maintains a safe level.

Absorption

The major site of absorption of fluoride in humans appears to be the stomach, although studies with experimental animals suggest that intestinal absorption also occurs. The soluble fluoride in drinking water is almost completely absorbed, whereas approximately 50 to 80% of the fluoride that naturally occurs in foods is absorbed.

Distribution

When compared with all other tissues and structures, the teeth and skeleton have the highest concentrations of fluoride because of the affinity of fluoride for calcium. In descending order, the highest levels are found in cementum, bone, dentin, and enamel. The fluoride content of teeth and bones increases rapidly during the early mineralization periods and continues to increase with age, but at a slower rate. Once it is deposited, fluoride is firmly bound to the tooth mineral for life.

Fluoride is found in both extracellular and intracellular fluids of soft tissues but at very low concentrations. Fluoride is also found in saliva at about 0.01 ppm. When fluoride is ingested, the salivary fluoride level increases after 5 to 15 minutes, reaches a maximum after about 30 minutes, and then decreases to normal levels in about 1 hour. This salivary level may play a part in the maintenance of fluoride concentrations in the outer layer of the tooth enamel.

Excretion

The principal route of excretion of fluoride is the urine (90 to 95%). The remainder (5 to 10%) is found in the feces. Sweat may also be a route of excretion of a minute amount of fluoride.

The outstanding characteristic of fluoride excretion is its speed. Fluoride derived from communal water supplies is excreted in part via the urine of normal human adults as quickly as 3 hours after ingestion. After 24 hours, as much as 50 to 60% of the 5 mg of fluoride will have been excreted. In individuals whose drinking water does not contain large amounts (2 ppm or more) of fluoride, the urinary excretion amounts to about 0.1 mg/hour (Fig. 11–1).[9]

The reason for the speed of excretion via the kidneys is that the reabsorption of fluoride from urine is less efficient than, for example, is the case with chloride (about 50% for fluoride compared with 99.5% for chloride).

The relatively low efficiency of the human kidney in the reabsorption of fluoride and the high affinity of the bones and teeth for fluoride are effective mechanisms for maintaining low concentrations of fluoride in the soft tissues and plasma. The amount of fluoride in urine is directly related to the degree of active bone growth. Fluoride excretion is lower when a child is growing rapidly and is actively depositing bone mineral than in adults with a mature bone structure and fully mineralized teeth. Zipkin et al. compared the amounts of fluoride in urine in children 5 to 14 years of age with the amounts in adults.[10] They found that it took 3 years for the urine of the children who were drinking fluoridated water (1 ppm) to reach excretion levels of 1 ppm of fluoride, whereas it took only 1 week for the urine of adults 30 to 34 years of age in the same communities to show this level of excretion.

In general, about half of the ingested fluoride is excreted in the urine each

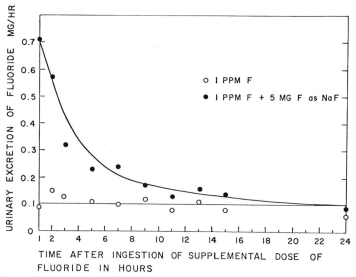

FIGURE 11–1. Urinary excretion of fluoride in eight normal individuals drinking water containing 1 ppm fluoride and receiving a supplement of 5 mg fluoride as sodium fluoride. (Modified from Zipkin. I.; Lee, W. A.; Leone, N. C. Am. J. Public Health 47:848, 1957.)

day. A steady state equilibrium in which the fluoride excretion almost precisely equals the fluoride intake occurs within a relatively short time in adults ingesting 1 ppm of fluoride per day, as shown by the classic studies of Machle et al.[11]

Storage

Fluoride tends to be deposited in calcified structures such as bones and teeth when they are in the active stage of mineralization.

Bone fluoride concentration increases steadily with water fluoride levels up to 4 ppm, but shows lower increases at 8 ppm. Skeletons of older persons contain more fluoride than those of younger ones because the amount of fluoride in bone gradually increases with age even though the rate and amount of fluoride deposition are greatest during the active growth years. The factors that attract fluoride to bones include (1) the presence of an active growth area at the ends of the long bones, (2) the small size of the bone crystals, and (3) the close contact between bones and the blood supply.

The mechanism of bone fluoride deposition from extracellular fluid involves the exchange of the hydroxyl ion in the hydroxyapatite lattice with the fluoride ion to form the compound fluorhydroxyapatite. The more active the bone mineralization process is, the more fluoride will be incorporated.

In the case of teeth, fluoride is deposited in the enamel via the systemic (affecting the body as a whole) route when the lattice is developing and maturing. Because mature adult tooth enamel has no cells, it is not affected directly by systemic fluoride. Rather, there is a local effect: fluoride in the mouth penetrates the enamel surface by diffusion through the minute spaces between the enamel crystals and through remineralization of the tooth surface. This local effect is increased when the crown is newly erupted into the mouth. Fluoride is continuously added to the enamel surface, but to a much lesser extent as the tooth ages and practically not at all when it is completely mineralized. The concentration of fluoride in the tooth enamel of individuals who regularly drink water containing 1 ppm of fluoride can reach 800 to 900 ppm in the outer layers.[12] In the developing enamel fluoride is deposited within the body of the crystal, whereas in the fully formed enamel fluoride is mainly deposited in the surface layer of the tooth.

Fluoride will also penetrate partly demineralized enamel, dentin, or cementum of new carious lesions. In fact, carious enamel may take up 10 times more fluoride than adjacent healthy enamel and thus help inhibit the expansion of the carious lesion.

Dentin may contain even more fluoride than enamel because it is chemically similar to bone. The highest concentration is found in the dentin adjacent to the pulp because it is so close to the blood supply and on the surface. The lowest concentration is usually at the dentin-enamel junction.

The body's built-in safety mechanisms—fluoride excretion and deposition in calcified tissues—prevent significant accumulation of fluoride in the circulating fluids (plasma, lymph, cerebrospinal fluid, and so forth).

RELATIVE SAFETY

Effect of Low and Moderate Intake of Fluoride on General Health

A number of large-scale studies have been made of the morbidity (rate of sickness) and mortality (death rate) of populations exposed to natural fluorides at low and high concentrations. For example, residents of Bartlett, Texas, who drank water with an 8 ppm fluoride content for 15 years were examined.[13] Their physical status was compared with that of the residents of Cameron, Texas, who drank water having a 0.4 ppm fluoride content. Ten years later the examinations were repeated on as many of these individuals as could be located. When the Bartlett residents were compared with the Cameron residents, no unusual cases of arthritis, bone fracture, healing of fracture, exostosis (benign bony projection), or hypertrophic bone change were found. In about 10 to 15% of the Bartlett group there was some increased bone density, but without any functional impairment. Thus, skeletal fluorosis may begin to appear with ingestion of 8 ppm of fluoride. There was one different physical sign in some of the Bartlett residents who had lived there during their childhood: they had mottled (marked with different spots) enamel. (Mottled enamel is discussed later in this chapter.)

Weidmann et al. have found no radiographic evidence of skeletal abnormality in persons who used a water supply throughout life that contained less than 4 ppm of fluoride.[14] However, cryolite (sodium aluminum fluoride) workers who were exposed to 20 to 80 mg of fluoride dust every day for 10 to 20 years did develop crippling skeletal fluorosis. This condition involves osteosclerosis (hardening or abnormal denseness of bone), exostoses (bony projections), and calcification of ligaments; it is so severe and crippling that the afflicted persons cannot work.[15]

Hodge saw no evidence of kidney or thyroid damage in persons who all their lives had been drinking water in which the fluoride concentration was 11 ppm.[16] Accounts of allergic reactions and other ailments have not been confirmed.[17]

In 1970 the World Health Organization (WHO) published a review of the scientific literature on fluoridation, its possible effects on different organs, and its alleged association with various diseases.[18] This review, which represented medical opinion throughout the world, revealed no evidence of harmful effects from ingestion of fluoridated water at the optimal level of around 1 ppm. In 1975 WHO released a statement that "the only sign of physiological or pathological change in lifelong users of optimally fluoridated water supplies, after two decades of the practice of fluoridation, is that they suffer less from tooth decay." In 1978 WHO reaffirmed its support for fluoridation, urging member states to consider fluoridation in their national planning for the prevention and control of oral disease.[19]

Myth of Cancer Linkage with Fluoridated Water

Erickson has reported on a comparison of cancer mortality statistics in cities in the United States with and without fluoridated water supplies for the years 1969 through 1971.[20] After adjusting for age, gender, and race differences of the residents of the fluoridated cities compared with those of the nonfluoridated cities and adjusting for city characteristics that influence mortality, he found no harmful effect of fluoridation. The death rate for all causes was 1123.9 and 1137.1 and that for malignant neoplasms was 195.3 and 196.9 in the cities with fluoridated and nonfluoridated water, respectively.

Neither the United States Centers for Disease Control[21] nor the National Heart, Lung, and Blood Institute[22] could find any evidence linking fluoride with cancer. Charges of a link between fluoridation and cancer have also been refuted in England. Doll and Kinlen of Oxford University reported that the American evidence from the National Cancer Institute[23] and from the University of Rochester[24] was consistent with the British evidence. It refutes any claims linking fluoridation to increases in cancer rates. They concluded, "None of it provides any reason to suppose that fluoridation is associated with an increase in cancer mortality, let alone causes it."[25] These reports and other studies of residents of communities with high and low fluoride show no evidence that fluoride has caused a greater incidence of fatal diseases[26] (Table 11–2).

Effect of High Intake of Fluoride on General Health

It is clear from the preceding discussion that the daily ingestion of fluorides in the range of 1 to 8 ppm is safe with respect to general health. However, it must be pointed out that fluoride, like other nutrients that are safe and beneficial at certain levels, can be toxic if ingested in unusually large amounts.

When ingested in excessive amounts over long periods, fluoride can be toxic. Under these circumstances, it can produce excessive mineralization of ligaments and bones. It should be noted, however, that doses of 25 to 150 mg of fluoride per day for up to 1 year have been used in therapy along with other types of treatment in the management of osteoporosis with no noticeable adverse side effects.[27]

Acute toxicity or death may occur from ingestion of a single dose of 2.5 to 5.0 g of sodium fluoride, which is 2500 to 5000 times greater than the amount contained in a quart of water having an optimal amount (1 ppm) of fluoride.

Early History of the Effect of Fluorides on Dental Health

A landmark epidemiological finding in public health dentistry was achieved when Dean reported that when dental fluorosis increased, the incidence of dental

TABLE 11–2. Mortality Rates Per 100,000 Population (Adjusted for Age, Race, and Gender)

Causes of Death	"Fluoride" Cities	Control Cities
Heart disease	354.8	357.4
Cancer	135.4	139.1
Intracranial lesions	111.5	104.8
Nephritis	21.9	26.9
Cirrhosis of the liver	6.6	8.2
All causes	1010.6	1005.0

From Hagan, T. L.; Pasternack, M.; Scholtz, G. C. Public Health Rep. 69:450, 1954.

caries decreased.[6] Indirectly related to this major discovery in preventive dentistry are a number of preliminary scientific observations dealing with fluorides and dental structures from the beginning of the nineteenth century. For example, in the early 1800s fluoride had been found to be one of the chemical constituents of teeth and bone by the reputable chemists Morichini,[28] Gay-Lussac,[29] and Berzelius.[30] In 1878, the great French investigator Magitot wrote in his treatise on dental caries that the resistance of enamel to acid decalcification was due in part "to the minute quantity of fluoride it [enamel] contains."[31] About 14 years later Crichton-Browne suggested that dental caries might be caused in part by a lack of fluoride.[32] He believed that the excessive intake of over-refined foods caused a fluoride deficiency, which, he hypothesized, was the reason for the large number of carious teeth that he observed.

At the turn of the century, J.M. Eager reported endemic discoloration of teeth in children who lived near Naples, Italy.[33] He described the dark markings on these children's teeth in a variety of ways: as *denti di Chiae* (after the Italian professor who originally noted this stain), *denti-neri* (black teeth), and *denti scritae* (writings of the teeth). Eager was prophetic in his suggestion that the cause of this condition was some unknown chemical in the drinking water, which came from subterranean streams that when analyzed later were found to have high concentrations of fluorides.

In 1916 Black and McKay noted that the teeth of children raised in the Colorado Springs area were stained brown (thus named Colorado brown stain).[34] They suggested the term *mottled enamel* for this condition. This dental disfigurement occurred only in children or in adults who as children drank the water drawn from deep artesian wells. Adolescents and adults who migrated to Colorado Springs after their teeth were fully matured did not develop this stain. Obviously, some chemical in relatively high concentration in the water supply interfered with the calcification of the unerupted, developing enamel but did not affect the posterupted mature, completely mineralized enamel. Furthermore, McKay reported that children with mottled enamel had a "curious absence of decay" and that certainly the incidence of caries in mottled enamel was no greater than that in normal enamel.[35] What was this chemical in the water supply?

H.V. Churchill, a chemist, demonstrated for the first time in 1931 that this chemical was fluoride.[36] McKay sent Churchill samples of water from six areas in which there was tooth mottling for fluoride analyses. Churchill compared the samples with the fluoride analyses of water from 30 areas in which tooth enamel was normal. The results confirmed the hypothesis that there was a correlation between high fluoride levels in water supplies and endemic mottled tooth enamel. This hypothesis was subsequently tested and confirmed in rats, which developed mottled incisors after ingesting excess fluorides.[37] Also, young children who drank from an unfluoridated water supply did not develop mottled enamel even though older brothers and sisters might have shown this defect, because the latter had drunk from fluoridated waters while their teeth were calcifying.[38]

In 1933 Dean began an extensive study of the relation of fluorides in community drinking water to tooth mottling or, as he termed it, "endemic dental fluorosis."[39] The results of these studies and others[40] not only proved this relationship but also provided the first scientific evidence that fluoride at an optimal level of 1 ppm in communal water supplies was a significantly effective caries-preventive nutrient.

ENDEMIC DENTAL FLUOROSIS OR MOTTLED ENAMEL

Mottled enamel is characterized clinically as white and/or brown spotty staining of the tooth enamel surfaces. Sometimes the teeth will have horizontal striations (stripes) (Fig. 11–2).

When compared histologically with developing normal enamel, developing mottled enamel is deficient in (1) the number of cells producing enamel, or ameloblasts (hypoplasia), which affects matrix formation and causes the pitting; and (2) mineral deposits (hypocalcification) accompanied by poorly formed rod substance, which causes the chalkiness.

Mottling occurs only in teeth that are being formed. If these developing teeth are exposed to high concentrations of fluoride (2 ppm or more), opaque spots will develop on the enamel. However, no mottling occurs if teeth are exposed to more than 2 ppm of fluoride only after eruption because all the ameloblasts have degenerated. ✓

Driscoll et al. assessed the prevalence of dental caries and fluorosis in children living in areas with a wide range of natural fluoride concentrations in drinking water.[41] The results are shown in Table 11–3. As can be seen, water fluoride levels above the optimal level all reduced the incidence of caries. But when severe fluorosis was found, the caries rate was higher than that for children without fluorosis. This agrees with other studies showing that the protection of fluoride is decreased by severe fluorosis.[42–48]

Leverett has suggested that fluorosis is increasing as a result of the use of fluoride in our food, toothpaste, and supplements.[49] Driscoll et al.[41] did not confirm this—only 2.9% of children and 1.3% of the teeth showed evidence of

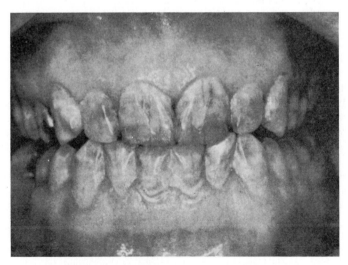

FIGURE 11–2. Mottled enamel due to fluorosis.

TABLE 11-3. Mean DMFS Scores According to Water Fluoride Level

Water Fluoride Level	No. of Children	Mean DMFS Per Child	Difference From Negligible (%)
Negligible	316	5.07	
Optimal	336	3.14*	38.1
Two times optimal	143	1.97†	61.1
Three times optimal	192	1.41†	72.2
Four times optimal	136	2.02†	60.2

From Driscoll, W. S., et al. J. Am. Dent. Assoc. 13:30, 1986. Copyright by the American Dental Association. Reprinted by permission.
*Significantly lower than negligible ($P = 0.001$).
†Significantly lower than negligible and optimal ($P = < 0.01$).

fluorosis in the optimal fluoride area.[41] The brown stains associated with fluorosis may be due to food, debris, or plaque.

The optimal systemic fluoride dosage to prevent caries is between 0.05 and 0.07 mg/kg per day. Mild fluorosis has been seen with oral intakes greater than 0.1 mg/kg per day. Because of this, children should avoid toothpaste ingestion because toothpaste contains 1 mg of fluoride per gram.

FLUORIDE AND DENTAL CARIES

Communal Water Fluoridation

Dean's classic surveys of children from 21 different cities with various amounts of fluoride in the water supplies showed that caries experience decreased as fluoride concentrations in communal water supplies increased from 0.5 to 1.5 ppm.[6, 39, 40] For example, the average dental caries experience was seven decayed, missing, or filled teeth (DMFT) for children living in cities where the water supply contained 0.5 ppm fluoride or less. However, children of similar ages who drank water with a fluoride concentration of 1.0 to 1.4 ppm had a caries experience of only three DMFT, a decrease of about 60% (Fig. 11–3).

The relation among levels of waterborne fluorides, the index of fluorosis, and the number of DMFT for 12- to 14-year-old children is shown in Figure 11–4. On the basis of this finding, Ast recommended that water supplies be artificially fluoridated with the amount of sodium fluoride that would provide 1 ppm of fluoride.[50]

In the northern United States, where water consumption and the mean temperature differ from those in the southern states, 1.0 to 1.2 ppm is desirable; in the southern states 0.6 to 0.7 ppm is appropriate.

In 1945 two well-designed studies of the effect of artificial fluoridation of public water supplies on dental caries incidence in children raised in Newburgh, New York,[51] and Grand Rapids, Michigan,[52] were carried out. These cities were compared with two cities with nonfluoridated water (Kingston, New York, and Muskegon, Michigan, respectively). The respective communities had similar socioeconomic, cultural, and environmental factors. Two other similar studies were conducted, one in Canada, with Brantford as the fluoridated city and Sarni

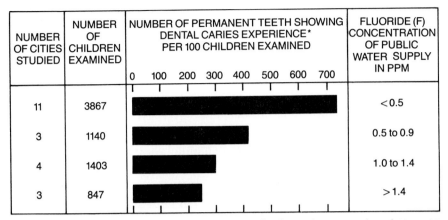

NUMBER OF CITIES STUDIED	NUMBER OF CHILDREN EXAMINED	NUMBER OF PERMANENT TEETH SHOWING DENTAL CARIES EXPERIENCE* PER 100 CHILDREN EXAMINED	FLUORIDE (F) CONCENTRATION OF PUBLIC WATER SUPPLY IN PPM
11	3867		<0.5
3	1140		0.5 to 0.9
4	1403		1.0 to 1.4
3	847		>1.4

FIGURE 11–3. *Amount of dental caries (permanent teeth) observed in 7257 selected 12- to 14-year-old white schoolchildren of 21 cities of four states classified according to the fluoride concentration of the public water supply. (From Dean, H. T., et al. Public Health Rep. 57:1155, 1942.)*

as the control,[53] and the other in the United States with Evanston, Illinois, as the fluoridated city and Oak Park, Illinois, as the control.[54]

After 10 years, dental examinations showed that children in Newburgh who drank the artificially fluoridated water experienced 40 to 60% less decay than the children of Kingston who drank the nonfluoridated water. Further, the children who drank the fluoridated water from birth enjoyed maximal protection against tooth decay (Fig. 11–5). In Newburgh the loss of teeth and the incidence of caries in children were less than half those of children in Kingston, and the

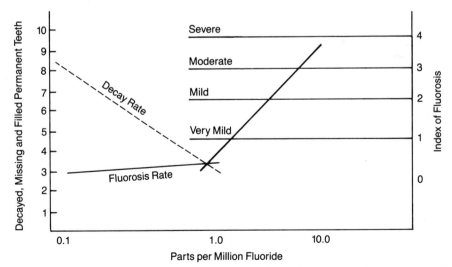

FIGURE 11–4. *The relation of the level of fluoride in the drinking water to the occurrence of various degrees of mottled enamel and to the dental caries experience in 12- to 14-year-old children. (From Sognnaes, R. F. Chemistry and Prevention of Dental Caries. Springfield, Ill., Charles C Thomas, 1962.)*

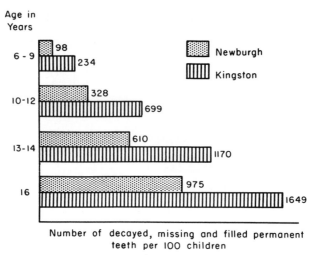

Age in
Years

FIGURE 11–5. *The relation of added fluoride in the water supply for 10 years to the incidence of dental caries in permanent teeth of children from 6 to 16 years of age. (From Sognnaes, R. F. Chemistry and Prevention of Dental Caries. Springfield, Ill., Charles C Thomas, 1962.)*

average cost of dental care in the first year was lowered by more than half ($13.86 for a Newburgh child compared with $33.73 for a Kingston child).[55]

From these results we learn that the greatest resistance to caries and the greatest amount of fluoride deposition are acquired by starting fluoride intake as early as possible and using it continuously. For the maximal effect, fluoride should be ingested throughout life, and systemic fluoride should be used together with topical application.

The great dental health benefits of communal fluoridated water programs were very clearly shown in Antigo, Wisconsin, where fluoridation was discontinued after 11 years.[56] Dental caries experience increased greatly in the subsequent 4½ years when communal water was not fluoridated. DMFT increased as much as 183% among children who were not exposed to the fluoride during the first 2 years of their lives. Fluoridation was re-established within a year after this finding.

Newbrun recorded the percentage of reduction in DMFT in children who were at the most caries-susceptible age (11 to 15) and who also had the benefits of drinking fluoridated water all their lives (Table 11–4).[57] There are nine studies reported here, and the range of caries reduction is 40 to 70%. From these studies, it would be reasonable to predict that a teenage person who has had lifelong exposure to water fluoridation might enjoy a 50% caries reduction when compared with a person of similar age, sex, and social status who did not drink fluoridated water.

There has been some attempt to determine whether drinking fluoridated water has significant lifelong benefits. Jackson found that adults did have significant protection against caries as a result of water fluoridation. He found that dentate persons aged 35 years or more who drank water in which the fluoride level was 1.5 to 2.0 ppm had 44% fewer caries than those who drank water with a 0.15 to 0.28 ppm fluoride level.[58] In a study of root caries in fluoridated vs. nonfluoridated communities, Stamm and Banting found a lower root caries rate in the fluoridated community.[59] This result stimulated research

**TABLE 11–4. Percent Reduction in DMFT Reported
in Various Fluoridation Studies**

Studies Site(s)	Years of Study*	Age Group	Percent Reduction in DMFT
Evanston, Ill.	1946–59	12–14	49
Grand Rapids, Mich.	1945–59	12–14	56
Brantford/Sarina, Ont.	—	12–14	57
Newburgh/Kingston, N.Y.	—	13–14	70
Hastings, New Zealand	1954–70	14–15	60
Karl-Marx-Stadt, G.D.R.	1959–72	11–15	59
Anglesey/Bangor, Wales	—	15	44
Tiel/Culemborg, The Netherlands	—	15	51
Toronto, Ont.	1964–75	11	40

From Newbrun, E. In Burt, B., ed. The Relative Efficiency of Methods of Caries Prevention in Dental Public Health, p. 33. Ann Arbor, University of Michigan Press, 1978.
*Years when before-after results were obtained from study sites without a control community.

on remineralization of adult caries with fluoride. Both in vitro and in vivo root caries have been remineralized with fluoride.[60–62]

The approximate per capita cost of water fluoridation is 6 to 80 cents per year, depending on the size of the community and the expected caries reduction of 50 to 60%.[63] If one assumes the caries increase of 2.0 decayed, missing, or filled surfaces (DMFS) per year in a nonfluoridated community and the cost of restoring a tooth surface at $10, the ratio of cost to benefit is 1:50; or, for every dollar spent on water fluoridation, each person in the community would save approximately $50 annually that would have been paid in dental fees for restoring decayed teeth.

Eight countries have reported a substantial caries reduction with fluoridation of the public water supply (Table 11–5).[64] It is interesting that Hong Kong, which has the lowest caries incidence and DMFT for 12-year-old persons, has had its water supply 100% fluoridated for more than 20 years. Conversely,

**TABLE 11–5. Effect of Fluoridation of Public Water Supply on
DMFT in Different Countries**

Country	Year Fluoridation Commenced	% Population in 1980	First DMFT	Second DMFT
Singapore	1958	100	5.4 (64)*	2.8 (79)
Hong Kong	1961	98	4.3 (60)	1.8 (80)
Australia	1953	65	3.8 (74)	2.6 (80)
Ireland	1964	60	8.0 (61)	3.9 (80)
New Zealand	1954	54	9.0 (73)	3.3 (83)
United States	1945	52	3.8 (74)	2.6 (80)
Columbia	1965	37	7.1 (65)	4.8 (80)
Brazil	1953	23	7.2 (75)	7.2 (80)

Adapted from Changing patterns of oral health and implications for oral health manpower. Part 1. Joint report Federation Dentaire Internationale and World Health Organization. Int. Dent. 35:235, 1985.
*Numbers in parentheses are years of measurement of DMFT (e.g., 64 = 1964).

Brazil, whose water supply had the lowest percentage of fluoridation, did not experience the decrease in caries seen globally. Brazil has now started fluoridating 45% of its water supply.

The World Health Organization suggested that the rapid spread of fluoride availability underlies the 30 to 50% decrease in the caries rate experienced by many children in highly industrialized countries during the past 20 years. Other factors contributing to this decline in caries were (1) greater dental health awareness, (2) expansion of dental resources, and (3) application of preventive dentistry including nutrition counseling, use of antibiotics, and herd (group) immunity.[64-66]

The following resolution was made and approved by the Council of the American Institute of Nutrition and by the Council of the American Society for Clinical Nutrition.[63]

Resolution

Tooth decay is one of the nation's most ubiquitous health problems in numbers of people affected and its persistence. Appropriate fluoridation of public water is a safe, economical, and effective measure to prevent dental caries. The most favorable and persistent benefits accrue to those who have had continuous exposure to optimum fluoride levels in drinking water. This public health measure is supported by the US Public Health Service and more than 60 health professional and technical associations including the American Medical Association and the American Dental Association. Therefore, the joint Public Information Committee of the American Institute of Nutrition and the American Society for Clinical Nutrition agrees that fluoridation of community water supplies to an optimum level wherever the natural level is less than optimum is a safe, economical, and effective measure to improve dental health by improving nutrition.

Thus, based on current knowledge, communal water fluoridation is the most effective, practical, feasible, and economical public health measure for preventing dental caries. The only shortcoming is that it can be implemented only in areas with central water systems. In some communities communal water fluoridation may not be feasible for engineering reasons or because of political opposition, so alternative methods of providing systemic fluoride, such as school water fluoridation or distribution of fluoride tablets at school, must be considered.

School Water Fluoridation

Of the U.S. population, 23% live in areas that lack central water systems.[67] Therefore, part-time availability of fluoridated water (i.e., in schools) has been suggested.

School water supplies have been fluoridated with levels of three times,[68] $4\frac{1}{2}$ times,[69] and seven times[70] the optimum for communal water fluoridation (1 ppm), resulting in a significant reduction in caries incidence. The caries reduction at each of these respective levels of fluoridation was 22, 40, and 40%.

It is projected that after 12 years of school water fluoridation one might expect a 40% reduction in caries at an approximate per capita cost of $1.50. The approximate cost to benefit ratio would be 1:5.3, that is, $1.00 invested in this fluoride program would save more than $5.00 in dental repair costs.

Dietary Supplements of Fluoride Tablets

The studies measuring the anticaries effectiveness of fluoride tablets can be summarized as follows: Most studies reported a caries reduction in deciduous teeth of approximately 50 to 80% when fluoride administration was begun before about 2 years of age and was continued for a minimum of 3 to 4 years. After the use of fluoride tablets for 2 to 4 years, caries reduction in the permanent teeth of children aged 9 to 13 years was approximately 20 to 40%. This means that when fluoride tablets are ingested daily beginning at around age 5 to 9 years (age during primary school), the permanent teeth can still be significantly protected from caries.[71] In an 8-year study with dietary fluoride supplements, Marthaler reported a dental caries reduction of 36%.[72]

A lozenge that is allowed to dissolve slowly in the mouth is preferred to a tablet or drops, because it can produce both topical and systemic effects. Fluoride tablets have an important advantage in that a specific and precise dose can be delivered. However, there are a number of disadvantages with fluoride lozenge or tablet usage when compared with water fluoridation. The assurance of continuous daily ingestion is much less and the cost is greater. Furthermore, fluorides taken once a day are excreted relatively rapidly. Thus it is difficult to maintain as constant a systemic and local fluoride level as when drinking fluoridated water several times a day.

The approximate cost to benefit ratio when fluoride tablets are distributed at schools is 1:17, that is, $1.00 of cost for fluoride tablets will save $17.00 in dental costs.

Prenatal Fluoride Supplement

On the basis of our knowledge of the chemistry of tooth maturation and mineralization, fluoride supplements are not recommended for adults, including pregnant women, for reducing dental caries. Also, there is not sufficient evidence to support a claim of significant caries prevention in children of women who took fluoride tablet supplements while pregnant. In fact, the U.S. Food and Drug Administration has banned the marketing of fluoride products that claim anticaries protection for these children.

Most investigators agree that fluoride ingested by the pregnant woman passes through the placenta and is incorporated into the developing bones and teeth of the fetus. However, the concentration of fluoride that actually reaches the fetus is generally lower than that in the maternal blood.[73] Fluoride uptake greatly increases in developing enamel with a small change in fluoride concentration in fetal extracellular fluids. Infants exposed prenatally will have higher plasma, skeletal, and developing enamel fluoride levels than those not exposed to prenatal fluoride.[74, 75] However, any dental health benefits that might result would affect the deciduous teeth only. Studies show that more proof of anticaries protection for the children is needed before fluoride supplements can be recommended for the pregnant woman.[76, 77]

Fluoride Supplements for Infants and Children

Daily administration of individualized dietary supplements of sodium fluoride is desirable for young children who live in areas where community or school water fluoridation is not practiced.

There has been some controversy about giving fluoride supplements to infants younger than 6 months of age, even when there is practically no fluoride in the water supplies. Because Aasenden and Peebles reported some mild dental fluorosis in children given 0.5-mg fluoride supplements from birth,[78] and because there is a wide range in the fluoride content of milk-based formulas, which more than 60% of infants drink, Adair and Wei recommended that no fluoride supplements be given to infants less than 6 months of age (with exception of breast-fed infants, who should be given 0.25 mg daily).[79] Singer and Ophaug stated that, in view of the wide range of fluoride intake in infants up to 6 months of age, only infants consuming breast milk or cow's milk and not milk-based formulas should be given 0.25-mg fluoride supplements if they live in nonfluoridated areas.[80] On the other hand, Driscoll and Horowitz suggested that in fluoride-free areas 0.25 mg (or 2 to 3 drops) of fluoride in solution be given daily from birth and continued until 2 years of age; then a 0.5-mg lozenge be given until the child is 3 years of age, up to 13.[81] (If the infant can manage a lozenge, it should be prescribed.) (See Table 11–8.)

This regimen of dietary fluoride supplementation has produced no objectionable dental fluorosis. Furthermore, beginning fluoride supplementation at birth probably gives some protection against caries to the deciduous teeth. Because calcification of the permanent dentition is just beginning during the first 6 months, very little if any fluorosis is likely to result from giving a 0.2- or 0.3-mg supplement. The Council on Dental Therapeutics of the American Dental Association endorses this regimen of fluoride supplementation of infants and children. Additional long-term research is necessary to establish optimum dosage, but the most suitable regimen now is that recommended by the American Dental Association.

Because fluoride is found everywhere, the natural level of fluoride in the drinking water should be determined before a fluoride supplement is prescribed. The following is a prescription for lozenges or tablets if there is no fluoride in the water supply. To avoid the possibility of dental fluorosis, the prescribed amount should be adjusted downward in proportion to the amount of fluoride provided in the water. For other appropriate doses, see the table of adjusted allowances (Table 11–6).

> Rx: Sodium fluoride tablets 2.2 mg
> Dispense 120 tablets
> Sig: One tablet each day to be chewed and swished before swallowing
> Caution: store out of reach of children

For the child between 2 and 3 years of age, the label directions can be changed to either one-half of a 2.2-mg tablet each day. More conveniently, a whole tablet containing 1.1 mg every day can be prescribed, if there is less than 0.2 ppm fluoride in the drinking water.

**TABLE 11–6. Adjusted Allowances of Sodium Fluoride Intake
Based on ppm Fluoride in Water Supply**

Water Fluoride (ppm)	Adjusted Allowance	
	Sodium Fluoride (mg/day)	*Provides Fluoride Ion (mg/day)*
0.0	2.2	1.0
0.2	1.8	0.8
0.4	1.3	0.6
0.6	0.9	0.4

The following is a prescription for fluoride solution:

Sodium fluoride 0.26 g
Distilled water to make 60 ml
Dispense in plastic dropper bottle that delivers 20 drops for each milliliter
Use each day, to be swished before swallowing
Caution: store out of reach of children

Each drop of this preparation will provide 0.1 mg of fluoride ion, and the appropriate number of drops is specified on the label. In fluoride-free areas, 3 drops or 0.3 mg is recommended.

Fluoride Rinses

Ripa et al. have shown that 3 years is necessary to achieve the maximum benefit from a rinse program for children.[82] This agrees with most other studies conducted. An additional year of rinsing did not reduce the caries rate further. Horowitz and Heifetz have reviewed the results of several studies showing caries reductions of 21 to 44%.[83] They concluded that the more frequent the use, the greater the inhibition of caries. DePaola et al.[85] found that ammonium fluoride reduces caries by 54%.[84] The lower incidence of caries on newly erupted teeth may have been due to a special effect of the fluoride ion.[85] A number of studies involving rinses once a week with high concentrations of fluoride (0.2%) showed caries reductions between 11 and 47%. Repeated use of 0.25% sodium fluoride twice daily or 0.5% fluoride gel daily over extended periods gave an 80% reduction. This level of fluoride is not recommended on a daily basis for a prolonged period because it may be toxic.

Bawden et al. found that fluoride mouth rinses were more effective in children with a higher caries baseline (normal level) than a low caries baseline.[86] The lower the incidence of caries, the more limited the effect of each preventive measure.

Ripa et al. found that combining 0.2% sodium fluoride rinses on a weekly basis with pit and fissure sealants increased the number of caries-free children and that the effects were cumulative.[87]

Sustained Release Delivery Systems

Several delivery systems have been developed for prolonged, precisely controlled fluoride release. The advantages of such systems are lower required dosage, reduced toxicity, release of a constant level of fluoride for a prolonged period, better use of fluoride at release site, and better patient compliance.[88] Clinical studies have shown that repeated exposure to low levels of fluoride is more effective in decreasing the incidence of caries than a single administration of fluoride gel at a high concentration[89] (most of which is lost in 36 hours).[90] The total effect is lost in one month.

Plaque has been shown to be a reservoir for fluoride's continuous release. A mechanism for providing the continuous release of fluoride or the reservoir may be the prolonged release systems. These include (1) sustained release fluoride tablets and (2) capsules and micro-encapsulated fluoride aerosols and control-release fluoride reservoirs. All of these produce high levels of fluoride in saliva and plaque without toxic or adverse side effects.

Sustained release dosage systems do not have uniform rates of release of fluoride, which minimizes their efficacy. The control release system has a potential for being an effective caries-preventing agent. This system could be useful in children who tend to get caries easily, patients with xerostomia (dry mouth), adults with rampant root or coronal caries, and mentally and/or physi-cally handicapped patients with newly exposed roots. Further evaluations should be made of these systems before they are widely used.[88]

Fluoridated Table Salt

Because table salt has been such an effective vehicle (carrier) for the addition of iodine to the diet, it was suggested that it be used for fluoride. There have been several studies with fluoridated table salt, but certain questions about the following have arisen: (1) determining the optimal concentration of fluoride in salt as related to the level of natural fluoride in water supplies; and (2) determining the amount of table salt that has to be ingested each day to produce a significant reduction in caries. It has been suggested that 200 to 300 mg[92, 93] of fluoride should be added to a kilogram of salt.[91, 92] The daily requirement for salt has not yet been determined, but the average adult consumes about 6 g.

When the effect of fluoridated salt on caries reduction was compared with that of fluoridated water, the salt was found to be about two-thirds as effective as the water (Table 11–7).[93] Studies in Latin America show that a 30 to 40% caries reduction was achieved when 90 mg of fluoride per kilogram of salt was used.[94]

TABLE 11–7. Caries Reduction in Permanent Tooth Surfaces of 9-Year-Old Children Who Used Fluoridated Table Salt or Fluoridated Water for 5½ Years

| | Percent Reduction in Carious Surfaces | | |
	Proximal	*Buccolabial*	*Occlusal*
Fluoridated salt	41	32	21
Fluoridated water	66	66	28

Fluoridated Milk

There have been studies in which milk has been used as a vehicle for fluoride administration. In one study, 1 mg of fluoride as sodium fluoride was added to a half pint of milk daily. The 80 children who drank this fluoridated milk for 4½ years had 80% less decay than did a control group.[95] In another study, fluoridated milk was found to be as effective as fluoridated water in reducing dental caries.[96]

Although several questions have been raised about the desirability of using milk as a vehicle for fluoride,[97] the same issues have been raised about water fluoridation and fortification of milk with vitamin D. For example, the consumption of both milk and water varies. Also, controlling the amount of fluoride added to milk is no more difficult than controlling the amount of added vitamin D. These types of problems have been discussed by several researchers.[98-101] Another question has been raised concerning the binding of the fluoride with the calcium and protein of the milk, thus making it unavailable to the tooth for anticariogenic action.[102] However, it has been demonstrated by a radioactive isotope technique that fluoride from milk is absorbed by the entire body, although more slowly than that from water.[103]

Thus it appears that long-term clinical studies would be appropriate to determine the efficacy of milk as a vehicle for fluoride.

SOME BIOCHEMICAL ASPECTS OF FLUORIDE ACQUISITION BY THE TOOTH

Fluoride uptake by the tooth via the pulp and other sources of blood supply takes place for the most part while the enamel is mineralizing. Under these circumstances the fluoride ion becomes incorporated within the body of the enamel crystal.

The salivary fluoride level is derived from systemic fluoride and exerts a topical effect on the tooth during the early posteruptive period when the enamel surface can be altered by the chemistry of the oral environment. Eating or drinking might speed up the clearance of fluoride from the mouth, and therefore should be postponed as much as possible after consumption or after topical application of fluoride. In this way, high levels of fluoride in saliva can be achieved for extended periods.

The enamel undergoes calcification starting as early as 12 to 16 weeks in utero for the first tooth that erupts, the deciduous central incisor. The calcification continues on until the last deciduous tooth erupts, namely, the second molar. This makes it possible for fluoride to affect the mineralization of the deciduous teeth if given early enough, that is, at birth in fluoride-free communities.

The first permanent tooth in which the enamel and dentin matrix is formed is the first molar. Some trace of mineralization occurs in this tooth as early as 28 weeks in utero. However, by 2½ to 3 years of age the enamel is usually completely formed. Therefore, fluoride ingestion must start some time before age 2, preferably at birth, in order to have the maximal benefit on the mineralization of the enamel (Fig. 11–6).

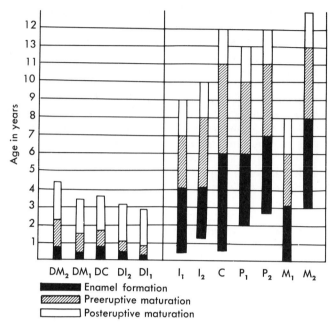

FIGURE 11–6. *Stage of formation and maturation of the enamel of each tooth type in the dentition at different ages. (From Brudevold, F. Fluoride therapy. In Bernier, J.; Muhler, J. C., eds. Improving Dental Practice Through Preventive Services, 3rd ed., p. 98. St. Louis, C. V. Mosby, 1975.)*

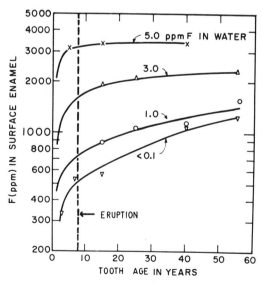

FIGURE 11–7. *Parts per million of fluoride in ash of surface enamel of teeth from areas with different levels of fluoride in the water supply. The dotted vertical line represents the time of eruption. (From Brudevold, F., et al., 1968.)*

The uptake of fluoride by enamel depends on the amount of fluoride ingested and on the age of the tooth at the time of fluoride exposure. The rate of uptake is very rapid during the first years and then tapers off (Fig. 11–7). Also, the higher the fluoride level in the water, the greater is the initial rate of deposition during tooth mineralization.

The ability of fluoride to be a cariostatic agent depends on genetic and environmental factors operating in the mouth (e.g., the degree of caries challenge by the amount of sugar-sweetened snacks and condition of the enamel). Thus great individual variation may be seen in the efficacy of fluoride in reducing the incidence of caries. DePaola et al. have shown a large disparity between fluoride concentration in enamel of individuals and caries experience.[84] Keene et al. have shown that caries-free subjects tend to have a higher fluoride level on the surface enamel and to live in fluoridated communities.[104]

MECHANISMS OF ANTICARIES ACTION OF FLUORIDE

For the last 4 decades, the element fluoride has been established as both the most used anticaries agent and the most useful agent in preventive dentistry. Since 1946, when Bibby first investigated the use of fluoride as a rinse,[105] it has been incorporated in a number of vehicles ranging from water to the more complex one, dentifrice. The ability of fluoride to help prevent tooth decay has been established by a vast number of clinical studies. Prescription drugs in the form of gels or rinses with high concentrations of fluoride have been used by dentists with excellent results.

There are three mechanisms by which fluoride inhibits caries, and usually more than one is involved.[60, 106, 107] These mechanisms are (1) an increase in the enamel's resistance to acid solubility as a result of a high concentration of fluoride in the outer enamel surface; (2) the ability of fluoride to remineralize demineralized or hypomineralized enamel; and (3) fluoride's antibacterial effects on plaque growth, glycolysis, glycogen synthesis, acid production, production of extracellular polysaccharides necessary for plaque adhesion to tooth surface, and solubility of calcium phosphate deposits within plaque.

The amount of caries protection a tooth will receive from fluoride depends on the extent and intensity of the challenge (sugar consumption, cariogenic plaque bacteria, deep fissures, and so forth). When the local challenges are very great, previous conditioning of the tooth with fluoride will not be able to overcome their destructive effects. Therefore it is likely that there is not a specific frequency of exposure or level of fluoride in enamel that can be expected to be 100% effective in the prevention of caries under all conditions.

Decreases in Acid Solubility

It has been shown that enamel formed in the presence of fluoride has more perfect and larger crystals, is less soluble in acid, and is less likely to develop caries. This happens because fluoride favors the formation of fluorapatite, a more acid-resistant apatite than the hydroxyapatite formed in the absence of fluoride.[108–110] The hydroxyl ion is replaced by the fluoride ion in the apatite lattice.

The apatite crystal is less stable and more soluble when it includes hydroxyl ions than when it contains fluoride ions because there are voids throughout the lattice where the hydroxyl ions cannot fit. The fluoride ion can enter and tighten the lattice and eliminate these voids, with the result that apatite becomes more stable and less soluble to acid. Thus a high concentration of fluorapatite on the outer surface of the enamel prevents or retards acid demineralization.

It has been noted that the rate of solubility to acid is relatively unimportant in protecting the tooth against caries.[109, 111]

Remineralization

Caries is believed to involve the intermittent dissolution of enamel. When carbohydrate is ingested, the pH drops because of acid formation, and there is some demineralization. During the interval between meals, the pH rises, which results in a certain amount of reprecipitation of minerals, or remineralization. Small amounts of fluoride enhance remineralization and reduce the amount of calcium and phosphate dissolution.[112] The greater the concentration of fluoride released from the dissolved enamel or already present in the plaque, the more will remineralization be favored and the more will the carious process be slowed.[113] However, Pigman et al.[114] and Kolourides et al.[115] have shown that fluoride levels as low as 1 ppm enhance remineralization.

Other studies have shown that enamel, cementum, and dentin remineralized in the presence of fluoride and saliva are more resistant to subsequent acid attack.[60, 61, 116–120] Zahradnik has shown in vitro that the use of fluoride rinses appears to favor greater deposition of mineral over the entire carious lesion in the presence of saliva by increasing subsurface remineralization.[121] When saliva is absent or diminished, or when rampant caries are present, the use of calcium phosphate remineralizing solutions in the presence of fluoride has been highly effective in promoting remineralization of both coronal and root caries.[60] Thus this type of oral health management system has been very effective in protecting those at high risk of dental caries, e.g., patients with head and neck radiation, patients with Sjögren's or other systemic diseases, and persons with drug-induced xerostomia (dry mouth).

A short-term intensive use of topical fluoride is used to raise the fluoride level of the tooth surface and underlying tissues to a level expected to protect against caries. (This level has been seen in moderately fluorosed teeth or remineralized enamel lesions.) The fluoride level is then maintained through daily use of fluoride toothpaste or the use of concentrated calcium phosphate-fluoride solutions at least twice daily to augment the physiological maintenance system and to provide new sites for mineral growth. This is done after meticulous oral hygiene (brushing, flossing, and cleaning with a cotton swab) to allow the chemicals to have direct contact with the tooth surface. Also salivary flow is mechanically stimulated through the use of an inert chewing gum.

Antibacterial Action

A third mechanism of action of fluoride in reducing caries is its antibacterial effect. It may have a bactericidal (destructive to bacteria) action and/or an antiplaque action. From a bactericidal standpoint, fluoride will inhibit many enzymes essential to cell metabolism and growth, such as enolase, an enzyme involved in carbohydrate metabolism. Specifically, the fluoride ion has an inhibitory effect on glycolysis (an enzymatic breakdown of carbohydrate), and the cells are unable to produce energy; therefore they die. From an antiplaque standpoint, it has been suggested that fluoride can lower the surface energy of the tooth, thereby making bacterial attachment and plaque formation difficult.[122] Also, fluoride can desorb (strip off) bacteria from hydroxyapatite because the fluoride can bind more effectively to positively charged areas on the apatite crystal than can the bacteria.

All these effects are likely to occur after a high topical dose of fluoride and are limited to the duration of fluoride's release from the tooth surface. Without reapplication of fluoride, the antibacterial effect will last from less than a day to a few weeks.[60, 61]

Although it has been claimed that children from areas with high fluoride levels accumulate less plaque than children from areas with low fluoride levels, a comprehensive microbiological study by Kilian et al. of plaque flora was unable to detect any significant difference between these children.[123]

CLINICAL CONSIDERATIONS IN SYSTEMIC FLUORIDE THERAPY

Dental Benefits

On the average, the consumption of fluoridated water is not a great concern because the amount of such water ingested varies with age and climate, a fact that is taken into account when communal waters are fluoridated. However, when fluoride supplements are used, the optimal dosage for different groups must be prescribed precisely. This was described in detail earlier in this chapter.

Fluorosis of the deciduous teeth is rarely seen and is not a problem. The first 2 to 3 years of life are the most critical period for the development of mottled enamel on the permanent anterior teeth and for this reason only 0.25 mg/day is prescribed from birth until 2 years of age, 0.5 mg/day from 2 to 3 years of age, and 1.0 mg/day from 3 until 13 years of age.

According to a report by Horowitz on school water fluoridation programs, no objectionable dental fluorosis resulted when 4.5 ppm of fluoride was consumed on a part-time basis (only during school hours) by children aged 5 or 6 and older.[124] He did find that the anticaries effect differed in teeth of different eruption ages. Canines, premolars, and second molars, which erupted at around 9 to 13 years of age, derived greater protection from caries than did the incisors and first molars, which erupted earlier (from 6 to 8 years of age).

The use of fluoridated water or fluoride supplements will enhance the formation of the relatively caries-resistant fluorapatite in the enamel surface during the pre-eruptive period of maturation and also—but to a lesser extent—in the early stage after eruption. Thus, the use of fluoridated water or fluoride supplements continuously from birth through age 13 will provide pre-eruptive and posteruptive anticaries benefits for the deciduous and the permanent teeth.

Fluoride dietary supplementation begun at 1 year of age should provide posteruptive benefits for the deciduous incisors, pre-eruptive and posteruptive benefits for the deciduous molars and cuspids, and full benefits for the permanent dentition. Supplementation at age 3 will provide benefits to the permanent teeth only. However, it would have a pre-eruptive as well as a posteruptive effect on all the permanent teeth. If fluoride supplements are delayed until the age of 6, the incisors and first molars will receive only partial benefits but significant benefits would be provided to cuspids, premolars, and second molars.[125]

A guide for fluoride therapy is shown in Figure 11–8. It will provide the dental health professional with the appropriate combination of systemic and topical fluoride therapies for different age-range groupings. It considers the availability of communal fluoridated water to the patient. The age-range groupings are based on the recommended fluoride dosage and the appropriate fluoride vehicles for the age period. The major objective of this guide is to provide a safe amount of fluoride during tooth formation and maturation in order to achieve maximal protection against dental caries. After selecting the section of the guide appropriate for age and the presence or absence of fluoridated water, one can make treatment decisions by referring to several blocks, in which check marks ($\sqrt{}$) indicate the specific therapy recommended and minus marks ($-$) indicate that the therapy is not recommended. IC means individual consideration related to a medical or dental problem.

Therapy for Osteoporosis and Effects on Periodontal Disease

Variable doses of fluoride (25 to 150 mg/day for up to 1 year) have been used therapeutically for osteoporosis.[126] These doses are given in combination

PATIENT'S AGE	0–2		2–3		3–6		6–9		9–14		14–17		17–+	
SYSTEMIC THERAPY Fluoridated communal H$_2$O (1 ppm) Equivalent of 4 glasses/day	YES	NO	YES	NO	YES	NO	YES	NO	YES	NO	YES	NO	YES	NO
Drops (0.1 mg F) daily	—	0.3	—	—	—	—	—	—	—	—	—	—	—	—
Lozenges (1.0 mg F) daily allow to dissolve slowly	—	—	—	0.5	—	1.0	—	1.0	—	1.0	—	—	—	—
TOPICAL THERAPY Professional (1.2% F) 60 mg F semiannual applications plus 4 weekly applications on newly erupted teeth	—	—	—	—	✔	✔	✔	✔	✔	✔	✔	✔	IC	IC
Dentifrice (0.1% F) 1 mg F brush for 3 minutes, twice a day	—	—	✔	✔	✔	✔	✔	✔	✔	✔	✔	✔	✔	✔
Oral Rinse (.02% F) 1 mg F daily or (0.2% F) 2 mg F weekly one teaspoon or tablespoon for 1–2 minutes	—	—	—	—	—	—	✔ t	✔ t	✔ T	✔ T	✔ T	✔ T	✔ T	✔ T
Custom Dental Tray (0.5% F) 3 mg F 10 drops for 30 daily consecutive 5 minute applications and once a week thereafter	—	—	—	—	IC	IC	IC	IC	IC	IC	IC	IC	IC	IC

FIGURE 11–8. Suggested guide for fluoride therapy to prevent and control dental caries. $-$ = Not recommended; ✔ = recommended; IC = individual consideration (cardiac, hemophilia, rampant caries); t = teaspoonful; T = tablespoonful.

with hormonal treatment, and special emphasis is placed on the intake of calcium, phosphorus, vitamin D, and protein. Also, physical activity is encouraged.

There is limited evidence that periodontal disease may occur less in communities with fluoridated water.[127]

SUMMARY

Water-borne fluorides, which originally were observed to cause an unattractive discoloration and deformity of tooth enamel (mottled enamel) when ingested at levels above 2 ppm, later were proved to be essential for dental health because they reduced the incidence of dental decay when ingested daily at optimal levels of 1 ppm. At this recommended level of intake, fluorides are safe. In addition, the efficiency of the kidney in eliminating fluoride and the affinity of calcified structures for fluoride provide a mechanism for maintaining a low, safe level of fluoride in body tissues and fluids. There is no scientific evidence of any allergy, cancer linkage, or other general health disability caused by using the optimally fluoridated water supply.

The best source of fluorides is fluoridation of communal water supplies. School water fluoridation and dietary fluoride supplements are alternatives, particularly if there are legal (political) or technical engineering reasons for not artificially fluoridating communal water supplies. Many different long-range studies have shown that the ingestion of artificially fluoridated water continuously from infancy throughout life will reduce the caries incidence within a range of 50 to 70%.

Systemic fluoride intake is recommended from birth through the early teens to enrich the enamel with apatite fluoride. This fluoride remains permanently and can effectively resist caries throughout life, given the usual and customary local cariogenic challenges.

Fluoride acts to reduce dental decay (1) by stabilizing the apatite lattice so that it has a more perfect structure, which increases its resistance to acid demineralization; (2) by prompting remineralization of carious lesions; and (3) by lessening bacterial acid formation and plaque formation.

Based on knowledge from epidemiological, clinical, microbiological, animal, and in vitro physiochemical studies, fluoride, even at low concentrations, is necessary in oral fluids to obtain maximal inhibition of caries. Thus continuous or frequent supplementation is necessary to combat caries at any age. A combination of systemic fluoride plus regular topical application is the most effective way to utilize fluoride.

Fluorides, in addition to providing significant protection against dental decay, should be considered as an adjunct in the management of osteoporosis in older people.

REFERENCES

1. Committee on Dietary Allowances, Food and Nutrition Board, National Academy of Sciences-National Research Council. Recommended Dietary Allowances, 9th rev. Washington, D.C., National Academy Press, 1980.

2. Messer, H.H.; Singer, L. Fluoride. In Present Knowledge in Nutrition: Nutrition Reviews, 4th ed., pp. 325–336. Washington, D.C., Nutrition Foundation, 1976.
3. Osis, D., et al. Dietary fluoride intake in man. J. Nutr. 104:1313, 1974.
4. Kramer, L., et al. Dietary fluoride in different areas in the United States. Am. J. Clin. Nutr. 27:590, 1974.
5. Hodge, H.C; Smith, F.A. Some public health aspects of water fluoridation. In Shaw, J.H., ed. Fluoridation as Public Health Measure. Washington, D.C., American Association for the Advancement of Science, 1954.
6. Dean, H.T. Endemic fluorosis and the relation to dental caries. Public Health Rep. 53:1443, 1938.
7. Ekstrand, J.; Ehraebo, M. Influence of milk products on bioavailability in man. Eur. J. Clin. Pharmacol. 16:211, 1979.
8. Hodge, H.C.; Smith, F.A. Minerals: fluorine and dental caries. In Gould, R.F., ed. Dietary Chemicals vs. Dental Caries, p. 93. Advances in Chemistry Series 94. Washington, D.C., American Chemical Society, 1970.
9. Zipkin, I.; Lee, W.A.; Leone, N.C. Role of urinary fluoride output in normal adults. Am. J. Public Health 47:848, 1957.
10. Zipkin, I.; Likins, R.C.; McClure, F.J., et al. Urinary fluoride levels associated with the use of fluoridated water. Public Health Rep. 71:767, 1956.
11. Machle, W., et al. Absorption and excretion of fluorides: normal fluoride balance. J. Ind. Hyg. Toxicol. 24:199, 1942.
12. Isaac, S.; Brudevold, F.; Smith, F.A., et al. The relation of fluoride in the drinking water to the distribution of fluoride in the enamel. J. Dent. Res. 37:254, 1958.
13. Leone, N.C.; Shimkin, M.G.; Arnold, F.A., et al. Medical aspects of excessive fluoride in water supply. Public Health Rep. 69:925, 1954.
14. Weidmann, S.M.; Weatherell, J.A.; Jackson, D. The effect of fluoride on bone. Proc. Nutr. Soc. 22:105, 1963.
15. Roholm, K. Fluorine Intoxication. London, H.K. Lewisand Co. Ltd., 1937.
16. Hodge, H.C. Safety factors in water fluoridation based on the toxicology of fluoride. Proc. Nutr. Soc. 22:111, 1963.
17. A statement on the question of allergy to fluoride as used in the fluoridation of community water supplies. J. Allergy 47:347, 1971.
18. World Health Organization. Fluorides and Human Health. Monograph Series 59, 1970.
19. World Health Organization. Thirty-first World Health Assembly F1-101, July 1978.
20. Erickson, J.D. Mortality in selected cities with fluoridated and non-fluoridated water supplies. N. Engl. J. Med. 298:1112, 1978.
21. Rogot, E., et al. Trends in urban mortality in relation to fluoridation status. Am. J. Epidemiol. 107:104, 1978.
22. Upton, A.C. Statement on relationship of fluoridation of drinking water to cancer. Intergovernmental Relations and Human Resources Subcommittee, House Committee on Government Operations, September 21, 1977.
23. Hoover, R.N., et al. Fluoridated drinking waters and the occurrence of cancer. J. Natl. Cancer Inst. 57:757, 1975.
24. Taves, D.R. Fluoridation and cancer mortality. Cold Spring Harbor Conf. Cell Prolif. 4:357, 1977.
25. Doll, R.; Kinlen, L. Fluoridation of water and cancer mortality in the U.S.A. Lancet 1:1300, 1977.
26. Hagan, T.L.; Pasternack, M.; Scholtz, G.C. Waterborne fluorides and mortality. Public Health Rep. 69:450, 1954.
27. Reuter, F.W., et al. In Vischer, T.L., ed. Fluoride in Medicine, pp. 143–152. Bern, Hans Huber Publishers, 1971.
28. Morichini, D. Analisi dello smalto di un dente fossile di elefante e dei denti umani. Mem. Mat. Fic. Soc. Ital. Sci. 12 (Pt. 2):73, 1805.
29. Gay-Lussac, J. Sur la présence de l'acide fluorique dans les substances animals et sur la pierre alumineuse de la Tolfa. Ann. Chim. 55:258, 1803.
30. Berzelius, J. Correspondenz Neues Allgem. J. Chem. 6:590, 1806.
31. Magitot, E. Treatise on Dental Caries, p. 151. Translated by Chandler, T.H. Boston, Houghton, Osgood and Co., 1878.
32. Crichton-Browne, J. Tooth culture. Lancet 2:6, 1892.
33. Eager, J.M. Denti di chiae. Public Health Rep. 16:2576, 1901.
34. Black, G.V.; McKay, F.S. Mottled teeth: an endemic developmental imperfection of the enamel of the teeth heretofore unknown in the literature of dentistry. Dent. Cosmos 58:129, 477, 627, 781, 849, 1916.
35. McKay, F.S. The establishment of a definite relation between enamel that is defective in its structure as mottled enamel, and liability to decay. Dent. Cosmos 71:747, 1929.
36. Churchill, H.V. Occurrence of fluoride in some waters of the United States. Ind. Eng. Chem. 23:996, 1931.
37. Smith, M.C.; Lantz, D.M.; Smith, H.V. The cause of mottled enamel; a defect of human teeth. Univ. Arizona Agric. Exp. Stat. Tech. Bull. 32:253, 1931.
38. McKay, F.S. Mottled enamel: early history and its unique features. In Moulton, E.R., ed. Fluorine

and Dental Health. Washington, D.C., American Association for the Advancement of Science, 1942.

39. Dean, H.T.; Jay, P.; Arnold, F.A., Jr., et al. Domestic water and dental caries. II. A study of 2832 white children, aged 12–14 years of eight suburban Chicago communities, including *Lactobacillus acidophilus* studies of 1761 of children. Public Health Rep. 56:761, 1941.

40. Dean, H.T.; Arnold, F.A., Jr.; Elvove, E. Domestic water and dental caries. V. Additional studies of the relation of fluoride domestic waters to dental experience in 4425 white children aged 12 to 14 years of 13 cities in 4 states. Public Health Rep. 57:1155, 1942.

41. Driscoll, W.S.; Horowitz, H.S.; Meyers, R.J., et al. Prevalence of dental caries and dental fluorosis in areas with negligible, optimal and above-optimal fluoride concentrations in drinking water. J. Am. Dent. Assoc. 113:29, 1986.

42. Ockerse, T. Endemic fluorosis in the Kenhardt and Gordonia districts, Cape Province, South Africa. J. Am. Dent. Assoc. 28:936, 1941.

43. Striffler, D.F. Fluoridation in New Mexico: its present status. N.M. Dent. J. 5:3, 1955.

44. Forrest, J.R. Caries incidence and enamel defects in areas with different levels of fluoride in the drinking water. Br. Dent. J. 100:195, 1956.

45. Forsman, B. Dental fluorosis and caries in high-fluoride districts in Sweden. Community Dent. Oral Epidemiol. 7:51, 1979.

46. Olsson, B. Dental findings in high-fluoride areas in Ethiopia. Community Dent. Oral Epidemiol. 7:51, 1979.

47. Tewari, A.; Joshi, J.L. Interrelationship of dental caries and different levels of fluoride in drinking water—an epidemiological study in an endemic fluoride area of rural northern India. Scientific Proceedings of the 10th Asian Pacific Dental Conference, Singapore Dental Association, p. 9, 1981.

48. Bronson, M.E. Dental health in an area of maximum water fluoridation. Dent. Hyg. 56:39, 1982.

49. Leverett, D.H. Fluorides and the changing prevalence of dental caries. Science 217:26, 1982.

50. Ast, D.B. The caries-fluorine hypothesis and a suggested study to test its application. Public Health Rep. 58:857, 1943.

51. Ast, D.B.; Smith, D.J.; Wochs, B., et al. Newburgh-Kingston caries-fluorine study. XIV. Combined clinical and roentgenographic dental finding after ten years of fluoride experience. J. Am. Dent. Assoc. 52:314, 1956.

52. Hayes, R.L.; Lilleton, N.W.; White, C.L. Posteruptive effect of fluoridation on first permanent molars of children in Grand Rapids, Michigan. Am. J. Public Health 47:192, 1957.

53. Hutton, W.L.; Linscott, B.W.; Williams, D.B. The Brantford fluorine experiment: interim report after 5 years of water fluoridation. Can. J. Public Health 42:81, 1951.

54. Blayney, J.R.; Hill, I.N. Fluorine and dental caries. J. Am. Dent. Assoc. 74:233, 1967.

55. Ast, D.B., et al. Time and cost factors to provide regular, periodic dental care for children in fluoridated and nonfluoridated areas: final report. J. Am. Dent. Assoc. 80:770, 1970.

56. Lemke, C.W., et al. Controlled fluoridation: the dental effects of discontinuation in Antigo, Wisconsin. J. Am. Dent. Assoc. 80:782, 1970.

57. Newbrun, E. Cost effectiveness and practicality features in the systemic use of fluorides. In Burt, B., ed. The Relative Efficiency of Methods of Caries Prevention in Dental Public Health. Ann Arbor, University of Michigan Press, 1978.

58. Jackson, D. An epidemiological study of dental caries prevalence in adults. Arch. Oral Biol. 6:80, 1961.

59. Stamm, J.W.; Banting, D.W. The occurrence of root caries in adults with a lifelong history of fluoridated water consumption. J. Dent. Res. 57:149, 1978 (Abstract).

60. Johansen, E.; Papas, A., et al. Remineralization of carious lesions in elderly patients. Gerodontics 3:47, 1987.

61. Featherstone, J., et al. Remineralization of artificial caries-like lesions in vivo by a self-administered mouth rinse or paste. Caries Res. 16:235, 1982.

62. Johansen, E.: Taves, D.R.; Olsen, T.O. Continuing evaluation of the use of fluorides. Am. Assoc. Adv. Sci. 11:61, 1979.

63. Committee on Nutrition. Fluoride supplementation. Pediatrics 77:758, 1986.

64. Changing patterns of oral health and implications for oral health manpower. Part 1, Joint report Federation Dentaire Internationale and World Health Organization. Internationale Dentaire 35:235, 1985.

65. Glass, R.L., ed. The First International Conference on the Declining Prevalence of Dental Caries. J. Dent. Res. 61:1304, 1982.

66. Brunelle, J.A.; Carlos, J.P. Changes in the prevalence of dental caries in U.S. school children. J. Dent. Res. 61:1346, 1982.

67. The United States Environmental Protection Agency's Contribution to the Adequate Supply of Safe Drinking Water for All Americans. Washington, D.C., GPO, 1972.

68. Horowitz, H.S., et al. Effect of school water fluoridation on dental caries in St. Thomas, V.I. Public Health Rep. 80:381, 1965.

69. Horowitz, H.S., et al. Effect of school water fluoridation on dental caries: final results in Elk Lake, Pa. after 12 years. J. Am. Dent. Assoc. 84:832, 1972.

70. Heifetz, S.B., et al. Effect of school water fluoridation on dental caries: results in Seagrove, N.C. after eight years. J. Am. Dent. Assoc. 97:193, 1978.
71. Driscoll, W.S. The use of dietary fluoride supplements in the prevention of dental caries. In Forrester, D.J.; Schulz, E.M., eds. International Workshops on Fluorides and Dental Caries Reductions, pp. 25–96. Baltimore, University of Maryland School of Dentistry, 1974.
72. Marthaler, T.M. Caries inhibiting effect of fluoride tablets. Helv. Odont. Acta 13:1, 1969.
73. Gedalia, I. Fluoride tablets. Int. Dent. J. 17:18, 1967.
74. Drinkard, C.R., et al. Enamel fluoride in nursing rats with mothers drinking water with high fluoride concentrations. J. Dent. Res. 64:877, 1985.
75. Parker, P.R.; Bawden, J.H. Prenatal fluoride exposure: measurement of plasma levels and enamel uptake in the guinea pig. J. Dent. Res. 65:1341, 1986.
76. Schutzmannsky, G. Fluorine tablet application in pregnant females. Dtsch. Stomatol. 21:122, 1971.
77. Driscoll, W.S. A review of clinical research on the use of prenatal fluoride administration for prevention of dental caries. J. Dent. Child. 100:9, 1981.
78. Aasenden, R.; Peebles, T.C. Effects of fluoride supplementation from birth on human deciduous and permanent teeth. Arch. Oral Biol. 19:321, 1974.
79. Adair, S.M.; Wei, S. Supplemental fluoride recommendation for infants based on dietary fluoride intake. Caries Res. 12:76, 1978.
80. Singer, L.; Ophaug, R. Total fluoride intake of infants. Pediatrics 63:460, 1979.
81. Driscoll, W.S.; Horowitz, H.S. A discussion of optimal dosage for dietary fluoride supplementation. J. Am. Dent. Assoc. 96:1050, 1978.
82. Ripa, L.W., et al. Supervised weekly rinsing with a 0.2% neutral sodium fluoride solution: results from a demonstration program after three school years. J. Am. Dent. Assoc. 100:544, 1980.
83. Horowitz, H.S.; Heifetz, S.B. The current status of topically applied fluorides in preventive dentistry. In Newbrun, E., ed. Fluoride and Dental Caries: Contemporary Concepts for Practitioners and Students, pp. 46–78. Springfield, Ill., Charles C Thomas, 1975.
84. DePaola, P.F., et al. Effect of high-concentration ammonium and sodium fluoride solution on dental caries in school children. Community Dent. Oral Epidemiol. 5:7, 1977.
85. DePaola, P.F., et al. A pilot study of the relationship between caries experience and surface enamel fluoride in man. Arch. Oral Biol. 20:859, 1975.
86. Bawden, J.W., et al. Effect of mouthrinsing with a sodium fluoride solution in children with different caries experience. Swed. Dent. J. 4:111, 1980.
87. Ripa, L.W., et al. The combined use of pit and fissure sealants and fluoride mouthrinsing in second and third grade children: one-year clinical results. Pediatr. Dent. 8:158, 1986.
88. McKnight, C.; Hanes, P.J. Effective delivery systems for prolonged fluoride release: review of literature. J. Am. Dent. Assoc. 113:431, 1986.
89. Mellberg, J.R.; Ripa, L.W. Fluorides in Preventive Dentistry, pp. 15–80. Chicago, Quintessence Publishing Co., 1983.
90. Mellberg, J.R., et al. The acquisition and loss of fluoride by topically fluoridated tooth enamel. Arch. Oral Biol. 11:1212, 1966.
91. Wespi, H.J. Experiences and problems of fluoridated cooking salt in Switzerland. Arch. Oral Biol. 6:33, 1961.
92. Muhlemann, H.R. Fluoridated domestic salt: discussion of dosage. Int. Dent. J. 17:10, 1967.
93. Marthaler, T.J.; Schenardi, C. Inhibition of caries in children after 5.5 years use of fluoridated table salt. Helv. Odontol. Acta. 6:1, 1962.
94. Carlos, J.J., ed. Prevention and Oral Health, p. 23. DHEW Public Health Series Publication no. 74–707. Bethesda, Md., National Institutes of Health, 1973.
95. Rusoff, L.L., et al. Fluoride addition to milk and its effect on dental caries in school children. Am. J. Clin. Nutr. 11:94, 1962.
96. Winz, R. Schweiz. Monatsch. Zahn. 74:767, 1964.
97. Pearlman, S. Untested alternatives to fluoridation of domestic water supplies. J. Am. Dent. Assoc. 46:287, 1953.
98. Stephen, K.W.; Boyle, I.T.; Campbell, D., et al. A 4-year double-blind fluoridated school milk study in a vitamin D–deficient area. Br. Dent. J. 151:287, 1981.
99. Banoczy, J.; Zimmerman, P.; Pinter, A., et al. Effect of fluoridated milk on caries: 3-year results. Community Dent. Oral Epidemiol. 11:81, 1983.
100. Legett, B.J.; Garbes, W.H.: Gardiner, J.F., et al. The effect of fluoridated chocolate flavored milk on caries incidence in elementary school children: two and three-year studies. J. Dent. Child. 54:18, 1987.
101. Zahlaka, M.; Metre, O.; Munder, H., et al. The effect of fluoridated milk on caries in Arab children: results after 3 years. Clin. Prev. Dent. 9:23, 1987.
102. Nikiforuk, G.; Fraser, D. Fluoride supplements for prophylaxis of dental caries. J. Can. Dent. Assoc. 30:67, 1964.
103. Ericsson, Y. The state of fluorine in milk and its absorption and retention when administered in milk; investigations with radioactive fluorine. Acta Odont. Scand. 16:51, 1958.
104. Keene, H.J.; Mellberg, J.R.; Nicholson, C.R. History of fluoride, dental fluorosis and concentrations

of fluoride in surface layer enamel of caries-free naval recruits. J. Public Health Dent. 33:142, 1973.

105. Bibby, B.G. Topical applications of fluorides as a method of combating dental caries. In Moulton, F.A., ed. Dental Caries and Fluorine, p. 93. Washington, D.C., American Association for the Advancement of Science, 1946.

106. Fejerskov, O., et al. Rational use of fluorides in caries prevention. A concept based on the possible cariostatic mechanisms. Acta Odont. Scand. 39:241, 1981.

107. Forrester, D.J.; Schulz, E.M., ed. International Workshop on Fluorides and Dental Caries Reductions. Baltimore, University of Maryland School of Dentistry, 1974.

108. Isaac, S., et al. Solubility rate and natural fluoride content of surface and subsurface enamel. J. Dent. Res. 37:254, 1958.

109. Brudevold, F.; McCann, H.G. Enamel solubility tests and their significance in regard to dental caries. Ann. N.Y. Acad. Sci. 153:20, 1968.

110. Larsen, M.J. Dissolution of enamel. Scand. J. Dent. Res. 81:518, 1973.

111. Brown, W.E., et al. Effects of fluoride on enamel solubility and cariostasis. Caries Res. 11 (Suppl.1):118, 1977.

112. Brown, W.E.; König, K.G., eds. Cariostatic Mechanisms of Fluorides. Caries Res. 11 (Suppl. 1): 1977.

113. Jenkins, G.N. Recent advances in work on fluorides and the teeth. Br. Med. Bull. 31:192, 1975.

114. Pigman, W.; Cueto, H.; Baugh, D. Conditions affecting rehardening of softened enamel. J. Dent. Res. 43:1187, 1964.

115. Koulourides, T.; Feagin, F.; Pigman, W. Remineralization of dental enamel by saliva in vitro. Ann. N.Y. Acad. Sci. 131:751, 1965.

116. Corpron, R.E., et al. In vivo remineralization of artificial enamel lesions by a fluoride dentifrice or mouthrinse. Caries Res. 20:48, 1986.

117. Koulourides, T.; Cameron, B. Enamel remineralization as a factor in the pathogenesis of dental caries. J. Oral Pathol. 9:255, 1980.

118. Ten Cate, J. M.; Arends, J. Remineralization of artificial enamel lesions in vitro. Caries Res. 15:60, 1981.

119. Gelhard, T., et al. Rehardening of artificial enamel lesions in vivo. Caries Res. 13:80, 1979.

120. Mellberg, J.R.; Chomicki, W. Fluoride uptake by artificial caries lesions from fluoride dentifrices in vivo. J. Dent. Res. 62:540, 1983.

121. Zahradnik, P.T. Effect of fluoride rinses upon in vitro enamel remineralization. J. Dent. Res. 59:1065, 1980.

122. Scholtaus, J.D.; Arends, J. Influence of fluoridating varnishes on dentine in vitro. Caries Res. 20:65, 1986.

123. Kilian, M., et al. Predominant plaque flora of Tanzanian children exposed to high and low water fluoride concentration. Caries Res. 13:330, 1979.

124. Horowitz, H.S. A review of systemic and topical fluorides for the prevention of dental caries. Community Dent. Oral Epidemiol. 1:104, 1973.

125. Brudevold, F. Fluoride therapy. In Bernier, J.L.; Muhler, J.C., eds. Improving Dental Practice Through Preventive Measures, 3rd ed. St. Louis, C.V. Mosby Co., 1975.

126. Reutler, F.W., et al. In Vischer, T.L., ed. Fluoride in Medicine, pp. 143–152. Bern, Hans Huber, 1971.

127. Adler, P. In Fluorides in Human Health, pp. 323–354. Geneva, World Health Organization, 1970.

12

Trace Minerals Other Than Fluorides

By definition, essential trace minerals, also known as trace elements or microminerals, are inorganic nutrients that are required by humans in very small amounts [from micrograms (0.001 milligram) to no more than a few milligrams—less than 100 mg/day for humans]. A trace mineral is essential for humans when it has a vital function and is required to avoid a deficiency disease.[1] Also, if the trace minerals (e.g., manganese, molybdenum, selenium, chromium, and cobalt) are concerned with enzyme actions and are identified in normal human enzyme systems, they are also considered essential. The trace elements for which there are recommended daily allowances are iron, iodine, and zinc.[2] For copper and fluorine, estimated safe ranges and adequate intakes have been ascertained.[2]

One of the major thrusts in nutrition research is an in-depth study of the human requirement of microminerals and of the roles they play in good health.

Some persons are quite concerned about a possible deficiency of a specific micromineral in their food intake. Yet, it is not recommended that individuals (1) use organically grown foods as a source for the microminerals that have not yet been found essential, or (2) take trace element pharmaceutical preparations as a supplement for these important reasons:

1. All microminerals can be toxic at a small increase over usual intakes; therefore supplements should be used only at recommended dietary allowance levels or at estimated safe and adequate daily dietary intake levels.

2. Microminerals are generally present in adequate amounts in a mixed diet consisting of a variety of foodstuffs and iodized salt.

3. Microminerals are not usually in short supply in farm soils. When they are, they can be added as inorganic fertilizers.

4. Theoretically, the compost or manure used in producing organically grown foods may provide more microminerals to foods than will chemical fertilizers. However, the organic (natural) fertilizers contain microminerals such as aluminum, antimony, and others that have not been proved essential for good health in plants and animals.

5. After a requirement for a micromineral has been established by nutrition scientists, it should be included in the food enrichment program. For example, iodine and iron have been added to one or more common foods.

Modes of Action

Trace elements act as catalysts either as metallo-enzymes (in which the trace element is an integral part of the enzyme molecule) or as metal-enzymes (in which the metal ion is loosely associated with the enzyme). Iron, zinc, copper, and molybdenum display the metallo-enzyme characteristic; for example, copper is firmly bound and incorporated in the protein molecule of the enzyme tyrosinase. An example of a metal-enzyme is arginase, which is physically separate from the manganese that activates it.

Trace elements also function as constituents and activators of hormones; examples are iodine, found in thyroid hormones, and chromium, which activates insulin. Cobalt is a trace element that acts as a structural center of the vitamin B_{12} molecule.

Dietary Sources and Classification

Meat, fish, and natural plant foods such as grains, beans, fruits, and vegetables are good sources of essential trace elements. On the other hand, the consumption of highly refined or processed foods substantially reduces the intake of essential micronutrients, unless these foods are fortified to concentrations at least equal to those naturally occurring in the product.

There are many trace elements. For convenience of discussion, the trace elements can be divided into two categories:

1. Those that have well-defined human requirements, namely, iron, zinc, iodine, copper and fluorine

2. Those that are integral constituents or activators of enzymes, namely, manganese, molybdenum, selenium, chromium, and cobalt

This chapter will deal briefly with the nutritional aspects of those trace elements for which there is a known human requirement.

Iron

Because iron in hemoglobin is involved in oxygen transport and cellular respiration, it is one of the most important minerals in nutrition. Although myoglobin has only one-quarter the iron of hemoglobin, it serves as an oxygen reserve in muscle metabolism. The total quantity of iron in the body averages about 4 g, and consists of two major fractions—70% essential body iron (hemoglobin, myoglobin, and intracellular enzymes such as cytochrome) and 30% mobilizable iron reserves (ferritin and hemosiderin).

PHYSIOLOGICAL FUNCTIONS

Absorption. Humans have difficulty in absorbing iron efficiently. Only 7 to 10% of the iron in cereals and vegetables and 10 to 30% of the iron in animal protein and soybeans can be absorbed.

Iron is absorbed in the reduced ferrous (iron in divalent form) state in the upper portion of the small intestine. Ascorbic acid, citric acid, and amino acids convert the less absorbable ferric (iron in trivalent form) iron present in foods to the more phosphoric absorbable ferrous form. On the other hand, if phytates (a salt of a phosphoric acid ester) present in bran or food phosphates are ingested in excess, the absorption of iron can be impaired. (An ester is a compound formed from an alcohol and an acid by the removal of water.)

The ferrous iron is initially taken up by the brush border of the intestinal wall, where it is passed into the intestinal mucosal cells. In the mucosal cells, it can be either bound to transferrin (an iron-binding protein for transport of iron in blood) and absorbed into the blood stream or combined with another protein, apoferritin. This protein-iron complex is known as ferritin (the storage form of iron), which remains within the cells and is released as needed. Control of iron absorption depends on the amount of iron deposited as ferritin in the mucosal cells.

The two most important factors determining the regulation of iron absorption are (1) the state of iron stores in the body (absorption is increased when iron stores are low and vice versa) and (2) the state of activity of red cell formation in the bone marrow. Absorption is increased in conditions that deplete or decrease body iron, for example, during growth or pregnancy when new red cells are being produced and during anemia resulting from hemorrhage.

Transport. In the plasma there is a special carrier protein, transferrin, designed for binding and transporting iron. Most of the plasma iron goes to the bone marrow, the site of red cell manufacture. The transferrin molecules attach themselves to the immature red cells and rapidly pass iron to them. Transferrin also attaches to the liver cells and transfers the iron to them, but more slowly.

The normal plasma iron concentration is about 100 micrograms (µg) per 100 ml. The total iron-binding capacity (TIBC) of transferrin is normally about 330 µg/per 100 ml. If one divides the plasma iron by the total iron-binding capacity, one can determine the percentage of transferrin saturation. Normally, transferrin is one-third, or 30%, saturated, plus or minus 15%.

A *drop* in the saturation of transferrin *below 10 to 15%* is indicative of *iron deficiency anemia.*

After 120 days, red cells are destroyed by the reticuloendothelial cells (large phagocytic cells) and the released iron is taken up by the transferrin molecules. Thus the transferrin is responsible for recycling the iron and transporting it to the bone marrow by production of new red cells. However, if there is an increased requirement for iron, e.g., during menstruation, iron is drawn both from food and from tissue iron stores in the liver and muscle.

IRON AND STORAGE OVERLOAD

Excess iron in the blood is deposited in all cells of the body but especially in the liver cells, where it is stored as ferritin. Ferritin is also found in the cells of spleen and bone marrow. When the amount of iron in the liver, spleen, and bone marrow exceeds the capacity of the cells to form ferritin, the excess is deposited as hemosiderin (an insoluble storage form of iron in the body). Hemosiderin occurs as a brown granular substance coarse enough to be visible under the microscope. In contrast, ferritin is distributed too diffusely to be seen microscopically. Excessive levels of hemosiderin, called hemochromatosis, occur in patients with iron overload. Common causes of hemochromatosis are (1) numerous transfusions in patients with hemolytic (separation of hemoglobin from red blood cells) anemias, (2) excessive intake of iron from food cooked in iron vessels, (3) drinking excessive amounts of inexpensive wines, or (4) failure of the body to regulate absorption, which occurs in alcoholics on low-protein diets and in patients with hereditary hemochromatosis, which is characterized by excess deposition of iron in the tissues, especially in the liver, and by pigmentation of the skin.

Iron metabolism is a well-regulated process. Exchange of iron between the body and food or medicinal sources is relatively limited. Under normal conditions, little iron comes in or goes out. Iron is dynamically balanced between the red cells and other tissues. It is rare to find intrinsic defects of iron utilization, transport, or storage. *Serious disturbances take place only when excessive blood loss or inadequate intake of food sources of iron over a long period of time occurs.*

RECOMMENDED DIETARY ALLOWANCES[2]

Usually, iron intake tends to be inadequate in the infant and child at some point during the first 2 years of life; the recommended dietary allowance (RDA) is 10 to 15 mg/day. For males aged 11 to 18, the recommended allowance is 18 mg daily, and for males aged 19 and older, 10 mg daily.

The recommended allowance for a woman of childbearing age is 18 mg of iron per day, which will allow her body to accummulate iron stores and thus help supply the increased needs for iron during menstruation and pregnancy. At present it is difficult and impractical to supply the needs of a pregnant woman for iron with ordinary food, so that daily iron supplementation (ferrous sulfate, one 300-mg tablet three times daily after food) is required. After menopause the RDA is 10 mg.

The amount of iron expected from a normal diet is about 6 mg/1000 kcal. Only 10% of iron from food is absorbed. Thus, this amount approximately replaces the 1 mg/day lost physiologically in a normal adult.

FOOD SOURCES

Iron in foods comes in three forms—heme (form of iron in hemoglobin and in myoglobin that is absorbed intact), nonheme, and additive iron. Heme iron is found in organ meats (liver, heart, kidney, spleen), red meats, veal, pork, poultry, fish, oysters, and clams, but not milk or milk products. About 40% of the iron in meat and fish is heme iron. However, only one-third can be assimilated by the body. Nonheme iron accounts for the other 60% of iron in animal protein and all the iron in molasses, fruits (figs, dates), green vegetables, dried beans, nuts, and grain products (wheat germ). Only 2 to 10% of this nonheme iron can be absorbed by the body. Additive iron is found in both enriched and fortified products. Enriched white bread, rolls, and crackers are a major source of iron in the United States—an even greater source than red meats.

The amount of iron that will be absorbed from the food depends on the need of the body for iron—the greater the need (as during rapid growth), the greater the absorption, even from foods that are modestly rich in iron.

IRON DEFICIENCY ANEMIA[3]

Iron deficiency anemia is due to inadequate intake or excessive loss of iron or both and is characerized by the production of small red cells that are deficient in hemoglobin. This is the commonest type of nutritional anemia. It leads to a loss of efficiency and impaired general health.

Iron deficiency anemia occurs most frequently in infants and children because they are undergoing rapid growth and therefore have rapid formation of red cells. Iron levels are often inadequate in infants because of the low iron content of milk and also because of low reserves of this mineral at birth. Iron deficiency anemia occurs in pregnant women because the rapidly growing fetus makes increasing demands on the mother's body iron. *Iron deficiency in adult males and postmenopausal women is usually the result of pathological blood loss. In premenopausal women, the physiological loss of blood because of menstruation is the usual cause of iron deficiency.*

Bizarre food habits (such as avoidance of meat and vegetables, as in some adolescents and food faddists) and inadequate intake among the elderly as a result of indifference or poverty are important contributory causes. Vomiting, diarrhea, and intestinal hypermotility will increase the loss of iron.

When losses of iron occur as a result of bleeding, the iron to manufacture new red cells is provided by the serum iron first, and then by the iron stores in the liver, spleen, and bone marrow. The functional nonhemoglobin iron found in enzymes is never affected by such a demand.

Clinical Manifestations. The clinical symptoms and signs of iron deficiency anemia are slow to develop, taking months or years. Anemia is characterized by weakness, fatigue, pallor, and numbness and tingling of the extremities. Epithelial changes can be early manifestations, e.g., nail changes characterized by dullness, brittleness, and a tendency to break at the edges. The fingernails may be flat instead of convex, taking on a distinctive spoon-shaped appearance with longitudinal ridges (koilonychia). Hair growth may be altered. Dysphagia (difficulty in swallowing) may occur in severe cases.

The oral manifestations of iron deficiency anemia are glossitis (inflammation of the tongue) and fissures (clefts or grooves) at the corners of the mouth. The papillae of the tongue are atrophied, thus giving the tongue a smooth, shiny, red appearance. The clinical appearance of the tongue in iron deficiency anemia resembles that in vitamin B complex deficiency. The oral mucous membranes may be atrophied and ashen gray. It is believed that oral tissues thus affected are more susceptible to carcinoma.

The combination of dysphagia (difficulty in swallowing), koilonychia (fingernails are concave or spoon shaped), angular stomatitis (cracks at corners of the mouth), and atrophic glossitis (inflamed smooth surface of the tongue because of reduced size and loss of number of papillae) is called the Plummer-Vinson syndrome.

Laboratory Findings and Diagnosis. In iron deficiency anemia the laboratory findings are as follows:

1. The red cells are small (microcytic) and pale (hypochromic).

2. The red cell count may be relatively normal (4.5 to 5.5 million/mm), but the hemoglobin value, instead of 14 g/100 ml for men and 11 g/100 ml for women, may be as low as 5 g/100 ml.

Zinc deficiency in pregnancy may result in abnormal taste sensations, prolonged gestation, protracted labor, and increased risks to the fetus.

Supplementation

People who take excessive amounts of zinc may be increasing their risk of cardiovascular disease, because high-density lipoprotein (HDL), which protects against heart disease, is lowered and low-density lipoprotein (LDL), which can lead to cardiac problems, is increased.

The common level of zinc in popular vitamin/mineral preparations is 15 mg, which is safe. But when zinc is sold by itself, the dosage may be higher than desirable.

Clinical Application

There is some evidence that zinc sulfate supplements will decrease wound-healing time significantly.[8]

When zinc peroxide powder was used topically on acute gingival lesions in acute necrotizing gingivitis, the soreness disappeared sooner than expected, and the mouth was quickly restored to normal health.[9]

Selenium

At physiological levels, selenium performs an antioxidant function. It is an essential component of the enzyme that catalyzes the oxidation of glutathione. Glutathione protects red blood cells through destruction of hydrogen peroxide, thus protecting hemoglobin from oxidative damage.[10]

It was discovered that selenium supplements are extremely effective in reducing the prevalence of Keshan disease, which is characterized by abnormalities in the heart muscle, first found in children in China.[11]

Estimated Safe and Adequate Intake and Food Sources. For adults the estimated safe and recommended daily intake of selenium is 0.05 to 0.2 mg. For infants, children, and adolescents, it is somewhat less.

Inclusion of animal protein in the diet will very likely ensure that humans receive adequate amounts of selenium.

The cariogenic property of selenium is described later in this chapter.

Molybdenum[12]

Molybdenum is part of the molecular structure of two enzymes, xanthine oxidase and aldehyde oxidase. Xanthine oxidase is responsible for the conversion of xanthine to uric acid. Therefore, it is an essential nutrient for humans.

Severe molybdenum toxicity in animals has been seen in areas in which the soil has a high molybdenum content. Symptoms include weight loss, growth retardation, and connective tissue changes.

Estimated Safe and Adequate Intake and Food Sources. For adults the estimated safe and adequate daily dietary intake is 0.15 to 0.5 mg (see

Appendix 3). Beef, kidney, some cereals, and legumes are considered good sources.

Chromium[13]

Trivalent chromium, which is the biologically active form of chromium, is required for the maintenance of normal glucose and energy metabolism in experimental animals; it may act as a cofactor in insulin, and it stimulates the synthesis of fatty acids and cholesterol in the liver.

The human body contains less than 6 mg, and this amount declines with age.

Chromium is not toxic in the forms and levels found in food, and excesses are rapidly excreted.

Estimated Safe and Adequate Intake and Food Sources. For adults the estimated safe and adequate daily dietary intake is 0.05 to 0.2 mg. Good food sources are fats (such as corn oil), meats, whole grains, and brewer's yeast.

Copper

FUNCTIONS

The normal amount of copper in the human body is 100 to 150 mg. The major functions of copper are to (1) aid in the synthesis of hemoglobin in the bone marrow, (2) form and maintain compounds having enzymatic activity, (3) influence central nervous system physiology, and (4) aid in the formation of pigments.

Even though copper aids in the formation of hemoglobin, it is not present in hemoglobin. Iron cannot be utilized by the bone marrow unless copper is present. However, the exact role of copper in causing increased hemoglobin synthesis is not known. It is postulated that copper in cytochrome oxidase might stimulate iron utilization.

Copper is a component of the enzyme that is necessary for the oxidation of the amino acid tyrosine. Traces of copper are also necessary for the oxidation of vitamin C. Copper may have a role in maintenance of the myelin sheath around the nerve tissue.

DEFICIENCY

Copper deficiency is seen in Australian lambs and is called swayback disease. It is characterized by demyelination and degeneration of the motor nerves in the central nervous system. This condition can be prevented by giving copper supplements to ewes (female sheep) during pregnancy.

Rats fed a diet consisting solely of milk developed an anemia. To cure it, in addition to pure iron salts, the rats were fed the ash of foods naturally rich in copper.

Although a frank copper deficiency has never been demonstrated in adults, some clinicians have found that the combined administration of copper and iron in treatment of hypochromic anemia is more effective than the administration of iron alone. In infants who develop anemia as a result of a diet limited to milk, iron supplemented with copper, rather than iron alone, is necessary to overcome the low hemoglobin.

There is no danger of a copper deficiency because adequate stores are present in the liver. There are good supplies in ordinary diets, and the amount needed for metabolism is minute.

EFFECTS OF EXCESS

In Wilson's disease, there is an accumulation of excess copper in the body tissues, probably because of a genetic absence of a liver enzyme. This disease is characterized by neurological degeneration and cirrhotic liver changes. A reduction in dietary copper may be useful in the treatment of this disease. It can also be arrested by giving chelating agents (penicillamine, 300 mg three times a day, orally) to mobilize copper from the tissues and promote its excretion in the urine.[14]

ORAL EFFECTS OF IMBALANCE

Copper has consistently been found in human saliva, but no relationship ___ established between its salivary level and dental caries.[15] However, copper concentrations in excess of the normal amounts found in human saliva appear to inhibit acid production.[16]

There have been conflicting reports on the ability of dietary supplements of copper to reduce dental caries. Some have noted no effect, whereas others have noted some caries reduction. At this time, nothing conclusive can be stated about any relationship between copper and dental caries.

ESTIMATED SAFE AND ADEQUATE INTAKE AND FOOD SOURCES

The estimate of the copper requirement of humans is based on balance studies. A daily copper intake of 2 to 3 mg is recommended for adults, which allows for a safety margin.

Foods high in copper are liver, kidney, oysters, chocolates, nuts, dried legumes, dried fruits, poultry, shellfish, and animal tissues.

Cobalt

Cobalt is considered an essential trace element because it is part of the vitamin B_{12} molecule. It may also be involved in the metabolism of sulfur-containing amino acids.

Inadequacies of cobalt can cause anemia, whereas in many species of animals, the feeding of relatively small amounts can bring on polycythemia (an increase in total red cell mass). Cobalt is essential for the adequate nutrition of sheep and cattle. A deficiency of this element in these animals will produce extreme emaciation and wasting.

Cobalt deficiency in humans is rare except (1) when no animal products are consumed, (2) if there is a lack of gastric intrinsic factor, (3) after a gastrectomy, or (4) during malabsorption syndrome.

High doses of cobalt can stimulate the bone marrow to produce excessive numbers of red cells (polycythemia) and a higher than normal hemoglobin level.

There is no danger of a dietary shortage of this mineral because traces of it appear in many foods, and the amount needed is very small.

Manganese[16a]

FUNCTIONS

Manganese is an essential nutrient for humans, even though the cinical signs and symptoms of a deficiency have not yet been clearly defined. It is needed for normal bone structure, for reproduction, and for the normal functioning of the central nervous system.

Manganese is an important catalyst and is a component of many enzymes in the body; examples are the enzyme (pyruvate carboxylase) involved in the synthesis of carbohydrates and the enzyme (superoxide dismutase) necessary for the protection of cells from high levels of oxygen. The enzymes (glycosyltransferases) necessary for mucopolysaccharide synthesis also appear to be affected by manganese deficiency.

EFFECTS OF DEFICIENCY AND EXCESS

Manganese deficiency produces skeletal abnormalities in animals. In fowl, a manganese-deficient diet proved to be the chief cause of a disorder called perosis, or slipped tendon disease, with enlargement and malformation of the tibial-metatarsal (between the foot and the leg) joint resulting in deformed legs. The basic defect is in cartilage or bone matrix formation.

Manganese excesses can produce profound neurological disturbances similar to those of Parkinson's disease. The successful treatment of parkinsonism with L-dopa seems to involve changes in manganese metabolism.

ESTIMATED SAFE AND ADEQUATE INTAKE AND FOOD SOURCES

The average adult estimated safe and adequate daily dietary intake appears to be between 2.5 and 5 mg. For infants, children, and adolescents it is somewhat less. Manganese is widely distributed in foods of plant and animal origin, especially nuts, seeds, whole grains, and fruits and vegetables. Manganese concentration in tea is exceptionally high. It is partially lost along with other trace elements in food processing.

Iodine

Historically, as already mentioned, iodine was one of the first trace elements to be recognized as essential for normal health.

Iodine is an integral part of the thyroid hormones thyroxine and triiodothyronine, whose function it is to maintain the control of the energy metabolism of the body. Most important in synthesis of thyroid hormone is the ability of the thyroid gland to trap and oxidize iodide molecules into free iodine. Without iodine, the gland can form no thyroid hormone.

The adult body normally contains about 15 to 30 mg of iodine; about 8 mg is concentrated in the thyroid gland and the rest occurs mostly in the circulating blood.

Iodine in food and water is quickly absorbed from the gastrointestinal tract as inorganic iodide. About 30% is removed by the thyroid, and the remaining is excreted in the urine. Depending on the activity of the thyroid gland, a portion of the iodine is taken up by the gland and combined with tyrosine. In the epithelial cells of the thyroid gland, the iodotyrosine compounds are converted to thyroxine that in turn combine with globulin to form thyroglobulin, the form in which it is stored in the thyroid gland. Triiodothyronine and thyroxine are called T_3 and T_4, respectively, and are the active hormones secreted by the thyroid gland. In primary hyperthyroid disease, there is an increased T_4—normal range, 4.5 to 11.5 mg/100 ml—whereas in hypothyroid disease there is decreased T_4.

Effects of Imbalance

Hypothyroidism. When a deficiency exists, goiter, a thyroid gland enlargement, develops as a swelling in the front of the neck in the area of the hyoid bone. In the absence of iodine, the thyroid gland increases its secretory activity to compensate. Before the iodization of salt, this condition was prevalent in certain geographic areas of the united States where iodine was lacking in the water and soils. The goiter belt included the Great Lakes regions, Wisconsin, Nebraska, the Dakotas, Colorado, Montana, Utah, Oregon, and Washington.

A classic experiment demonstrated that potassium iodide in small doses could completely eliminate the incidence of goiter in children. Of 1800 untreated girls (controls), 26% developed goiter, whereas no goiter developed in any of the 800 girls given small doses of potassium iodide during two 10-day periods.[17]

This study led to the commercial iodization of salt. The current level of enrichment furnishes 76 mg of iodine per g of salt.

Cretinism and myxedema are pathological conditions resulting from low thyroid activity. When the hypothyroidism is due to physiological atrophy from advancing age, or to neoplasia or surgery or other causes, myxedema (nonpitting type of swelling) results with puffiness and edema of the face and a slowed metabolism. The skin is dry and coarse and the tongue is thick. Patients move, think, and talk slowly. Treatment involves administration of thyroid hormone until a euthyroid (normal) state is achieved.

When hypothyroidism affects the fetus prior to birth, cretinism develops. It is characterized by a low basal metabolism, enlarged tongue, thick lips, arrested skeletal development, and severe mental retardation.[18]

Hyperthyroidism. The excessive activity of the thyroid gland that is brought on by a deficiency of iodine produces an enlarged excretory gland as a result of hyperplasia of the cells lining the follicles (small excretory glands) along with increased colloidal (particles that are larger than crystalline molecules and do not pass through a membrane) material. It produces a hypermetabolic state, which is characterized by increased pulse rate, temperature, and blood pressure, with extreme nervousness, irritability, increased sweating, dyspnea, weight loss, and tiredness. Patients with diffuse primary thyroid hyperplasia may develop exophthalmos (abnormal protrusion of the eyeball).

Oral Effects of Imbalance. In severe hypothyroidism, the jaws are small and the rate of tooth eruption is retarded. These patients suffer from a deficiency of thyroid activity and have a predisposition to root resorption.

On the other hand, hyperthyroid patients can conceivably develop caries rapidly because of their increased need for calories and the possible use of excessive sugars to satisfy this need.

RECOMMENDED DIETARY ALLOWANCE AND SOURCES

The adult requirement for iodine is 0.15 mg daily. The amounts recommended for children and pregnant and lactating women can be found in Appendix 2.

Seafoods such as clams, lobsters, oysters, sardines, and other fish are rich sources of iodine. The amount of iodine in vegetables depends on the amount of iodine in the soil in which they were grown. Dairy products and eggs may be good sources if the cows and chickens that produce them are fed iodine-rich rations. The iodine needs of most people can be easily met by the use of iodized salt.

Even though iodized salt will prevent the formation of goiter, iodine supplements will not decrease the size of the thyroid gland in adults once it has enlarged.

TRACE ELEMENTS OTHER THAN FLUORIDES: EFFECTS ON DEVELOPMENT OF DENTAL CARIES

Geographic Variation in Caries Prevalence

The prevalence of dental caries in the United States seems to follow a definite geographic pattern. For example, the natives of New England, middle Atlantic, and the Northwest have significantly greater caries experience than natives of the South Central states.[19] There has been a consistent finding in dental surveys conducted from the time of the Civil War until now. It is assumed that the mineral content of the food grown in the different soils, the mineral content of the respective communal water supplies, some other environmental factor (hours of sunshine, dietary habits), or all of these may influence this distribution of caries in the United States.[20]

No doubt one major reason for this geographic difference is the presence of natural fluorides in concentrations about 1 part per million (ppm) in the water supplies of communities in Texas, Arkansas, New Mexico, and other South Central states compared with the approximately 0.1 to 0.2 ppm level of this nutrient in the water of the communities in New Hampshire, Vermont, Massachusetts, and other New England states. But optimal fluoride levels in community water supplies are only one part of the total answer to the prevention of this complex disease. For example, in his original epidemiological surveys of the effect of fluorine in dental caries, one research scientist noted that fluoride was

further investigation. The following list is arranged in the order of cariogenicity, with the elements that are thought to belong to each category:

1. Caries-promoting elements: selenium, magnesium, cadmium, platinum, lead, silicon

2. Elements that are mildly cariostatic: molybdenum, vanadium, strontium, calcium, boron, lithium, gold

3. Elements with doubtful effect on caries: beryllium, cobalt, manganese, tin, zinc, bromine, iodine

4. Caries-inert elements: barium, aluminum, nickel, iron, palladium, titanium

5. Elements that are strongly cariostatic: fluorine, phosphorus

POSSIBLE MECHANISM OF TRACE ELEMENT ACTION ON DENTAL CARIES

If trace elements influence susceptibility to caries, it would seem likely that they do so by altering the resistance of the tooth itself or by modifying the local environment at the plaque–tooth enamel interface.

Like fluoride, other elements can modify the chemical and physical composition of the teeth, especially the surface layers of the enamel. They may alter the size of the enamel crystals available to acid exposure, thus influencing the solubility of the enamel. A group of smaller crystals have a greater surface area and therefore are more exposed to acid solubility than a group of larger crystals in enamel rods of similar size.

The trace elements may also influence the microbial ecology of plaque to either inhibit or promote the growth of caries-producing bacteria.

SELENIUM AND DENTAL CARIES

One of the commonest problems occurring in persons who ingest foods grown in soils that are rich in selenium is a higher than usual dental caries experience. Other symptoms of high selenium intake are dermatitis, gastrointestinal disturbances, and abnormal fingernails.

In a survey of the teeth of children reared in seleniferous areas west of the Cascade Mountains in Oregon, it was found that these children experienced a higher incidence of caries than did children reared east of the Cascades, where there is no selenium in the soil.[29] The findings of the Oregon study were corroborated by a study in Wyoming, but not by a similar study in New Zealand.[30]

In animal studies, it was found that the ingestion of selenium during the period of active tooth development increased the incidence of caries significantly, and that the increase was proportional to the amount of selenium in the diet of the animals. It is speculated that incorporation of selenium during formation of teeth changes the protein components of the enamel and makes it more prone to caries. However, the threshold value of intake below which selenium does not increase caries is not known. It appears that the margin between the beneficial and the harmful amounts of selenium intake may be quite narrow.

Hadjimarkos made the valid point that effects of trace elements that promote caries as well as of those that reduce caries should be investigated to determine how to prevent dental caries.[29]

MOLYBDENUM AND DENTAL CARIES

An epidemiological study in Hungary[31] concluded that high molybdenum content of water was responsible for the lower caries incidence among children born and reared in the town of Devavanya compared with the incidence in children from a neighborhood town, Gyoma, which had only traces of molybdenum in its water supplies. Hadjimarkos reviewed the data on this study and commented that the conclusions were questionable because data were incomplete.[29]

In another study in New Zealand, the number of caries was found to be low in natives of Napier. These people ate vegetables in which the ash content was higher in molybdenum, aluminum, and titanium but lower in copper, manganese, barium, and strontium compared with the same vegetables produced in Hasting, where the number of dental caries was high.[32] The conclusion of the investigators was that an increased amount of molybdenum was responsible for the 21 to 57% fewer caries in the Napier children.

There have been conflicting reports of the relative caries-inhibiting property of molybdenum when used as a dietary supplement in animal-feeding experiments. It is possible that the administration of combined molybdenum and fluoride enhanced the beneficial effects of fluoride in reducing caries development, but this has not been confirmed.

In general, the action of molybdenum as a mildly cariostatic agent needs further testing.

VANADIUM AND DENTAL CARIES

Vanadium resembles phosphorus in chemical behavior.

From the epidemiological studies of Tank and Storvick there appears to be an inverse correlation between the vanadium content of water supplies and dental caries; that is, with increased amounts of vanadium, there is a decreased number of caries.[33] When vanadium was administered either in food or by injection to hamsters and rats, the number of caries was decreased. However, the opposite results have been reported by others.[29]

In general, the data are still too meager to arrive at any firm conclusion that vanadium is a significantly cariostatic trace mineral.

STRONTIUM AND DENTAL CARIES

Trace elements in tooth enamel from natives of New England, the area highest in caries, were compared with those from natives of Texas, the area lowest in caries, as shown by data from many epidemiological caries studies of military personnel.[20] The strontium concentration in the teeth of the New Englanders was found to be low, whereas the concentration in the Texans was comparatively high.[34]

Another group of investigators found that increases of both fluorine and strontium in tooth enamel were associated with a lower caries incidence in the teeth that they analyzed. They compared enamel samples from teeth of natives of New England and South Carolina and found that fluorine and strontium levels were about 82 and 104 ppm, respectively, for the New England group (high number of caries) and about 125 and 184 ppm, respectively, for the South Carolina group (low number of caries).[35]

It appears that high concentrations of fluorine and strontium may work together to enhance the resistance of enamel to dissolution.

CONCLUSIONS

On the basis of the several studies completed to date, it may be postulated that a mixture of trace elements such as fluorine, strontium, boron, and molybdenum may work together to retard caries. Conversely, selenium, lead, and manganese, either alone or in combination, may increase caries.

Importantly, it may not be possible to find another single mineral element that will exert as great an anticaries effect as fluoride. In future research on the effect of minerals on dental caries, our efforts should be directed to developing mixtures of elements at optimal levels and in ratios to maximize their possible combined inhibitory effects on caries. Also, it is equally important to identify those mixtures of microminerals in foods or water supplies that exert a cariogenic effect.

REFERENCES

1. Mertz, W. The essential trace elements. Science 213:1332, 1981.
2. Committee on Dietary Allowances, Food and Nutrition Board, National Research Council-National Academy of Sciences. Recommended Dietary Allowances, 9th rev. ed. Washington, D.C., National Academy Press, 1980.
3. Finch, C. A.; Cook, J. D. Iron deficiency. Am. J. Clin. Nutr. 39:471, 1984.
4. Waldravens, P.A., et al. Linear growth of low income school children receiving a zinc supplement. Am. J. Clin. Nutr. 38:195, 1983.
5. Buzina, R., et al. Zinc nutrition and taste acuity in school children with impaired growth. Am. J. Clin. Nutr. 33:2262, 1980.
6. Oberleas, D.; Prasad, A. S. Adequacy of trace minerals in bovine milk for human consumption. Am. J. Clin. Nutr. 22:196, 1969.
7. Shah, B. G.; Belonje, B. Zinc bioavailability in infant formulas and cereals. In Inglett, G. E., ed. Nutritional Bioavailability of Zinc. American Chemical Society Symposium Series 210. Washington, D.C., American Chemical Society, 1983.
8. Pories, W. J., et al. Acceleration of wound healing in man with zinc sulphate given by mouth. Lancet 1:121, 1967.
9. Nizel, A. E.; Rubin, S. Zinc peroxide's role in the treatment of Vincent's stomatitis. Military Surg. 93:49, 1943.
10. Schwarz, K. Essentiality and metabolic functions of selenium. Med. Clin. North Am. 60:745, 1976.
11. Mertz, W. The significance of trace elements for health. Nutr. Today 18:26, 1983.
12. Schroeder, M. A., et al. Essential trace metals in man: molybdenum. J. Chronic Dis. 23:481, 1970.
13. Hambridge, K. M. Chromium nutrition in man. Am. J. Clin. Nutr. 27:505, 1974.
14. Davidson, S., et al. Human Nutrition and Dietetics, 6th ed. New York, Churchill Livingstone, 1975.
15. Dreizen, S.; Spies, H. A.; Spies, T.D. The copper and cobalt levels of human saliva and dental caries activity. J. Dent. Res. 31:137, 1952.
16. Forbes, J. C.; Smith, J. D. Studies of the effect of metallic salts on acid production in saliva. J. Dent. Res. 31:129, 1952.
16a. Hurley, L. S. Manganese. In Present Knowledge in Nutrition: Nutrition Reviews, 5th ed., p. 558. Washington, D.C., Nutrition Foundation, 1984.
17. Marine, D.; Kimball, O. P. Prevention of simple goiter in man. JAMA 77:1068, 1921.
18. Robinson, C. H., et al. Normal and Therapeutic Nutrition, 17th ed., p. 128. New York, Macmillan Publishing Co., 1986.
19. Dunning, J. M. Incidence and distribution of dental caries in the United States. In Johansen, E., ed. Symposia on Dental Caries. Dent. Clin. North Am. July: 291:1962.

20. Nizel, A. E.; Bibby, B. G. Geographic variations in caries prevalence in soldiers. J. Am. Dent. Assoc. 31:1619, 1944.
21. Arnold, F. A. Fluorine in drinking water: its effect on dental caries. J. Am. Dent. Assoc. 36:28, 1948.
22. Ockerse, T. Dental Caries, Clinical and Experimental Investigations. Department of Health, Pretoria, 1949.
23. Rothman, K. J., et al. Dental caries and soil content of trace metals in two Colombian villages. J. Dent. Res. 51:1686, 1972.
24. Glass, R. L., et al. The prevalence of human dental caries and water-borne trace elements. Arch. Oral. Biol. 18:1099, 1973.
25. Sognnaes, R. F.; Shaw, J. H. Experimental rat caries: IV. Effect of a natural salt mixture on the caries-conduciveness of an otherwise purified diet. J. Nutr. 53:195, 1954.
26. Nizel, A. E.; Harris, R. S. Cariostatic effects of ashed foodstuffs fed in the diets of hamsters. J. Dent. Res. 32:672, 1953.
27. Harris, R. S.; Nizel, A. E. Effects of food ash and trace minerals, especially phosphorus, upon dental caries in hamsters. J. Dent. Res. 38:1142, 1959.
28. Navia, J. M. Effect of minerals on dental caries. In Gould, R. F., ed. Dietary Chemicals vs. Dental Caries, p. 141. Advances in Chemistry Series 94. Washington, D.C., American Chemical Society, 1970.
29. Hadjimarkos, D. M. Effect of trace elements on dental caries. Adv. Oral Biol. 3:263, 1968.
30. Hadjimarkos, D. M., et al. Selenium and dental caries: an investigation among school children of Oregon. J. Pediatr. 40:451, 1952.
31. Adler, P.; Straub, J. Water-borne caries-protective agents other than fluorine. Acta Med. Acad. Sci. Hung. 4:221, 1953.
32. Ludwig, T. G., et al. An association between dental caries and certain soil conditions in New Zealand. Nature 186:695, 1960.
33. Tank, G.; Storvick, C. A. Effect of naturally occurring selenium and vanadium on dental caries. J. Dent. Res. 39:473, 1960.
34. Steadman, L. T., et al. Distribution of strontium in teeth from different geographic areas. J. Am. Dent. Assoc. 57:340, 1958.
35. Curzon, M. E. J.; Losee, F. L. Dental caries and trace element composition of whole human enamel: eastern United States. J. Am. Dent. Assoc. 94:1146, 1977.

13

Food Composition, Preparation, Processing, Preservation, Fabrication, and Labeling

FOOD COMPOSITION[1]

Food can be defined as an edible substance made up of a variety of nutrients that nourish the body. Essentially, there are two broad categories of food: plant and animal.

Plant Foods

All the food eaten by human beings, including meat, originates from plant food. Livestock graze on grasses—plant food—to sustain themselves. But plants can manufacture their own food by the process of photosynthesis. Thus plant food is a basic requirement for human survival.

The current trend of humans to eat more plant foods and to decrease their intake of animal foods has three very good reasons: plant foods are more readily available, more economical, and, under certain circumstances, more healthful.

CEREALS

Cereals are essentially derived from the seeds of grasses. The important cereal grains are corn, wheat, rice, barley, rye, and oats. Economics, cultural and ethnic practices, environmental conditions (sunshine, rainfall, soil, and so forth) and adaptability of the plants determine local choices of crops. For example, wheat is grown in temperate climates, whereas rice is grown in tropical or semitropical areas.

The most truly American cereal is corn, or maize, which was first grown by the American Indians. More than half of the world production of 230 million metric tons of corn is grown in the United States. Some varieties developed by hybrid breeding, called sweet corn, are of high quality and suitable for human consumption. These represent only about 1% of the harvested corn. The other 99% is grown primarily for feeding pigs, chickens, and cattle. Yellow corn is rich in carotene (a provitamin A), zein (an incomplete protein of low biological value), and starch. Hominy grits, a favorite southern food, is corn from which the nutrient-rich bran and germ are removed, leaving the starchy inner endosperm.

Rice is the principal cereal food commodity of Asians, who make up more than half the world's population. It is grown in moist tropical or semitropical climates. When the bran of the rice is removed by polishing or milling to make the rich kernel more palatable, the nutritional value of rice is significantly lowered; the bran is rich in thiamin. This vitamin can be preserved only if the unhusked rice is parboiled (steamed or boiled after preliminary soaking). However, in this country, refined rice, like other refined cereal grains, is enriched with vitamins and minerals.

Wheat is grown in the temperate climates of countries such as the United States, Russia, Canada, Argentina, Australia, Egypt, and northern India. (In the United States, Kansas is famous for its seemingly endless fields of ripe, golden wheat.) It contains gluten (a highly nutritious protein) whose sticky texture makes it the preferred grain for yeast breads.

Barley, a hardy plant, is the oldest known cereal. Natives of Canada and the northern European countries eat the dark bread made from barley. In the United States, barley is used in soups and as flour for infants who may be allergic to wheat. It is also used as malt and as a food for livestock.

Rye is grown in cold northern climates; rye bread is commonly used in Germany and the Scandinavian countries.

Oats, eaten in the United States mostly in the form of cooked oatmeal, contain slightly more protein, calcium, and fat than any other cooked cereal. Oats are mainly used as food for livestock.

LEGUMES

Legumes are pods, the seed case of peas, beans, or lentils, for example. Legumes resemble cereal grains but have almost twice as much protein. Dried peas contain about 22% protein because of their low moisture content; however, the protein content of fresh peas or cooked dried ones is only 6 to 8%. Legumes are used as meat substitutes in Central and South America and the Middle East.

An average serving of a legume furnishes only about one-third as much protein as an average serving of meat. It is also an incomplete protein unless it is combined with at least another complementary protein such as corn or rice, not another legume. Rice and beans, for example, will provide all the essential amino acids necessary to make a complete protein. But two or three times as much of this combination is required to equal the complete protein of animal food (see Complementary Proteins, Chap. 5).

The peanut is not a true nut but a beanlike legume, rich in oils and protein. One pound of peanuts provides more protein (but it is incomplete) than a pound of steak, more carbohydrate than a pound of potatoes, and approximately as much fat as a pound of butter. Peanuts have a double virtue; they are high in food value and they also have a long shelf-life in comparison with meat, which spoils quickly if not frozen.

The soybean is perhaps the most important legume in the world. It has been cultivated for hundreds of years in China and Japan. The dry, whole bean contains 40% protein and 20% fat. Soy forms the basis of both a great variety of cooking sauces that many Asians use to garnish their foods and a cheeselike product, tofu or bean curd. Soy can be used as a flour in bread or as a breakfast food. Well-processed soy protein products have a protein nutritional value that closely approaches or equals that of high quality animal protein sources.

FRUITS

Fruits, which are usually attractive and pleasant tasting foods, are defined as the edible, more or less succulent, products of seed-bearing plants. Fleshy fruits, such as apples and pears, have numbers of seeds in the center of their pulp, whereas stone fruits, such as peaches, cherries, and apricots, contain a single stone or pit.

Tomatoes, peppers, okra, squash, and avocados are popularly known as vegetables but really are fruits and are often called "fruit-vegetables." The tomato, originally known as the love apple, was long considered poisonous and was grown only for ornamental purposes.

Such fruits as the banana, fig, coconut, date, and breadfruit (a pulpy fruit of a tree found in the tropics, which has a texture like that of bread when baked) are staple articles of food for people of the tropics and are as important to them as meat is to us.

The most popular fruit is the apple. Second in popularity are the citrus fruits—oranges, lemons, limes, and grapefruit.

Besides vitamin C, in which citrus fruits are especially rich, fruits are good sources of cellulose, which decreases the time for passage of waste products through the large intestine. Some fruits consisting of from 5 to 20% carbohydrate also contain pectin, which assists in the formation of jelly. Fructose and glucose are found in equal proportions in most fruits. The sourness of unripe fruits is due to the presence of organic acids such as citric, malic, and tartaric acids. Citrus fruits and peaches yield an alkaline ash, whereas plums and cranberries yield an acid ash. The alkaline ash fruits are fully oxidized in the body. Acid ash foods may be used in conjunction with a low-calcium dietary regimen to create a urinary environment less conducive to formation of renal (kidney) stones.

VEGETABLES

Vegetables may be any part of the plant, the leaf stalk (e.g., celery), the leaves (e.g., spinach), or the root (e.g., carrots). The greatest part of many vegetables is water; therefore, vegetables are sensitive to weather changes and tend to spoil quickly. Most vegetables have a high vitamin and mineral content. Ascorbic acid, the B complex vitamins, and provitamin A carotenoids (marked by a yellow color resembling that of carotene) are the vitamins most commonly found in vegetables: calcium and iron, the minerals most commonly found.

Potatoes are the plant's swollen underground root stems. The botanical term for these underground stems is *tubers*. Plants usually store starch in stems (as in the white potato), in roots (as in the sweet potato), and in bulbs or seeds. The white potato, known as the Irish potato, for many years was the staple food in Ireland. The sweet potato, which belongs to a different species, is found in warm climates. Potatoes yield more calories per acre than any of the cereal crops. They contain 75 to 80% water and yield 70 to 90 kcal/100g, most of which is from starch. Potatoes also contain small amounts of protein, minerals, and B complex vitamins. They are not rich in ascorbic acid but if eaten in large quantities can contribute a significant amount of ascorbic acid to the diet.

Other starchy vegetables from different tropical regions of the world are the cassava (found in South America), taro (a tuberous plant), and sago (a starch obtained from certain palms).

SUGARS

Bees probably were the first collectors of sugar. They gathered nectar from flowers and made it into honey long before any human knew of the existence of sugar. For a long time, humans obtained sweetening from honey. Then they learned to squeeze out the juices of certain plants, such as sugar cane and sugar beet, and evaporate the water by boiling until sugar remained.

The name sugar is derived from a Persian word shakar, which was derived from a Sanskrit word meaning small grains or pebbles. Sugar was not used as a food in ancient times but rather as a food preservative. It had an important place in the pharmacopeia of Arab physicians of the eighth and ninth centuries.

Plants manufacture sugar from water and air by the process of photosynthesis. The extra supply of sugar is converted into starch and stored for future use (e.g., potato), converted into fats and oils (e.g., nuts), or converted into protein (e.g., beans).

Sucrose is found in extracts from sugar cane, sugar beets, sorghum (a cereal grass from which a syrup is made), and sugar maples. All fruits contain at least fructose and glucose, and some even contain sucrose in varying amounts. Fruits that are especially rich in sugar are apples, pineapples, strawberries, watermellons, grapes, raisins, dates, prunes, and figs.

OILS

The growing plant manufactures extra food, and some of this is stored as fats and oils. Oils are found in the fruits and seeds of plants: for example, poppy and sunflower seeds, soybeans, corn, cotton, peanuts, coconuts, and olives.

In the Western world the best- and earliest-known vegetable oil is olive oil. For Italians and Spaniards, olive oil takes the place of butter and animal fat.

In the United States, the largest source of vegetable oil (cottonseed oil) is the cotton plant. Corn oil and safflower oils have become popular because, like cottonseed oil, they are good sources of unsaturated fatty acids, which are desirable in reducing elevated serum cholesterol levels. A great deal of peanut oil is also used for shortening. Oils not only have nutritional value but are also the source of food odors; the strong odor of onions is a good example.

Animal Products

Animal products such as meat, fish, milk, other dairy products, eggs, and poultry products provide two-thirds of the protein and two-fifths of the calories consumed in the United States. Animal products are the best source of protein of high biological value.

The addition of various hormones or hormonelike products, antibiotics, minerals, vitamins, and chemicals to animals' diets is known to increase the weight of the animals, to increase milk and egg production, and in some instances to improve efficiency of feed utilization. Some persons who consume animal foods that contain the residue of antibiotics may be allergic to them, or these residues may result in a bacterial resistance when the individual is being treated for an infection. Although the American Council on Science and Health does not recommend yet restriction of low-dose antibiotics, this matter should be reviewed on a regular basis.[2] These additives do not change the quality of the product. The law requires that their residues not be present in harmful amounts in the products that the consumer eats.

Meat

Because meat consists not only of muscle and connective tissue but also of fat, it is also an important source of energy. Meat is rich in phosphorus, niacin, and riboflavin. Red muscle meat is a good source of iron. Pork is especially rich in thiamin.

The organ meats such as liver and kidneys have significant nutritional value; for example, liver contains more vitamins and more iron than muscle meat.

Adding vitamin and mineral supplements other than carotene to the feed of livestock does not materially increase the amount of these nutrients in the meat produced. Their inclusion in the ration can prevent deficiencies and improve feed conversion efficiency and thus lower the cost of production. With all types of livestock, feeding practices have a great influence on the rate of growth and the efficiency of production. The amount of feed and the balance of nutrients in the feed influence the cost of production.

Processed meat is meat that is changed from the original fresh state to another form by curing, smoking, seasoning, cooking, or any combination of these processes. The purpose is to preserve the product and enhance flavor, texture, and convenience of the item. Cooking concentrates the protein, mineral, and vitamin content and reduces the fat. Some cured meats are allowed for a nonrestricted, moderate sodium level of 300 mg or less per serving. Cereal, soybean products, and milk products may be incorporated in limited amounts in processed meats to improve binding qualities.

Milk

Milk is a complete food (the exception is its minimal vitamin C and iron contents) that is readily digested and absorbed by most people (except those with lactose intolerance).

The important nutrients in milk are its proteins—casein and lactalbumin. Milk fat consists of short-chain fatty acids that are easily digested. The carbohydrate in milk is lactose. Milk is the best single food source of calcium. The calcium in milk is generally more readily absorbed than that in other foods because it is present chiefly in combination with caseinogen. An equal amount of phosphorus, but very little iron, is present in milk. It is a good source of the B complex vitamins, especially riboflavin, and vitamin A. It serves as the best food vehicle for the addition of vitamin D.

Cows tend to secrete milk of uniform composition even if their ration is low in nutrients. There is, however, a direct relationship between vitamin A value of the butterfat in milk and the amount of carotene (the deepness of the green and yellow pigment) in the forage of cows.

EGGS

Eggs supply complete protein, most of which is albumin, found in the white portion. Eggs also contain calcium and iron. Yolks are a rich source of fat, some protein, significant amounts of vitamin A, and some thiamin, niacin, and riboflavin.

FISH

On the average, fish supplies 5 to 10% of the animal protein consumed by humans. However, fish serves as the major source of animal protein for a few island population groups. Fish contains about 18% complete, well-balanced protein that is almost entirely digestible. The fat content varies according to the type of fish: from 1% in cod and haddock to 20% in salmon and mackerel. Some fish have large amounts of unsaturated fatty acids (e.g., linoleic, linolenic, and arachidonic acids) that can reduce, or at least not increase, the level of cholesterol in the blood stream.

The vitamin content of fish varies. An average serving of salmon or mackerel, for example, will provide the following percentages of the adult daily requirements: 10% of vitamins A and D, 10% of thiamin, 15% of riboflavin, and 50% of niacin.

The minerals found in the edible parts of most fish are magnesium, phosphorus, iron, copper, and iodine. The softened edible bones of canned fish are good sources of calcium and phosphorus. A serving of six average-sized oysters supplies more than the minimum daily need for iron and cooper.

About half of the fish that are caught are used for human consumption. The rest become meal for chickens, canned food for pets, or bait to catch still more fish. Some fish oil has industrial use.

The fish taken in greatest volume is menhaden, a herringlike fish used mostly for animal feed. The average person in the United States eats about 10 lb of fish a year, of which 57% is fresh or frozen; 40% canned; and 3% salted, smoked, or otherwise preserved. Canned tuna; fillet of cod, haddock, and ocean perch; canned salmon; and shrimp are the most popular fish in the United States and are eaten in this order of preference.

Small amounts of fish eaten regularly may be beneficial in that they can protect against heart disease. However, knowledge of where the fish were caught is advisable because of possible contamination of some fishing areas with chemicals such as polychlorinated biphenyls (PCBs). The allowable level of PCBs in fish is 2 parts per million. Lean white fish such as cod, haddock, and pike do not usually contain as high levels as do oily fish such as trout, salmon, mackerel, smelt, and carp. One or two meals per week that include fish are recommended to minimize the risk of heart disease.[3]

Quality of Nutrients from Plants and Animals

The nutritional quality of plant food depends on (1) the genetic characteristics of the seed produced by hybridization, (production of plants from parents belonging to two different species); (2) favorable climate; (3) adequate ripening on the tree or vine; and (4) consumption of the fruit or vegetable soon after it is picked (preferably the same day).

The influence of genetics on the nutrient quality of plant food is illustrated by the finding of agronomists that the vitamin C and carotene contents of tomatoes have been doubled and the niacin content of corn has been increased by selective crossbreeding of different genetic strains of plants. The same is true for animals; for example, plump chickens and meaty hogs can be produced by selective breeding.

Other factors that can influence nutrient composition of plants are environmental: e.g., light intensity, temperature, and the particular season of the year when the fruits or vegetables are harvested. For example, the orange-yellow color of carrots develops most rapidly at 60 to 70°F (14 to 21°C) and the carotene content of broccoli is highest in plants harvested in the spring and is lowest in plants harvested in the fall and winter. On the other hand, potatoes harvested in the spring have the lowest ascorbic acid content. Sunlight affects the vitamin D content of milk and eggs, and seasonal changes influence the composition of beef, eggs, and milk.

Size and maturity are two other factors that influence the nutritional value of plants. For example, small cabbages are richer in ascorbic acid than large ones. Small fruits and vegetables are generally richer in nutrient content per pound, especially when these nutrients are located in the surface layers. The B complex vitamins are highest in the youngest leaves of vegetables because metabolism is at a maximum there. As the leaf matures, the vitamin content decreases, and the cellulose increases. The relationship of the stage of a plant's maturity to its nutritive value differs among plants. For example, snap beans have their highest nutritive value when still immature, whereas broccoli is most nutritious when it is a little overripe.[4]

FOOD PREPARATION

Trimming, Peeling, and Chopping

When foods of plant origin are trimmed or peeled, the nutrient losses generally exceed the weight losses, because these nutrients are usually found in higher concentrations in the outer leaves of vegetables and in the outer layers of seeds, tuber roots, and fruits. For example, vitamin C is present in highest concentration in the potato skin. The outer green leaves are often richer in mineral salts than the inner leaves. The leaves of many vegetables contain from two to more than six times as much vitamin C as the stems.

Preliminary washing and soaking of vegetables and tubers before cooking may cause the loss of water-soluble constituents, but except for potatoes, these losses are generally insignificant. The vitamin C content of potatoes drops after thorough washing. However, since potatoes are not the only nor the major source of vitamin C in our diets, the benefits of sanitation outweigh that of its vitamin C contribution.

Chopping vegetables does not cause much loss of vitamin C. Nevertheless, when vegetables are minced or chopped, some nutrients become much more unstable, and vegetables should be eaten promptly, frozen, or stored under refrigeration.

The chopped and sliced vegetables at salad bars, popular in restaurants and supermarkets, are perishable. Therefore these prepared vegetables should preferably be eaten the day they are chopped or sliced. Also, these prepared vegetables should be kept on ice and protected by a plastic or glass cover to prevent bacterial growth and spoilage.

Also, bulk foods should be kept in shallow bins that have plastic doors. Scoops or tongs must be kept in the bins for the removal of the foods that are then placed in plastic bags.[5]

Boiling, Steaming, Roasting, Baking, and Frying

Nutrient losses that occur when foods are boiled can be minimized if the water barely covers the vegetables; it should then be allowed to boil briskly. For best results, green vegetables are usually added to boiling water, and root vegetables are started in cold water.

If sodium bicarbonate is added to help preserve the green color of the vegetables or if the saucepan is left uncovered, the alkali-sensitive nutrients such as ascorbic acid or the light-sensitive nutrients such as riboflavin will be destroyed.

It has been shown that nutrient losses were two to six times greater when foods were boiled in a copper vessel (which accelerates oxidation of ascorbic acid) than when they were boiled in Pyrex or aluminum ware.

The loss of nutrients is considerably less during pressure cooking of vegetables than during boiling at atmospheric pressure. For example, potatoes cooked in a pressure cooker can retain as much as 80% of their ascorbic acid; normal cooking leaves about 30 to 50%. There is also less extraction of nutrients during steaming than during boiling. Destruction of ascorbic acid is minimal when fruits and vegetables are immediately placed in boiling water but maximal when they are placed in cold water and slowly brought to a boil.

Most of the nutrients lost from vegetables during cooking are present in the cooking water, so losses can be reduced considerably by limiting the volume of cooking water.

The nutrient losses from cooking vegetables and fruits occur because the water leaches out the water-soluble nutrients and the heat destroys some sensitive vitamins. Essentially, this means that the greatest losses are of ascorbic acid and thiamin, because ascorbic acid is readily oxidized and thiamin is unstable when heated. Fat-soluble vitamins, such as carotene, are not so readily affected by heat. Vegetable cooking water contains significant quantities of starch, vitamins, minerals, and amino acids and should therefore be used as a base for soup stock rather than discarded.

When foods are roasted or baked in an electric, gas, or coal-burning oven, the heat-sensitive nutrients are lost, particularly in the surace layers of the food.

The amount of nutrient loss that occurs during frying depends on the length of cooking time—the longer the frying time, the greater the loss of nutrients.

Leftover cooked foods lose significant amounts of critical nutrients as a result of cooling, refrigeration storage, and reheating.

Optimum retention of nutrients during food preparation requires a short cooking time such as ocurs when using a microwave oven, a minimum addition of water, and a brief holding time before serving. Only food that will be consumed at each meal should be prepared, because the cooking, refrigeration, reheating, and boiling of leftover foods seriously reduce their vitamin content.

FOOD PROCESSING[6]

The term *food processing* as used here refers to the industrial processing of foods through preservation techniques, the use of additives, and nutritional enhancement.

Food processing has increased the number of available food products. Fresh foods are not able to withstand long transportation distances and not all foods can be shipped rapidly enough from the farm to the metropolitan areas before they decay. Because of the great distance between grower and consumer there is a need for the prevention of aging and of microbial and chemical decay of foods.[7] By preserving foods through various food-processing techniques—e.g., milling, pasteurization, freezing, canning—the consumer can buy safe food with a high nutritional value. Also, out-of-season foods are available as a result of processing.

Biotechnology may have some impact on agriculture and traditional food processing through the potential for genetic improvement of plants and animals.[7]

Food Preservation Techniques

MILLING OR REFINING OF CEREALS

Whole wheat is milled to yield white flour because whole-grain products have comparatively poor keeping qualities; they are subject to infestation and rapid decay from action of bacteria.

Each kernel of wheat consists of (1) fibrous (cellulose and hemicellulose) outer husks, the bran layer; (2) a brownish layer just below the bran called the aleurone layer, containing some protein, niacin, and iron; (3) the inner portion, or endosperm, consisting chiefly of starch and some protein; and (4) the small germ at one end of the kernel that contains B complex vitamins, iron, and vitamin E.

In the refining process, the bran and aleurone layers and the germ are removed to prevent development of rancidity and to prolong storage time. In this process of making white wheat flour, a large part of the protein, iron, B complex vitamins, and vitamin E is lost. To compensate for this loss, refined white flour is now required by law to be restored to specific standards with thiamin, riboflavin, niacin, and iron. Minor quantities of other nutrients, such as vitamin E, which might be lost during processing are widely available in other foodstuffs.

Essentially, the refined wheat flour has a 70 to 80% starch content and a moderate content of protein, 7.5 to 14%. The following percentages of recommended dietary allowances (RDA) for these nutrients are added to one loaf of bread as a result of the restoration and enrichment program: thiamin, 40%; niacin, 20%; riboflavin, 15%; and iron, 25%. It costs less than one-tenth of one cent to enrich a loaf of bread with these nutrients. As a result of flour enrichment with these B complex vitamins, nutrition surveys in the United States have shown that the incidence of a frank deficiency in thiamin, niacin, or riboflavin is rare. Restoration, enrichment, and fortification are discussed in Chap. 15.

REFINING OF SWEETENERS

Honey, raw sugar, brown sugar and white sugar are practically the same nutritionally. Honey and raw and brown sugar may have a more pleasant taste than white sugar and there may be traces of minerals and vitamins because of the presence of molasses, but this minor nutrient contribution is of no real significance. Both natural and refined sugars are equally detrimental from a dental caries-producing standpoint. Therefore, honey should not be condoned nor considered to be safer for teeth than refined sugar.

PASTEURIZATION

Pasteurization consists essentially of heating raw milk to 60°C in order to destroy any pathogenic microorganisms that may be present. The high risks of contracting undulant fever or tuberculosis outweigh the small benefits to be derived from the enzymes and vitamin C in raw milk, and thus it would seem prudent from a health standpoint to use the pasteurized milk. Actually, the enzymes present in milk are of no use to humans in any event. Since enzymes consist of protein, they are denatured and probably destroyed by stomach acid. Milk is not considered a good source of vitamin C; other foods in a balanced diet provide sufficient amounts of this vitamin to more than satisfy the RDA.

CANNING

Nutrient losses can be minimized in the canning of food, if the manufacturer uses a heat-processing time based on microbial death. Excessive nutrient destruction is avoided by mathematical determinations of a minimum safe cooking time. The increased value that the consumer now places on the nutrient value of foods (rather than on flavor and texture only, as in the past) has caused food canners to increase the nutrient value of processed foods by enrichment or restoration. Canners are using newer methods for improving the quality of heat-processed foods; for example, in the aseptic canning of peas, they are heated for only 2 minutes at 350°F instead of 35 minutes at 240°F. The higher temperature, shorter time technique destroys less than 5% of the vitamin C in the peas, compared with the 25% lost with the lower temperature and longer heating method.

FREEZING

The principle behind the use of refrigeration and freezing for the preservation of foods is that low temperatures slow the growth of microorganisms and the chemical reactions within the foods. For example, tomatoes may lose 40% of their vitamin C within 3 days after picking if they are not refrigerated.

Frozen foods have a higher nutritional quality than canned and dehydrated foods and have a high consumer acceptance rating. The highest nutrient quality is preserved in a frozen food when it is subjected to a fast freezing method. Use of liquid nitrogen ($-280°F$) is currently the best method for freezing fruits and vegetables on a commercial basis. In liquid nitrogen, these foods are frozen in a matter of minutes, whereas a home freezer requires more than 6 hours to freeze a similar amount of food. In addition, faster thawing gives better nutritional quality than thawing at room temperature. It is suggested that turkeys and chickens be roasted directly from the frozen state in order to maintain the maximal nutritional quality.

DEHYDRATION

Another good method for preserving foods is dehydration, which involves the removal of most or all of the water. The resulting product has excellent keeping qualities and can later be reconstituted by the addition of water.

For example, dried milk, which is the least expensive and most transportable form of milk solids, is made by blowing small droplets of liquid milk into a heated chamber where they dry almost instantly to a fine powder. Partial dehydration of milk produces condensed and evaporated milks.

Foods such as fruits and vegetables may be dehydrated by cutting them in thin slices and passing the slices on a conveyor belt through an oven, or they may be finely mashed and placed on a perforated tray or mat. A current of heated air is blown through the perforations.

New methods include quick drying in a vacuum with controlled temperatures (lower than formerly used) and fans for removal of water vapor.

Dehydrated foods, precooked or raw, are extremely convenient when only minimal storage space is available.

ADVANTAGES AND DISADVANTAGES OF PRESERVATION TECHNIQUES

In conclusion, the advantages of food preservation techniques are (1) increased storage time; (2) decreased home preparation time; (3) ensured food safety; and (4) enhanced overall product appeal and edibility.

The disadvantages are (1) destruction of some nutrients; (2) increased cost; and (3) decreased taste appeal for some persons.

Nutrient losses resulting from modern industrial food processing and storage are generally less than those that occur during normal home preparation procedures. Improved methods of processing have resulted in attractive food products with improved properties that stimulate sensory organs. These factors can ultimately provide more utilization.[8]

Food Safety

The Food Safety and Inspection Service of the U.S. Department of Agriculture (USDA) oversees the safety and accurate labeling of meat and poultry products.

The USDA food safety activities complement those of the Food and Drug Administration (FDA). The FDA oversees the safety of food additives. USDA determines the type and quantity of additives that can be used in meat and poultry products and may decide that an FDA-approved additive is not appropriate for use in meat and poultry products.[9]

FABRICATED AND FORMULATED FOODS

Fabricated foods are complex mixtures of ingredients specifically designed for a particular use and may or may not closely resemble existing foods. Such items include, for example, dairy substitutes such as nondairy creamers and imitation milk, which consist of water, sugar, vegetable fat, emulsifiers, stabilizers, and casein or soy. This fabricated milk is nutritionally inferior to cow's milk. (The protein content of imitation low-fat dry milk is about half that of regular milk.[9, 10]) Other examples of fabricated foods are egg substitutes without cholesterol and many of the saturated fats; meat substitutes without cholesterol and many of the saturated fats; meat substitutes, from a soybean base, that resemble hot dogs, ground beef, or bacon; and meal-replacement beverages and bars used for weight reduction.

Formulated foods are mixtures of two or more foodstuffs or ingredients other than seasoning, for example, liquid meals and prepared breakfast foods. Snack foods may be formulated from conventional foods and become important when they displace quantities of nutrients in the diet.

To ensure the nutritional quality of formulated foods, the American Medical Association Council on Foods and Nutrition and the National Research Council Food and Nutrition Board have established relevant guidelines.[11, 12]

- Formulated foods are significant in the diet if they contribute 5% or more of any recommended nutrient or energy requirement or if they are substituted for other foods.
- Unless developed for a specific dietary reason, substitute products should contain nutrients similar to those of the foods they are formulated to resemble.
- The quantity of protein and fat should be nutritionally appropriate to the food and its use.
- Foods that are meal replacements should provide 25 to 50% of the actual or estimated RDA.
- The caloric content should be determined by the intended use.

FOOD LABELING[9, 12, 13]

The purpose of the food-labeling program designed by the FDA is to provide nutrition information that will help consumers make informed choices by providing (1) a way to compare store brands of a food item with those of national or regional brands for possible savings, (2) information about the nutrient content of new foods for planning varied and balanced diets, (3) information to make it easier to count calories, and (4) information for selecting foods for special health needs such as low-sodium or low-cholesterol foods. (In the near future, labels may also list the amount of added sugar.)

Ingredient Labeling

All food labels must have the following basic information:

- Legal name of the product, which includes a description of the product such as "whole tomatoes," "cream style" corn, or "waffled" potato chips
- Net contents or net weight, including the packaging medium, such as water in canned vegetables
- Name and location of the manufacturer, packer, or distributor
- Ingredients listed in descending order by weight, including any functional additives

Colors and flavors do not have to be listed by name but can be listed simply as "Coloring" or "Flavoring." However, if the colors or flavors are artificial, they must be so described.

About 300 foods have a standard of identity. These foods include catsup, mayonnaise, margarine, ice cream, peanut butter, macaroni, and noodle products. Their container labels do not have to list ingredients because of the FDA standard for these products. The name of the product therefore describes the ingredients.

Some food labels are based on specific qualities of the product, for example a USDA "Grade A" label. There may be such labels as, for example, "Inspected for wholesomeness by the U.S. Department of Agriculture." Milk and milk products may carry a grade A label based on FDA-recommended sanitary standards for the production and processing of these products. Eggs are graded according to size and quality (freshness).

Nutrition Labeling

In addition to ingredient information, a nutrition information panel must appear on the label giving the size of one serving (for example, 1 or 2 oz or 1 tablespoon), the number of servings, and the number of calories, followed by the amount of protein, carbohydrate, and fat (in grams) per serving. Also, all additives must be listed on the label.

The label contains the percentage of the U.S. Recommended Daily Allowance (USRDA) fulfilled by eight indicator nutrients: protein, vitamins A and C, thiamin, riboflavin, niacin, calcium, and iron. Information for 12 other vitamins and minerals and for cholesterol, fatty acids, and sodium content is optional. For example, a label may state the following:

	Percentage of USRDA:
Protein	30
Vitamin A	35
Vitamin C	10
Thiamin	15
Riboflavin	15
Niacin	25
Calcium	2
Iron	25

USRDA

The USRDA represents the amounts of nutrients needed every day by healthy people plus an excess of 30 to 50% to allow for individual variations. The USRDA is a standard that is used to evaluate the contents of a food container. Thus many adults need only two-thirds to three-fourths of the USRDA for several nutrients, and children about half.

The USRDAs (Table 13–1) have three categories. The best-known and -used for conventional foods is the one for adults and children over 4 years of age. The second category is for infants and children under 4. It is used for baby foods and vitamin-mineral supplements for infants and small children. The third category is for pregnant or lactating women. To be certain that almost everyone's needs are amply covered, the FDA uses the highest recommended allowance in each category for almost every nutrient in the USRDA.

Consumption of less than 100% of the USRDA does not necessarily result in a deficient diet because of the excess added in allowances. Nor does eating 100% of the USRDA for the eight listed nutrients absolutely ensure an adequate diet, because there are about 40 or more other nutrients essential for humans.

PRACTICAL APPLICATIONS OF NUTRITION LABELS

When shopping, compare net weight, size, and price of products, and see which product or size offers the best value.

Some stores have unit pricing, that is, cost of products per ounce, pound, or other unit of measurement.

Some foods are labeled as imitation so the word imitation is used on the label when the product is less nutritious than the original. If a product is similar to another and is as nutritious, it is given a new name. For example, the name *margarine* instead of imitation butter is used for a product as nutritious as butter.

The words *artificially flavored*, in for example, *artificially flavored vanilla pudding*, are used only if the artificial flavor predominates. If the pudding contains mostly natural vanilla flavor but also some artificial flavoring, it is called *vanilla flavored pudding*. If the pudding contains only natural vanilla flavor, it is simply called *vanilla pudding*.

To ascertain whether a frozen food has the same amount of protein, vitamins,

TABLE 13–1. United States Recommended Daily Allowances (USRDAs)

	Used for Conventional Food or "Special Dietary Foods"	Used for "Special Dietary Foods" Only	
	Adults and Children 4 or More Years of Age	*Infants and Children Under 4 Years of Age*	*Pregnant or Lactating Women*
Nutrients That Must Be Declared on Label*			
Protein†	45 g high-quality protein		
	65 g proteins in general		
Vitamin A	5000 IU	2500 IU	8000 IU
Vitamin C (ascorbic acid)	60 mg	40 mg	60 mg
Thiamin (vitamin B_1)	1.5 mg	0.7 mg	1.7 mg
Riboflavin (vitamin B_2)	1.7 mg	0.8 mg	2.0 mg
Niacin	20 mg	9 mg	20 mg
Calcium	1.0 g	0.8 g	1.3 g
Iron	18 mg	10 mg	18 mg
Nutrients That May Be Declared on Label			
Vitamin D	400 IU	400 IU	400 IU
Vitamin E	30 IU	10 IU	30 IU
Vitamin B_6	2.0 mg	0.7 mg	2.5 mg
Folic acid (folacin)	0.4 mg	0.2 mg	0.8
Vitamin B_{12}	6 μg	3 μg	8 μg
Phosphorus	1.0 g	0.8 μg	1.3 g
Iodine	150 μg	70 μg	150 μg
Magnesium	400 mg	200 mg	450 mg
Zinc	15 mg	8 mg	15 mg
Copper	2 mg	1 mg	2 mg
Biotin	0.3 mg	0.15 mg	0.3 mg
Pantothenic acid	10 mg	5 mg	10 mg

*These figures are utilized for label information on any food that is enriched to provide more than 50% of the RDA of any given nutrient, plus any food that is said to be a special dietary food. If the dietary food is for young children or pregnant or lactating women, RDAs from the appropriate columns are used. (From the Food and Drug Administration, USDHEW.)

†"High-quality protein" is defined as having a protein efficiency ratio (PER) equal to or greater than that of casein (a milk protein). "Proteins in general" are those with a PER less than that of casein. Proteins with a PER less than 20% that of casein are considered "not a significant source of protein" and may not be expressed on the label.

and minerals it contained when the food was fresh, look for the statement: "Provides nutrients in amounts appropriate for this class of food as determined by the U.S. Government."

In summary, food labels help consumers to understand the nutritional value of the foods they are buying and give directions on how to use them.

REFERENCES

1. Hansen, R. G. An index of food quality. Nutr. Rev. 31:1, 1973.
2. Antibiotics in Animal Feed: A Threat to Human Health? (report). New York, American Council on Science and Health, November 1983.
3. Benefits of eating fish. Tufts Univ. Diet Nutr. Lett. 3(5): 1985.

4. Harris, R. S. The effect of processing on the nutritional values of foods. In Nizel, A. E., ed. The Science of Nutrition and Its Application in Clinical Dentistry, 2nd ed., pp. 208–210. Philadelphia, W.B. Saunders Co., 1966.
5. Self-service salads: how safe are they? Tufts Univ. Diet Nutr. Lett. 2(8):7, 1984.
6. Labuza, T. P. Food for Thought. Westport, Conn., Avi Publishing Co., 1974.
7. Chichester, C. O.; Lee, T. C. Nutrition and food processing. In Rechcyl, M., ed. Nutrition and World Food Problems, p. 310. Basel, S. Karger, 1979.
8. Harlander, S. K. Biotechnology in the food processing industry. Contemporary Nutrition, General Mills Nutrition Dept., Vol. 11, no. 3, 1986.
9. Gast, L. L. A response to today's food safety concerns. Nutr. News 48:9–10, 1985.
10. Kotula, K.; Briggs, G. M. The nutritional aspects of imitation and substitute foods. Nutr. News 46:9–11, 1983.
11. Council on Foods and Nutrition. Improvement of the nutritive quality of foods. JAMA 225:1116, 1973.
12. Nutrition labeling. Nutr. Rev. 31:36, 1973.
13. Food and Drug Administration. We Want You to Know About Labels on Foods. Health, Education, and Welfare Publication no. (FDA) 73-2043 and no. (FDA) 74-2039, Washington, D.C., GPO, 1973.

14

Recommended Dietary Allowances; Food Groups; Dietary Goals

In the preceding chapters, the qualitative and functional nature of nutrients and foods, their preparation, processing, and labeling were discussed. In this chapter, the amounts of nutrients and foods recommended for daily intake are discussed. Information from earlier chapters plus the amount of foods from the basic four essential food groups, namely, milk, meat, fruit-vegetable, and bread-cereal plus a fifth group consisting of fats, sweets, and alcohol, which provide calories but few essential nutrients, can provide a suitable framework upon which to base an acceptable nutrition guidance service for most patients with dental/oral health disorders that are caused in part by improper food and nutrient choices.

The U.S. Recommended Daily Allowances (USRDAs) (discussed in Chap. 13) are used for labeling the nutritional contents of packaged foods. In this chapter, three other nutrition guides—(1) Recommended Dietary Allowances (RDAs), (2) the Food Group Guide, and (3) Dietary Goals—are discussed.

RECOMMENDED DIETARY ALLOWANCES

Since 1943, the Food and Nutrition Board, a group of nutrition scientists, has published at approximately 5-year intervals revised and updated editions of the Recommended Dietary Allowances. The 1980 edition is the ninth and the most recent one. The RDAs are sets of values for levels of intake of the nutrients currently considered essential. These should meet the physiological needs of nearly all individuals in the United States. The RDAs are primarily designed for planning and procuring nutritionally adequate food supplies for population groups rather than for individuals. If the foods consumed contain the amounts of nutrients that meet the RDA, the probability of developing nutritional deficiencies is negligible.

In addition to providing standards for the USRDA nutrition labeling, the RDA also serves as the basis for (1) the food guides, (2) the development of diets and products for therapeutic uses, (3) the formulation of new food products, and (4) a guide for foods provided by community resources for nutrition such as senior centers, home-delivered meals, and food stamps, which increases the probability of purchasing foods from the four essential food groups.

A number of dentists use the RDA as a basis for evaluating their patients' nutrient intake recorded in a 7-day food diary. This may be considered a higher than necessary goal because the RDA exceeds by 30 to 50% the requirements of most persons. The RDA for each vitamin and mineral is determined on the basis of the *entire range of normal human needs plus the aforementioned safety factor.* Since the individuals with either low or high requirements cannot be distinguished from one another, the RDAs do not provide a specific means for identifying the point at which individual nutrient intakes become inadequate. According to Harper, "If intake is equal to or greater than the RDA, the risk of nutritional inadequacy is remote. When intake falls below the RDA, however, all that can be said is that the further the intake falls below the RDA, the greater the risk of nutritional inadequacy."[2] Since dietary standards in general cannot directly be related to individual requirements, statistical methods for estimating the probability of a nutrient deficiency may be the most satisfactory solution to this problem (Fig. 14–1).[3]

RDA and Estimated Safe and Adequate Intake Tables

The 1980 Recommended Daily Dietary Allowances in Appendix 2 are recorded in a table that lists definitive amounts of protein, three fat-soluble vitamins, seven water-soluble vitamins, and six minerals that should be ingested daily. These amounts vary according to individuals' sex, age, weight, and height; and during pregnancy and lactation. In Appendix 3, Estimated Safe and Adequate Daily Dietary Intakes of Selected Vitamins and Minerals, there is a subsidiary table of ranges for three vitamins, six trace minerals, and three electrolytes recommended as safe and adequate. For the latter group of nutrients, ranges rather than specific amounts are given because less than desirable

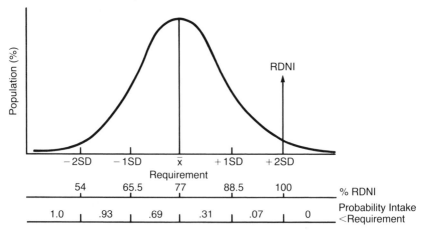

FIGURE 14–1. Description of distribution of nutrient requirements and the probability of intakes being less than the individual's requirement within given intervals below the Recommended Daily Nutrient Intake (RDNI—Canadian dietary standard). (Reprinted with permission from Nutr. Res., vol. 2, Anderson, G. H.; Peterson, R. D.; Beaton, G. H. Estimating nutrient deficiencies in a population from dietary records. The use of probability analyses, Copyright 1982, Pergamon Press plc.)

scientific data were available as a basis. The estimates are limited to broader age categories than those for the definitive allowances. Estimated safe and adequate intakes have been established because the increased availability of formulated foods, food analogs (similar foods), and vitamin and mineral supplements may increase the risks of deficiency and toxicity. Guidelines are needed both for the manufacturers who formulate these food products and for the public who consumes them. In order to avoid toxicity, it is recommended that the upper limits of intake for the six trace elements in this category not be habitually exceeded.

The RDAs are recommendations for the average daily amounts of nutrients that will meet nutritional requirements of most people. The RDAs are considered adequate for healthy persons in the United States. The allowances take into consideration the presence of precursor nutrients, such as beta-carotene, which is converted to vitamin A. It also takes into consideration differences in the efficiency of absorption and use of nutrients. For example, iron is poorly absorbed; and possible inefficient use of an ingested mixture of amino acids was taken into consideration when protein allowances were recommended.

The amount by which the allowance is set above the average requirement varies from nutrient to nutrient. When these margins of safety (which vary with each nutrient) were determined, it was appreciated that storage of nutrients by the body varies and that excessive intake of certain nutrients can produce toxicity. For example, Herbert believes that taking vitamins A, D, E, or K at five times the RDA on a regular basis is dangerous. He also believes that no more than 10 times the recommended amount of the water-soluble B and C vitamins should be taken, and that mineral levels should not exceed 3 times the RDA.[4]

Only the energy requirements were not set at a value above the average requirement. Calorie needs, described in Chap. 1, depend upon the age, body size, and physical activity of each person and should be calculated accordingly.

Applications of the RDA

RDAs are used in the planning of menus for the armed services, for hospitals, for mental and penal institutions, for school lunches, and by a variety of public and private organizations concerned with feeding large groups of people.

Because RDAs are standards for the amounts of nutrients that should be consumed, allowance must be made for losses of nutrients that occur during food preparation.

The RDAs are not considered absolute requirements and should be regarded as flexible recommendations because the specific amounts recommended by the Food and Nutrition Board are purely judgmental. There is a "minimum risk level" that is above the actual need of practically every one in the group. Thus the RDAs should be used as rough guides.

Individuals should not be assumed to be suffering from malnutrition if they do not receive the full RDA, nor should diets be judged poor on the basis of an arbitrary figure (such as a computerized analysis of nutrients in the diet) compared with the RDA. Only the total nutritional status and health picture can determine the presence of a dietary deficiency. Since the requirements of individuals are not known, the recommendations are high enough to ensure that they meet the needs of those with the highest requirements. Therefore, the RDAs exceed the essential nutrient requirements of most members of the population. To repeat, the final evaluation of the nutritional status of an individual must be determined by the condition of the person consuming the diet, not by comparison of the calculated nutrient intake against standards that are not necessarily applicable to an individual. The RDA can be used only as a relative index of adequacy.

Limitations of the RDA

Hegsted suggested that a single set of standards such as the RDA is not adequate both for telling people how to eat and for evaluating dietary data.[5]

Munro stated, "Lack of unanimity by experts and a long history of revision should warn the user that dietary recommendations, although based on the most reliable data available, are not infallible."[6] For example, he pointed out that we do not yet have enough solid information about the needs of adolescents and the elderly. In addition, there is not sufficient information to set specific allowances for a number of essential trace elements. However, some estimated safe and adequate ranges have been recommended in the ninth edition of the RDA.[1] Also, other essential nutrients may be discovered in the future. The changing pattern of food selection and availability may also affect the RDA because of interactions between nutrients—for example, the ability of ascorbic acid to increase iron absorption if both nutrients are consumed at the same meal; the role of phosphates and proteins in determining calcium balance; and the effect of energy on protein use. Thus it is best for the consumer to select a varied diet of natural foods, because there is no guarantee that the RDAs represent all of a person's nutrient needs.

In conclusion, RDAs are

- Acceptable levels of intake for population groups
- Goals at which to aim when providing for the nutritional needs or assessing the nutritional status of groups
- Allowances and estimates of nutrients that should meet the needs of nearly all healthy individuals within a group
- In excess of nutrient requirements except for energy needs, and they ensure growth and maintenance of health of most people

On the other hand, RDAs are not

- Intended for evaluation of the nutritional status of an individual
- Recommendations for an ideal diet
- Average requirements
- Adequate to cover the special needs of such problems as inherited metabolic disorders, infections, chronic diseases, and traumas

For the world population as a whole, the World Health Organization (WHO) and Food and Agriculture Organization (FAO) have established "safe levels of intake" that are somewhat lower than those of the U.S. Food and Nutrition Board. For example, the international calcium allowance is 400 to 500 mg/day (in contrast with the U.S. allowance of 800 mg). FAO/WHO standards, however, conform to the expectation of a smaller body size and a limited degree of adaptation to habitually lower intakes.

FOOD GROUP GUIDES

Purpose

The objective of national food guides for the United States has been to translate dietary standards into simple and reliable devices for the nutrition education of the lay person.[7] The factors that were taken into consideration in the development of food guides were the customary food patterns, the availability of food, food economics, and the nutritive value of foods in a particular locale. For the RDA to be understandable and useful to the lay person, it had to include familiar names of foods categorized into a limited number of food groups. The food group guides serve as a practical and workable plan for helping the homemaker select the kinds and amounts of food that need to be included in each day's meals in order to provide a balanced diet. Since people think in terms of foods rather than nutrients, these food guides make good sense.

Food group guides have been devised for each culture and country. The United States has had food guides with as few as 2 or 3 food groups and with as many as 11 to 13. The Basic Seven food groups was the National Food Guide in 1946, and the Basic Four food groups was suggested by the Institute of Home Economics of the U.S. Department of Agriculture (USDA) in 1957.[8] The percentage of nutrients contributed by the four food groups is shown in Table 14–1. In 1979, the USDA recommended a five–food group daily food guide (see Fig. 4–1).[9] In the five–food group guide a Fats, Sweets, and Alcohol group was added to the Basic Four.[10]

When the food groups were designed, the foods were categorized on the basis of their similarity in composition or nutritive value or both. For example, the group that includes meat, poultry, fish, and beans is the principal source of protein, phosphorus, and vitamins B_6 and B_{12}. Certainly, other foods also contribute some of these nutrients but are not necessarily the principal contributors.

The Daily Food Guide[9]

The USDA Daily Food Guide divides commonly eaten foods into five groups according to their respective nutritional contributions: (1) vegetable-fruit, (2) bread-cereal, (3) milk-cheese, (4) meat, poultry, fish, and beans, and (5) fats, sweets, and alcohol. Suggested numbers of servings are recommended for the first four groups. No servings are recommended for the fifth group. If an adult were to eat the recommended four servings each from the vegetable-fruit and bread-cereal groups and two servings each from the milk-cheese and the meat, poultry, fish, and beans groups, he or she would consume daily about 1200 calories and be provided with adequate amounts of protein and most of the vitamins and minerals needed daily. Twelve hundred calories will usually meet

TABLE 14–1. Nutrient Contributions to Diets of Adults*

Food Group†	10 to 25% of Diet	25 to 50% of Diet	50 to 75% of Diet	75% or More of Diet
Milk	Calories Vitamin A Thiamin	Riboflavin Protein	Calcium	
Meat	Calories Vitamin A (if liver chosen)	Protein Thiamin Iron Riboflavin	Niacin	
Fruits and vegetables	Calories Calcium Iron Thiamin Riboflavin Niacin			Vitamin A Ascorbic acid
Bread	Calories Protein Iron Riboflavin Niacin	Thiamin		

From Hertzler, A. A.; Anderson, H. L. J. Am. Diet. Assoc. 64:19, 1954.
*Based on minimum number and size of servings recommended for the adult.
†In the fifth group of the five food groups, Fats, Sweets, and Alcohol, the only recommended nutrients are 2 to 4 tablespoons of polyunsaturated fats, which supply essential fatty acids.

the basal metabolic needs of an adult but are not enough to meet the energy requirements for physical activity.

VEGETABLE-FRUIT GROUP

Vegetables and fruits are important because they contribute vitamins A and C and fiber as well as trace amounts of other nutrients.

In general, the color of the vegetable or fruit is a guide to its food value. Dark green and deep yellow vegetables are good sources of vitamin A; for example, carrots are better than corn because they are of a deeper yellow color, and spinach is better than celery because it is a darker green than celery. The specific foods, in alphabetical order, that are good sources of vitamin A are apricots, broccoli, cantaloupe, carrots, chard, collards, cress, kale, mangoes, persimmons, pumpkins, spinach, sweet potatoes, turnip greens, and winter squash. Table 14–2 lists the foods that are the best sources of vitamin A and those that contain about half as much. Most dark green vegetables, if not overcooked, are also reliable sources of vitamin C as well as riboflavin, folacin, iron, and magnesium. Certain greens—collards, kale, mustard greens, turnips, and dandelions—provide calcium.

As can be seen in Table 14–3, in choosing foods for vitamin C content, it takes smaller quantities of good sources of vitamin C to fill the daily need. Therefore it would seem wise to emphasize orange juice, cantaloupes, grapefruit, broccoli, and strawberies rather than tomato juice, for example, unless the latter

TABLE 14–2. Sources of Vitamin A (from Carotenes in Plants)

Best	About Half as Much*
1 raw or ⅓ c cooked carrots	½ c broccoli
½ c cooked greens	½ c pumpkin
½ c winter squash	3 raw apricots
½ medium sweet potato	1 wedge (4- × 8-inch) watermelon
½ medium cantaloupe	

*Smaller but important amounts may be obtained from asparagus, endive, tomatoes, canned apricots, yellow peaches, chili peppers.

is enriched with vitamin C. In addition, the contribution of a generous serving of cabbage salad or potato baked or cooked in its skin should not be overlooked.

The food guide recommends four basic servings daily from this group. This includes one good vitamin C source each day and a dark green and a deep yellow vegetable at least every other day and more frequently if possible. And, to ensure adequate fiber, unpeeled raw fruits and vegetables and edible seeds such as berries should be eaten when possible.

A serving is one-half cup of a vegetable or fruit, or a portion as ordinarily served, such as one medium-size apple, orange, or potato; one bowl of salad; or half of a medium-size grapefruit or cantaloupe.

BREAD-CEREAL GROUP

The bread and cereal group is the most economical source of nutrients in our daily diets. A wide variety of cereal grains is available, including wheat, rice, corn, rye, oats, and barley.

Whole-grain or enriched bread and cereals contain substantial amounts of the B vitamins and iron. The purpose of restoration is to return to refined flour and bread made from it the original nutritive value of whole grain before refinement with respect to iron, thiamin, riboflavin, and niacin. Bread and cereals also provide protein, and are a major source of this nutrient in vegetarian diets. Whole-grain products also contribute magnesium, folacin, and fiber.

Many breakfast cereals are enriched at nutrient levels higher than those that occur in natural whole grain. In some cases, fortification adds vitamins, such as A, B_{12}, C, and D, not normally found in cereals (which is not desirable or recommended, especially the addition of vitamins A and D). However, fiber and other still unidentified vitamins and trace minerals that may normally be

TABLE 14–3. Sources of Vitamin C

Best	About Half as Much
1 medium orange	1 medium tomato
½ c orange juice	½ to ⅔ c tomato juice
½ medium grapefruit	1 medium tangerine
½ c grapefruit juice	1 wedge (4- × 8-inch) watermelon
½ cantaloupe	¼ raw pepper
⅔ c fresh strawberries	1 medium to large potato
½ c broccoli	½ c cooked asparagus
	½ c cooked kale or other greens
	½ c coleslaw

present in whole grain are not replaced in the usual restoration process of the refined cereals. Therefore it is strongly recommended that natural whole-grain products be included in the diet whenever possible.

In a society that eats as many sugar-sweetened products as frequently as this one, it is impossible to demonstrate in clinical experiments the relative contribution of a single food item, such as presweetened breakfast cereals, to dental caries development. However, there is not much doubt that presweetening of any food item, including cereals, helps compound and perpetuate the taste for sweets. The habit of eating sugar-sweetened foods is as undesirable for the development of dental caries as the smoking habit is for development of lung cancer or as the heavy drinking of alcoholic beverages (liquor) is for development of cirrhosis of the liver.

Four servings daily of breads and cereals, especially of whole-grain products, are recommended. By checking the labels on bread wrappings or cereal packages, one can note the presence of whole-grain products. Counted as one serving are 1 oz of ready-to-eat cereal, ½ to ¾ c of cooked cereal, corn meal, grits, macaroni, noodles, spaghetti, or rice, and one slice of bread. Even for weight-conscious individuals, some whole-grain or enriched flour, bread, or cereals should be included in the daily diet to ensure adequate amounts of B vitamins and iron.

MILK-CHEESE GROUP

In the United States, milk products are an important part of the diet. Milk and milk products provide about two-thirds of the calcium, one-half of the riboflavin, and one-fourth of the protein in the foods normally eaten. Milk is low in vitamin C and iron, but it supplies more of the other essential nutrients in significant amounts than any other single food.

Nonfat milk solids cost about one-third as much as a quart of fresh milk, but they are low in fat and vitamin A. However, adequate amounts of fat and vitamin A can be economically obtained by using fortified margarine.

Evaporated milk is also economical. It can be used in cooking or in coffee or tea; it is less expensive than cream and contains more calcium and protein. Evaporated milk is whole milk from which more than half the water has been removed by an evaporating process. It differs from condensed milk in that the latter is prepared by adding about 42% sugar to the milk before the water is evaporated.

Those who prefer fermented milk can choose either buttermilk or yogurt. Buttermilk is equal to skim milk in food value; yogurt is equivalent to whole milk. Yogurt has no special health values greater than those of whole fresh milk, and costs more. But for some people with lactose intolerance, it is the milk product of choice. Buttermilk, on the other hand, usually costs less than regular milk. For those who enjoy it, it can be used in place of some or all of the regular milk.

Cheese is the curd (solids) of milk separated from the whey (liquid) by coagulation; it contains most of the protein, calcium, and riboflavin. Cheddar cheese is a whole-milk cheese product that has been cured (preserved by salting). Processed cheese is pasteurized and is made by blending different cheeses and adding emulsifier. Cottage cheese is made from pasteurized skim milk and provides high-quality protein and a few calories. Cream cheese is made from whole milk; cream is added. Cream cheese contains a high percentage of fat and vitamin A and much less protein than cottage cheese; therefore, it is usually placed in the fifth food group with the fats.

Since cheese and ice cream can be used to replace milk and to supply calcium, it is of interest to tabulate their milk equivalent in calcium:

1-inch cube Cheddar cheese = ⅔ c milk
½ c cottage cheese = ⅓ c milk
½ c ice cream = ¼ c milk

An average serving is one 8-oz c of milk or about a 1-inch cube of cheddar cheese. Children and adolescents should have the equivalent of 3 to 4 c daily; adults, 2 c daily; and women over age 50 (who may be candidates for osteoporosis), 3 to 4 c daily.

MEAT, POULTRY, FISH, AND BEANS GROUP

The choices within this group are many: beef, lamb, veal, pork, fish, poultry, eggs, dried beans or peas, and nuts. These foods are valued for protein, phosphorus, niacin, vitamin B_{12}, and iron. Only foods of animal origin provide vitamin B_{12}.

Foods in this groups are usually the most expensive items in the diet. The cost of a specific cut of meat is not related to its food value. The less expensive grades and cuts are just as high in protein and iron as is tenderloin of beef. In this group, the organ meats (liver, heart, and kidneys) deserve special mention for their high nutritional value in relation to cost.

There is relatively little difference in the protein and iron content of beef, veal, lamb, and pork, although pork is richer in thiamin. Fish, poultry, and eggs are complete protein foods and can be used as meat equivalents.

Dried beans and peas (lentils) are economical. Although their protein is not complete, when they are used with other vegetables, such as corn, or with complete proteins such as milk or cheese or small amounts of meat, they can be used to help meet the amino acid requirements of the body. Such dishes as chile con carne, pea soup with ham, or frankfurters with beans, which combine meat and dried legumes, are excellent both nutritionally and economically. Nuts and their products, such as peanut butter, can be included in the diet for variety.

It is strongly recommended that the choices among the above-mentioned foods be varied, because each has distinct nutritional advantages. For example, red meats and oysters are good sources of zinc. Liver and egg yolks are valuable sources of vitamin A. Dry beans, dry peas, soybeans, and nuts are worthwhile sources of magnesium. Fish and poultry are low in saturated fat. Sunflower and sesame seeds contribute polyunsaturated fatty acids.

Cholesterol is found in high concentration in organ meats and egg yolks, whereas fish and shellfish except shrimp are relatively low in cholesterol.

To obtain full advantage of the protein from the foods in this group, it is preferable to have an occasional egg for breakfast, a fish or meat sandwich at noon, and some meat, fish, poultry, or beans at night rather than to have a large serving at only one meal and no food from this group at other meals.

Suggested daily amounts from this group of foods are 2 or more servings. Count 3 to 4 oz of lean, cooked meat, poultry, or fish filet as a serving. One-half to ¾ c cooked dry beans, dry peas (split peas), soybeans, or lentils; 2 tablespoons peanut butter; and ¼ to ½ c nuts, sesame seeds, or sunflower seeds count as 1 oz of meat, poultry, or fish. Two eggs are equivalent to about 3 oz of meat.

FATS, SWEETS, AND ALCOHOL GROUP[9]

This group of foods provides mostly calories. Included in the group are butter, margarine, mayonnaise, other salad dressings, and other fats and oils; candy, sugar, jams, jellies, syrups, sweet toppings, and other sweets; soft drinks and other highly sugared beverages; and wine, beer, and liquor. Refined flour products that are not restored or enriched used as ingredients in prepared foods are also included in this group. Vegetable oils supply vitamin E and essential fatty acids. Margarine and butter provide some vitamin A. These are the most desirable foods in this group. Two to four tablespoons of polyunsaturated oil daily are recommended.

In general, with the exception of the fats just mentioned, these foods provide practically no essential nutrients such as vitamins, minerals, and protein. Therefore no serving sizes are defined.

Limitations of the Food Group Guide

The Daily Food Guide has oversimplified and perhaps overgeneralized the eating plan, because it suggests that there are only a few key nutrients that should be monitored. It is assumed that the nutrients not being monitored will be automatically ingested if the diet is varied. This assumption should be tested. For example, legumes are accepted alternatives for meat, fish, or poultry. But the animal products contain vitamin B_{12}, and legumes do not. However, foods from the milk-cheese group will supply the vitamin B_{12} requirement. Seventy percent of the vitamin B_{12} is supplied by meats, poultry, and fish; 20% by dairy products excluding butter; and 9% by eggs.[10]

The high amounts of iron required by pregnant, lactating, and premenopausal women cannot be met by these five food groups.

Ready-to-eat processed and fabricated foods, such as formulated fruit drinks and breakfast bars, cannot be classified into a food group because they do not necessarily follow the nutrient pattern of any one food group. Potato chips cannot, for example, be included in the vegetable group because overprocessing destroys the vitamins, especially vitamin C. Combinations of foods, such as casseroles and pizza, make group classification difficult.

NEW DIETARY GOALS AND THE MAJOR DEGENERATIVE HEALTH PROBLEMS

These past few years, consumers, researchers, and health professionals have expressed concern about the contribution of dietary practices to the relatively high incidence of obesity, diabetes, dental caries, atherosclerosis, and particularly coronary heart disease and hypertension in the United States. The United States

Senate responded to this public concern about food consumption practices by inviting recognized authorities in nutrition and public health to investigate this problem and provide some recommendations for dealing with it. These experts reviewed the scientific knowledge from basic research on animals, from metabolic studies and clinical trials, and from epidemiological surveys. On the basis of the consultants' review and evaluation of the scientific data, the Senate Select Committee on Nutrition and Human Needs proposed a national nutrition policy that they believed would support more healthful food consumption than is now current. They documented the dietary goals and the methods for achieving these goals in a committee report, "Dietary Goals for the United States," published in February 1977. This publication provoked negative as well as positive reactions. In response to the criticisms, a second edition, containing some revisions, was published in December of the same year.[11] This last edition clarified the controversial issues and rectified the omissions in the earlier edition by adding sections (e.g., on obesity and alcohol consumption).

This report cited a number of risk factors that should be recognized and dealt with: controllable risk factors (poor diet, lack of exercise, eating too many sweets) and uncontrollable ones (genetics, age, gender) associated with a higher-than-average incidence of health problems. Consumers can do something about controllable factors such as diet selection and eating behaviors.

The major purpose of this report was to provide guidelines for the proper amounts of macronutrients in the diet. The RDAs deal mainly with allowances of micronutrients. Thus one guide complements the other, and together they give consumers an objective measure of the excess, adequacy, or deficiency of their diet.

The Dietary Goals are stated in terms of specific levels or percentage ranges of total carbohydrates, fat, protein, cholesterol, and sodium. In order to achieve these goals most of the population probably should modify their eating behaviors.

THE DIETARY GOALS

The following dietary goals (Fig. 14–2) and changes in food selection and preparation are recommended:

1. To avoid overweight, consume only as many calories as expended; if overweight, decrease energy intake and increase energy expenditure.

2. Increase the consumption of complex carbohydrates and naturally occurring sugars from about 28% to about 48% of calorie energy intake.

3. Reduce the consumption of refined and processed sugars by about 45% to account for about 10% of total energy intake.

4. Reduce overall fat consumption from approximately 40% to about 30% of energy intake.

5. Reduce saturated fat consumption to account for about 10% of total energy intake, and balance that with polyunsaturated and monounsaturated fats, which should account for about 10% each of total energy intake.

6. Reduce cholesterol consumption to about 300 mg/day.

7. Limit sodium intake by reducing salt to about 5 g/day.

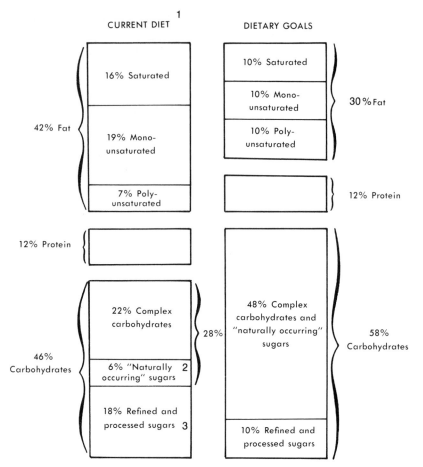

FIGURE 14–2. *Current diet percentages are based on calories from food and nonalcoholic beverages. Alcohol adds approximately 210 calories per day to the average diet of drinking age Americans. Naturally occurring sugars are those that are indigenous to a food, as opposed to refined (cane and beet) and processed (corn sugar syrups, molasses, and honey) sugars, which may be added to a food product. In many ways alcoholic beverages affect the diet in the same way as refined and other processed sugars. Both add calories (energy) to the total diet but contribute few or no vitamin or minerals. (Sources for Current Diet: Changes in Nutrients in the U.S. Diet Caused by Alterations in Food Intake Patterns. Agricultural Research Service, USDA, 1974. Proportions of saturated versus unsaturated fats based on unpublished Agricultural Research Service data. Dietary goals from U.S. Congress. Senate Select Committee on Nutrition and Human Needs, Report on Dietary Goals for the United States, 2nd ed. Washington, D.C., GPO, December 1977.)*

Changes in Food Selection and Preparation Suggested by the Dietary Goals

1. Increase consumption of fruits and vegetables and whole grains.

2. Decrease consumption of refined and other processed sugars and foods high in such sugars.

3. Decrease consumption of foods high in total fat, and partially replace saturated fats, from animal or vegetable sources, with polyunsaturated fats.

4. Decrease consumption of animal fat, choosing meats such as veal or poultry and fish to reduce saturated fat intake.

5. Except for young children, substitute low-fat and nonfat milk for whole milk, and use other low-fat dairy products.

6. Decrease consumption of butterfat, eggs, and other sources high in cholesterol. Some consideration should be given to easing the cholesterol goal for premenopausal women, young children, and the elderly in order to obtain the nutritional benefits of eggs in the diet.

7. Decrease consumption of salt and foods high in salt content.

Two important points concerning the interpretation of these goals are that (1) the specific percentages recommended should be considered the center of a range and (2) these dietary recommendations will increase the probability of improved protection from the six common degenerative diseases previously mentioned (obesity, atherosclerosis, diabetes, coronary heart disease, hypertension, and dental caries), but they do not guarantee it.

To achieve these goals, it was recommended that there be a public health education program in classrooms and cafeterias of schools and an extensive use of television and other educational approaches. It also was recommended that Congress require labels to be placed on foods to show their fat, sugar, cholesterol, salt, and additive content.

In order to implement these goals effectively, they must be linked to an easily understood food guide, such as the 1979 Daily Food Guide, which divides the foods commonly eaten into the five groups described earlier.[9] Even with its limitations, there is not at this time an equally simple, equally workable alternative food guide for people in the United States. One way to improve the value of the five–food group guide is to select a variety of foods from the alternative foods in each group.

How to Implement the Goals

In summary, to achieve the Dietary Goals and assure selection of a prudent diet one should[11]

- Eat a variety of foods
- Avoid consuming too much fat, saturated fat, and cholesterol by drinking more skim milk and less whole milk and eating more fish, poultry, and beans and less meat
- Eat foods with adequate starch and fiber, such as whole-grain bread, cereals, raw vegetables, and fruits
- Eat a minimum to moderate amount of sugar
- Eat a minimum to moderate amount of sodium
- Consume alcohol only in moderation
- Achieve and maintain ideal weight

The following statement, by one of the nutrition consultants to the Senate committee on the development of the U.S. dietary goals, provides an appropriate summary[12]:

"There will undoubtedly be many people who will say we have not proven our point; we have not demonstrated that the dietary modifications we recommend will yield the dividends expected. We would point out to those people that the diet we eat today was not planned or developed for any particular purpose. It is a happenstance related to our affluence, the productivity of our farmers, and the activities of our food industry. The risks associated with eating this diet are demonstrably large. The question to be asked, therefore, is not Why should we change our diet? but Why not? What are the risks associated with eating less meat, less fat, less saturated fat, less cholesterol, less sugar, less salt, and more fruits, vegetables, unsaturated fat and cereal products—especially whole grain cereals. There are none that can be identified and important benefits can be expected."

The desire to identify dietary goals that lead to good health and to reduce the incidence of illness is shared by all nutritionists. However, according to the Food and Nutrition Board, more research is needed to establish the dietary guidelines for energy, sodium, lipids, carbohydrates and fiber, and protein.[14] The Board noted that "no single recommendation to the public regarding appropriate intakes" can be made because needs "vary with age, sex, physiological state, heredity, and physical activity." Moreover, individuals vary greatly in their susceptibility to chronic degenerative diseases. Thus the justification for making changes in the national diet is being debated. This issue will probably not be resolved to the satisfaction of all until the recommended research is completed.

REFERENCES

1. Committee on Dietary Allowances, Food and Nutrition Board, National Academy of Sciences-National Research Council. Recommended Dietary Allowances, 9th rev. ed. Washington, D.C., National Academy Press, 1980.
2. Harper, A. E. Recommended Dietary Allowances in perspective. Food Nutr. News 58(2):7, 1986.
3. Anderson, G. H.; Peterson, R. D.; Beaton, G. H. Estimating nutrient deficiencies in a population from dietary records: the use of probability analyses. Nutr. Res. 2:409, 1982.
4. Special report on Recommended Dietary Allowances. Tufts Univ. Diet Nutr. Lett. 4(2):4, 1986.
5. Hegsted, D. M. Dietary standards. Nutr. Rev. 36:33, 1978.
6. Munro, H. N. How well recommended are the Recommended Dietary Allowances? J. Am. Diet. Assoc. 71:490, 1977.
7. Hertzler, A. A.; Anderson, H. L. Food guides in the United States. J. Am. Diet Assoc. 64:19, 1974.
8. Page, L.; Phipard, E. Essentials of an Adequate Diet. Facts for Nutrition Programs. USDA Home Economics Research Report no. 3, Washington, D.C., GPO, 1957.
9. Davis, C. A., et al. Food. USDA Home and Garden Bulletin no. 228. Prepared by Science and Education Administration. Washington, D.C., GPO, September 1979.
10. Marston, R. M.; Welsh, S. O. Nutrient content of the U.S. food supply. 1982. Natl. Food Rev. (Winter):7, 1984.
11. USDA-DHHS Nutrition and Your Health: Dietary Guidelines for Americans, 2nd ed. Washington, D.C., GPO, 1985.
12. U.S. Senate Select Committee on Nutrition and Human Needs: Dietary Goals for the United States, 2nd ed. Washington, D.C., GPO, December 1977.
13. Food and Nutrition Board. Research Needs for Establishing Dietary Guidelines for the U.S. Population. Washington, D.C., National Academy Press, 1980.

15

Health Foods, Additives,
Food Facts and Fallacies,
Megavitamin Therapy, and
Vegetarianism

HISTORICAL HIGHLIGHTS OF "HEALTH" FOOD FADS

"Health" foods have been popular for many years. Concerns about health, safety, and the protection of the environment have increased their popularity. Mistakenly, some of the public have developed a distrust of scientists; consequently, "food mythology" has been substituted for food science. Many popular books and magazines have aided and abetted this distrust of food science and technology.

Historically, food mythology began when primitive humans used some foods and herbs for their pharmacological, not nutritional, effects. In addition, some ancient religions bestowed magical powers on certain foods during their ritual dances and prayers. The individual who is credited with being the first food faddist is Cato, a Roman, living in the second century, A.D., who selected cabbage as the perfect food and thought it to be the panacea for all ailments. A number of food faddists have become popular since then, as described in R. Deutsch's book, The New Nuts Among the Berries.[1] A few of the more popular food faddists offered a variety of "cures." They originated graham flour, bread, and crackers, opposed including meat in the diet because it made people too aggressive, advocated that food should be chewed until it was liquefied in the mouth before swallowing, advocated wheat germ and blackstrap molasses as miracle foods, and recommended a concoction of vinegar and honey products for any health problem.

DEFINITIONS OF HEALTH, ORGANIC, AND NATURAL FOODS[2]

The terms *health foods, organically grown foods*, and *natural foods* are used interchangeably by most people. But if accurately defined, they mean different things.

Health foods are supposed to possess health-giving, curative properties beyond their ordinary nutritive action.

Organically grown foods are foods grown without the use of any manufactured agricultural chemicals and fertilizers (insecticides, pesticides, herbicides, antibiotics, hormones). These foods are processed without the use of food chemicals or additives (synthetic sweeteners, preservatives, dyes, emulsifiers, stabilizers). Even the fertilizers and pesticides used in the production of organically grown foods are from animal and vegetable sources.

Natural foods are foods in their original state, such as raw fruits and vegetables, with minimal refinement and minimal processing.

MAIN ISSUES IN THE HEALTH FOOD MOVEMENT[3]

The main issues that concern the health food users are the following:

- Chemical fertilizers compared with organic fertilizers, produce a nutritionally inferior food.
- Foods are poisoned by inorganic fertilizer.
- Food processing reduces the nutritional value of foods (see Chap. 13).
- Some foods have miraculous curative properties and functions.
- Megavitamins are not only useful but even essential in the prevention and treatment of some common medical problems such as colds, heart disease, and schizophrenia.

As an example, the following answer might be given when the first issue is raised.

The major purpose of fertilizing soil is to increase the quantity or yield per acre of the fruit, vegetables, or grains. Fertilizers do not affect the nutritional quality of plant foods. The nutritional quality of a food depends on (1) the genetic characteristics of the seed produced by hybridization (the process of producing plants from parents of two different species), (2) favorable climatic conditions, (3) adequate ripening on the tree or vine, and (4) consumption of the fruits or vegetables immediately after being harvested.

For organically grown foods, manure and compost are used as fertilizers; most commercially grown foods are fertilized by inorganic, synthetic chemicals (potassium, nitrogen, and phosphorus).

Organic fertilizer advocates claim that organically grown crops have a higher vitamin content than those grown with inorganic fertilizers. According to Beeson and Brandt of the U.S. Plant, Soil, and Nutrition Laboratory in Ithaca, New York, it is not the type of fertilizer that influences the vitamin content of a fruit or vegetable but the quantity and intensity of sunlight.[4] For example, sunlight has much more influence on the concentration of vitamin C in tomatoes than any variation in the type of fertilizer applied to the plant. Further, they have shown that high humidity produces a plant with a higher carotene content; high soil temperature results in high concentration of B vitamins and minerals; and high rainfall increases the concentration of a number of vitamins and minerals.

Only the size of the crop yield is influenced by soil fertility; the quantity of output, not the quality of the plant, is affected by fertilization. Neither organic nor inorganic fertilizers influence the nutritive value of the food.

Scientific data indicate that there is no significant nutritional difference between crops grown with organic or chemical fertilizers. The fact is that any organic matter must be broken down by the soil bacteria into inorganic nutrients before a plant can use them. The three mineral elements recognized as prime factors in the nourishment or fertilization of plant foods are nitrogen (N), phosphorus (P), and potassium (K). Nitrogen aids in the growth of the plant and in the depth of green color of the leaves. Phosphates give color to flowers and fruits and assist in their development, and potassium strengthens the stems and roots of the plant.

The plant is unable to distinguish between the phosphate, nitrate, and potassium that result from the decomposition of organic fertilizer and those from synthetic chemical fertilizers. It is impractical to supply these elements in organic form because it would take 10 tons of farm manure per acre and 1 lb of bone meal per 100 square feet to provide the 140 lb of nitrogen, 140 lb of phosphorus, and 140 lb of potassium usually needed per acre to produce a satisfactory crop.

The superior flavor often attributed to organically grown produce is really due to the fact that these fruits and vegetables are allowed to ripen on the vine or tree, are harvested at the peak of quality, and are used promptly. The same advantages would occur in these circumstances even if chemical fertilizers were used.

Although there are no significant nutritional, health, or taste advantages, there are sound ecological reasons for returning organic materials to the soil when possible. There is a risk, however, that manure, moldy leaves, and other organic material used in organic gardening may be infected with fungal toxins such as aflatoxin, an extremely potent poison and carcinogen. Also, there is a possibility of *Salmonella* contamination.

FOOD ADDITIVES[5, 6]

Food additives are substances that are combined with food to (1) prevent growth of microbes or spoilage; (2) improve their nutrient quality, or (3) enhance texture, flavor, color, and odor. In general, additives are used to keep food safe and edible.

Chemical and Microbial Inhibitors

Sodium chloride and sucrose are two of the oldest and probably are the most used microbial inhibitors. Because they absorb water, they make it less available for chemical reactions and microbial growth. This is one of the reasons for using sucrose in making jams, jellies, and cured hams.

Citric acid, acetic acid, and phosphoric acid lower the pH of food to an acid state in which organisms cannot grow.

Other bacterial growth inhibitors are calcium propionate (added to bread) and sorbic acid (added to beverages).

As fresh fruits, vegetables, and processed foods age, they change in color, flavor, and texture as a result of oxidation. Antioxidants are added to foods to reduce this spoilage. For example, sprinkling some vitamin C powder on sliced apples or potatoes will prevent browning through action of enzymes. This antioxidant is acceptable because it is a natural food component. On the other hand, BHT (butylated hydroxytoluene) and BHA (butylated hydroxyanisole) are synthetic antioxidants that are added to polyunsaturated acids to prevent formation of toxic substances. These compounds have been found to be acceptable at the levels used but are suspect, because they are toxic when fed to rats at levels equal to 5% of the diet. When baboons were used as the experimental animal for testing the safety of BHA and BHT, these compounds were found to be harmless. In human foods, BHA and BHT are consumed at only 100 parts per million.

Other antioxidants are metal-chelating agents (EDTA and citric acid), which bind trace metals and prevent them from catalyzing the oxidation of lipids.

Enhancers of Nutrient Quality

Some vitamins, minerals, and proteins are added to foods to increase the nutritional value of the product and in fact have been responsible for overcoming many acute nutritional deficiencies seen in the early part of the twentieth century.

Three processes are used for improving the nutrient quality of food: restoration, enrichment, and fortification. Each process serves different objectives.

1. Restoration. Selected nutrients are added to a food to restore nutrients lost through processing (e.g., adding vitamin C to sterilized fruit juice).

2. Enrichment. Nutrients are added to a food to conform to standards established for certain nutrients (e.g., iron, niacin, thiamin, riboflavin, calcium, and vitamin D added to flour or bread).

3. Fortification. Selected nutrients not normally present in that particular food (e.g., vitamin D in milk or vitamin A in margarine) are added.

Agents Essential for Food Processing

A few of the additives that are used in food technology to satisfy the consumer's taste and the acceptability of the appearance and texture of foods are

- Leavening agents (yeast, baking powder), which cause baked goods to rise
- Emulsifiers (lecithin), which keep oil- or fat-containing ingredients mixed with a water base and give baked goods a light texture
- Thickeners (gelatin), which give foods a smooth thick texture or prevent ice crystal formation in frozen foods such as ice cream
- Humectants, which prevent foods such as marshmallows from absorbing water
- Artificial flavors and colors, which impart the expected flavor and color to a food (margarine is colored yellow to resemble butter)
- Foaming agents that cause bubbles in such beverages as instant hot chocolate mix.

Although use of these and other additives is questioned by health food advocates, the Food and Drug Administration (FDA) protects the food purchaser by enforcing the National Pure Food and Drug Law, which requires that chemicals used in food production must be shown to be safe before they may be used commercially. It would be impossible to provide enough food for the people in this country without additives.

Generally Recognized as Safe

Chemical additives generally recognized as safe (GRAS) are considered harmless when added to the food supply under normal manufacturing processes and are nontoxic in normal use. Anything, including water, ingested in large enough amounts can cause death. All the chemicals on the GRAS list are repeatedly being reexamined under stringent criteria to reaffirm their safety. Additives that produce cancer in any species of experimental animals, although fed at a much higher dosage than is usually ingested by humans, are banned from the food supply in accordance with the Delaney Amendment of the Pure Food and Drug Act.

Before additives can be used in food they are evaluated on the basis of risk versus benefits. For example, without adding calcium propionate, bread would mold rapidly. The risk is that calcium propionate can be toxic if added at much higher levels than normally used. When used at recommended levels, the benefit is increased shelf life and reduced waste. As long as the benefits of increased quality, nutritional value, shelf life, and so forth exceed the risk of toxicity from the accepted tolerance level, the additive is acceptable.

Unacceptable and Questionably Safe Additives

The following chemical additives have been removed, or use at low levels has been allowed:

1. Diethylstilbestrol (DES), a synthetic growth hormone that was used in animal feeds, has been removed.

2. FDC Red dye #2, a coloring agent used in lipstick and beverages, has been under study for mutagenic effects. Permits have been granted for its use at lower levels. The FDC Red dye #3, used in plaque disclosing tablets, is acceptable.

3. Violet dye #1, used for stamping the grades of meat into beef carcasses, is suspected of being carcinogenic and is undergoing further testing. However, the exposure is so low that it is not considered a significant risk.

4. Synthetic sweeteners such as cyclamates and saccharin are still used but are being periodically reassessed regarding their safety.

5. Monosodium glutamate (MSG), a flavor enhancer, has been shown to cause tissue damage to the brain in immature rats. MSG has been removed from baby food.

We can conclude from present scientific knowledge that although there are some food additives that should not be permitted, other additives have proved safe when subjected to stringent testing. If all additives were forbidden, the variety and palatability of our foods would be drastically reduced, the nutritional and preservation quality of foods sharply curtailed, and the price of foods considerably higher.

Continued rigorous testing and vigilance by the FDA should help make additives in the food supply safe for human consumption.

FOOD FACTS AND FALLACIES[7]

Over the years, a number of myths, fallacies, and false claims relating to food have created confusion in the minds of consumers.

Dairy Products

Fallacy: Any milk other than cow's milk is desirable. Goat's milk, which is nutritious, is recommended with the consent of the pediatrician in case there is a question of allergy.

Fact: The fact that goats are not susceptible to tuberculosis, whereas cattle are, may have been the origin of this particular belief. Pasteurization destroys the tuberculosis germ and makes the cow's milk safe.

Fallacy: Yogurt is nutritionally superior to ordinary milk.

Fact: Yogurt is fermented whole milk evaporated to two-thirds of its original volume making it thick enough so that it can be eaten with a spoon. It has the same nutritive value as whole milk. It is true that a few people (those with lactose intolerance) find yogurt more digestible. Its chief value is that it provides a source of milk in other forms. Its taste is pleasant to many people. Commercial yogurt is often presweetened and is an expensive form of milk.

Fallacy: Milk and cheese are constipating.

Fact: Milk and cheese are easily digested and leave little residue. If constipation does occur, it is because the diet lacks food that contains bulk.

Fallacy: Pasteurized milk is "dead" milk.

Fact: Pasteurization does not alter the nutritional value of milk except to reduce the vitamin C content slightly (milk is a poor source of vitamin C). Pasteurization destroys bacteria that can cause undulant fever and tuberculosis.

Bread and Cereal Products

Fallacy: Gluten, protein bread, and dark bread are less fattening than white bread.

Fact: Breads vary little in caloric content. Thus one is not superior to another from the standpoint of weight loss.

Fallacy: White bread and white flour are unfit for human consumption because all the vitamins and minerals have been removed and the bleaching process is poisonous.

Fact: Almost all commercial white breads and white flours are restored and enriched, according to law, with iron, niacin, thiamin, and riboflavin, which makes them nutritious. Chlorine dioxide, a harmless compound, is currently used to bleach flour.

Meat, Fish, and Eggs

Fallacy: Eggs with brown shells are more nutritious than white shell eggs.
Fact: The color of the shell does not indicate the nutritive value of the egg. The color of the shell is determined by the breed of hen.

Fallacy: The characteristics of the type of meat are transmitted by consumption: for example, eating heart makes one courageous.
Fact: This of course is not true.

Fallacy: Meat that is raw or cooked rare is more nourishing than well-done meat.
Fact: This is not true; proteins are not damaged by cooking. Also, cooking protects the individual against bacterial infections and disease such as trichinosis.

Fallacy: Fish is brain food.
Fact: This belief may have originated from the fact that the brain contains phosphorus and fish is a rich source of this mineral. But this reasoning is erroneous.

Vegetables

Fallacy: Drink your vegetables.
Fact: Vegetable juices make an excellent contribution to the diet but do not contain the bulk necessary in the diet.

Fallacy: Tomatoes clear the brain; onions will cure a cold; and lettuce is soothing to the nerves.
Fact: There is no scientific evidence to substantiate these claims.

Sugars

Fallacy: Blackstrap molasses cures practically every affliction, from restoring color to gray hair to restoring youth.
Fact: This dark, thick syrup represents the leavings of sugar manufacture. It contains small amounts of iron, calcium, and B complex vitamins. The iron present comes from contact with the factory machinery. The calcium comes from the limewater used in processing.

Condiments

Fallacy (ancient): Spices and condiments have the power to prevent disease.
Fact: The belief that diseases originated in foul-smelling air may have led to the conclusion that the pungent odor of spices warded off disease.

Fallacy: Hot spicy foods have a reputation for being cooling and for that reason are eaten in tropical countries.
Fact: The real reason for eating spicy foods in the tropics is that hot weather

and a natural increase in water intake cause appetites to lag. Spices tend to stimulate a desire for food. Spices and condiments have no food value, and no health-promoting qualities can be attributed to them.

Water

Fallacy: Drinking water with meals will dilute the gastric juice and interfere with digestion.
Fact: This is untrue. Water stimulates the flow of digestive juice.

Fallacy: Large amounts of water are said to thin the blood.
Fact: There is no evidence for this.

Fallacy: Drinking water will increase weight.
Fact: Water drunk in excess of body needs is eliminated.

Lecithin

Fallacy: Lecithin is an important dietary supplement for people with coronary heart disease; it removes fat deposits.
Fact: Lecithin is a phospholipid present in many foods, especially in egg yolk and meats. Phospholipids are essential parts of living cells and are used in the transport and utilization of fats and fatty acids. There is no good evidence to indicate that lecithin lowers serum cholesterol levels or that it has a role in the treatment of coronary heart disease. Nor can combinations of lecithin, kelp, cider, vinegar, and vitamin B_6 remove fat deposits in obese subjects.

MEGAVITAMIN THERAPY[8]

Use of megadoses of vitamins for improvement of health is based on the concept that if a little is good, more must be better; which is not true. Use of megavitamins for conditions other than those known to be acute vitamin deficiencies is not scientifically sound.

Most vitamins (at least the water-soluble ones) function as coenzymes. Vitamins are relatively small molecules that when combined with associated proteins form active enzymes that facilitate the metabolic reactions in the body. Since the quantity of protein is limited, vitamins in excess of the amount of protein available do not serve the vitamin function. To the contrary, excessive doses of vitamins may have a pharmacological or toxic effect, or both.

Only two major groups of disorders are corrected or alleviated by large doses of specific vitamins. These include the malabsorption syndrome and some inborn errors of metabolism.

Megadoses of vitamins used over a long time can create tissue dependency by raising the metabolic level of body cells, so that they adapt to functioning with maximal amounts of both the specific vitamins ingested and the biochemically related vitamins (e.g., water-soluble B complex and C). Although the cells still can receive only a limited amount, that amount may be considerably more than that they need. Thus, a return to normal doses can cause a transient or temporary deficiency not only of the individual vitamin but also of related ones. Megadoses of vitamin C taken by pregnant women can create a dependency affecting the newborn infant, who could develop scurvy, with bleeding tendencies, when fed the normal amount of vitamin C. It is vital that the pregnant woman consult a physician or nutritionist before taking megadoses of any vitamins.

Justifications for megadoses of vitamins include providing optimal health and individual variability. That megavitamins will produce optimal health is not supported by the facts. The truth is that large doses of fat-soluble vitamins, such as A and D, which can be stored, are actually toxic when high levels accumulate.

The argument that individuals vary is based on the allegation that the Recommended Dietary Allowances (RDAs) do not take into account individual variation in need for vitamins. Actually, the RDA is deliberately set at a level above the range of normal human variability. However, there is individual variability in vitamin toxicity. For example, a dosage of a vitamin 10 times higher than the RDA may not be toxic to patient A but may be toxic to patient B.

Megadoses of Vitamin C

There is no evidence that vitamin C kills the cold-carrying virus. There is some preliminary evidence that vitamin C may have an antihistaminic effect. If this finding is corroborated, then some people with colds may have reduced symptoms if they take vitamin C. Clinical data relating to the safety and effectiveness of pharmacological doses of ascorbic acid in the prevention and treatment of the common cold were reviewed. The conclusion was that the unrestricted use of ascorbic acid for these purposes could not be advocated on the basis of the evidence.[9]

Megadoses of vitamin C can cause acidic urine, with accompanying burning sensations on urination. Inaccurate glucose tests in diabetes can result from megadoses, because vitamin C is related chemically to glucose. Massive doses of vitamin C may also cause kidney problems; overproduction of oxalate can result in formation of oxalate stones. If vitamin C is taken as a supplement, the recommended daily dose is 60 mg for an adult.

Megadoses of Vitamin E

Vitamin E acts as an antioxidant, an organic compound occurring in minute amounts in food that protects other molecules from combining with oxygen to form toxic substances.

It has been asserted that megadoses of vitamin E will improve human sexual function, and prevent and cure heart disease, acne, ulcers, habitual abortion, muscular dystrophy, and certain menstrual disorders. Most of these assertions stem from observations in experimental animals. That the same effects occur in humans has not been proved. Nor is there clear proof that extra quantities of vitamin E have any significant effect on plasma cholesterol or low-density lipoprotein concentrations.

Research over a considerable number of years has not proved the virtues claimed for large doses of vitamin E. To the contrary, vitamin E excess, like excesses of other fat-soluble vitamins, may be toxic to some extent. Interference with vitamin K activity (prolongation of coagulation time) as a result of large doses of vitamin E has been reported. Vitamin E may not be tolerated in large doses, as shown in a report stating that the development of "flu-like" symptoms in humans taking 800 mg of vitamin E per day disappeared when the dose was reduced to half that amount.

VEGETARIANISM[10]

A vegetarian is a person whose diet is composed predominantly of plant food and who abstains from the consumption of meat, fowl, or fish, but may eat eggs and dairy products. A pure vegetarian, or vegan, consumes only plant foods. A lacto-ovovegetarian consumes dairy foods and eggs, in addition to plant foods. A lactovegetarian eats dairy products, as well as plant foods. A fruitarian is a person whose diet consists chiefly of fruits.

The motives for adopting a type of vegetarian diet may be health concerns (avoidance of additives and use of natural "organic" foods), religious or philosophical beliefs (respect for animal life), or both.

Some of the possible nutritional risks of a vegetarian diet, particularly for infants, children, pregnant and lactating females, and the elderly, are as follows:

- Caloric needs are sometimes difficult to meet, particularly in children, because the diet is so high in bulk.
- Diminished caloric intake would require increased bodily use of protein, which may not be abundant in the diet, as an energy source.
- There may be low calcium, vitamin D, and riboflavin intake, especially for children, unless some forms of dairy foods are included in the diet. On the other hand, a lacto-ovovegetarian diet is quite safe for children. Although green, leafy vegetables are high in calcium content, absorption of calcium may be impeded by the metal-binding properties of high-fiber diets.
- A vitamin B_{12} deficiency may develop, because the best sources of vitamin B_{12} are animal products.
- Such a diet may cause iron deficiency in infants, young children, and pregnant women—those who have the greatest need for iron.
- A vegetarian diet may cause zinc deficiency because the best sources of zinc are animal products.

Some of the positive health benefits from a vegetarian diet are the following:

- Less likelihood of atonic constipation
- Lower incidence of atherosclerosis
- Reduced blood pressure
- Lower death rates from cancers of breast, intestines, lungs, and mouth (as demonstrated in studies of Seventh Day Adventists—although their abstention from tobacco, alcohol, and coffee may be equally or more important than their vegetarian diet)

- Low blood levels of cholesterol and triglycerides, fewer low-density lipoproteins, and more high-density lipoproteins, which may help prevent atherosclerosis and the consequence of coronary heart disease

Vegetarian diets offer both risks and benefits. However, the health risks can be avoided and the benefits maximized when dietary planning is based on (1) Milk Group (2 servings): milk, cheese, yogurt, fortified soy milk; (2) Protein Group (2 servings): tofu, eggs, nuts, legumes; (3) Fruit and Vegetable Group (4 servings): especially the fresh raw type rich in fiber; and (4) Bread and Cereal Group (4 servings): whole-grain bread, cereal, and flour products. If more calories are necessary, the fifth group (fats, sugars, and alcohol) may be used prudently, with the approval of your physician.

Some vegetarian diets, especially the lacto-ovovegetarian, may improve health because they introduce formerly neglected foods, such as milk and eggs. They may help to develop a more regular (i.e., 3 meals per day) pattern of eating. Note, however, that foods used by vegetarians are usually more expensive when bought in health food stores.

Studies of vegetarians show them to have a lower serum cholesterol concentration than a comparable meat-eating group. This may be a reason for a comparatively low incidence of coronary artery disease in vegetarians.[11]

The FDA has called attention to the possible hazard of consuming some herbal teas in excessive amounts. Some herbs contain nicotine and digitalis.[12]

CONCLUSION

Accurate, sound nutritional information can be obtained from qualified nutritionists at your local hospitals, community college or state university, state agricultural extension service, publications of the U.S. Department of Agriculture, and the district office or the headquarters of the Food and Drug Administration (5660 Fishers Lane, Rockville, Md. 20852).

REFERENCES

1. Deutsch, R. M. The New Nuts Among the Berries. Palo Alto, Calif., Bull Publishing Co., 1977.
2. McBean, L. D.; Speckman, E. W. Food faddism: a challenge to nutritionists and dietitians. Am. J. Clin. Nutr. 27:1071, 1974.
3. Margolius, S. Health Foods, Facts and Fallacies, pp. 6–9. New York, Walker & Co., 1973.
4. Beeson, K. C.; Brandt, C. S. Influence of organic fertilization on certain nutritive constituents of crops. Soil Sci. 71:449, 1951.
5. Kermode, G. O. Food additives. Sci. Am. 226:15, 1972.
6. Hall, R. L. Food additives. Nutr. Today (July/August):10, 1973.
7. Fleck, H.; Munves, E. Modern Diet and Nutrition, pp. 242–258. New York, Dell Publishing Co., 1955.
8. Herbert, V. The rationale of massive-dose vitamin therapy. In White, P. L.; Selvey, N., eds. Western Hemisphere Nutrition Congress IV Proceedings, pp. 84–91. Acton, Mass., Publishing Sciences Group, 1975.
9. Dykes, M. H. M.; Meier, P. Ascorbic acid and the common cold. Evaluation of its efficacy and toxicity. JAMA 231:1073, 1975.
10. Dwyer, J. T. Vegetariansism and alternative life style diets. In Rechcigl, M., Jr., ed. CRC Handbook Series in Nutrition and Food. Cleveland, Oh., CRC Press, 1979.
11. Eastwood, M. Dietary fiber. In Present Knowledge in Nutrition: Nutrition Reviews, 5th ed., pp. 162–163. Washington, D. C., Nutrition Foundation, 1984.
12. Larkin, T. Herbs are often more toxic than magical. FDA Consumer 17:15, 1983.

16

Nutritional Management of Diet-Related Problems of the Oral Mucosa and Tooth Enamel

The abnormal appearances and functions of dental-oral structures, especially the corners of the mouth, the tongue, the palate, and the teeth, may serve as important clues to underlying systemic nutritional deficiency and/or psychological problems. Inadequate food choices, excessive intake of acidic fruit, or regurgitating gastric acid as seen in an eating disorder may be responsible. For example, glossopyrosis or glossodynia (a burning sensation in the tongue) may be an oral symptom of a nutritional deficiency such as pernicious anemia, which results from a dietary iron deficiency. Erosion of the lingual enamel surfaces of the upper anterior teeth may be attributed to the acidic oral environment of an eating disorder such as bulimia or anorexia nervosa. Thus the dentist should inform the patient's physician about the dental-oral pathology as a result of a thorough history and examination.

EFFECTS OF NUTRITIONAL DEFICIENCIES ON ORAL HEALTH

There are two major reasons for the relatively great sensitivity of the oral mucosa to physiological or anatomical changes resulting from nutritional deficiencies. First, the oral epithelial cells probably grow and are replaced more rapidly than almost any other type of cell in the body. In fact, the epithelial cells lining the gingival sulcus completely renew themselves every 3 to 7 days. This means that DNA, RNA, and the formation of protein, which contribute to tissue synthesis and cellular turnover in the oral mucosa, are extremely rapid. Therefore intake of appropriate foods of suitable nutrient density in adequate amounts is needed daily. Second, a healthy oral epithelium can act as an effective barrier against the invasion of toxic substances into the underlying collagenous (insoluble fibrous protein) connective tissue. But this protective property can easily be compromised or even negated—for example, by a vitamin C deficiency. In fact, inadequate nourishment can cause the oral epithelium to break down and become infected readily, which may manifest itself as an oral mucosal ulceration.

Nutritional deficiencies are no longer considered to be only an acute lack of individual vitamins, as in beriberi, pellagra, scurvy, or rickets. Currently, a nutritional deficiency is thought to be an expression of a metabolic malfunction caused by lower than desirable intake and use of essential interacting nutrients from the daily diet.

No nutrient can carry out its function without adequate supplies of other, related nutrients. The interaction of several nutrients is usually necessary for optimal food metabolism and bodily homeostasis (stability). For example, several of the B complex vitamins are involved in the intermediary metabolism of carbohydrates, which ultimately provide the body with energy. Therefore when the requirements for carbohydrates are increased, it is best to increase the concurrent intake of several of the energy-releasing B complex vitamins (niacin, riboflavin, and thiamin) rather than a single one, such as thiamin, which is usually mentioned as the essential B vitamin for carbohydrate metabolism. Another example is the interdependence of protein and riboflavin. Cracked lips or lesions at the corners of the mouth (angular cheilosis), usually associated with riboflavin deficiency, will not clear up when treated with riboflavin supplements if the patient is also protein deficient. Both an adequate protein diet and a riboflavin supplement must be prescribed simultaneously to effect a cure.

Although the coexistence of multiple deficiencies has been emphasized, a deficiency of any nutrient alone can produce characteristic manifestations. Each nutrient has one or more primary functions and often has a predilection (partiality) for particular cells, tissues, or structures. Therefore its deficiency may often be associated with one part of the body (e.g., vitamin C deficiencies with vascular integrity and vitamin B complex deficiencies with disorders of the oral mucous membranes).

The classification of nutritional diseases into acute and chronic types is useful because the speed of response to treatment can be anticipated.[1] Some deficiencies may be rapid in onset and severe in intensity, and may become florid (fully developed) in a short period of time; these are acute deficiencies. Others are insidious (have a more serious effect than is apparent), mild in intensity, and slow to develop; these are chronic deficiencies. In acute deficiencies in which tissues are drastically depleted of their nutrients and cellular metabolism is markedly altered, a rapid, dramatic response can be expected once therapy is instituted. Conversely, chronic deficiencies will respond slowly to therapy because oral tissue changes take place gradually over a long time.

PRIMARY AND SECONDARY NUTRITIONAL DEFICIENCIES

Malnutrition can be caused directly by a faulty selection of foods—a condition called primary nutritional deficiency—or it can be due to a conditioning factor such as a systemic disorder that can interfere with the ingestion, digestion, absorption, transport, and use of nutrients—referred to as a secondary or conditioned nutritional deficiency.[2] More frequently, malnutrition is produced by a combination of primary and secondary factors.

Primary nutritional deficiencies arise because people do not select or eat enough of the proper foods. There can be many reasons, such as:

- Lack of knowledge of what constitutes an adequate diet
- Fad diets

- Poor food habits
- Food likes and dislikes
- Lack of availability of proper foods in the local market
- Poverty
- Lack of facilities to prepare food
- Lack of desire for or interest in food
- Emotional prejudices
- Physical incapacities and handicaps, such as blindness or confinement to a wheelchair

In a dental practice, candidates for a primary nutritional deficiency may be seen. Age, income, and education may singly or in combination contribute to the production of malnutrition. For example, college students living in an apartment often have limited time and money for preparing adequate nutritious meals. The poor may select inexpensive foods that may be low in nutrient density or provide only empty calories. Alcoholics may have little or no desire for food. Food faddists, who severely limit their own food choices, are also candidates for nutritional disorders. The elderly who live alone may lack the energy for planning and preparing meals or lack the money to buy adequate amounts of the desirable nutritious foods. All of these persons may develop a primary nutritional deficiency disease.

Secondary nutritional deficiencies, as the name implies, occur because even though the food is available, the body is not healthy enough to ingest, digest, metabolize, or use the nutrients provided by the food. The patient usually has a previous history of some systemic disorder.

These are some of the conditioning factors that can cause secondary nutritional deficiencies:

- Factors that interfere with food intake—anorexia (loss of appetite), fever, infection, nausea, vomiting, allergy, neurological disorders, or poor dentition that impairs chewing
- Conditions that interfere with digestion of food—e.g., gastrectomy (removal of part of the stomach) or pancreatic insufficiency, which can cause calcium, fat-soluble vitamin, calorie, or protein deficiencies
- States that interfere with absorption of nutrients—long-term ingestion of antibiotics, colitis (inflammation of the colon), diarrhea, celiac (abdominal) disease, achlorhydria (lack of hydrochloric acid in the stomach), liver and gallbladder diseases
- Factors that interfere with metabolism—e.g., use of chemotherapy (methotrexate, a neoplastic depressant) in some leukemias, producing a folic acid deficiency
- Conditions that interfere with utilization of nutrients—diabetes, alcoholism, liver failure
- Factors that increase nutritional requirements—physical exertion, hyperthyroidism, fever, growth, pregnancy, lactation
- Factors that cause excessive excretion—sweating or polyuria in diabetes, Addison's disease (which leads to sodium depletion), dehydration

STAGES IN THE DEVELOPMENT OF NUTRITIONAL DEFICIENCIES

Primary dietary inadequacies coupled with systemic conditioning factors that interfere with nutrient utilization can lead to a sequence of events that may result in the death of cells and tissues.

1. A deficiency begins after the gradual tissue depletion of the nutrient

reserves. This can be measured biochemically by determining the *level of the nutrients in the blood, urine, or tissues.* For example, a patient with iron deficiency anemia will have a reduced serum ferritin (water-soluble storage form of iron in the body) level.

2. As the tissue depletion progresses, there will be *increased enzyme activity.* For example, an increased serum alkaline phosphatase might indicate a disturbance in calcification or a vitamin D deficiency.

3. This is followed by *physiological or functional abnormalities,* which are reversible when the deficiency is treated. For example, the eyes of a patient who has a vitamin A deficiency are unable to adapt to darkness until the patient is given therapeutic doses of vitamin A.

4. If the nutritional deficiency continues for a long enough time, classic *anatomical lesions* appear. The deficiency progresses to the point at which cells die, and the tissue begins to break down. Unless dead cells can be replaced, the damage is irreversible. For example, bowlegs resulting from rickets are a lifelong stigma of vitamin D deficiency during childhood.

Although each of these stages—the biochemical, physiological, and anatomical—have been described as separate time periods in the development of the nutritional deficiency, in reality they overlap.

In the United States today most nutritional deficiencies are of the preclinical or subclinical type. The physician does not necessarily see gross signs, but the combination of the patient's complaints, history of the illness, and laboratory tests may provide clues to the presence of a subclinical nutritional deficiency. For example, a symptom such as tiredness and a laboratory report that the patient has a low hematocrit (volume percentage of erythrocytes in whole blood) may suggest the possibility of an anemia. However, in order to establish the presence of a nutritional deficiency, more information than laboratory tests or the patient's complaints must be obtained. The following comprehensive approach is an acceptable method of assessing a patient's nutritional status.

ASSESSMENT OF A PATIENT'S NUTRITIONAL STATUS[3, 4]

Nutritional status is defined by Christakis as the "health condition of an individual as influenced by his intake and utilization of nutrients determined from the correlation of information from physical, biochemical, clinical, and dietary studies."[5]

No single criterion, such as a diet history or laboratory test, can measure nutritional status properly. What is required is a collection of data from four sequential routes of inquiry: (1) the patient's complaints and medical and social histories, (2) dietary history and evaluation, (3) physical examination, including anthropometric (dealing with size, weight, and body proportion) measurements, and (4) pertinent laboratory tests. Therefore the determination of nutritional status is done by measuring, compiling, and interpreting the findings from each of these four diagnostic considerations.

Also, dietary excesses as well as deficiencies can and do cause nutritional problems in developed countries. Most of the current nutritional problems in the United States are associated with degenerative diseases produced by excessive caloric intake (e.g., obesity, coronary heart disease, and diabetes); (2) sodium intake (e.g., hypertension); and (3) sugar intake (e.g., dental caries). The excessive intake of some nutrients can cause a concurrent deficiency of others.

Complaints

Some of the more common complaints heard from individuals who may have a nutritional deficiency are general weakness, chronic fatigue; loss of appetite; loss of weight; painful bleeding gums; sore lips, tongue, or oral mucous membranes; diarrhea; chronic nervousness; irritability; loss of ability to concentrate; confusion; memory loss; apathy; dizziness; lethargy; photophobia (intolerance of light); loss of manual dexterity; pains in legs; and skin problems.

Medical and Social Histories

In children, a general retardation of growth and development is indicative of malnutrition.

In adults, a history of chronic debilitating diseases, alcoholism, digestive disturbances, ulcerative colitis, diarrhea, or diuria (frequency of urination during the day) should alert the clinician to the possibility that a secondary nutritional deficiency might result.

Emotional or personal problems or quitting smoking are often the basis for overeating, and resultant obesity. Excessive weight loss may be due to anorexia nervosa (a nervous condition in which the patient loses his/her appetite, takes little food, and becomes emaciated), bulimia (food binges followed by vomiting), food fads, or medically unsupervised quick weight-reduction diets.

Social factors that may influence a patient's food selection, food habits, and eating schedule include type of employment; hobbies and recreation; and family, economic, and cultural influences.

Dietary History and Evaluation

An individual's eating habits determine the dietary patterns that affect his or her nutritional status.

There are a number of ways in which information can be collected for a dietary history. Some of these include 24-hour recall or a 3-, 5-, or 7-day record of food intake. The method of choice depends on the amount of detail required.

The 24-hour recall is the most rapid method (15 to 20 minutes) for recording current food intake in a superficial fashion. The problem with this procedure is that quantities consumed may be over- or underestimated and that food intake on a single day may not be representative of the usual intake. Plastic models of an average serving of different foods and examples of various portion sizes— water glass, juice glass, cup, bowl, spoons, and so forth—can help the patient estimate the quantities consumed.

The 3-, 5-, or 7-day record is a food diary that the patient keeps on a day-by-day basis. After each meal, each dish or food eaten is recorded giving the amounts in household measures and the method of preparation (e.g., baked, steamed) is described. It is important for the counselor to review the food diary with the patient and to refine the information provided. A detailed, accurate food diary is essential for a proper dietary evaluation.

For the 24-hour recall, the Dental Health Diet Score (see Chap. 17) can provide a rapid but superficial food intake overview with respect to the adequacy of the patient's diet during that 24-hour period. If the score is barely adequate or not adequate, the patient needs a detailed diet evaluation and counseling.

To assess the adequacy of food intake over a 3-, 5-, or 7-day period, a quantitative calculation of each of the nutrients consumed can be made from the Nutritive Value of Foods table in Appendix 1. This total daily nutrient intake can be compared with the Recommended Daily Dietary Allowances in Appendix 2. Theoretically, the difference between the recommended and actual intake would be none, excess, or deficient. The calculations involved in this type of analysis are very time-consuming. Computer analysis of dietary records would be a more rapid means of performing the calculations. However, there are several negative aspects to both of these diet analysis techniques. First, the Food and Nutrition Board specifically warns against the use of the Recommended Dietary Allowance as a reference point for determining the adequacy of an individual's diet.[6] Second, the nutrient contents of food can vary considerably, depending on the genetics of the plant seeds, the geographic location of the crop, the method of preparation, and other factors. Third, considerable time must be spent in calculating or in preparing the dietary record information for computer processing. Fourth, and most important, there is no physiological or biochemical need for such a detailed nutrient analysis for the prevention or control of the usual dental-oral problems.

In our opinion, a simpler and more practical approach to diet evaluation is to classify the foods consumed into the appropriate food groups and then compare the average number of actual servings from each of the food groups with the amounts recommended. The recommended size and number of servings from each food group vary with the age grouping (child, adolescent, or adult) and for the adolescent, his or her frame size. For example, a large-frame adolescent should have 4 or 5 8-oz glasses of milk a day or the equivalent, whereas 2 8-oz glasses or the equivalent is adequate for an adult. A sample diet evaluation form that can be used for this purpose is shown in Figure 16–1.

The fact that a person does not drink as many glasses of milk or eat the number of suggested ounces of meat recommended does not necessarily signify that he or she is nutritionally deficient. It merely suggests that the patient is consuming less than the amounts of nutrients that are considered desirable for maintaining good nutrition in most healthy persons in the United States. These amounts represent goals rather than requirements. If these standards are maintained, a nutritional disorder probably will not occur as long as there are no secondary conditioning factors to interfere with bodily use of the food consumed.

A dietary history and evaluation not only should provide information on the amounts of food ingested, it should also provide information about the patient's eating habits and attitudes about food and health.

SUGGESTED DAILY AMOUNTS

FOOD GROUP	PORTION SIZE CONSIDERED ONE SERVING	1ST DAY	2ND DAY	3RD DAY	4TH DAY	5TH DAY	AVER.	CHILD	SMALL FRAME	MED. FRAME	LARGE FRAME	ADULT	DIFF.
									ADOLESCENT				
FRUITS and VEGETABLES (including citrus fruits, dark green and deep yellow vegetables)	1/2 c. cooked 1 medium raw 1/2 medium grapefruit or cantaloupe 6 oz. (1/2 c.) fruit juice							4 or > serv.	4-5 serv.	5-6 serv.	6 or > serv.	4 or > serv.	
BREADS and CEREALS (enriched or whole grain)	1 slice bread 3/4 c. dry cereal 1/2 c. cooked cereal, rice, noodles, macaroni							4 or > serv.	4-5 serv.	5-6 serv.	6-8 serv.	4 or > serv.	
MILK (milk & cheese)	8 oz. (1 cup) milk 1 1/2 oz. Cheddar cheese 1 1/2 slices American cheese 1 1/2 c. cottage cheese							3-4 serv.	2-3 serv.	3-4 serv.	4-5 serv.	2 serv.	
MEAT (meat, fish, poultry, nuts, dry beans)	2-3 oz. lean cooked meat, fish, or poultry 2 eggs 4 T peanut butter 1 c. cooked dry beans or lentils							2 or > serv. (2-3 oz. each)	2 serv. (3-4 oz. each)	2 serv. (4-5 oz. each)	2 serv. (5-6 oz. each)	2 or > serv. (3-4 oz. each)	
FATS, SWEETS ALCOHOL	No serving sizes defined												

FIGURE 16–1. Diet evaluation score sheet based on five food groups. Instructions: For each food item, place a mark (卌) in the appropriate block.

Clinical Examination

The clinical examination should begin with a general inspection. This will enable the examiner to ascertain whether the person is grossly overweight or underweight, or has excessive pallor, generalized skin lesions, or other indications of unsatisfactory health related to diet. A physician would, of course, be in a position to do a more extensive physical examination, as outlined in Table 16–1. However, for those areas that are accessible to the dentist, such as weight, height, skin, eyes, neck, and oral cavity, some significant clues with respect to the possibility of an undesirable nutritional state can be discovered (Table 16–2).

Weight-Height Relationship and Fat-Fold Thickness

For children, useful anthropometrical measurements include head and upper arm circumference as well as weight, height (growth charting), and fat-fold thickness.

Simple inspection will show whether a patient is thin or fat. However, the amount of variation from normal can best be ascertained by comparing the patient's weight with the desirable weight for the height for adults shown in Table 1–1. If there is some question about weight for height for boys or girls, consult with the patient's family physician.

The fat-fold thickness is important because it indicates whether the increased weight is due to fluid accumulation, muscular development, or fat deposits. Pinching a double fold of skin over the outer surface of the upper arm

TABLE 16–1. The Physical Examination

General appearance—obese? skinny?
Head—bossing, deformities, craniotabes (under 1 year old)
Eyes—ophthalmoplegia, cataracts, xerosis keratomalacia, Bitot's spots, retinal
 hemorrhage, papilledema
Mouth—glossitis, gingivitis, caries, periodontal disease, cheilosis, ageusia, dysgeusia
Nose—Anosmia, dysosmia, nasolabial seborrhea
Skin—pallor, abnormal pigmentation (carotenemia, hemochromatosis), follicular
 hyperkeratosis, bruises, perifollicular petechiae, pellagrous dermatitis, flaky-paint
 dermatitis, fistulas, status of wound healing, subcutaneous fat and skin-fold thickness,
 edema
Hair—easy pluckability, sparseness, depigmentation
Nails—friability, bands and lines
Neck—goiter
Heart—enlargement, high-output failure, resting tachycardia
Lungs—emphysema? Use of accessory muscles to breathe?
Abdomen—enlarged (fatty) liver, distended loops of bowel, ascites, varices
Genitourinary—secondary sexual characteristics, hypogonadism, delayed onset of
 puberty
Skeletal—epiphyseal thickening, bowing, rachitic rosary, osteoporosis, frog leg position,
 tenderness
Muscle—atrophy, wasting, hemorrhage, pain
Joints—effusions, arthralgia
Neural—foot drop, confabulation, improper position and vibratory sense, hyperreflexia,
 hyporeflexia, irritability, convulsions

TABLE 16–2. Physical Signs and Causes of Malnutrition

Body Area	Signs Associated with Malnutrition	Nutrition-Related Causes
Hair	Lack of natural shine; dull, dry, sparse, straight, color changes (flag sign); easily plucked	Protein-calorie deficiency; often multiple coexistent nutrient deficiencies
Face	Dark skin over cheeks and under eyes (malar and supraorbital pigmentation), scaling of skin around nostrils (nasolabial seborrhea)	Inadequate caloric intake; lack of B complex vitamins, particularly niacin, riboflavin, pyridoxine
	Edematous (moon face)	Protein deficiency
	Color loss (pallor)	Iron deficiency, general undernutrition
Eyes	Pale conjunctivae	Iron deficiency
	Bitot's spots,* conjunctival and corneal xerosis,* soft cornea (keratomalacia)	Vitamin A deficiency
	Redness and fissuring of eyelid corners (angular palpebritis)	Niacin, riboflavin, pyridoxine deficiency
Lips	Redness and swelling of mouth or lips (cheilosis),* angular fissure and scars	Niacin or riboflavin deficiency
Tongue	Red, raw and fissured, swollen (glossitis)*	Folic acid, niacin, B_{12}, pyridoxine deficiency
	Magenta color	Riboflavin deficiency
	Pale, atrophic	Iron deficiency
	Filiform papillary atrophy	Niacin, folic acid, B_{12}, iron deficiency
	Fungiform papillary hypertrophy	General undernutrition
Teeth	Carious or missing	Excess sugar (and poor dental hygiene)
	Mottled enamel (fluorosis)	Excess fluoride
Gums	Spongy, bleeding, may be receding	Ascorbic acid deficiency
Glands	Thyroid enlargement (goiter)	Iodine deficiency
	Parotid enlargement	General undernutrition, particularly insufficient protein
Skin	Follicular hyperkeratosis,* dryness (xerosis) with flaking	Vitamin A deficiency; insufficient unsaturated and essential fatty acids
	Hyperpigmentation*	B_{12}, folic acid, niacin deficiency
	Petechiae*	Ascorbic acid deficiency
	Pellagrous dermatitis*	Niacin or tryptophan deficiency
	Scrotal and vulval dermatosis*	Riboflavin deficiency
Nails	Spoon nails (koilonychia), brittle or ridged	Iron deficiency

*From Butterworth, C. E.; Blackburn, G. L. Nutr. Today 10:8–18, 1975.

or just below the rib cage and applying the calipers to measure this thickness can indicate whether a patient is thin, fat, or normal. About 25 mm (1 inch) indicates overweight; below 10 mm suggests underweight.

Skin

Changes in the skin can be brought about by unfavorable environmental conditions, inadequate nutritional status, or both. Rough, dry, scaly skin with follicular hyperkeratosis (hypertrophy of the horny layer of the skin) resulting from keratotic plugs protruding from hair follicles can be associated with lack of vitamin A or with insufficient unsaturated fatty acids. Poor hygiene, aging, uremia (presence of urinary constituents in the blood and the toxic conditions produced thereby), and local vascular insufficiency can also produce dry skin and must be considered when making a differential diagnosis.

Bruising at pressure points may be caused by lack of vitamin C or vitamin K, but it also can result from several non-nutritional blood disorders.

Tiny hemorrhages around the hair follicles may be associated with vitamin C deficiency.

Skin lesions that occur in symmetrical areas exposed to the sun or over pressure points and that are dark brown and rough may be caused by niacin or tryptophan deficiency or both. The skin in the affected areas becomes dry, scaly, and shrunken. Acute lesions are red, macerated (softened) and abraded (worn away), with superimposed infection in skin fold areas.

In protein deficiency, the feet and lower legs as well as the arms show a marked edema that pit on pressure. A dermatosis (skin disease) characterized by follicular hyperkeratosis, xerosis (dryness), and flaking of the skin may be caused by a vitamin A deficiency as noted in Table 16–2.

Eyes

Xerophthalmia, or dryness of the conjunctiva (the delicate membrane that covers the eyeball), may be due to a vitamin A deficiency. There may also be conjunctival translucence or opacity as well as a decrease in tear production. Bitot's spots, which are grayish yellow, frothy, foaming, superficial patchy lesions on the exposed conjunctiva, are usually associated with xerophthalmia. Softening of the eye (keratomalacia) and blindness can result from a prolonged vitamin A deficiency.

Redness and fissuring of eyelid corners can be due to a B complex (particularly niacin, riboflavin, and pyridoxine) deficiency.

Neck

A swelling in the front of the neck may be the result of an enlarged thyroid gland; this condition, which is called goiter, is caused by an iodine deficiency. The enlargement can be seen and palpated when the head is in a normal position or when it is thrown back.

ORAL CAVITY

Oral tissues can undergo three major changes as reactions to a nutritional deficiency, an irritant, or a change in the oral environment (e.g., xerostomia or dryness of the mouth). They can change functionally or anatomically; their color may also change.

A *functional change* noted in the mouth is a burning sensation caused by irritation of the nerves in the tongue or the roof of the mouth. The sensation is nonspecific because it may be a manifestation of a nutrient deficiency (e.g., lack of iron, folic acid, vitamin B_{12}, or niacin), uncontrolled diabetes, or an allergy.

In contrast with functional changes, which may be reversed within a few days after the basic dietary deficiency or insufficiency has been corrected, the *anatomical changes* of chronic disturbances can exist for weeks or even months. The time factor is an important difference between functional and anatomical changes.

Color changes in the tissues can result from several different factors. The color of the mucous membranes of the mouth is that of the underlying vascular bed seen through the surface epithelial tissues. The combination of epithelial thickness and texture and the amount of the vascularity of the underlying tissue can produce variations in light transmission and color generation.

There may be several reasons for changes in this color. If the surface epithelium becomes keratinized (horny), thickened, or less translucent, the color will appear pale, not because there has been any change in the vascular underlying bed but because there has been a blockage in the transmission of light or color from the underlying structures. Conversely, if there has been a loss of surface epithelial tissues, the color may appear deep red because the surface opacity has been lost, allowing the underlying color of the vascular bed to be more perceptible.

However, if the epithelial surfaces are normal, the color of the tongue may be pale as a result of vasoconstriction, or it may be red as a result of vasodilation. The important questions are these: Are these epithelial changes or vascular changes? What are the mechanisms that produce them? The mechanism, rather than the visible change, is the more positive indicator of the nature of the problem.

Inflammation of the Lips (Cheilosis) and of the Corners of the Mouth (Angular Stomatitis). Cheilosis and cheilitis are synonymous terms describing inflammation of the entire upper and lower lip surfaces. Angular cheilitis (also called angular stomatitis) involves cracks at the corners of the mouth; inflammation and infection at the junction (commissures) of the upper and lower lips and the adjoining skin are characteristic.

The lips are readily affected by metabolic disturbances, local irritants, or both. The inflammatory changes seen in the mucosa of the lips, particularly at the commissures, may be a sign of a deficiency of one or more of the following nutrients: riboflavin, niacin, pyridoxine, folic acid, vitamin B_{12}, protein, and iron.

—Usually, patients develop lip lesions in an ordered pattern. The lesions begin with pallor of the mucosa at the commissures. Erythema (redness), macerations (softening), and fissuring (clefts and grooves) of the corners of the lips follow in that order. Eventually, the moist, white membranous exudate of the lesions dries; secondary bacterial infection often follows, producing a yellowish white crust.

The other surfaces of the upper and lower lips tend to be excessively dry and wrinkled. There is vertical fissuring (rhagades) and peeling (desquamation) of the vermilion border of the lips (Fig. 16–2). The contact area of the lips is intensely reddened and encrusted and will bleed readily if traumatized.

A differential diagnosis between non-nutritional and nutritional etiological factors must be considered. For example, an overclosure of the jaw resulting from a loss of vertical dimension can cause a folding of the skin and mucosa at the angles of the lips, thus producing cheilitis. This type of angular cheilitis is seen in edentulous patients, in those who wear old or ill-fitting dentures with missing or worn down teeth, and in those with marked attrition of the incisal and occlusal surfaces of their natural teeth, which also produces overclosure.

Other possible non-nutritional causes of angular cheilitis are allergies, excessive salivation with drooling, and the habit of licking the lips.

Inflammation of the Tongue (Glossitis). The tongue may undergo a variety of changes, in color, size, topography, and sensitivity. The tongue is sensitive to nutritional aberrations because the rapid growth of the epithelial cells covering the dorsum (upper surface) requires high amounts of nutrients. A nutritional deficiency may actually reduce the thickness of the epithelial protection of the tongue. Color or topographic changes in the dorsum may be confined to a single area or may include many localized, well-demarcated areas.

Color changes may be diffuse, following a sequential pattern that starts at the anterior border and gradually proceeds posteriorly. Changes in color range from a pale pink through deep red to bluish purple. As previously discussed, pallor may be associated with a low blood hemoglobin, as in iron deficiency anemia, or it may be the result of keratinized epithelium from a vitamin A deficiency. Conversely, abnormal redness is caused either by increased vascularity (number of blood vessels) or by atrophy of the papillae (small projections on the upper surface of the tongue). Reddening of the tongue at the tip and lateral margins may be associated with sprue or vitamin B complex deficiency, especially of niacin. A purple or magenta color probably results from a slowing of the circulation and a stagnation of the blood flow, which is often seen in riboflavin deficiency.

Topographically (with respect to the surface configuration), the papillae may undergo the following sequential changes: hypertrophy (enlargement), flattening, atrophy (diminution in size), and complete loss. Usually there is some enlargement of the fungiform papillae (those shaped like a mushroom and found mostly

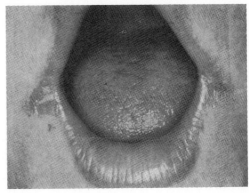

FIGURE 16–2. Vertical fissuring (rhagades) of lips and angular cheilosis. (Courtesy of Dr. G. Shklar.)

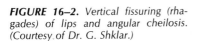

at the edges and apex) and some atrophy of the filiform (smallest threadlike) papillae, which occur in greatest numbers, so that the surface of the tongue appears reddened and smooth, with prominent spots representing the fungiform papillae. The surface of the tongue may have patchy, atrophic, ulcerated areas, and deep fissures (the latter are usually a developmental anomaly). The ulcerated lesions may be caused by a vitamin deficiency or an infection superimposed upon the normally fissured tongue, or both. In ariboflavinosis (riboflavin deficiency), the dorsum of the tongue takes on a pebbly or granular appearance. However, in most chronic deficiencies of vitamin B complex, iron, or protein, the main feature is atrophy of both the fungiform and filiform papillae, so that the dorsum of the tongue is slick, shiny, and red (Fig. 16–3).

The tongue size is influenced by edema (accumulation of fluid) or dehydration. With edema (from excessive sodium intake, for example), the tongue becomes swollen (a condition called macroglossia) and the sides have a scalloped appearance caused by indentations from the pressure of the teeth. In contrast, during dehydration the tongue is dry and shrunken, with smooth borders.

Sensitivity changes (e.g., burning and soreness) can be early symptoms of folic acid or vitamin B_{12} deficiency. Diminution of taste sensation is not unusual in elderly persons, particularly those who are malnourished.

Inflammation of the Oral Mucosa. A patient with an acute vitamin B complex deficiency, as seen in alcoholism, will develop a markedly red and inflamed oral mucosa that sometimes has a patchy appearance as a result of isolated spots of grayish green pseudomembrane (false membrane). The epithelial layer very often becomes detached from the underlying tissue, leaving raw red, readily infected patches.

Pallor of the oral mucosa is a characteristic sign in patients with anemias, such as those caused by iron, folic acid, or vitamin B_{12} deficiency.

There may also be aphthae (small ulcers or canker sores) with fiery red borders. Allergy to certain foods has been suggested as a cause of these lesions, but this has not been proved. The most likely causes are stress, hormone imbalance, and local injury.

Gingivitis. Gingivitis, which is an inflammation of the gingival collar around the neck of the tooth, is initiated by local irritants, such as dental plaque, and may be intensified by various systemic factors, such as nutritional deficiencies.[7] For instance, a niacin deficiency can predispose the gingiva to a fusospi-

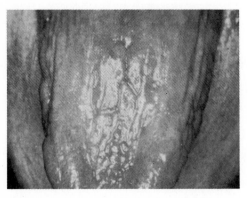

FIGURE 16–3. Complete atrophy of tongue papillae.

rochetal (fusiform bacillus and spirochetes) bacterial infection, called Vincent's infection, or acute ulcerative necrotic gingivitis, that results in characteristically wedge-shaped, punched-out ulcers in the interdental papillae of the marginal gingiva. The lesions, which are necrotic, exudative, foul smelling, and extremely painful, are covered by a grayish white pseudomembrane that when peeled off leaves a raw bleeding tissue surface.

An acute vitamin C deficiency in the presence of local gingival irritants, such as plaque and calculus, will cause the gums to become inflamed. Vitamin C deficiency contributes to the gingivitis through defects in capillary walls produced by a failure in collagen formation. The engorgement of the blood vessels of the gingiva can produce a swollen gingiva that is fiery red, smooth and glazed, and devoid of stippling. The congested gingiva may become infected and undergo ulceration, necrosis, and sloughing. Histologically, the gingiva shows hyperemia (excess blood), diminution of fibroblasts, and deficiency of collagen fibrils. Gingival manifestations of scurvy will not develop in the absence of teeth, because the initiating local factor must be an irritant on the gingival third of the teeth and affect the periodontal connective tissue membrane.

In severe ascorbic acid deficiency, the teeth may exfoliate (fall out) because of the extensive destruction of the supporting structures (peridontal ligament and alveolar bone), which are derived from collagen.

Sensitive, friable (crumbling) gingiva can also occur in advanced stages of pernicious anemia and folic acid deficiency. In iron deficiency anemia, the gingiva is characteristically quite pale.

Significance of Signs and Symptoms. From a practical standpoint, it is important to emphasize that no single clinical indicator is of any significance by itself; at least two or three different indicators, all pointing in the same direction, are necessary. Only in association with other aspects of the nutritional assessment, such as confirmed insufficiency of certain foods and laboratory tests, can one come to a bona fide diagnosis of a specific nutritional deficiency. A single tissue change may be caused by local irritant and may be in no way related to a nutritional deficiency.

Laboratory Tests

Laboratory tests provide an objective means of monitoring one aspect of a patient's nutritional status. In the development of a nutritional deficiency, these tests may detect subclinical deficiencies before the onset of overt clinical signs. This allows for early treatment for those at risk and the probability of more rapid recovery from treatment than if the nutritional deficiency had proceeded to the anatomical, or clinical, stage. The signs of clinical deficiency usually appear after there is a decreased urinary excretion and/or plasma concentration, which means that the nutrient or its metabolite is being conserved.

Urinary excretion levels fluctuate more than plasma levels and reflect immediate rather than prior intake. However, a functional test that measures the metabolism, or cellular use, of a nutrient provides a more reliable indication of a patient's nutritional status with respect to that nutrient. For example, the ascorbic acid level in leukocytes is the most dependable biochemical measure of an individual's vitamin C status. It is better than either urinary ascorbic acid excretion levels or plasma concentrations, which really only measure transient vitamin C levels.

Some of the routine laboratory tests used in establishing the biochemical nutritional status of a hospitalized patient are serum protein and albumin; total urinary nitrogen:creatinine and creatinine:height ratios; serum iron and iron binding capacity (transferrin saturation); plasma ascorbate; and serum electrolytes.

These are some of the more reliable laboratory methods for determining the presence of adequate body levels of the following nutrients[8]:

Iron. The serum iron and the percentage of transferrin saturation are more reliable indicators of iron for nutritional status than is blood hemoglobin or hematocrit. Non-nutritional conditions can also cause a reduction in blood hemoglobin. However, the mean corpuscular hemoglobin concentrates (MCHC), calculated from hemoglobin and hematocrit data, are acceptable because of their simplicity but are not as good indicators of iron nutritional status as the serum iron and transferrin saturation.

Folic Acid. The most reliable method is by direct measurement of its concentration in the serum.

Vitamin B_{12}. The Schilling test, which measures the amount of radioactive cobalt uptake, is best.

Ascorbic Acid. The level of plasma or serum ascorbic acid is commonly used, but ascorbic acid concentrations in the white blood cells–plateletes (20 μg/10^8 leukocytes) is the most reliable index of vitamin C adequacy. According to a number of laboratories, the lingual ascorbic acid test based on decolorization of a dye placed on the tongue is not a reliable indicator of ascorbic acid status. Many agents in the tissues or on the surface of the tongue may interfere with this test.

Vitamin A. The serum levels of beta-carotene usually reflect recent dietary intake, whereas the levels of vitamin A in the serum appear to be related to the liver stores. Measurement of vitamin A in the serum (or plasma) appears to be the best method. More than 100 mg/100 ml of vitamin A is indicative of hypervitaminosis. A plasma vitamin A level of less than 10 μg/100 ml is indicative of a deficiency.

Vitamin K. The prothrombin time of Quick is used more widely in clinical situations than is the measurement of serum vitamin K levels.

Vitamin D. There is no direct measurement. Indirect methods—blood levels of calcium, phosphorus, and alkaline phosphatase—are used. In vitamin D deficiency (rickets or osteomalacia), there is generally an increase in serum alkaline phosphatase, a decrease in serum inorganic phosphorus, and, perhaps because it is closely regulated, a slight decrease in serum calcium. Paget's disease also causes an increase in serum alkaline phosphatase, but in osteoporosis a normal serum alkaline phosphatase level is found. Vitamin D toxicity is evidenced by hypercalcemia (more than 12 mg of calcium/100 ml of serum).

Vitamin E. Serum levels are most often used in estimating the vitamin E status of a patient.

Thiamin. Erythrocyte activity of transketolase is best for determining thiamin status.

Riboflavin. The level of glutathione reductase in red blood cells is the desirable indirect functional test for riboflavin status.

Pyridoxine. A red blood cell transaminase level is used to ascertain pyridoxine status.

Protein. The ratio of creatinine to height and the ratio of total urinary nitrogen to creatinine appear to be of some value in evaluating the protein status of the patient.

Summary

Assessment of a patient's nutritional status involves a consideration of both the environmental and the bodily factors that contribute to the malnourishment of cells: (1) the primary dietary inadequacies influenced by educational, social, psychological, cultural, and economic factors and (2) the secondary constitutional factors that interfere with the body's utilization of the nutrients or increase the requirement for nutrients.

The dietary history and evaluation is only one facet of the total appraisal of a patient's nutritional status. This assessment must include medical history, subjective and functional symptoms, body measurements, clinical signs, and laboratory tests.

Finally, because neither primary dietary failure nor conditioning factors are limited to a single nutrient, every patient suspected of having a nutritional deficiency is a potential victim of multiple deficiencies, with a few outstanding criteria that point to the predominant deficiency or deficiencies. For example, finding edema, skin pigmentation, hair changes, apathy, and anorexia in a child would suggest severe protein deficiency (kwashiorkor), although concomitant deficiencies of vitamin A, vitamin C, iron, and so forth, may also be present. Similarly, the occurrence of pigmented lesions in areas of skin exposed to sunlight suggests a primary niacin deficiency, as in pellagra, although experience has demonstrated that treatment with thiamin and riboflavin in addition to niacin is usually necessary for satisfactory recovery. In fact, treatment with niacin alone will often precipitate signs of acute thiamin or riboflavin deficiency.

NUTRITIONAL MANAGEMENT OF ACUTE PROBLEMS OF THE ORAL MUCOSA

The major consideration in the nutritional management of patients with acute problems of the oral mucosa is to provide an adequate and varied well-balanced diet in a physical form and at a temperature that is not only comfortable but also soothing to sensitive oral tissues. Between eating periods, if there are isolated painful mucosal lesions that need to be treated, a topical application of corticosteroid gel, such as Kenalog in Orabase, will be helpful.

Since appetite in general is usually poor, the doctor may recommend several small meals daily rather than the customary three full meals. Because of general oral discomfort, patients should rinse their mouth with a pain-relieving mouthwash such as Dyclone solution before eating. Use of a straw, when possible, to drink a nutritious liquified diet consisting of eggnogs, milkshakes, fruit juices, instant breakfast preparations, soups, and regular foods liquified in blenders is helpful. Patients must avoid the irritation of spicy or sharp-tasting foods.

Puddings, custards, ice cream, and gruels are other bland nutritious foods that can be included. The obvious purpose of this liquified diet is to satisfy the nutritional needs of patients during this initial period of illness when they cannot chew comfortably. Usually, this liquid diet is necessary only for the first 24-hour period. Patients should then change to a soft diet consisting of a variety of foods from the food groups:

- Vegetable-fruit group, e.g., cooked or canned fruits, cooked and mashed vegetables
- Bread-cereal group, e.g., pastas, rice, cooked cereals
- Milk group, e.g., cottage cheese and other soft cheeses
- Meat group, e.g., hamburger, boiled or ground chicken, cooked fish, and legumes

It should be added that a patient with acute necrotizing ulcerative gingivitis is often febrile. Fever does not preclude prescribing a full diet. In fact, the nutrient requirements for a satisfactory recovery are increased during this febrile stress period, and patients should eat enough food to overcome the negative nitrogen balance that might occur if they are underfed. Underfeeding will interfere with the normal defense mechanisms of the body and delay healing and convalescence.

On the basis of the increased nutrient requirements during the period of stress, and because some of the vitamin reserve has probably already been used, vitamin supplementation is indicated. Therapeutic doses (three to five times the maintenance doses) of a multivitamin preparation consisting of vitamin B complex and vitamin C are recommended.

MANAGEMENT OF VITAMIN DEFICIENCIES

Supplementation of the diet with vitamins is useful when a person is unable or unwilling to consume an adequate diet.[9] Vitamin supplementation should augment the diet, not replace it. However, other situations for which this supplementation is indicated include the following:

- In physiological stress periods, e.g., during children's growth-spurt periods and during pregnancy and lactation
- When poor eating habits are likely—in the elderly, food faddists, and alcoholics
- When a person is unable, for example, to chew foods because of sensitive oral tissues
- During emotional or physical illness, such as anorexia, allergies, chronic gastrointestinal upsets, and prolonged illness

Types of Vitamin Therapy

There are two major types of vitamin therapy: supportive and therapeutic.

The purpose of supportive doses of vitamins is to protect the individual against the development of vitamin deficiency states during stress periods such as pregnancy or illness. This supplementation is preventive. It can be justified by the argument that the optimal biochemical requirements for each individual is unknown, so that supplementation may meet a personal need and provide the support necessary for maintaining a state of well-being.

Therapeutic vitamin preparations are indicated for the treatment of specific vitamin deficiencies and for maintaining good nutritional status in patients with severely debilitating diseases. They can also aid in establishing a nutritional diagnosis when used in a therapeutic trial.

In both supportive and therapeutic vitamin supplementation it is recommended that polyvitamin preparations be used. These combinations of vitamins have complementary functions, as in the energy-releasing B complex vitamins— thiamin, niacin, riboflavin, pyridoxine hydrochloride, and calcium pantothenate. Other combinations include two groups of vitamins—(1) the five B complex vitamins just mentioned plus vitamin C or (2) a combination of the fat-soluble vitamin, D, with calcium and phosphorus. Also, the combination of both the major fat-soluble (A and D) and water-soluble (B complex and C) vitamins, with or without minerals, is commonly used as an all-purpose preparation.

If the specific cause of anemia has been found to be a deficiency of a single nutrient such as vitamin B_{12} or folic acid or iron, the single supplement should be given, rather than a combination of all three.

Dosage of Vitamin Supplements

The dosages of the supportive supplemental vitamin preparations should be the amounts recommended by the Food and Nutrition Board as the desirable daily allowance (Table 16–3). Although generic preparations are usually less expensive, trade name brands for vitamin B complex and C in maintenance doses, such as Cebefortis, or for a multivitamin preparation in maintenance doses, such as Unicaps, may be easier to prescribe.

TABLE 16–3. Formulas of Supportive Multivitamin Preparations

Vitamin	Daily Dosage (Range)
Basic formula*	
Vitamin A (synthetic or natural)	1500–5000 U.S.P. units
Vitamin D	400 U.S.P. units
Thiamin (hydrochloride or mononitrate)	1.0–2.0 mg
Riboflavin	1.0–3.0 mg
Niacinamide	5.0–20.0 mg
Ascorbic acid	50.0–100.0 mg
Expanded formula (add to basic formula)†	
Pyridoxine hydrochloride	0.5–2.0 mg
Calcium pantothenate	5.0–15.0 mg
Folic acid	0.05–0.10 mg
Vitamin B_{12}	1.0–2.0 µg
Vitamin E	5.0–10.0 mg
Preparations of water-soluble vitamins Remove vitamins A, D, and E from the expanded formula	

From Goodhart, R. S.; Wohl, M. G. Manual of Clinical Nutrition. Philadelphia, Lea & Febiger, 1964.
*This formula contains all the vitamins for which the Food and Nutrition Board has recommended a daily dietary allowance.
†Vitamin K is given separately when indicated.

The dosage of therapeutic vitamins should be three to five times the recommended daily dosage (Table 16–4). If, for example, a specific vitamin deficiency, such as scurvy, has been diagnosed by clinical and laboratory means, then a therapeutic polyvitamin preparation plus additional ascorbic acid (1 g/day) should be prescribed. The point is that multivitamin preparations are always preferable to single vitamin types. A trade name preparation used for therapeutic doses of B complex and C vitamins is Allbee with Vitamin C; another is Navogran. For the multivitamin preparation in therapeutic doses, Theragran may be prescribed.

Toxicity

Vitamin A. Acute toxicity from accidental intake of a single dose of vitamin A concentrate has been observed in children who have ingested 175,000 to 350,000 IU. Adults taking a daily dose of 50,000 to 100,000 IU over a prolonged period (5 years) may develop toxic signs of desquamation (peeling) and scaly skin, hair loss, cheilosis, hyperostosis (hypertrophy of bone; exostosis) and joint pains. In addition, anorexia, weight loss, nausea, vomiting, and diarrhea may be present.

Vitamin D. Toxic effects from vitamin D have been observed in adults receiving 100,000 IU or more daily and in children given 40,000 IU daily. The serum calcium and phosphorus levels are increased. Calcium may be deposited in the aorta, the renal tubules, and the lungs. Renal failure and hypertension may develop.

TABLE 16–4. Formulas of Therapeutic Multivitamin Preparations

Vitamin	Daily Dosage (Range)
Basic therapeutic formula*	
Vitamin A	10,000–25,000 U.S.P. units
Vitamin D	400 U.S.P. units
Thiamin	5.0–10.0 mg
Riboflavin	7.0–15.0 mg
Niacinamide	50.0–150.0 mg
Ascorbic acid	150.0–400.0 mg
Water-soluble vitamins (stress formula)	
Thiamin	5.0–10.0 mg
Riboflavin	7.0–15.0 mg
Niacinamide	50.0–100.0 mg
Pyridoxine	5.0–10.0 mg
Calcium pantothenate	20.0–50.0 mg
Folic acid	0.05–0.10 mg
Vitamin B_{12}	2.0–5.0 μg
Ascorbic acid	50.0–400.0 mg
Expanded therapeutic formula† (add to stress formula)	
Vitamin A	10,000–25,000 U.S.P. units
Vitamin D	400–1000 U.S.P. units
Vitamin E	30.0–100.0 mg

From Goodhart, R. S.; Wohl, M.G. Manual of Clinical Nutrition. Philadelphia, Lea & Febiger, 1964.
*This formula contains all the vitamins for which the Food and Nutrition Board has recommended a daily dietary allowance.
†Vitamin K is given separately when indicated.

Folic Acid. Any preparation containing more than 0.1 mg of folic acid in the daily recommended dose is a prescription item. This precaution reduces the possibility of masking pernicious anemia by the administration of a multivitamin preparation that might contain sufficient folic acid to cause a red blood cell formation response but without protecting against the neurological effects of vitamin B_{12} deficiency.

Ascorbic and Nicotinic Acids. Ascorbic acid taken orally in an amount of 0.5 g or larger may have a mild diuretic effect. This does not appear to be associated with any significant lesion. The "flushing," or vasodilating, effect of nicotinic acid (which does not occur with niacinamide) is well known and protects against the administration of excessive quantities of this vitamin without specific indication.

DENTAL PROBLEMS ASSOCIATED WITH BULIMIA AND ANOREXIA NERVOSA[10-14]

Bulimia is a cycle of food binges followed by self-induced vomiting, as well as laxative or diuretic abuses. The dental pathology that results in the bulimic who chooses to throw up the food that has been saturated with the hydrochloric acid of the stomach is a slow destruction of both enamel and dentin, particularly of the palatal surfaces of the anterior teeth. This process is called perimolysis. These exposed surfaces become extremely sensitive to hot or cold liquids and foods. Even the enamel of the occlusal surfaces of the posterior teeth may be eroded and become extremely sensitive to temperature changes. Furthermore, restorations "stand out" from the adjacent deteriorated enamel and dentin.[10-13]

Acid decalcification of the lingual surfaces of the upper anterior teeth may also be due to excessive use and intake of acidic foods such as oranges, lemons, or their juices.

Anorexia nervosa is seen in individuals who want to maintain an extreme thinness.[14] The dental problems are not only acid decalcification of the teeth, but also extensive tooth decay. The high caries index is usually due to a high fermentable carbohydrate food intake and poor oral hygiene.

In addition to providing the patient with nutritional guidance concerning substitution of cariogenic foods with nuts, cheese, and firm fruits and vegetables, it is vital that these patients be referred at the outset to their physician to deal with their emotional problems. Fluoride rinses and topical application of fluoride gels on the areas of eroded enamel should also be provided to remineralize the exposed dentin.

REFERENCES

1. Goldsmith, G. A. Curative nutrition: vitamins. In Schneider, H. A.; Anderson, C. E.; Coursin, D. B., eds. Nutritional Support of Medical Practice, pp. 101–127. Hagerstown, Md., Harper & Row, 1970.
2. Robinson, C. H., et al. Factors contributing to malnutrition. In Robinson, C. H.; Lawler, M. R.; Chenoweth, W. L., et al., eds. Normal and Therapeutic Nutrition, 17th ed., pp. 348–349. New York, Macmillan Publishing Co., 1986.
3. Krehl, W. A. The evaluation of nutritional status. Med. Clin. North Am. 48:1129, 1964.
4. Scrimshaw, N. S.; Ascoli, W. The clinical evaluation of nutritional status. In Nizel, A. E., ed. The

Science of Nutrition and Its Application in Clinical Dentistry, 2nd ed., pp. 235–246. Philadelphia, W. B. Saunders Co., 1966.

5. Christakis, G. Nutritional assessment in health programs. Am. J. Public Health 63:80, 1973.
6. Committee on Dietary Allowances, Food and Nutritional Board, National Academy of Sciences-National Research Council. Recommended Dietary Allowances, 9th rev. ed. Washington, D.C., National Academy Press, 1980.
7. Dreizen, S.; Stone, R. E.; Spies, F. D. Oral manifestations of nutritional disorders. Dent. Clin. North Am. July:429, 1958.
8. Drummond, J. F. Clinical and laboratory diagnosis of nutrition problems. Dental Clin. North Am. 20:593, 1976.
9. Darby, W. J. The rational use of vitamins in clinical practice. In Nizel, A. E., ed. The Science of Nutrition and Its Application in Clinical Dentistry, 2nd ed., p. 393. Philadelphia, W. B. Saunders Co., 1966.
10. Carni, J. D. The teeth may tell: dealing with eating disorders in the dentist's office. J. Mass. Dent. Soc. 30:80, 1981.
11. Rosenthal, R. H., et al. Diagnosis and management of persistent psychogenic vomiting. Psychosom. Med. 21:722, 1980.
12. Wolcott, R. B.; Yager, J.; Gordon, G. Dental sequelae to the binge-purge syndrome (bulimia): report of cases. J. Am. Dent. Assoc. 109:723, 1984.
13. Kleier, D. J.; Aragon, S. B.; Auerbach, R. E. Dental management of the chronic vomiting patient. J. Am. Dent. Assoc. 108:618, 1984.
14. Stege, P.; Visco-Dangler, L.; Rye, L. Anorexia nervosa: a review including oral and dental manifestations. J. Am. Dent. Assoc. 104:648, 1982.

17

Dietary Counseling for the Prevention and Control of Dental Caries

During the preeruptive periods of development of both deciduous and permanent teeth, foods exert a *nutritional* (i.e., systemic) effect on the formation of the dental matrix and its mineralization. However, during the posteruptive period, when the deciduous or permanent teeth are fully erupted, foods exert a *dietary* (i.e., topical) effect.

Dentists sometimes see highly caries-prone patients with erupted teeth whose enamel surfaces are partly covered with dental plaque bacteria. These bacteria degrade the ingested carbohydrate-rich foods that adhere to the tooth enamel to organic acids, producing a carious lesion. In these instances, dietary counseling to inhibit the carious process rather than systemic nutritional counseling for developing a caries-resistant tooth is appropriate.

When giving dietary counseling, some food choices and eating habits merit attention. These include (1) frequency of between-meal snacking, (2) physical form and retentiveness of sugar-sweetened snacks on and between the teeth, and (3) the amount of sugar added to food or beverages for sweetening.[1, 2] Sugar in liquid form can be as damaging to the teeth as sugar in sticky foods, according to some researchers.[3] However, other researchers have demonstrated that starch-containing foods, e.g., bread, may be more cariogenic than foods with a high sugar content because the mixture of bread and sugar is retained around the teeth for a longer time than highly sugared foods that are cleared rapidly from the mouth.[4] From these findings, it can be concluded that it is the length of intimate contact of fermentable carbohydrate with plaque bacteria that determines the relative cariogenic potential. However, from the studies mentioned, it is evident that sugar-sweetened foods in both solid and liquid form combined with dental plaque bacteria can produce tooth decay. Shaw states, "the frequency of eating, the amount of food retained in the mouth particularly on tooth surfaces, and the length of time that food residues are retained in critical areas are more important than the total amount of sugars consumed."[5]

The sequence of intake of foods during a meal can influence dental caries incidence. Eating cheese or peanuts before or after sugar-containing foods reduces the cariogenicity of the latter.[6, 7] Furthermore, meats, eggs, some types of nuts, and some dairy products do not produce an acidic plaque pH. Findings from human dental plaque investigations suggest that milk and certain cheeses (Cheddar, Swiss, blue, Monterey jack, mozzarella, Brie, and Gouda) produce little or no plaque acid.[8] The mechanism by which dairy foods decrease the development of dental caries needs further investigation.

The diet counselor should incorporate into the diet prescription whenever possible: (1) a nutritionally balanced varied diet from the high-density nutritious basic four food groups; (2) eliminate high-sugar snacks, whenever possible; (3) if sugar-containing foods must be included for providing the energy needs, restrict them to mealtime when the organic acids formed may undergo neutralization; and (4) recommend hard cheeses and nuts as between-meal snacks.

DIET COUNSELING

A basic prerequisite for accomplishing dietary change is the advice that the patient not the counselor bears the responsibility for making the change. The counselor should explain candidly the need for full cooperation and a sincere effort by the patient to modify the diet, and the patient should agree.

Minimal requirements for a successful dietary counseling service include (1) enrolling active patient involvement in planning, implementing, and evaluating the diet before and after counseling and (2) insisting on a series of follow-up visits to tailor the diet to the patient's needs and likes, and to avoid if possible dislikes without jeopardizing the dental-oral health status.

A simple initial screening that shows a typical 24-hour food intake can disclose possible dietary inadequacies, excesses, or both that may exert a negative influence on an individual's dental health—a potential cariogenic diet.

Diet counseling involves giving advice on food selection based on the individual's reasons for liking or not liking certain foods. Counseling requires obtaining information as to why, where, when, and what specific foods (e.g., sweets) are eaten, how frequently, and what feelings are experienced.

Patient Selection

Diet counseling will not succeed with every dental patient. Persons who need counseling must also want information about their potential dental caries problem and must be willing to improve current undesirable food selections and eating habits. Potential candidates for counseling should give high priority to preventive dentistry and should be willing to expend long-term efforts to maintain their natural dentition in good health for a lifetime.

In addition to a positive attitude, potential candidates for counseling should have a demonstrable need for dietary improvement, based on their current food intake regimen. The Dental Health Diet Score is a screening device to achieve this objective. It is a simple scoring procedure that can disclose a potential dietary problem that is likely to adversely affect a patient's dental health.

Essentially, the Dental Health Diet Score gives points earned as a result of an adequate intake of foods from each of the food groups plus points for ingesting foods especially recommended because they are the best sources of the ten nutrients essential for achieving and maintaining dental health. From this sum, points are subtracted for frequent ingestion of foods that are overtly sweet—whose sweetness is derived from added refined sugar or concentrated natural sugars. The difference is the Dental Health Diet Score.

A score of 60 to 100 is acceptable, and dietary counseling is not usually given unless the patient requests it. If the score is 56 or less, dietary counseling is both indicated and recommended as a part of a comprehensive preventive dentistry service to patients.

Instructions for Calculating a Dental Health Diet Score

STEP 1

To ascertain the average daily intake, list everything you eat and drink on an ordinary weekday including snacks. Record the time when the meal or snacks were eaten, the amount ingested (in household measures), how the food was prepared, and the number of teaspoons of sugar added (Fig. 17–1).

STEP 2

Circle the foods in the diary that have been sweetened with added sugar or are concentrated natural sweets (honey, raisins, figs, and so forth). Classify the uncircled foods or mixed food dishes into one or more of the appropriate food groups (Fig. 17–2).

For each serving of these foods listed in the food intake dairy, place a check mark in the appropriate food group block.

Add the number of checks and multiply by the number shown. The maximum number of points credit for the milk and meat groups is 24 each and for the fruit-vegetable and bread-cereal groups is 24 each.

Add the points. The sum is the Food Group Score (96 is the highest score).

Average Daily Intake

LIST ALL THE FOODS THAT YOU EAT ON ONE ORDINARY WEEKDAY, INCLUDING SNACKS.

Example:

Lunch (12:00 Noon)	4 oz tomato juice 1 chicken (3 oz) sandwich on rye bread 1 slice of chocolate cake with fudge icing 1 cup of coffee with 1 tsp of sugar
P.M. Snack (2:00 P.M.) (3:00 P.M.)	1 breath mint 1 piece of sugarless gum

BREAKFAST (Time:)	A.M. SNACK (Time:)
LUNCH (Time:)	P.M. SNACK (Time:)
DINNER (Time:)	ANY OTHER SNACKS (Time:)

FIGURE 17–1. Dental Health Diet Score: 24-hour intake diary.

Step 3

How many of the foods listed contain one or more of the ten nutrients essential for dental-oral health? In the Nutrient Evaluation Chart (Fig. 17–3) are listed the foods that are good sources of the nutrients essential for good health in general and dental-oral health in particular.

In each of the eight columns of foods, check the one or more eaten on this usual weekday. If a food is checked, circle the number 7 beside the nutrient that heads this column. The same food, such as broccoli, may be found in several columns. Also, in a column more than one food may be checked. Regardless of the number of foods checked in the column, only seven points is given per nutrient (56 is a perfect score).

Add the circled numbers to obtain the Nutrient Score.

Step 4

List the sweets and sugar-sweetened foods and the frequency with which they are consumed in a typical day.

Classify each sweet into either the liquid, solid and sticky, or slowly dissolving category (Fig. 17–4).

Place a check mark in the Frequency column for each item as long as they are eaten at least 20 minutes apart.

Add the number of checks. If the sweets are liquid, multiply by 5; if solid, multiply by 10; if slowly dissolving, multiply by 15.

Write the products in the Points column and total them. This is the Sweet Score.

Scoring the Four Food Groups
Look at what you ate and circle the empty-calorie foods (sugar-sweetened, saturated fat, and alcoholic beverages).

- Separate the foods into appropriate food groups.
- Leave out the sweet or sweetened foods (except for fresh fruit and juices).
- Put a check mark (✔) for each serving.
- Add up the number of checks, multiply by the number provided, and write down the points.
- If the total score for a food group is greater than the highest possible score, record the highest possible score.

	Food Group	Portion Size Considered One Serving	Number of Servings	Points
Example: 2 c milk 1½ oz Cheddar cheese	MILK (milk and cheese)	8 oz (1 c) milk 1½ oz Cheddar cheese 1½ slice American cheese 1½ c cottage cheese 8 oz (1 c) yogurt	✔✔✔ ×8 =	24 (highest possible score = 24)

FIGURE 17–2. Food Group Evaluation Chart.

Food Group	Recom-mended Adult Servings	Portion Size Considered One Serving	Number of Servings	Points
MILK (milk and cheese)	3	8 oz (1 c) milk 1½ oz Cheddar cheese 1½ slice American cheese 1½ c cottage cheese 8 oz (1 c) yogurt	___ × 8 =	___ (highest possible score = 24)
MEAT (meat, fish, poultry, dry beans, nuts)	2	2-3 oz lean cooked meat, fish, or poultry 2 eggs 4 tbsp peanut butter 1 c cooked dry beans or lentils	___ × 12 =	___ (highest possible score = 24)
FRUITS AND VEGETABLES Vitamin A: (dark green and deep yellow fruits and vegetables)	1	½ c cooked fruit or vegetable 1 medium raw fruit or vegetable ½ medium grapefruit or melon 4 oz (½ c) juice	___ × 6 =	___ (highest possible score = 6)
Vitamin C: (juice and citrus fruits)	1		___ × 6 =	___ (highest possible score = 6)
Other	2		___ × 6 =	___ (highest possible score = 12)
BREAD AND CEREALS (enriched or whole grain)	4	1 slice bread ¾ c dry cereal ½ c cooked cereal, rice, noodles, or macaroni	___ × 6 =	___ (highest possible score = 24)

TOTAL SCORE = ___
(highest possible score = 96)

Figure 17–2 Continued

STEP 5

Now put it all together (Fig. 17–5). Transfer the 4 Food Group Score and the Sweet Score to the Totaling the Scores page. If the 4 Food Group Score is barely adequate or not adequate and/or the Sweet Score is in the "Watch Out" zone, nutrition counseling is indicated.

Nutrient Score

In each nutrient column check the foods you recorded in Figure 17–1.
At the top of each column that has a checked food, circle the number 7.

Example:

	Protein ⑦	Ascorbic Acid 7	Calcium ⑦
3 oz hamburger on roll 8 oz milk 1 medium apple	cheese milk ✔ meat ✔	broccoli grapefruit greens	broccoli eggs milk ✔

Protein and Niacin 7	Vitamin A 7		Iron 7	Folic Acid 7

cheese
dried beans
dried peas
eggs
fish
meat
milk
nuts
poultry
	apricots
	broccoli
	butter
	cantaloupe
	carrots
	collards
	eggs
	greens
	liver
		margarine
		milk
		peaches
		squash
		spinach
		sweet pota-
		   toes
			beef
			broccoli
			eggs
			green leafy
			   vegetables
			liver
			oysters
			sardines
			shrimp
				asparagus
				broccoli
				cereals
				kidney
				liver
				spinach
				yeasts

Riboflavin (Vitamin B₂) 7	Ascorbic Acid (Vitamin C) 7		Calcium and Phosphorus 7	Zinc 7

broccoli
chicken breasts
eggs
ham
liver
milk
mushrooms
pork
okra
spinach
	broccoli
	brussels sprouts
	cantaloupe
	grapefruit
	green peppers
	greens
	oranges
	raspberries
	strawberries
	tomatoes
			broccoli
			cheese
			eggs
			green leafy
			   vegetables
			milk
			oranges
			string beans
				beef
				liver
				lobster
				oysters
				shrimp
				(other red
				   meats and
				   shellfish)

Add the circled numbers. The total is your NUTRIENT SCORE. _____

FIGURE 17–3. *Nutrient Evaluation Chart.*

Scoring the Sweets

Using the dietary recall of an ordinary weekday . . .
- Classify each sweet into liquid, solid and sticky, or slowly dissolving.
- For each time a sweet was eaten, either at the end of a meal or between meals (at least 20 minutes apart), place a check in the frequency column.
- In each group add up the number of sweets eaten and multiply by the number provided. Write down the number of points.
- Add up all the points for the total score.

Example:

10:00 A.M. 1 jelly donut
12:00 NOON ham and
  cheese sandwich
  1 c milk
  1 cupcake
3:00 P.M. 1 coke
5:00 P.M. 1 cough drop

Form	Frequency	Points
Liquid	✔ × 5 =	5
Solid and sticky	✔✔ × 10 =	20
Slowly dissolving	✔ × 15 =	15

TOTAL SCORE = 35

Decay-Promoting Potential

Form	Frequency	Points
Liquid soft drinks, fruit drinks, cocoa, sugar and honey in beverages, nondairy creamers, ice cream, sherbet, gelatin dessert, flavored yogurt, pudding, custard, popsicles	____ × 5 =	
Solid and Sticky cake, cupcakes, donuts, sweet rolls, pastry, canned fruit in syrup, bananas, cookies, chocolate candy, caramel, toffee, jelly beans, other chewy candy, chewing gum, dried fruit, marshmallows, jelly, jam	____ × 10 =	
Slowly Dissolving hard candies, breath mints, antacid tablets, cough drops	____ × 15 =	

TOTAL SCORE = ____

FIGURE 17–4. *Sweets Evaluation Chart.*

Communication Techniques

Communication is a basic tool in the practice of preventive dentistry. It can create motivation for change. Communication is the giving and receiving of information; it involves the knowledge, thoughts, and opinions of the counselor and patient. Because it is not a service performed in the operatory, some dentists and dental hygienists have been reluctant to provide the service on a fee-for-time basis. This attitude is faulty, unrealistic, and should be changed. Dentists, because they are doctors, are expected to teach, advise, and counsel patients. (The word *doctor* means teacher. It is derived from the Latin verb *docere*, which means to teach.) Both the dentist and the dental hygienist, by virtue of their education and training, should recognize that they render a vital dental health service when they advise patients on diet and nutrition as well as on other preventive dentistry home care procedures. Diet counseling is an important preventive and supportive service. Because faulty diet and inadequate nutrition

Totaling the Scores

4 Food Group Score: ____

72–96	Excellent
64–72	Adequate
56–64	Barely Adequate*
56 or less	Not Adequate*

Sweet Score: ____

5 or less	Excellent
10	Good
15 or more	"Watch Out" Zone†

*If your score is barely adequate or not adequate you need nutrition counseling (perhaps from your dentist or nutritionist).
†If your sweet score is in the "Watch Out" Zone your dentist will talk with you about what improvements you might make.

FIGURE 17–5. Dental Health Diet Scorecard.

can be major etiological factors in dental-oral health problems, it is necessary that the dentist or dental hygienist give diet counseling when indicated. Thus prevention of future dental-oral problems related to dietary factors contributes to the lasting beneficial effects of restorative or periodontal therapy or both.

There are three rules for achieving effective communication with a patient:

1. During a face-to-face interview, keeping eye contact with the patient is a persuasive and powerful device for motivating behavioral change.

2. Communications can be both verbal and nonverbal. Words transmit information. The interviewer's tone of voice, facial expression, and gestures convey sincerity, enthusiasm, and empathy. These nonverbal actions can be influential in helping the patient to change his or her behavior.

3. The message must be adapted to the patient's needs and level of understanding. Personalization of the message is more likely to result in a sustained change in behavior.

To communicate with a patient, a combination of interviewing, teaching, counseling, and motivating is used.

Interviewing

PURPOSES

The purpose of an interview is to obtain information and to give help. The first and basic goal in interviewing is to understand (1) the problem, (2) the factors that contribute to it, and (3) the personality of the patient.

Why should a dental health professional elicit information concerning the food and dietary intake and habits of patients?

First, the dietary interview can serve as a valuable diagnostic aid. Food selection and eating habits may affect a person's dental or general health or both. Appraisal of an individual's dietary status may provide a clue to potential difficulties. For example, eating many sweet foods daily for a long period at the expense of nutritious food will probably result in clinically detectable carious lesions within 6 to 18 months in addition to poor general health.

Second, knowledge of a person's daily routine is important for adapting the caries-preventive diet to an individual's lifestyle. This adaptation may help a patient adhere to the newly prescribed diet, the basis for achieving the health goals and rewards from diet counseling.

Third, many practical research contributions could be made if data from nutritional assessments could systematically be gathered to correlate dental, periodontal, or oral mucosal problems with such factors as food habits, dietary intake, physical conditioning factors, and socioeconomic status, among others.

PHYSICAL SETTING

Privacy and a comfortable, relaxed atmosphere are important. The interview should not take place chairside in the dental operatory for the very good reason that this is a threatening atmosphere that may engender fear and withdrawal. Rather, it should take place in a separate counseling room that contains a small conference table, some chairs, a blackboard, and visual aids. Discussing food habits is a personal matter. Therefore using a private counseling room will indicate that you respect the patient's feelings. Furthermore, distractions and interruptions are unlikely. The patient will probably talk more freely, and as a result, the interviewer will be able to provide better advice.

THE DIET INTERVIEWER

Good dietary interviewing requires skill, time, and some background knowledge of the science and practice of nutrition, including familiarity with ways in which food habits are formed and the factors that affect these habits. The interviewer should also have some background and updated information in oral medicine and oral pathology, particularly cariology and periodontology. The people who are most likely to have this dual educational background are dentists and dental hygienists. Certainly nutritionists can readily qualify with some extra course work in the nature of dental caries and periodontal disease and in preventive dentistry.

Ideally, as the professional authority, the dentist should be the diet interviewer, but it is probable that he or she will not be able to give adequate time to this phase of preventive services. Consequently, clinical dental nutrition services probably will be assigned to a dental hygienist or a nutritionist. In any event, the dentist is the responsible professional who must reinforce the advice given by the dental hygienist or nutritionist at the check-up visits.

HOW TO INTERVIEW A PATIENT[9, 10]

First, the interviewer should be relaxed and should help the patient to relax and feel comfortable.

Start with a brief introductory statement about the purpose of the interview. Ask questions that will encourage the patient's expression of feelings about his or her current dental health condition and the importance of preserving the natural dentition. It is important to allow the patient to talk freely, thus giving the interviewer leads for additional questions. The interviewer can thereby become better acquainted with the patient's personality and language skills. These observations can guide the phrasing of questions, comments, and suggestions and will allow the interviewer to communicate at the patient's level.

An important advantage to listening before speaking is that the patient may reveal answers to many questions without being asked. Sometimes the patient provides a direction for the course of action that should be taken. The interviewer need only confirm and strengthen the patient's suggestion. Such recommendations are more likely to be followed.

Allowing the interviewee to speak first may change the interviewer's views about the cause of the problem and may reveal the causes of the dental decay problem from the patient's point of view. It is the patient who must act; therefore it is best to start from her or his understanding.

Cross-examination may make the patient defensive. In general, questions that require reflection or extended answers are preferable to questions that can be answered Yes or No. In general, the interviewer should be encouraging and sympathetic and should not assume an adversary position.

The interviewer should unobtrusively direct the interview, deciding when to listen and when to speak and observing responses. When a person is inclined to ramble, the interviewer must gently and sympathetically redirect the patient to the immediate situation. The interviewer must decide what information is needed and the best way to obtain it. Once the person's confidence is obtained and rapport is established, the underlying basic factors of the specific dental problem can be investigated.

Do not make decisions for the person. For a better follow-through, allow the patient to make choices based on what has been learned and with which the patient can cooperate.

When closing an interview, it is usually a good plan to end by recapitulating what the patient has learned and the future action that you have agreed on.

A new appointment for reinforcement, answering questions, and taking further action, such as referrals to other specialists, may be in order. For example, a patient with a deep-seated emotional problem or a patient with a serious economic problem would best be advised to consult a psychologist or a social worker, respectively.

Teaching and Learning

Patient education is more than simply giving information: it requires the presentation of information with sufficient impact to stimulate action by the learner.

A number of teaching aids may be used, including booklets on nutrition and dental health, which can be purchased at little cost. Three of the best available sources of these materials are the American Dental Association, The National Dairy Council, and the U.S. Department of Agriculture (USDA) Human Nutrition Center.

The American Dental Association has available such pertinent pamphlets as "Diet and Dental Health," "Kick the Sweet Snack Habit," and "Nutrition and Dental Disease." The National Dairy Council provides a poster, "Guide to Good Eating," and a booklet, "Guide to Wise Food Choices," that deal with the use of food groups and nutrition labeling in planning nutritionally sound daily diets. The Public Documents Distribution Center in Pueblo, Colorado, will provide booklets such as "Food Is More Than Just Something to Eat" and "The Confusing

World of Health Foods." Many other publications from other sources are also available for waiting room use or for reading at home by the patient.

Visual aids include ivorine tooth models depicting dental caries or peri-odontal disease and plastic or rubberlike food models to help the patient visualize what you are teaching. The National Dairy Council has life-size cardboard models of foods that can be used to show how to plan well-balanced and varied meals. Also, samples of different types of food containers should be available so that nutrition labeling and ingredient listing can be explained.

In our hands, the best teaching aids have been a blackboard with chalk or a pad of paper and pencil for drawing sketches or diagrams. Explaining while one draws and labels the parts of a tooth, for example, always holds the patient's interest.

Even with these various aids available, teaching will not be effective if the information is not presented in small increments. If the patient does not understand the explanation, it should be repeated. The next level should not be attempted until the previous level is fully understood.

Using analogies with everyday experiences may help to explain biological facts in simple language.

The more the patient is involved in the educational process the greater is the extent of learning. People learn least well by hearing; they learn better what they can also see; and they learn best by doing, because they are totally involved. Any time the patient participates in evaluating his or her diet and writes his or her own diet prescription with guidance from the counselor, optimal learning and adherence to the new regimen will result.

Counseling

Approaches to counseling may be directive or nondirective. In directive counseling, the role of the patient is passive and the decisions are made by the counselor for the patient. In nondirective counseling, the counselor's role is merely to aid the patient in clarifying and understanding his or her own situation and to provide guidance so that the patient can make his or her own final decision as to the type of action that should be taken. The nondirective counseling approach is recommended.

GUIDELINES FOR COUNSELING

A prerequisite for successful nutrition counseling is a realistic and honest statement that the patient, not the counselor, bears the responsibility for making changes in food selections and eating habits. The patient should accept respon-sibility for the dietary modifications.

The guidelines for counseling are as follows:

1. *Gather information*—personal identifying data, likes and dislikes, and the patient's perception as to the cause(s) of the problem.

2. *Evaluate and interpret information*—relative adequacy of the diet, eating habits, and the indirect environmental or systemic factors that contribute to the dietary problem—to find the reasons for the patient's dental problem.

3. *Develop and implement a plan of action*—a patient-prescribed diet consisting primarily of gradual, qualitative modifications of the diet using acceptable food exchanges. Be realistic in the types and amounts of changes made initially. The dietary frequency chart may help in determining what changes might be made (Fig. 17–6).

4. *Seek active participation of the patient's family* in all aspects of dietary change. Whenever possible, include them in the counseling session.

5. *Follow up to assess the progress made.* The major purposes of this session are to clarify problems encountered in following the diet prescription and to reinforce and encourage making and maintaining the changes. Set up visits for periodic checkups.

MOTIVATION

Motivation stimulates or is an incentive for action. To modify a patient's diet, the clinician can only seek and encourage the patient's own motivation. However, the counselor's positive attitude and conviction as to the necessity and effectiveness of nutrition counseling can stimulate the patient to initiate an improved dietary pattern.

According to Garn, the basic factors that motivate people are self-preservation, recognition, love, and money.[11] The order of importance varies from one individual to another, but all four factors influence the desires of each person. If clinicians can help patients understand that a healthy mouth and teeth and a nice-looking smile can help them achieve one or more of these four goals, patients will be inclined to adopt a diet that will promote better oral health.

MOTIVATING PATIENTS TO MODIFY FOOD HABITS[12]

A person passes through four preliminary decision stages in changing a dietary pattern—awareness, interest, involvement, and action. The fifth stage involves forming a new habit.

1. *Awareness* is recognition that a problem exists, but without an inclination to solve it.

2. *Interest* is a greater degree of awareness but still with no inclination to act.

3. *Involvement* is an interest and a definite intention to act.

4. *Action* is a trial performance.

5. *Habit* is a commitment to perform this action regularly over a sustained period of time.

If giving up hard candy to prevent dental decay is used as an example, the stages can be illustrated as follows:

1. Awareness—Hard candies produce acid, which can cause my teeth to decay.

2. Interest—Maybe I should give up the hard candies; I don't want any more sensitive or painful teeth.

3. Involvement—I definitely will give up hard candy.

4. Action—I have given up hard candies and chew sugarless gum instead to prevent the dry feeling in my mouth.

5. Habit—I haven't had a hard candy in six months.

For each food group for which you scored less than the recommended number of servings in Figure 17–2, check how often you use foods from that group.	*Weekly Frequency of Consumption*		
	FREQUENT 5× OR MORE	SELDOM* 2–5×	RARELY* 2× OR LESS
Food Groups			
MILK GROUP—FOR CALCIUM, PROTEIN, AND B VITAMINS *1 c of:* milk, buttermilk, skim milk, yogurt, collard leaves *2 c of:* broccoli; *1½ c of:* kale, cheese sauce; *1½ oz of:* cheese *3 c of:* soybeans; *4 oz of:* tofu			
MEAT GROUP—FOR PROTEIN, ZINC, IRON, AND B VITAMINS *2 oz of:* beef, liver, heart, kidney, pork, poultry, fish *1 c of:* beans, peas, lentils, soybeans, peanuts; *2:* eggs			
FRUIT AND VEGETABLE GROUP—FOR VITAMINS A & C AND FIBER *Vitamin A sources:* *1 large:* raw carrot, sweet potato *1 c of:* cooked carrots, yellow squash, spinach, greens; *1½ c of:* kale; *2 c of:* cantaloupe; *2 med.:* papaya; *12–15 med:* apricots			
Vitamin C sources: *4 oz of:* orange, grapefruit, or tomato juice; *½ med.:* orange, grapefruit, cantaloupe, raw red or green pepper; *1 med.:* cooked green or red pepper; *2 med.:* tomatoes; *½ c of:* broccoli, kale, greens, strawberries; *1 c of:* cooked cabbage, spinach, cauliflower, kohlrabi; *2 c of:* raw cabbage.			
	FREQUENT 10× OR MORE	SELDOM* 4–10×	RARELY* 4× OR LESS
All other fruits and vegetables: (usual serving size = ½ c)			
	FREQUENT 15× OR MORE	SELDOM* 7–15×	RARELY* 7× OR LESS
BREAD AND CEREAL GROUP—FOR B VITAMINS AND FIBER *1 slice of:* bread; *½ of:* bagel, english muffin, hamburger roll, hot dog roll; *1:* dinner roll, 6-inch tortilla, muffin, pancake, waffle; *2:* graham crackers; *6:* saltines; *½:* 4×6 inch square matzoth; *¼ c of:* wheat germ; *½ c of:* hot cereal, noodles, spaghetti, macaroni; *¾ c of:* dry cereal			

*If you scored Seldom or Rarely for any group you need to increase your consumption of foods from that group if possible.

FIGURE 17–6. *Diet Frequency Chart.*

Although there is no sure way to motivate all patients to alter their food habits, we have had some success by

1. Helping patients to understand the source of their dental problems
2. Helping patients to understand why they have rejected certain foods
3. Allowing patients to prescribe their own dental caries–reduction diet, which they can follow without difficulty

By appealing to patients' reason and by explaining both the undesirable consequences without self-help and the desirable consequences with it, assisting patients to modify food habits is possible.

The clinicians who have never actually counseled patients are the ones who say that food habits are impossible to modify. However, food habits have been changed and the health professionals who have actually counseled are confident that in most instances, they can help patients make behavioral modifications. It is rewarding for the diet counselor when a patient says, "Why didn't someone take the time to give me this advice about my food habits before? It doesn't seem that difficult to make some changes."

Principles of Diet Management: Application to Caries Prevention

A rational nutrition program for dental caries prevention based on the effects of various nutrients and food practices on the production or inhibition of dental caries coupled with some basic dietetics principles can be formulated.

The fundamental principle that applies to all supportive diets is that they are simply slight modifications of a normal or adequate diet pattern. A normal diet is one that provides all the nutrients essential for good health by using a variety of foods from the USDA Daily Food Guide (Chaps. 4 and 15). A combination of foods from each of the food groups in the amounts recommended will fulfill almost completely, with the exception of calories, the recommended daily allowances of all the essential nutrients. Furthermore, if a food from each of the food groups for which servings are recommended is eaten at each meal, the diet will not only be adequate but will also be balanced. The importance of a balanced meal is that the nutrition of the human organism is most efficient when there is an interaction of complementary nutrients at the same meal. For example, the protein in bread is more efficiently used by the body if milk or meat is eaten with it.

Therefore these four rules should be adopted when making dietary modifications:

1. Maintain overall nutritional adequacy by conforming to the USDA Daily Food Guide for at least the recommended number of servings from each of the food groups.

2. The prescribed diet should vary from the normal diet pattern as little as possible.

3. The diet should meet the body's requirements for the essential nutrients as generously as the diseased condition can tolerate.

4. The prescribed diet should take into consideration and accommodate the patient's likes and dislikes, food habits, and other environmental factors as long as they do not interfere with the objectives.

Dietary modifications are made with respect to frequency of eating; quantitative increase, decrease, or elimination of one or more nutrients; or alteration of the physical consistency of the food. These general principles may be applied to the prevention or control of caries as follows:

- Limit the number of eating periods to three regular meals per day, stressing the need to avoid between-meal snacks.
- Increase the intake of protective foods such as vegetables and fruits, milk and cheese, meat, fish, and legumes, which are rich in minerals, vitamins, and protein.
- Decrease the total amount of carbohydrates so that they provide no more than 50% and no less than 30% of the calories. (This is further explained in the next paragraph.)
- Ideally, it is best to wean the patient from the taste of sweets. Next best is to restrict the consumption of sugar-containing foods to meals. The complete elimination of sticky, concentrated sweets such as candy, cakes, pastries, and dried fruits, especially between meals, is a requirement. The dental health professional should direct preventive efforts to at least minimizing sugar intake if elimination of sugar is not feasible.
- Recommend the liberal use of firm detergent (tooth-cleansing) foods such as raw fruits and raw vegetables so that there will be some oral clearance of food debris and stimulation of salivary flow. These and other nutritious snacks should be recommended as suitable alternatives for the sugar-rich, sticky, retained foods.
- Recommend drinking and cooking with fluoridated water or the ingestion of fluoride supplements if the patient lives in a nonfluoridated area from birth to 13 years of age; also recommend the use of a fluoride dentifrice and mouth rinse.

Since there is a tendency to limit carbohydrate intake when giving dietary advice for caries prevention and control, it is wise to be mindful of some of the problems that may arise from the overzealous restriction of carbohydrate intake. The Food and Nutrition Board of the National Research Council recommends that a normal adult ingest about 500 calories (125 g) per day from carbohydrates to meet the biological needs of the body.

As discussed in Chap. 2, some of the important functions of carbohydrates besides providing a readily available inexpensive source of energy are to conserve water and electrolytes and to spare protein for body building. Also, if not enough dietary carbohydrates are available, the body will not be able to oxidize fat efficiently to one of its end products, carbon dioxide, which may cause an accumulation of ketones and organic acids, a condition known as acidosis or ketosis.

STEP-BY-STEP DIETARY COUNSELING PROCEDURE FOR CARIES PREVENTION

The following step-by-step counseling procedure is recommended. Keep in mind the facts about motivating the patient as already discussed and the application of the principles of dietary management that apply to the prevention of dental caries.

INSTRUCTIONS FOR KEEPING A FOOD DIARY

An accurate, complete record of food intake is best achieved by having the patient keep a running daily record of meals and between-meal snacks. Recording from memory details concerning the kinds, amounts, and preparation of the foods eaten is not reliable and should be discouraged.

A FIVE-DAY FOOD INTAKE DIARY

Name: *John Doe*

Date: *July 11, 1987*

INSTRUCTIONS

1. Please record in detail everything you eat or drink in the order in which it is eaten

2. The frequency of eating is an important consideration; therefore, include not only meals but between-meal snacks, candies, gum, etc.

3. The following information is essential:
   a. The amount in household measurements such as 8 oz , 1 serving, 1/2 cup, 1 teaspoon
   b. The food and how it is prepared such as fried chicken, baked apple, raw carrots, etc.
   c. The addition of sugar, syrup, or milk to cereal, beverages, or other foods such as 1 bowl of cornflakes with 2 t of sugar and 1/2 c of milk

4. Example:

Wrong	Right
juice	1/2 c tomato juice
sandwich	1 chicken sandwich with
dessert	lettuce
coffee	1 slice chocolate cake
	1 cup coffee with milk
	and 2 t sugar

A.E. NIZEL D.M.D.   (NOT TO BE REPRODUCED WITHOUT PERMISSION)

FIGURE 17–7. Part I.

FIRST DAY

BREAKFAST:

4 oz orange juice
2 slices of toast
1 pat butter
1 cup coffee with milk

A.M. Snack:

1 donut
1 cup coffee with milk

LUNCH:

1 baloney sandwich
(2 slices bread)
(2 slices baloney)
1 glass milk

P.M. Snack

1 cola
1 pkg (4) crackers
with peanut butter

DINNER:

1/4 cantaloupe
2 servings roast turkey
1 baked potato
salad - lettuce and tomato
1 cup tea

Extras:

1 slice apple pie
1 cup of milk
1-oz bar chocolate
1 apple

FIGURE 17–7 Continued. Part II.

A 5-Day Food Intake Diary similar to the one shown in Figure 17–7 is recommended. The diary is kept for 5 consecutive days, including a weekend day or holiday, to provide a more representative sample of food intake. Stress the importance of detail. The instructions shown in Figure 17–1 will help the patient record food intake accurately.

The patient is asked not to make any changes in the usual dietary pattern during this week of diary keeping because that diet may be perfectly acceptable and may be unrelated to the dental caries problem. For this reason, do not discuss at this time the mechanism of caries production or the role that food can play.

The demonstration and discussion of keeping a food diary take only 5 to 10 minutes and can be done as part of any dental visit.

THE INTERVIEWING AND COUNSELING VISIT

This visit is scheduled for at least 5 days after the food diary is given to the patient to complete. It is strongly advised that this visit be devoted exclusively to interviewing and counseling and that it not include other dental procedures, even oral prophylaxis or x-rays, for two reasons: first, a useful diet counseling service takes from 45 to 60 minutes, depending on the experience of the counselor and the patient's comprehension. Second, reserving this office visit solely for diet counseling gives the counseling session the identification and importance it deserves, with the result that the patient is more likely to heed the prescribed diet. Furthermore, a fee for the time spent and the counseling rendered is less likely to be questioned.

ARRIVING AT A DIAGNOSIS

Chief Complaint and Present Illness. After the conversation opens with introductions and pleasantries, the first question might be: Are you having some problems with your teeth? This gives the patient an opportunity to state his or her chief complaint. (A case history outline is shown in Fig. 17–8.)

The follow-up questions relating to the present illness might be: When did you first notice this problem? When did you visit the dentist last? Did you have your teeth completely restored at that time? How many cavities have you developed since your last dental check-up? The answers to these questions will give the counselor a fairly good picture of the rapidity of the carious process. As a rule of thumb, the occurrence of a half dozen or more new carious surfaces after having completed all of the necessary dental work 6 months previously should be of some concern. If this relatively rapid rate of new cavity formation is interpreted by the dentist as rampant caries, it is advisable to use a nutrition-counseling procedure including behavior modification.*

Personal and Social History. This aspect of the case history can provide some important clues to the reasons the patient chooses a particular diet. It is accomplished by ascertaining the patient's daily routine, interests, and habits (lifestyle).

---

* See A. E. Nizel. Nutrition and Preventive Dentistry: Science and Practice, 2nd ed., pp. 455–458. Philadelphia, W. B. Saunders, 1980, or refer patient to a nutritionist.

DATE_____

Name_____Occupation_____Height_____Weight_____

Address_____Age_____Desirable weight_____

Nationality_____   Religion_____

General Appearance: (Alertness, Gait, Posture, Muscular and Skeletal Development,
          Overweight or Underweight, etc.)

Chief Complaint: The dental problem in the patient's words
          and

Present Illness: When was the problem first noted?
          How rapidly has it progressed?

Personal and Social History:
   1. Grade in school_____
   2. Number of hours per day watching TV_____
   3. Other spare time activities and interests_____
   4. Emotional status_____

Family History:
   1. Father's occupation_____Mother's Occupation_____
   2. Number and ages of brothers_____sisters_____
   3. If both parents are working, who looks after the children?_____
   4. Dental status of other family members_____
   5. Any special diets followed in family?_____
   6. Does this affect patient's food intake? Yes_____ No_____

Medical History:
   1. Food allergies_____
   2. Medical problems: anemia, diabetes, etc._____
   3. Diet supplements_____
   4. Medications (with particular emphasis on antisialogogues such as atropine, Ban-
      thine, belladonna, sleeping pills, antihistamines, etc.)_____
      _____
   5. Mouth breathing (due to nasal obstruction, smoking)_____

Diet History:
   1. Appetite: Good_____Fair_____Poor_____
   2. Person responsible for food preparation_____
   3. Eat with family or alone?_____
   4. Is there a craving for sweets?_____
   5. Religious or ethnic dietary practices_____
   6. Is there a candy dish or cookie jar always full at home?_____
   7. Bedtime snacks_____
   8. Is food diary typical of patient's usual food habits?_____
      If not, what circumstances altered usual pattern?_____
   9. Fluorides: In communal water supply?_____; tablets?_____

Diet Evaluation:
   1. Adequacy in type and amount of 4 Food Groups (are foods from the 4 Food Groups
      eaten in the recommended amounts?)_____
   2. Balance of meals: Good_____Poor_____
   3. Frequency of eating including snacks_____
   4. How many plaque-forming sweets?_____
   5. How many nonplaque-forming foods at each meal?_____

Clinical Observations:
   1. Skin changes_____
   2. Lips, tongue and oral mucous membrane changes_____
   3. Periodontal health_____
   4. Amount of dental plaque_____
   5. Teeth – Caries: number, prime location and distribution (occlusal, buccal, inter-
          proximal of anteriors, etc.)_____
          Alignment and occlusion:_____
   6. Salivary flow_____

Laboratory Tests:
Color of Synder's medium after incubating: 24 hours_____ 48 hours_____

Impressions:
   1. Dental caries incidence Rampant_____High_____Low_____
   2. Food deficiencies or excesses_____
   3. Reasons for food selection_____

Other comments:

FIGURE 17–8. Nutrition case history outline for a caries-susceptible patient.

The counselor may say to a teenage patient: I'd like to be better acquainted with you and what you do. The easiest way may be by your telling me your routine for a typical day—yesterday, for example. What time do you get up? Do you have enough time to eat breakfast? Who makes breakfast? When do you brush your teeth, before or after breakfast? How long do you spend at brushing your teeth? Do you take lunch to school? What grade are you in? Do you like school? What is your favorite subject? What hobbies do you have? Do you belong to a club? How much time do you spend watching TV? How much reading do you do? Do you snack while reading, studying, or watching TV?

These are examples of questions that a counselor might ask to start the conversation. Usually, the direction and extent of the questioning depend on how much and how soon rapport is established. Some patients are outgoing and need little stimulation to speak freely of their daily activities. Others may need to have their conversation guided by specific questions. As a rule, however, if the counselor uses patience some common point of interest can be found that will cause the conversation to flow spontaneously. The patient will probably automatically include information about environmental factors (economic, cultural, religious, social personal stresses and anxieties) that influence food selection and food habits.

Information concerning the dental health status of the parents or siblings or special diets for other members of the family is elicited at the same time as the personal and social history is developed. Relating information about other members of the family is almost automatic because involvement with them is part of everyday activities.

Medical History. As part of the conversation about daily routine, questions about both general and dental health are always asked. The importance of systemic conditioning factors in contributing to malnutrition has already been discussed in detail in Chap. 16. Physiological stresses, such as the spurt growth period, diabetes, allergies, and gastrointestinal problems, are examples of common medical problems that can influence nutritional status.

The foregoing information will provide the basic causes of and the behavioral reasons for the patient's food habits.

Diet History and Evaluation. The patient's 5-day food diary is analyzed for (1) adequacy of intake of foods from the food groups and (2) the amount and type of foods sweetened with sugar and the frequency of eating them.

The patient is asked to do the following:

STEP 1. Circle in red all the foods recorded in the 5-day food diary that are sweetened with sugar. This means soft drinks, coffee with sugar; cookies, cakes, and pastries; jam; hard candies; cough drops and cough syrup; fruits canned in syrup, and other foods that have an overtly sweet taste. (So many foods contain added sugar that it would not be practical to circle all of them. Our major goal is to try to wean the patient from the readily detectable sweet flavor.) Dried fruits such as figs, dates, prunes, apricots, and raisins should also be circled, because they are highly concentrated sweets. However, fresh fruits with high water and fiber content, such as apples, oranges, or pears, are not.

This circling foods in red will point out and separate the protective, noncariogenic, high–nutrient density foods from the empty calorie, cariogenic types. Usually, the patient is surprised at the number of circled foods.

Explain the causes and process of dental decay and that certain foods, especially sugars, and certain eating habits can contribute to initiating and developing carious lesions. A simplified explanation of the carious process is as follows:

$$\text{Bacteria } + \text{ sugar} \rightarrow \text{acid}$$

The acid produced in this plaque attacks the enamel and weakens it by a process called demineralization, which means the acid withdraws minerals from the tooth, creating a weak spot, or defect, in the enamel. This can be expressed as

$$\text{Acid } + \text{ tooth} \rightarrow \text{demineralization} \rightarrow \text{beginning of tooth decay}$$

STEP 2. The total number of exposures of the teeth to sweets, the form of the sweets (solid or liquid), and when they were eaten (at meals or between meals) are determined. On the Plaque-Forming Sweets Chart (Fig. 17–9), the patient classifies and tallies the foods circled in red in the diary according to their physical nature and how frequently they were eaten. The significance of the total number of check marks becomes clear if the patient multiplies that number by a factor of 20. The factor 20 represents approximately the number of minutes that the plaque pH remains at a tooth demineralization potential when concentrated sweets in liquid form come into contact with dental plaque. If the sweets are retained, as are hard candies, toffees, and cookies, then the number of minutes of acid production may be doubled. After the patient has calculated the number of hours each day that the teeth have been exposed to acid demineralization, he or she usually recognizes the problems and wants to solve them.

STEP 3. The adequacy of the diet in terms of the desirable number of servings of each of the food groups is readily determined as follows: each food or mixture of foods is classified and tallied in one of the food groups—(1) vegetable-fruit, (2) bread-cereal, (3) milk, and (4) meat. The amount of a food considered an average serving is credited by one stroke in the appropriate block (Fig. 17–10). A conversion table in Appendix 3 classifies foods and mixed dishes into their proper food groups and also lists the amount commonly considered one serving.

For example, a lunch consisting of a bowl of fish chowder, a serving of macaroni and cheese, and half a cantaloupe is classified as follows: The fish chowder equals one-half a meat serving and 1 cup of milk, the macaroni and cheese is listed as 1 serving of bread and 1 cup of milk. The half cantaloupe is considered 2 servings of fruit.

The average daily intake is calculated by dividing the number of strokes for the 5 days by 5 and recording the result in the average column (see Fig. 17–9). The actual average intake is then compared with the suggested daily intake, which depends on the individual's age and size. If the average actual intake is less than is suggested, the amount is recorded as a minus quantity (e.g., -2) in the difference column. However, if the average actual intake is equal to or more than the suggested daily intake then OK is written in the difference column.

With these work sheets, the diet can be qualitatively evaluated for its adequacy, and the amount of the sugar-sweetened foods with their cariogenic potential is clearly shown.

Form of Sugar	When Eaten	1st Day	2nd
LIQUID	with meals	✓	✓
(soda, sugar in coffee etc.)	between meals	✓	O
SOLID	with meals	O	O
(cookie, candy)	between meals	✓✓	✓

Total for day: 4

Minutes ($\times$ 20):   80

FIGURE 17–9. Part I. Plaque-forming sweets. Make one check for each item eaten, and add zeros to the unmarked blocks. To find the minutes (or hours) your teeth are potentially exposed to acid in a day, add the number of checks for a day and multiply by 20.

Clinical and Oral Examination. In order to assess a patient's nutritional state, it is necessary to determine whether there are any clinical signs suggestive of malnutrition; for example, overweight, underweight, pallor, excessive dryness or multiple bruises of the skin. The lips, gingivae, and oral mucosa may suggest a nutritional anemia if they are pallid. Cheilosis, stomatitis, swollen interdental gingival papillae, and papillitis (inflamed papillae) of the tongue are other oral manifestations of possible malnutrition. Mouth breathing, which tends to produce a dry mouth, should be noted. The cause of mouth breathing in many children is nasal obstruction. Extreme dryness of the mouth may also occur in older women, perhaps as a result of menopause or other hormonal changes. Presence or absence of significant amounts of saliva is an important sign from the standpoint of dental caries and should always be noted.

Diagnosis. The diagnosis developed from the history and examination consists of three parts: (1) the relative amount (e.g., moderate or slight) of dental caries, (2) produced by faulty food habits that are caused by (3) lack of knowledge or by psychological, social, economic, or systemic problems. (Of course, the dentist must decide if referral to a physician, psychologist, or nutritionist is indicated.)

NUTRITIONAL MANAGEMENT

Managing the Causes of Improper Diet

It is important to deal with the basic causes first. Some of the more common reasons for eating an excessive amount of sweets, for example, are as follows:

3rd	4th	5th	Total
O	✓	✓	4
✓	✓✓	O	4
O	O	O	O
✓✓	✓	✓✓✓	9

FIGURE 17–9 Continued. *Part II.*

- Eating sweets is an accepted household dietary practice of the family—grandparents, parents, and siblings.
- Sweets are a compensation for psychosocial stress (a domineering parent, parental rejection, adolescent rebellion, sibling rivalry, or domestic discord).
- Sweets are used as breath sweeteners after smoking.
- Sweets moisten a dry mouth or soothe throat irritation.

Each minor psychological problem will probably be managed in a different way. The major function is to make patients aware that it exists. Then if patients are allowed to vent their feelings, they usually begin to find their own answers.

Economic problems are managed best by advising the patient that low-cost foods such as milk powder, margarine, and lean hamburger are as nutritious as their more expensive counterparts, whole milk, butter, and steak. Noting newspaper advertisements, using discount coupons, and noting unit-pricing labels for comparable generic brand foods will all help save money on food bills.

A patient with dry mouth syndrome caused by nasal obstruction should, of course, be referred to a nose and throat specialist. If there is need for stimulation of salivary flow, chewing firm fibrous fruits and vegetables or softened paraffin wax can be very helpful.

How to Assist the Patient to Select an Adequate Noncariogenic Diet

Step 1. Commend the Patient. It is important to commence a counseling procedure on a positive note. Patients do not like to be criticized at the very outset. Since the food evaluation chart will probably show that the recommended allowances were met in at least one or two food groups, a good starting point is to commend the patient for this and urge continuance of this good practice.

Step 2. Allow the Patient to Suggest Improvements and Write His or Her Own Diet Prescription. Again refer to the evaluation chart. It can readily be seen (and may even be commented on by the patient) that an intake of only two

Food Group	Portion Size Considered one serving	1st Day	2nd	3rd	4th
MILK (milk & cheese)	8 oz (1 cup) milk 1½ oz Cheddar cheese 1½ slices American cheese 1½ c cottage cheese	\	\\	\\\	\
MEAT (meat, fish, poultry, nuts, dry beans)	2-3 oz lean cooked meat, fish or poultry 2 eggs 4 T peanut butter 1 c cooked dry beans or lentils	\\	\	O	\\
FRUITS and **VEGETABLES** (including citrus fruits, dark green and deep yellow vegetables)	½ c cooked 1 medium raw ½ medium grapefruit or cantaloupe 4 oz (½c) fruit juice	\\	\	\\\	⊬⊦⊦
BREADS and **CEREALS** (enriched or whole grain)	1 slice bread ¾ c dry cereal ½ c cooked cereal, rice, noodles, macaroni	⊬⊦⊦	⊬⊦⊦ \\	\\\\	⊬⊦⊦ \

FIGURE 17–10. Part I.

FOUNDATION FOODS

Instructions: For each food item, place a chit mark (卅十) in the appropriate block

SUGGESTED DAILY AMOUNTS

5th	Average	Child	Adolescent Small Frame	Medium Frame	Large Frame	Adult	Diff.
\\	2	3–4 Serv.	2–3 Serv.	3–4 Serv.	4–5 Serv.	2 Serv.	OK
\	\+	2 or > serv. (2–3 oz each)	2 serv. (3–4 oz each)	2 serv. (4–5 oz each)	2 serv. (5–6 oz each)	2 or > serv. (3–4 oz each)	–\
O	2	4 or > serv.	4–5 serv.	5–6 serv.	6 or > serv.	4 or > serv.	–2
\\\	4	4 or > serv.	4–5 serv.	5–6 serv.	6–8 serv.	4 or > serv.	OK

FIGURE 17–10 Continued. *Part II.*

or three food groups is insufficient. For improvement, positive recommendations for increasing the amounts to the recommended levels in order to achieve an adequate diet should be made in IA, Figure 17–11. There is a wide variety of foods in each food group, and it is rare that the food likes of the patient cannot be satisfied by judicious substitution. To achieve a balanced diet, selecting a variety of foods is helpful. In fact, including a variety of foods is the best practical means of consuming a nutritious diet.

Not only should the adequacy of the total diet be improved, the nutrient balance of each meal probably needs improvement. A balanced diet is one in which a food from each of the food groups for which recommended servings are suggested is present in each meal. A balanced diet provides at one meal all the nutrients necessary for the optimal functioning of the human machine. This type of food mixture provides for the most efficient use of the nutrients. Thus the patient can complete IB of Figure 17–11.

Step 3. Allow the Patient to Delete from the Diet Plaque-Forming, Sugar-Sweetened Foods. By reexamining the sweets intake chart, the patient will note the grand total of the number of exposures to sweets, the type of sweets most often consumed, and the frequency with which they were eaten. Since the form of sweets and the frequency of their use are the two most pressing factors in caries production, it must be emphasized that there can be absolutely no compromise with respect to the deletion from the diet of sweets that tend to be retained in the mouth. The sweets the patient is honestly willing to give up should be recorded under IIA in Figure 17–11.

Step 4. Allow the Patient to Select Non-plaque–Promoting Snack Substitutes. If snacking is a habit of long standing, realize that it is futile and unrealistic to expect total immediate abandonment of between-meal nibbling. Acceptable alternatives include raw fruits, raw vegetables, Cheddar cheese, or nuts. Provision of suitable noncariogenic snack substitutes is one of the major reasons for the success of this counseling. These should be recorded in Figure 17–11. However, if the patient is consistently reminded that increasing the total food intake at each meal will satisfy appetite and hunger, it is possible that the number of between-meal snacks will eventually be reduced.

Step 5. Allow the Patient to Select Menus. Starting with the existing menu as a nucleus, encourage the patient to examine each meal and make deletions, substitutions, or additions with which he or she can comfortably live. The rule is to improve the quality, not the quantity, of the food so that acceptance will be more likely. The menu is recorded in III of Figure 17–11. For example, if the patient is accustomed to eating doughnuts and coffee sweetened with sugar, suggest as a substitute coffee sweetened with an artificial sweetener (or no sweetener at all) and muffins or toast. Do not list a five-course breakfast and expect cooperation if for years the patient has eaten only one or two food items for breakfast. Gradual improvement is a more realistic goal than drastic change. Evolution, not revolution, should be the objective of this dietary prescription.

The same procedure, suggesting gradual change, is used for lunch menus. If the patient's lunch has been a jelly sandwich and coffee, do not prescribe vegetable soup, tuna casserole, tossed salad, bread and butter, milk, and fruit. Merely suggest that, instead of jelly, tuna fish or a luncheon meat be the sandwich filler, include milk as a beverage (or perhaps coffee or tea without

1

I. EVALUATION of your diet suggests that

A. The QUALITY of your diet can be IMPROVED by including:

more milk

more fresh fruit

B. The BALANCE of your meals can be IMPROVED by including:

fruit juice at breakfast

milk at lunch

salad at dinner

2

II. DENTAL PLAQUE and the **DECAY-PRODUCING POTENTIAL** of your diet can be **DECREASED** by

A. ELIMINATING these SUGAR-CONTAINING items:

1. Jelly doughnut
2. Hard candies and cough drops

B. SUBSTITUTING the following NON-PLAQUE-PROMOTING items*

1. Toasted bread + butter
2. Nuts, cheese curls, apples, oranges

* For further suggestions refer to **Acceptable Snack List** on Page 5.

FIGURE 17–11. *Parts I and II. Diet prescription to aid in dental caries prevention and control. (A. E. Nizel, D.M.D., Tufts University School of Medicine.)*

Illustration continued on following page

3

III. A realistic eating pattern for you that improves the QUALITY and VARIETY of your diet is

<u>Breakfast</u>

or

<u>Lunch</u>

or

4

<u>Dinner</u>

Extras*

The FREQUENCY of EATING BETWEEN MEALS should be MINIMIZED and LIMITED to:

For further suggestions, see the lists on Page 5.

FIGURE 17–11 Continued. *Parts III and IV.*

5

I.   Acceptable Snacks
from the Four Food Groups

Milk Group: milk, cheese — hard or soft varieties

Meat Group: turkey, chicken, nuts of all kinds,
                         sunflower seeds

Fruit &
Vegetable Group: raw fruits like oranges, grapes,
                         grapefruit, peaches, pears
                         raw vegetables like carrots, celery,
                         cucumbers, lettuce, salad greens
                         and tomatoes
                         unsweetened fruit juices, tomato or
                         vegetable juices

Bread & Cereal   crackers, toast, pretzels
Group:

II. Snacks to Include		III. Snacks to Avoid
pizza	popcorn	candy, mints
pretzels	cheese dips	cake, cookies
corn chips	submarine	pie, pastry
corn curls	sandwiches	ice cream sundaes
cheese curls		caramel popcorn
		candy apples
		candy-coated gum

FIGURE 17–11 Continued. *Part V.*

sugar), plus some carrot strips for a final food. Let that be the first change. In the weeks that follow, a gradual build-up of quantity and variety can be attained.

The patient should also make a commitment about the frequency of snacks between meals and of what they will consist. This is recorded in Figure 17–11 under Extras. Some snacks that will help to provide a varied and interesting diet are shown in Figure 17–11, as are foods and food preparations to include and to avoid. Using these alternatives to vary the menu is the key to motivating patient cooperation.

Compare the New Diet with the Old. Encourage the patient to evaluate the adequacy of the new, self-prescribed diet, and also to note in it the number, form, and frequency of concentrated sweets and sugar-rich foods having an overtly sweet taste. The patient usually compares the new diet with the old one with a sense of satisfaction that the substitutions were so easily made. The patient is pleasantly surprised and grateful to the counselor that an easily acceptable and less cariogenic alternative diet was so easy to design.

Reinforcement by Follow-up Reevaluation. Schedule a follow-up visit for 2 weeks later. The patient is asked to complete a second 5-day food diary in the same manner first just before returning.

Evaluate the new food diary and compare the results with the original plan to note whether recommendations have been followed. Discuss misinterpretations, misunderstandings, and problems that have arisen during this period. Menu changes are recommended if necessary.

Patients' misconceptions of food composition can sometimes be surprising. For instance, a patient with high caries susceptibility mentioned that she had been constipated, and, rather than use a laxative, had been nibbling on "some natural dried fruits that do not contain refined sugar." Unfortunately, the patient had not realized that the natural sugars of dried fruits are just as cariogenic as refined sugar and sugar products. She was advised to increase her roughage and bulk with bran and cellulose foods and to eliminate the dried fruits.

Continuing reinforcement of dietary advice is just as important as continuing review of toothbrushing and flossing practices. Self-help preventive measures should be discussed at each dental visit. Repetition, clarification, and encouragement are the keys to success in long-term maintenance of the new, acceptable, less cariogenic and more nutritious diet.

CONCLUSIONS

1. The dietary guidance advocated here can improve general as well as dental health.

2. Personalized dietary counseling added to other caries-preventive measures should reduce caries recurrence significantly.

3. The daily ingestion of a balanced and varied selection of foods from the 4 food groups, avoidance of sweets that are retained next to tooth enamel, and discontinuance of between-meal snacking are the basic elements in achieving a diet that produces few caries.

4. To realize maximum patient acceptance and cooperation with the diet prescription, determine and manage the reasons for the original diet, and suit the new diet to the patient's daily routine and lifestyle.

5. The objectivity, personalization of the diet, and the time spent in counseling are rewarded both financially and by the satisfaction of performing a useful health care and preventive dentistry service.

SUMMARY GUIDELINES, DIETARY COUNSELING FOR CARIES PREVENTION AND CONTROL

Before Counseling

I. Explain to the patient the *reason* for counseling
   For example: "Usually we deal with the *effects* of dental decay by restorative procedures. We would also like to find the *cause* in order to prevent cavities rather than to *treat* them in the future; this is a complex disease

in which diet plays one of the important roles. We would like to rule out diet as a factor in your tooth decay problem."
II. Dental Health Diet Score: Below 56 indicates a need for diet counseling
III. Food Intake
Obtain a representative food intake pattern by asking the patient to keep a 5-day diary (preferably including a weekend)

The Counseling Visit

IV. Reasons for the Diet
To develop rapport with the patient, ask him or her to describe a typical days activities
   A. This description provides clues to the *reasons* for *food selection*
   B. The description makes possible *personalization of the diet*, which will *maximize patient cooperation*
V. Education about the role of diet in the development and prevention of dental caries
   A. Caries: explain the interaction of teeth, plaque, and sugar

$$\text{Plaque bacteria} + \text{sugar} = \text{acid}$$
$$\text{Tooth} + \text{acid} = \text{decay}$$

   B. Ask patient, "Which is easiest for you to control—sugar, teeth, or bacteria?"
VI. Cariogenic potential of the diet (if applicable)
   A. Have the patient circle in red all foods listed in the food diary, that are sweetened with sugar
   B. Stress the difference in cariogenic potential between retained and nonretained sweets
   C. Explain the importance of *frequency* of eating as an important factor in cariogenicity
      1. State that the reaction of bacterial enzymes (in the plaque) on sugar is to change it to acid within 20 *SECONDS*. The acid continues to form for about 20 *MINUTES*
      2. Multiply: number of sugar exposures multiplied by 20 minutes equals total minutes of acid production (convert to hours)
         a. When the sugar is eaten (with or between meals)
         b. Form (solid or liquid)
VII. Adequacy of diet listed in food dairy
   A. Explain the importance of an adequate diet
   B. Have patient transpose individual combinations of foods and dishes into appropriate food groups
   C. Determine the adequacy of the diet by comparing the patient's intake with the amounts recommended (place OK or minus in the Difference column; the patient can see the several causes of tooth decay and inadequacies of his or her diet)
VIII. Diagnosis of the problem
Determine with patient any possible nutritional or dietary implication in the oral problem

IX. Diet prescription
  A. Allow the patient to write his or her own diet prescription for
    1. Diet quality
    2. Nutrient balance
    3. Cariogenic potential
X. Compare new and old diets
  A. Compare the total exposure of sweets in the two diets
  B. Compare the adequacy of new and old diets
XI. Summary
  Allow the patient to summarize the decisions for changes and the reasons for them
XII. Follow-up
  Two or 3 weeks later, ask patient to complete a new 5-day food diary; compare it with the original; clarify misunderstandings

REFERENCES

1. Burt, B. A. What recommendations should dentists make to their patients regarding the effect of diet and nutrition on their oral health? What kind of diet and consumption patterns promote better oral health and what kinds are less consistent with good oral health? In Jukush, J., ed. Diet, Nutrition and Oral Health: A Rational Approach for the Dental Practice. J. Am. Dent. Assoc. 109:21, 1984.
2. Jensen, M. E. What factors, such as retention or clearance, are important in the cariogenic potential of food? Are some foods anticariogenic? Which ones? Should food product labeling include information about the cariogenicity of the food? In Jukush, J., ed. Diet, Nutrition and Oral Health: A Rational Approach for the Dental Practice. J. Am. Dent. Assoc. 109:30, 1984.
3. Ismail, A. J.; Burt, B. A.; Elkund, S. A. The cariogenicity of soft drinks in the United States. J. Am. Dent. Assoc. 109:241, 1984.
4. Bibby, B. G.; Mundorg, S. A.; Ziro, D. T., et al. Oral food clearance and the pH of plaque and saliva. J. Am. Dent. Assoc. 112:233, 1986.
5. Shaw, J. H. Causes and control of dental caries. N. Engl. J. Med. 317:996, 1987.
6. Schachtele, C. F.; Harlander, S. K. Will the diets of the future be less cariogenic? J. Can. Dent. Assoc. 50:213, 1984.
7. Edgar, W. M.; Bowen, W. H., et al. Effects of different eating patterns on dental caries in the rat. Caries Res. 16:384, 1982.
8. Schachtele, C. F.; Jensen, M. E.; Harlander, S. K., et al. Placement of dairy products in a food ranking system, based on changes in human dental plaque pH. J. Dairy Sci. 66(Suppl.):65, 1983.
9. Palmer, C.; Rounds, M. Nutrition counseling. In Clinical Preventive Dentistry. Student Manual. Boston, Mass., Tufts University School of Dental Medicine, 1986.
10. Rogers, C. Client-Centered Therapy. Cambridge, Mass., The Riverside Press, 1965.
11. Garn, R. The Magic Power of Emotional Appeal, p. 49. New York, Prentice-Hall, 1960.
12. Cassidy, R. J. Psychological factors in preventive denistry. Ala. J. Med. Sci. 3:358, 1968.

18

The Role of Nutrition in Prevention and Management of Periodontal Disease

It is generally acknowledged that gingivitis and periodontitis are the result of an accumulation of supra- and subgingival plaque or calculus or both. However, the extent and the intensity of the gingival inflammatory process are directly affected by both the number and the virulence of dental plaque bacteria around the supra- and subgingival margins of the teeth; it is indirectly affected systemically by the relative innate resistance of the periodontal tissues to infection. The dental health professional therefore has a responsibility not only to remove the local gingival plaque and calculus irritants by scaling, polishing, root planing, and curettage accompanied by a meticulous daily home plaque control program (e.g., thorough toothbrushing and flossing) but also to help the patient increase the systemic resistance of the periodontal tissues by nutrition counseling.[1-3] The latter process includes evaluating the diet, determining the reasons for food selection, and prescribing a diet that uses an adequate, well-balanced food intake as a foundation. The objectives of this chapter therefore are twofold: (1) to update the clinician on the current scientific knowledge concerning nutrition–periodontal health interrelationships; and (2) to provide a practical method for implementing this information by using an orderly, easily understood nutrition counseling service that will appeal to the patient.

FACTS ABOUT NUTRITION–PERIODONTAL HEALTH INTERRELATIONSHIPS

Food and nutrition can affect periodontal disease at three levels by[4, 5]
1. Contributing to microbial growth in the gingival crevice
2. Affecting the immunological response to bacterial antigens
3. Assisting in the repair of connective tissue at the local site after injury from plaque, calculus, and so forth

The microbial growth in the gingival crevice is enhanced by the degradation of retained food in and around the teeth.[6] It is possible that these bacteria produce lytic enzymes that contribute to the breakdown of the periodontal structures.

During a state of protein malnutrition, for example, activity of phagocytes (cells that ingest bacteria) in the patient's immune system may be impaired and other immune responses may be defective.[7] Thus adequate protein nutrition is important for reducing the severity of periodontal disease infections.

The repair and defense mechanisms of the patient may be jeopardized not only by marginal nutritional deficiencies in protein but also by deficiencies in vitamins such as ascorbic acid,[8] folic acid,[9] and vitamin A[10] or in minerals such as iron,[11] zinc,[12] and calcium (see Chaps. 9 and 10).[13] Nutritional deficiencies can thus contribute to periodontal disease by interfering with the (1) integrity of the gingival epithelial barrier, (2) tissue repair processes, and (3) resistance mechanisms of the body.

Nutrition and the Epithelial Barrier

The rapid rate of the turnover (i.e., short life span) of the epithelial cells of the gingival sulcus indicates the need for continuous synthesis of DNA, RNA, and tissue protein. This means that the sulcular epithelium (surface tissue) has a high requirement for such nutrients as folic acid and protein, which are involved in cell formation. Further, if malnutrition does occur, the gingival sulcular tissue may be among the first to be affected adversely.

To maintain the integrity of this epithelium, vitamin A is also needed. At the base of the sulcular epithelium is a narrow basement membrane made up of collagen. This basement membrane acts as a barrier against the entrance of toxic materials into the underlying connective tissue.[2] Since collagen is the major biochemical component of the basement membrane, adequate amounts of ascorbic acid, iron, and zinc are important for collagen synthesis and ultimately for wound healing.

Nutrition and the Repair Process

Protein and ascorbic acid are intimately involved in connective tissue formation and zinc hastens the repair process. Zinc seems to have the property of accelerating wound healing, which may be due to its anti-infective action. Since epithelial tissue contains about 20% of the body's zinc and since zinc is involved in the healing process, it follows that an adequate intake of foods that are good zinc sources could be helpful.

Calcium and phosphorus are important nutrients for promoting the density of the alveolar bone, which surrounds the roots of the teeth. There is, however, no proof that a calcium deficiency causes periodontal disease. It has *not* been shown that the two major signs of periodontal disease—decrease in alveolar bone height and the migration of the epithelium of the gingival crevice—are produced by a low calcium, high phosphorus ratio (see Chap. 10). Therefore if calcium supplements are supplied, it should be with the intent of overcoming the possible osteoporosis of the edentulous alveolar bone, particularly in postmenopausal women, rather than that of the periodontal disease status.

Nutrition and Immune Mechanisms

Protein deficiencies impair the body's immune mechanisms; they interfere with antibody formation, activity of the cells that ingest bacteria, and nonspecific resistance factors. Protein-deficient diets interfere with the body's formation of immunoglobulins that act as antibodies to infectious agents or their toxins.[14] Consequently, infection will not be readily controllable unless the diet contains an adequate amount of protein.

In summary, to maximize periodontal health, one must eat a diet that is varied, adequate, and balanced, including foods rich in protein from animal (meat, fish, poultry, hard cheese) or vegetable (nuts, beans, soybeans) sources. In addition, good food sources of vitamin A (carrots, squash, greens, cantaloupe) and vitamin C (oranges, spinach, broccoli, peppers) and folacin (asparagus, broccoli, liver, salmon) are some of the specific foods recommended for patients with periodontal disease. Finally, good sources of the minerals calcium (milk, cheese, greens and soybeans), iron (beef, liver, peas, beans, lentils), and zinc (red meats and shellfish) should be included in these patients' diets.

Effects of Food Textures on Periodontal Health

Ever since a critical review of the literature in 1947[15] on the effect of the physical consistency, or textures, of food on periodontal health, it has been assumed that firm, fibrous foods may be beneficial to periodontal health and that eating soft, sticky foods might tend to have an adverse effect. These basic tenets still seem to have some validity, but perhaps for different reasons from those originally suggested.

The evidence seems to deny that chewing fibrous foods exerts a natural cleansing action, particularly with respect to the removal of the plaque from the gingival half of the tooth.

Sreebny believed that the major functions of chewing fibrous foods are "to increase the salivary flow [volume] and the total protein and amylase activity of stimulated saliva." The oral clearance of food debris is evidently enhanced by the increased volume of saliva that occurs when chewing firm foods as opposed to soft, sticky foods.[16] In conclusion, it seems that oral food retention, not plaque, may be lessened by chewing on fibrous foods.

Also, it has never been demonstrated that firm foods promote gingival keratinization. However, chewing foods of firm physical consistency may promote the formation of a fibrous structure in the periodontal ligament that may help stabilize the teeth.

Another important positive effect of including fibrous foods in the diet is that these foods can replace empty-calorie, sugar-rich sweets that are retained in the mouth and that may provide the substrate for increased formation of supragingival bacterial plaque.

The following conclusions can be drawn from the currently available evidence about the local effects of the physical consistency of food on periodontal health:

- Fibrous foods do not remove plaque at the gingival level of the tooth.
- Chewing on fibrous or firm foods stimulates salivary flow and can therefore aid in the oral clearance of food debris.
- Chewing fibrous or firm foods does not increase gingival keratinization, but it does produce a type of local exercise that can stimulate and strengthen the periodontal ligament and perhaps may also increase the density of alveolar bone adjacent to the roots.

DIETARY MANAGEMENT OF ACUTE NECROTIZING ULCERATIVE GINGIVITIS (ANUG)

Acute necrotizing ulcerative gingivitis (Vincent's infection) is an acute bacterial infection of the gingiva that is usually initiated locally as a result of poor oral hygiene and/or third-molar periocoronitis superimposed on a generalized lowered systemic resistance to infection.

History

The general complaints associated with ANUG are a very sore mouth, with easily bleeding and extremely painful gums, a bad taste, and bad breath accompanied by a generalized malaise and fever. As a rule, food intake is minimal because of poor appetite and inability to bite or chew. Usually, the diet is grossly inadequate and consists of empty-calorie, sugar-rich foods such as soft drinks, cakes, pastries, and candy.

A history of the patient's general and oral hygiene habits, daily routine, socioeconomic status, and food likes and dislikes is necessary to understand the reasons for food choices and dietary practices. This history shows the reason for the diet and serves as a guide for recommending a personalized diet that the patient will be able to realistically follow.

Dietary Screening

A simple initial method of screening the adequacy of the diet is to use the Dental Health Diet Score (see Figs. 17–1 to 17–5). It separates the desirable high-nutrient density foods from the empty-calorie soft foods. Any patient scoring less than 64 on the Food Group Score should have nutrition counseling. If the Sweet Score is 15 or more the dentist should recommend healthier alternatives from the dietary frequency chart (Fig. 17–6). Figure 18–1 may also be used to evaluate undesirable foods in the diet for periodontal health.

Dietary Prescription

The dietary prescription should include (1) a daily food pattern; (2) meal plan; and (3) suggested menus.

DAILY FOOD PATTERN (QUALITATIVE AND QUANTITATIVE CONSIDERATIONS)

In order to ingest the minimal recommended intake of the nutrient-rich four food groups, 4 servings of fruits and vegetables, 4 servings of breads and cereals, 3 servings of milk, and 2 servings of animal or vegetable protein—foods that are good sources of protein, calcium, vitamins A and C, folacin, iron, and zinc—should be stressed. Examples of the foods rich in these nutrients can be found in Table 18–1.

Evaluation of Nonfibrous, Soft, and Empty-Calorie Foods

Classify the circled foods in Figure 17–2 into nonfibrous and empty–calorie foods. Place a checkmark in the frequency column for each time one of the foods was eaten. Add the number of checkmarks. If it is a soft food, multiply by 6; if an empty-calorie food, multiply by 3. Write the products in the point column and total.

Example:

	Types	*Frequency*	*Points*
9 A.M. cream cheese on soft bread coffee with sugar	NONFIBROUS cream cheese, soft bread	√√ × 6	12
3 P.M. 8-oz soft drink 6 P.M. 8-oz can of beer	EMPTY-CALORIE coffee with sugar, soft drink, beer	√√√ × 3	9

Types	*Frequency*	*Points*
FOODS OF SOFT CONSISTENCY THAT ARE ALSO AVAILABLE IN FIRM OR FIBROUS FORM soft bread without crusts, cooked cereals, cream cheese, cooked or canned fruits or vegetables, ground meat, salmon, tuna and peanut butter	× 6	
EMPTY-CALORIE FOODS (LOW-NUTRIENT DENSITY), ALCOHOLIC BEVERAGES, SUGAR-RICH SWEETS, SATURATED FATS Beer, wine, liquor Bacon, butter, lard, sausage, cream cheese Apricots, candies, cakes, chocolates, cookies, cough drops, figs, fruit in syrup, honey, ice cream, jams, jellies, mints, pies, prunes, raisins, sherbet, sugar-sweetened beverages and yogurt	× 3	

Add the points. The total is the amount of undesirable food types you ate during a typical day.   Total _____

FIGURE 18–1. *Undesirable foods for maintaining periodontal health.*

TABLE 18–1. Foods That Are Good Sources of Nutrients

Nutrient	Sources
Protein	
Animal	Meat (beef, lamb, pork, organ meats, veal)
	Luncheon or canned meats
	Poultry (chicken, turkey, duck)
	Fish or shellfish
	Eggs
	Cheese, milk
Vegetable	Nuts, peanuts, peanut butter
	Dried split green peas
	Pea beans, pinto beans, red beans
	Soybeans, tofu
Mixed Protein Dishes with Starch	Pot pies, pizza, spaghetti with meat
Calcium	Milk, yogurt, buttermilk, skim milk
	Cheese, cheese dishes
	Collard leaves, broccoli, kale, greens, okra
	Bokchoy, soybeans
Vitamin A	Carrots, yellow squash, sweet potatoes
	Kale, greens, spinach
	Apricots, cantaloupe, papaya
Vitamin C	Orange, grapefruit, tomato
	Strawberries, cantaloupe
	Cabbage, spinach
	Broccoli, greens, kale
	Kohlrabi, mung bean sprouts
	Green or red pepper
Folacin	Asparagus, broccoli, spinach
	Peanuts, pecans, soybeans
	Cod, haddock, tuna, salmon
Iron	Beef, liver, heart, kidney, pork
	Eggs, poultry, fish
	Beans, peas, lentils, soybeans, peanuts
Zinc	Red meats (beef, organ meats)
	Shellfish (oysters, lobster, shrimp)

FREQUENCY OF MEALS

The patient should fulfill the daily food intake requirements by eating six to eight small meals instead of the usual three. Only one or two foods need to be eaten at each meal, but a large enough variety of foods should be selected so that the eating experience will be pleasant and will satisfy the recommended daily allowance of each food group, which, as previously stated, is 4 servings of vegetable-fruit, 4 of bread-cereal, 3 of milk-cheese, and 2 of meat, poultry, fish, or beans.

MENU PLAN (TEXTURAL CONSIDERATIONS)

Menus should be planned so that the general consistency of the diet is liquid or soft. Spicy or sharp-tasting foods are omitted during the acute period. Foods should be chosen to suit the patient's individual taste and food budget. For variety, some of the following food exchanges in each food group are suggested:

Vegetable-Fruit Group. Fruits and vegetables puréed and liquified by a blender may be used. Strained fruits may be used with milk as a drink, and strained vegetables may be cooked with milk, butter, and other seasonings as soup.

Bread-Cereal Group. Strained gruels (thin, boiled cereals).

Milk-Cheese Group. Milk in all forms may be used. For extra nourishment, nonfat milk solids may be added to regular milk. Add 2 tbsp of milk solids to each 8 oz glass of whole milk. Soft, plain ice cream is also soothing. Milk shakes and malted milks are recommended. Cream may be added to milk if desired.

Meat, Poultry, Fish, and Bean Group. Eggs in the form of eggnog or baked custard may be eaten. Chicken soup, pea soup, meat broth, or fish chowder is recommended.

The following are sample menus for a liquified diet using these suggested foods:

Breakfast: Pineapple-grapefruit juice, strained oatmeal gruel, coffee, with cream and sugar if desired
Midmorning: Orange eggnog
Noon: Strained cream of tomato soup, custard with cream, tea or coffee
Midafternoon: Chocolate milk shake
Evening: Strained pea soup, spanish cream (or any custard pudding)
Bedtime: Cocoa

The obvious purpose of this diet is to satisfy the recommended dietary allowances for all nutrients in a form that requires no chewing. It is to be hoped that this type of diet need be used for only a day or so. The patient should then change to a soft diet consisting of a balanced and varied selection of the following foods:

Vegetable-Fruit Group. Cooked or canned fruits and ripe bananas; vegetables without skins or seeds, mashed potatoes

Bread-Cereal Group. Soft bread, macaroni, noodles, rice, spaghetti, cooked breakfast cereals with milk, and ready-to-eat flaked and puffed cereals, such as wheat or corn flakes or puffed wheat or puffed rice

Milk-Cheese Group. Soft cheese such as cottage cheese in addition to milk and ice cream

Meat, Poultry, Fish, and Bean Group. Tender or ground meats, chicken, fish without bones, and cooked legumes

Even without being specifically told, the patient will gradually change to foods of regular texture as the soreness of the mouth lessens. The important point is that a diet can be adequate if sufficient servings of liquid or soft foods or both from the four food groups are eaten each day.

Vitamin Supplementation

Because nutrient requirements are increased during periods of physiological stress and the mouth is sore, the patient has not been able to chew fruits and vegetables and instead has probably used empty-calorie foods and beverages— cakes, pastries, and soft drinks—to meet calorie needs. Vitamin supplementation, in addition to a nutritious soft or liquid diet during the acute phases of necrotizing gingivitis, is indicated.

The type of multivitamin preparation most often indicated is a combination of the B complex vitamins and vitamin C. The B complex vitamins in most commercial preparations usually include thiamin, riboflavin, niacin, folic acid, pyroxidine, and calcium pantothenate. The therapeutically effective dosage that is recommended is three to five times the recommended dietary allowance. Remember that the recommended dietary allowance for riboflavin or thiamin under normal circumstances is about 2 mg and that a multivitamin preparation should be considered therapeutic if it contains 6 to 10 mg of each of these listed vitamins, plus the other water-soluble vitamins in corresponding therapeutic doses. Two such vitamin capsules twice a day, once before breakfast and one before the evening meal for the first week tapered off to one a day for the next 2 weeks should be all that are usually necessary. In fact, as soon as adequate amounts of foods from the four food groups can be ingested, vitamin supplementation is unnecessary.

NUTRITION COUNSELING FOR A PATIENT WITH CHRONIC PERIODONTAL DISEASE

Based on our recent knowledge of nutrition-periodontal health relationships discussed in earlier sections, it is clear that maintenance of periodontal health may be helped in part by sound nutritional advice, especially for those who have poor food selection and eating habits.

The following is a step-by-step office procedure for giving personalized nutritional guidance to a patient with chronic periodontitis.

Step 1: Ascertain the Dental Health Diet Score and If Necessary, Demonstrate the Method for Keeping a Food Intake Diary

As a means of justifying the need for nutrition counseling and stimulating a patient's interest in improving his or her diet, the Dental Health Diet Score (Figs. 17–1 to 17–5) is most helpful as a preliminary, rapid procedure to determine whether the patient's current diet is satisfactory (64 or above). If the patient scores below 64, a detailed nutritional assessment and nutrition counseling service should be provided.

The patient should be asked to list the customary food intake for 5 consecutive days, including a weekend. Every meal and between-meal snack should be recorded. The amounts and preparation of the foods and the order in which they are eaten should be detailed (see Fig. 17–6).

It is advisable for the dentist or dental hygienist to demonstrate how the diary should be kept by recording as an example the patient's previous 24-hour food intake.

Step 2: Explain the Nutrition-Periodontal Relationship

In order for the patient to understand the reason for this nutritional guidance service, an explanation of the role of proper foods and diet in the promotion of periodontal health should be given. Patients tend to be more cooperative if the nature of the problem and the rationale for making some improvement in their dietary pattern are explained. The conversation might proceed as follows:

"Because your 24-hour dental health nutrition score was less than desirable, we will analyze your 5-day food intake to see if it is adequate in foods that are good sources of the nutrients that we know can help fight infection and strengthen your periodontal tissues.

"The major factors responsible for initiating your gum problem are local irritants, particularly dental plaque and calculus. Dental plaque is an accumulation of bacteria and other cells that adhere to each other and produce a film over the surface of the teeth. Dental plaque is not a food residue. When the minerals from the saliva mix with the plaque, calculus, or tartar, is formed. In turn it causes gum irritation and infection.

"If you eat less sugar-rich foods, or better still try to avoid them, your diet will tend to be richer in the more desirable nutritious foods.

"In order to decrease the possibility of inflammation, we not only should eliminate the gum irritants, we also should strengthen the tooth supporting tissues from a nutritional standpoint to make them resistant to infection. This can be done by eating recommended amounts of the nutrients essential for optimal periodontal health. For example, the outer 'skin' of the gum may be made more resistant to infection by adequate amounts of *vitamin A*; the latter is found in deep green and yellow vegetables. The connective tissue ligament that joins the tooth to the bone can be strengthened by the *vitamin C* found in oranges, grapefruit, and other citrus fruits. Strong bones require adequate amounts of *calcium, phosphorus, and vitamin D* found in milk and hard cheeses. All of these tissues are nourished by blood; so we recommend foods rich in *iron*, such as liver, red meats, and enriched cereals. *Folacin*, a vitamin found in leafy green vegetables, contributes to new cell formation, and *zinc* found in meat and shellfish helps speed tissue repair.

"Thus we would like you to improve your diet by (1) reducing sugar intake, (2) replacing sweets and other empty-calorie foods with nutritious firm and fibrous foods that will stimulate and strengthen the periodontal tissues, and (3) selecting a well-balanced, varied, adequate diet to provide all the essential nutrients and to support overall health, in general, and the health of tooth-supporting structures, in particular."

Step 3: Assess Nutritional Status

Follow the format suggested in Figure 18–2 to obtain the information necessary for arriving at clinical nutritional diagnosis:

Chief Complaint. Record the patient's problem by a mark in the appropriate column, or if necessary write in the complaint.

Medical History. Ask if the patient has had or presently is experiencing any medical problems (listed under Medical History) that may influence food selection or assimilation.

Social and Diet Histories. In order to prescribe a diet that the patient will be able to fulfill with ease, it is necessary to ascertain his or her daily routine, food likes and dislikes, food purchases, food preparation, and eating habits. Have

Name _____ *M,S,W Age* _____

Address _____

_____ *Home Phone* _____

Occupation _____ *Business Phone* _____

Complaints

GENERAL	+	−	ORAL	+	−	OTHER
Loss of weight			Thirst			
Loss of appetite			Bleeding			
Apathy			gums			
Tiredness			Loose teeth			
Nervousness			Sore lips			
Gastrointestinal			Burning			
problems			tongue			
			Breath odor			

Medical History

PERSONAL	+	−	FAMILY	+	−	OTHER
Allergy			Diabetes			
Atherosclerosis			Coronary			
Diabetes			heart			
Hyperthyroidism			disease			
Liver disease			Hypertension			
Gallbladder disease			Osteoporosis			
Osteoporosis						
Hypertension						

Personal and Family Dental History

Social History
Daily routine
Hobbies and physical exercise

Diet History
FOOD PURCHASING

How often?	By whom?
Food List?	Influenced by price?
by advertising?	by food labels?

FIGURE 18–2. Nutritional case record for patient with periodontal disease.

FOOD PREPARATION
By whom?   How?
Eat with whom?   Where?   How many meals?
between meals?   Fast, average, slow
FOOD INTAKE   eater?
  Special diet?
  Vitamin or mineral supplements?
  Three types of favorite and least liked foods:
  Types of snack foods?
  Use of sugar, salt, and fats or oils?

Diet Evaluation
  Milk-cheese
  Protein
  Vegetable-fruit
  Bread-Cereal
  Fats-Oils

Clinical Nutritional Findings
Actual weight   Desirable Weight
Posture   Gait
Skin health
Lips   Tongue   Oral mucous membrane

PERIODONTAL HEALTH
Gingival color   Tone   Consistency
Plaque index   Gingival bleeding index Periodontal index
Tooth mobility
X-ray findings

Laboratory Tests
  Benedict's fasting blood sugar, hemoglobin, hematocrit
  Serum albumin, serum folate, serum carotenoid, plasma ascorbic acid, serum
    alkaline phosphatase

Diagnosis
DENTAL
Possible medical and/or nutritional conditioning factors
Dietary excesses
Dietary deficiencies

Management of Nutritional Problem
Diet prescription
Recommended behavioral changes

FIGURE 18–2 Continued

FOOD GROUP	PORTION SIZE CONSIDERED ONE SERVING	PHYSICAL CONSISTENCY	DAY 1	DAY 2	DAY 3	AVERAGE	RECOMMENDED MINIMUMS			DIFFERENCE
							13-19 yr.	20-60 yr.	60+ yr.	
	Vitamin C-Rich 4-6 oz citrus juice ½ grapefruit, cantaloupe 1 medium orange	whole or raw juice or cooked					1-2	1	1-2	
VEGETABLE-FRUIT	*Vitamin A-Rich* ½ c carrots, broccoli, spinach, corn and other deep green & yellow types	whole or raw juice or cooked					2	2	1	
	Other ½ c potatoes, peas, string beans 1 medium apple	raw cooked					1	1	1	
BREAD-CEREAL	1 sl bread 1 oz (¾ c) dry cereal ½-¾ c cooked cereal, pasta	firm soft					4	3-4	2-3	
MILK-CHEESE	1 c (8 oz) milk, yogurt 1-1½ oz Cheddar, processed cheese 1-1½ c cottage cheese						3	2	2	
MEAT, POULTRY, FISH, AND BEANS	2-3 oz cooked lean meat, fish, poultry 2 eggs 4 T peanut butter 1 c cooked dried peas, beans or lentils	whole or firm ground or soft					2	2	2	

FIGURE 18-3. Food intake evaluation. A method for assessing the adequacy and physical consistency of a diet (especially for patients with periodontal disease). Instructions: For each serving of food eaten, place a checkmark (√) in the appropriate block.

the patient begin by describing a typical day's routine from the time of arising in the morning until retirement at night. This information will provide an insight into the patient's eating pattern and will help suggest a diet modification that can be tailored to the patient's lifestyle.

Diet Evaluation: Adequacy and Physical Consistency. A Food Intake Evaluation Chart (Fig. 18–3), in which all foods are classified into the four food groups, is used to determine the adequacy and physical consistency of the diet. Credit each serving of the uncircled foods in the appropriate food group block by the use of one checkmark. Add the number of servings for each group and divide the total by three; record the average daily intake in the Average column. Subtract the actual average daily intake from the recommended daily intake. If the difference is equal to or more than the recommended intake, write OK in the Difference column. If the difference is less than the amount recommended, record it as a minus quantity (-1, -2, and so forth). Summarize this information under Diet Evaluation (Fig. 18–2).

Use the Dietary Frequency Chart to ascertain how often (frequently, sometimes, or never) the patient ingests food sources rich in the nutrients that are especially helpful in relieving periodontal disease (Fig. 18–4).

Examine for Clinical Signs of Malnutrition. Observe whether there are any clinical or oral manifestations of malnutrition, such as pallor, dry skin, overweight, underweight, skin petechiae (tiny hemorrhages), cheilosis, or glossitis. Record the findings in Figure 18–2 under Clinical Nutritional Findings.

Diagnosis. From the complaints, medical and dietary histories, and clinical findings, a nutritional diagnosis that includes the primary and secondary nutritional factors can be made.

Step 4: Prescribe a Diet

GENERAL CONSIDERATIONS

1. Systemic Factors. On the basis of the history, particularly the medical history, one should be able to determine the possibility of any systemic factor that might interfere with nutrient use. If a systemic problem is suspected, refer the patient to his or her physician for a more detailed examination and medical advice.

2. Reasons for Food Habits. When prescribing a diet, keep in mind the behavioral factors or environmental cues and stimuli (why, when, where, with whom) that determine food habits and eating patterns. If the diet takes these factors into account, it will be individualized, ensuring a more cooperative patient and a better chance for a successful outcome. In short, radical dietary changes should be avoided initially. Modifications that the patient is willing to make can contribute to a successful improvement of the diet.

3. Patient's Prescription. The specific diet prescription should be completed by the patient (Fig. 18–5, p. 3) with the guidance of the nutrition counselor, as has been done in the figure. In a sense, this represents an agreement that the prescribed diet can be followed.

Text continued on page 329

	F	S	N
Protein Sources			
ANIMAL			
Meat (beef, lamb, pork, organ meats, veal)			
Luncheon or canned meats			
Poultry (chicken, turkey, duck)			
Fish or shellfish			
Eggs			
Cheese, milk			
VEGETABLE			
Nuts, peanuts, peanut butter			
Dried split peas (green)			
Pea beans, pinto beans, red beans			
Soybeans, tofu			
PROTEIN DISHES MIXED WITH STARCH			
Pot pies, pizza, spaghetti with meat			
Calcium Sources			
Milk, yogurt, buttermilk, skim milk			
Cheese, cheese dishes			
Collard leaves, broccoli, kale, greens, okra			
Bokchoy, soybeans			
Vitamin A Sources			
Carrots, yellow squash, sweet potatoes			
Kale, greens, spinach			
Apricots, cantaloupe, papaya			
Vitamin C Sources			
Orange, grapefruit, tomato			
Strawberries, cantaloupe			
Cabbage, spinach			
Broccoli, greens, kale			
Kohlrabi, mung bean sprouts			
Green or red pepper			
Folacin Sources			
Asparagus, broccoli, spinach			
Peanuts, pecans, soybeans			
Cod, haddock, tuna, salmon			
Iron Sources			
Beef, liver, heart, kidney, pork			
Eggs, poultry, fish			
Beans, peas, lentils, soybeans, peanuts			
Zinc Sources			
Red meats (beef, organ meats)			
Shellfish (oysters, lobster, shrimp)			

FIGURE 18–4. Dietary Frequency Chart. Key: F = frequently or daily; S = sometimes (once or twice a week); N = never.

A. To IMPROVE the QUALITY of your diet include:

more vegetables and fruit

B. To IMPROVE the BALANCE of your meals include:

_____ *fruit* _____ at breakfast

_____ *milk* _____ at lunch

_____ *salad* _____ at dinner

C. To INCREASE the RESISTANCE of your PERIODONTAL
    TISSUES emphasize the following foods rich in:
    (Put a line through those you dislike)

PROTEIN	IRON	VITAMIN A	VITAMIN C
meat, fish	~~organ meats~~	carrots, winter	oranges,
poultry	lean meat	squash, sweet	grapefruit,
eggs, ~~dried~~	~~shell fish~~	potato, apricots	tomatoes,
~~peas,~~ dried	egg yolk	peaches,	strawberries,
beans	whole grain	~~spinach,~~	~~broccoli~~
	or enriched	asparagus,	green peppers
CALCIUM	breads & cereals	~~broccoli~~	orange juice
milk	green leafy		grapefruit juice
cheese	vegetables		

FIGURE 18–5. Part I. Diet prescription for promotion of periodontal health.

Illustration continued on following page

D. ELIMINATE these PLAQUE-FORMING SWEETS and other SOFT and STICKY foods:

jelly sandwiches cookies)

E. SUBSTITUTE these NON-PLAQUE PROMOTING Foods:

Raw fruits and vegetables	Firm foods	Liquids
oranges	steak	water
grapefruit	chops	milk
cantaloupe	toast	fruit juice

FIGURE 18–5 Continued. *Part II.*

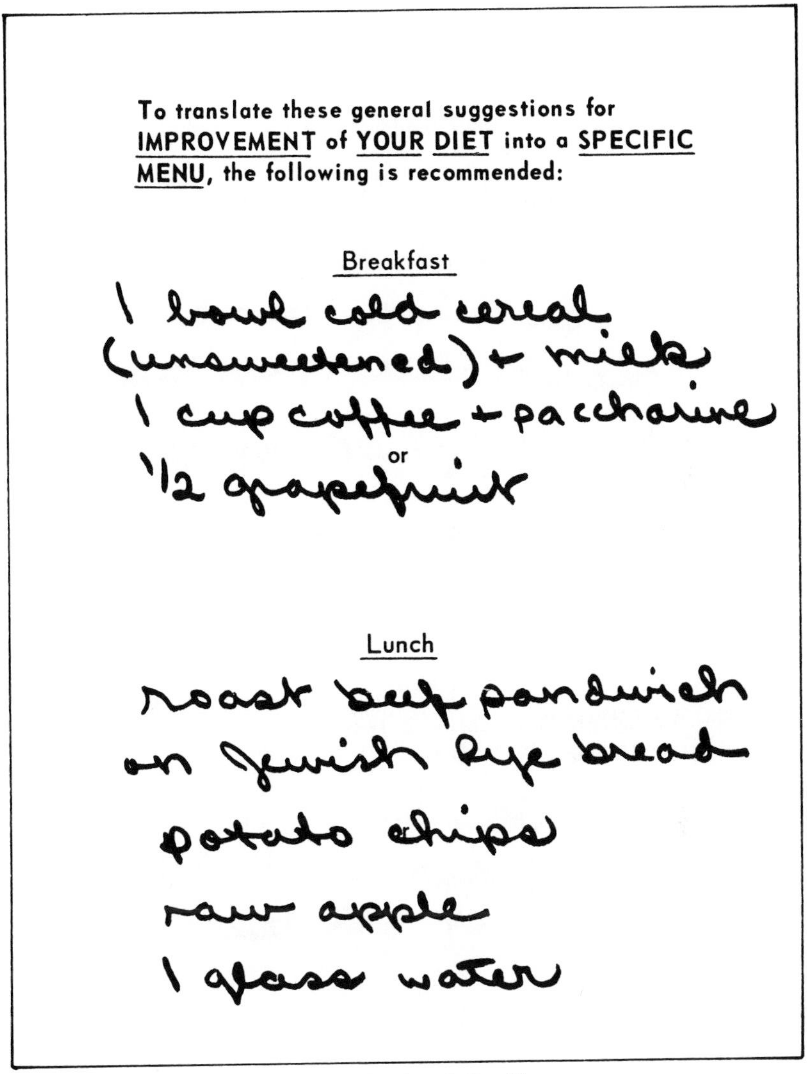

To translate these general suggestions for
IMPROVEMENT of **YOUR** **DIET** into a **SPECIFIC**
MENU, the following is recommended:

Breakfast

1 bowl cold cereal
(unsweetened) + milk
1 cup coffee + saccharine
or
1/2 grapefruit

Lunch

roast beef sandwich
on Jewish rye bread
potato chips
raw apple
1 glass water

FIGURE 18–5 Continued. *Part III.*

Illustration continued on following page

Dinner

2 pork chops
1 baked potato
1 serving peas
hard roll with butter
or
fresh fruit compote
1 cup tea + saccharine

Extras

The **FREQUENCY** of eating between meals should be **MINIMIZED** and **LIMITED** to:

milk
cheddar cheese + crackers
carrot stick

FIGURE 18–5 Continued. Part IV.

A VARIETY of Foods
to INCLUDE and AVOID
for maintaining
Optimal Gingival and Periodontal Health

MEAL	INCLUDE	AVOID	
		Sugar containing Foods	Soft or Mushy Foods
Breakfast			
Fruit	FRUIT or JUICE (FRESH, FROZEN, or CANNED, UNSWEETENED ORANGE OR GRAPEFRUIT)	fruits dried or sweetened with sugar syrup, fruit drinks, applesauce	banana
Eggs	ANY STYLE	—	—
Bread whole grain or enriched	ENGLISH MUFFIN, HARD ROLL, TOAST	Sweet roll, jam, jelly, preserves, syrup	soft bread or rolls
or			
Cereal	DRY FLAKES, SHREDDED, PUFFED	sugar coated or sugar added	cooked or gruel
Beverage	MILK, COFFEE, or TEA	syrup or sugar added	

FIGURE 18–5 Continued. *Part V.*

Illustration continued on following page

Lunch			
Sandwich (whole grain or enriched bread)	MEAT, FISH, OR POULTRY, HARD CHEESE, LUNCHEON MEATS, AND EGG FILLING	raisin or cinnamon bread, jam, jelly, or honey fillings	soft bread, peanut butter, cheese spreads
Dessert	FRESH FRUIT, CHEDDAR CHEESE AND CRACKERS, OR JELLO	cakes, cookies, pastry pie, pudding	applesauce, pureed fruits
Beverage	COFFEE, TEA, MILK, JUICE, DIETETIC SOFT DRINKS	soda pop, sugar added to drinks, sodas, frappes	—
Dinner			
Soup	FRESH OR CANNED	added sugar	—
Meat	ANY CHEWY MEAT, FISH, OR POULTRY	glazes or sugar sauces	soft, ground, boiled, casseroles, sauces, gravies
Vegetables	RAW or LIGHTLY COOKED, DARK GREEN or DEEP YELLOW also POTATO,	candied carrots, Harvard beets, and candied sweet potato	soft cooked like squash or turnip mashed potato, white sauces, and
Bread	HARD ROLL		creamed vegetables
Salad	ANY COMBINATION OF FRUITS AND VEGETABLES	raisins and sugar in dressings	—
Dessert	FRESH FRUIT, CHEESE AND CRACKERS	cakes, cookies, pies, pastry	pureed fruits, et. applesauce; cheese spreads
Beverage	COFFEE, TEA, MILK, JUICE, DIETETIC SODA	soda pop, sugar added to drinks	—

FIGURE 18–5 Continued. *Part VI.*

A SAMPLE MENU PLAN

Breakfast	1/2 grapefruit
	Whole wheat cereal with milk
	Coffee (milk and saccharine)
Lunch	Roast beef sandwich
	on hard roll
	Sour pickles Potato chips
	Milk Fresh apple
Dinner	Pork chops
	Baked potato Peas
	Tossed salad
	Hard roll with butter
	Fresh fruit compote
	Coffee (milk and saccharine)
Bedtime	Cheddar cheese and crackers

FIGURE 18–5 Continued. *Part VII.*

PROCEDURE

1. Improve Adequacy of Diet. The patient should be able to readily ascertain the food groups that have been shown to be deficient from the Diet Evaluation. The number of foods in each food group should be increased to at least the recommended amounts. (The two food groups most often deficient are the milk and the vegetable-fruit groups.)

The patient records the food groups that must be added to the daily intake in order to improve the quality of the diet, then the types and amounts of foods from each of the 4 food groups for each of the three meals should be decided.

2. Emphasize Foods That Are Particularly Beneficial to Periodontal Tissues. Because the function of the periodontium is unique, certain nutrients—protein, vitamin C, vitamin A, folic acid, calcium, iron, and zinc—need to be emphasized in order to increase the resistance of the periodontal tissue to infection and to speed its repair.

The patient is asked to cross out those foods under each nutrient category that are disliked. The remaining foods are emphasized and recommended.

3. Encourage the Elimination of Plaque-Forming Sweets and the Substitution of Fibrous Foods. So far, nutritional guidance has dealt with the endogenous (internal or systemic) nutritional factors in periodontal health. The next step deals with the exogenous (external or local) effects of the composition (sweets) and consistency or texture (firmness and retention) of food on the gingiva.

Instead of sweets, any raw fruit or vegetable can be suggested. Fruits include: raw apples, cherries, grapefruit, grapes, melons, oranges, pears, pineapple, and tangerines. If possible, raw vegetables—carrots, cauliflower, celery, cucumbers, tossed salads, and cole slaw—should be consumed in liberal amounts during the last part of the meal. Raw vegetables such as carrot or celery strips can be used as snacks between meals.

4. Allow the Patient to Prescribe Meals. Meal planning consists of translating the food groups into various foods and combinations of foods that are appropriate for each meal. Using the patient's usual diet pattern as a point of reference, let the patient substitute foods that are liked and that will satisfy the nutritional objective, which is a varied, balanced, adequate, and low plaque-forming diet that can also provide physical stimulation to the periodontal tissues.

The patient should also remember to limit the number of between-meal snacks, particularly if toothbrushing, flossing, and oral irrigation are not possible immediately after eating.

Let the patient make a commitment as to how many between-meal snacks there will be and what they will include.

Step 5: Follow-up

Just as home care oral hygiene procedures must be constantly reinforced and checked for proficiency, so should the patient's prescribed diet be periodically reviewed.

Obviously, the best method of review is not to ask the patient, "How are you doing on your diet?," because the answer usually will be, "OK" or "Pretty good," even if it is not. To assess the success of diet counseling, ask the patient to keep a second 5-day food diary for reevaluation. Verbal histories of food consumption based on memory are never as accurate as written records.

After the patient has completed the second food diary, it can be evaluated for nutrient adequacy from a periodontal health standpoint. A comparison of the second diet evaluation with the first will show how much progress the patient has made. If there are any problems, they can be clarified at this point.

Motivate patients by repeated commendation of the good points in their diet and by describing the benefits from a good diet. But in the final analysis, the practice of good nutrition, like that of plaque control, depends on the patient's motivation and perseverance.

Conclusions in Nutrition and Periodontal Disease

Usually, the role of diet and nutrition in the management of gingival and periodontal disease is primarily that of prevention and maintenance.

The benefits from good nutrition are local oral physiotherapeutic action and systemic support, especially with respect to increasing the capacity of the periodontal tissues to (1) resist infection, (2) strengthen and maintain the epithelial barrier, and (3) promote the repair of damaged periodontal tissues.

The potential benefits are great enough that judicious use of nutritional guidance should be as much a routine periodontal preventive office procedure as instructing the patient on oral hygiene home care measures.

DIET BEFORE PERIODONTAL SURGERY

When prescribing a diet before periodontal surgery, the goal is to enable the patient to meet the stress of surgery. Furthermore, a well-nourished state is optimal for wound healing; it also increases resistance to infection and hastens convalescence and recovery.

If the periodontal surgery is elective, it may be best to delay it until the patient's nutritional status is optimal.

If the patient is malnourished, a diet high in protein (120 g/day) and enough carbohydrate and fat to provide about 2500 kcal should be prescribed for 7 to 14 days before surgery (Table 18–2). Or nutritionally complete proprietary supplements such as Sustacal or Ensure (Table 18–3) can be prescribed. Adequate amounts of carbohydrates need to be ingested for protein sparing.

A well-planned, balanced diet will supply foods rich in water-soluble vitamins. However, it may be necessary to prescribe a multivitamin capsule to be certain that adequate amounts of ascorbic acid, for example, are ingested. If the patient drinks a pint of orange juice (two 8-oz cups—equal to 200 mg of ascorbic acid) every day for at least 1 week before oral surgery, the tissues will be

TABLE 18–2. High Energy, High Protein Diet

Approximate Composition:
  2500 kcal (10.5 MJ)
  345 carbohydrate
  110 g protein
  120 g fat
  Protein is increased by addition of high caloric, high protein supplements, e.g.,
    Sustacal*
Nutrients for a 50-kg female, 23 years of age, 2 weeks postoperative:
  50 kcal (210 kJ)/kg body weight
  (approx) 2 g protein/kg body weight
  (approx) 25 nonprotein calories/g of protein

Sample Menu	
Breakfast	**Lunch**
½ c orange juice	½ c cream of asparagus soup
1 slice white toast with butter and jelly	½ c salmon with mayonnaise
1 soft-boiled egg	2 saltines, butter
tea, 2 tsp sugar	coffee ice cream
	vanilla wafers
	tea, ½ c milk, 2 tsp sugar
10:00 A.M. snack	**2:00 P.M. snack**
250 ml Sustacal*	250 ml Sustacal*
2 Uneeda biscuits, jelly	4 arrowroot biscuits
Supper	**Bedtime snack**
2 oz baked meatloaf with plain gravy	Cornflakes with 1 c milk, sliced
mashed potato	peaches, and 2 tsp sugar
baked hubbard squash with butter and brown sugar	
cottage cheese with French dressing	
fruited gelatin dessert	
Sanka, cream, 1 tsp sugar	

From Goldstein, S. Surgery, stress, burns and nutritional care. In Howard, R. B.; Herbold, N. H., eds. Nutrition in Clinical Care, p. 512. New York, McGraw-Hill Book Co., 1978.
*Reduced lactose = 6 g/12 fl oz.

TABLE 18–3. Proprietary Supplements

Brand (Major Ingredient)	Carbo-hydrate (g/l)	Protein (g/l)	Fat (g/l)	kcal/l (kJ/l) Estimate	Comments
Sustacal (liquid) (sucrose, corn syrup, soy oil, sodium and calcium caseinate, soy protein plus vitamins and minerals)	138	60	23	1000 (4200)	6 g lactose/12 fl oz 14.4 mEq Na/12 fl oz May be used as a tube feeding
Meritene (liquid) (concentrated sweet skim milk, corn syrup solids, vegetable oil, sodium caseinate, sucrose), vitamins, minerals	115	60	33	1000 (4200)	May be used as a tube-feeding formula
Eggnog (egg, milk mixture)	129	52	30	994 (4175)	Delmark brand made with whole milk
Sustagen (powder) (powdered whole milk solids, calcium caseinate, Dextrimaltose, dextrose, vitamins, iron)	300	105	15	1750 (7350)	3 c Sustagen powder + 3 c water = 1 qt (1 l) May be used as a tube feeding
Carnation Instant Breakfast (powder) (similar design to Sustagen)	140	70	36	1200 (5040)	4 packages powder, plus 1 qt whole milk
Controlyte (powder) (enzymatic hydrolysate of cornstarch; polysaccharides, vegetable oil)	143	0.08	48	1008 (4234)	Concentrated source of kcal (kJ); essentially protein-free; low in electrolytes
Ensure (soy and casein isolate, corn oil, corn syrup solids, vitamins, minerals)	145	37	37	1060 (4452)	460 mosmol May be given orally (variety of flavors: orange, vanilla, cherry, strawberry, etc.) or as tube feeding; lactose-free

From Goldstein, S. Surgery, stress, burns and nutritional care. In Howard, R. B.; Herbold, N. H., eds. Nutrition in Clinical Care, p. 529. New York, McGraw-Hill Book Co., 1978.

conditioned to heal well. Other good food sources of ascorbic acid can also be recommended—grapefruit, tomatoes, strawberries, cantaloupe, and green peppers, for example.

If, because of a vascular problem, the patient is taking an anticoagulant that cannot be stopped for a few days before periodontal surgery or if there is a history of repeated postoperative bleeding after surgery or tooth extraction because of an elevated prothrombin time (10 to 15 seconds is normal), consideration should be given to vitamin K supplementation.

It is of utmost importance that adequate fluids (six to eight glasses of liquids) be drunk every day.

POSTOPERATIVE DIETARY MANAGEMENT FOR HOSPITALIZED PERIODONTAL SURGERY PATIENTS

During periodontal surgery under general anesthesia, intravenous infusions are administered to maintain water and electrolyte balance and glucose levels. A solution of 0.45% saline with 5% dextrose in water (D5W) contains 500 ml of water, 25 g of glucose, and 38.5 milliequivalents (mEq) of sodium. Usually, the intravenous infusion is terminated in the recovery room if the patient is in good health. However, if the patient seems dehydrated, it may be wise to continue the infusion until the patient is fully reactive and can take fluids by mouth. When fully recovered from the anesthesia, the patient should be given clear fluids as tolerated. In addition to water, beverages such as cola drinks, ginger ale, apple juice, and orange juice in addition to clear broths or bouillon, clear tea or black coffee with sugar, and flavored gelatin are usually well tolerated. Preferably, the patient should sit up to drink.

On the first postoperative day, in addition to the beverages mentioned, sherbets, junkets, custards, and ice cream may be advised. If the patient is hungry, gruels or cereal topped with sugar and milk as well as milk, egg or eggnog, or some type of strained chicken, pea, or vegetable soup can be suggested. Frequent small feedings are tolerated better than a few large ones. These liquid diet suggestions should be ordered in the same way as other routine postoperative instructions. A meal plan and a menu are shown in Tables 18–4 and 18–5.

If adequate amounts of the foods cannot be tolerated, supplementary feeding of proprietary nutritional supplements should be given. These supplements are usually milk based (e.g., Meritene) or casein and/or soy protein based (e.g., Ensure or Sustacal) with additional carbohydrate, fat, vitamins, and minerals. Many are designed for use as the sole source of nutritional support. They provide a sound balance of energy and protein and are easily digested. However, they are much more expensive than skim milk powder (which is approximately 35% protein of high biological value) added to a flavored milk drink. Eggnogs and frappés (egg, milk, ice cream, and orange juice) and commercial preparations used in some weight reduction diets, such as Instant Breakfast drink, Nutriment, and Slender, can also be suggested.

On the second postoperative day, the patient may supplement the diet with the following:

- Vegetable-fruit group: citrus juices such as orange and grapefruit are highly recommended, as are tomato juice and other fruit and vegetable juices. Blended

TABLE 18–4. Liquid Diet

Total Food for the Day	Sample Meal Plan	Your Diet
Milk 1 quart As beverage, cocoa, with cereal, in soups; dry skim milk may be added	**Breakfast** Fruit juice, strained Gruel, with butter, milk Coffee, cream, sugar	**Breakfast** Orange juice Farina with milk Coffee with cream and sugar
Eggs 2–3 serv. Soft custard, eggnog	**Midmorning** Milk drink	**Midmorning** Eggnog
Vegetables 2–4 tbsp. Strained, with meat, in cream soup, strained juice	**Lunch** Strained cream soup Custard Milk Hot beverage	**Lunch** Split pea soup Chocolate custard Milk Tea with lemon and sugar
Fruit 1 pint Strained juice		
Cereals 2 serv. Gruel	**Midafternoon** Vegetable juice	**Midafternoon** Gevral frappé
Fats as tolerated Cream; butter in soups, cream soups	**Dinner** Strained meat and vegetable soup Eggnog	**Dinner** Chicken noodle soup Hamburg and tomato Vanilla pudding
Desserts 2–3 serv. Custard, junket, gelatin, ice cream, sherbet	Dessert Hot beverage	Eggnog Coffee with cream and sugar
Soups 1–2 serv. Clear broth, strained meat or vegetable soup, cream soup	**Bedtime** Milk drink Dessert	**Bedtime** Eggnog Strained pears and ice cream
Miscellaneous as desired Tea, coffee, gingerale, sugar		

fruits and vegetables may be used and may even be mixed with milk as drinks. Strained vegetables may be cooked with milk and butter and other seasonings and used as soups.

- Bread-cereal group: use strained gruels such as cream of wheat with milk.
- Milk group: supply milk in all forms. Nonfat milk solids may be added to regular milk for increased protein (add 3 tbsp of milk solids to each 8-oz glass of whole milk). Ice cream is soothing; milk shakes and malted milks are recommended. Cream may be added to milk if desired.
- Meat group: eggs in the form of eggnogs may be used in a liquid diet. They may also be used in soft, baked custards. Bouillon or meat broths can be recommended.

Table 18–6 outlines a full liquid diet that furnishes 2000 calories and 80 g of protein per day.

POSTOPERATIVE DIETARY MANAGEMENT FOR OFFICE SURGERY PERIODONTAL PATIENTS

One of the first questions the patient will ask after the periodontal surgical procedure is, "What can I eat?" A general answer, such as, "Whatever you can

TABLE 18–5. Additional Sample Menus for Liquid Diet

Breakfast	**Breakfast**	**Breakfast**
Orange juice	Prune juice	Grapefruit juice
Strained oatmeal with milk	Farina with milk	Wheatena with milk
Coffee with cream and sugar	Coffee with cream and sugar	Coffee with cream and sugar
Midmorning	**Midmorning**	**Midmorning**
Frappé	Vanilla pudding	Frappé
Lunch or Supper	**Lunch or Supper**	**Lunch or Supper**
Cream of chicken soup	Cream of mushroom soup	Split pea soup
Custard	Ice cream	Tapioca pudding
Milk	Milk	Milk
Tea or coffee	Tea or coffee	**Midafternoon**
Midafternoon	**Midafternoon**	Jello
Tomato juice	Vegetable soup	**Dinner**
Dinner	**Dinner**	Tomato juice
Vegetable soup	Beef broth	Chicken noodle soup
Applesauce	Jello with whipped cream	Strained pears
Milk	Milk	Milk
Tea or coffee	Tea or coffee	**Bedtime**
Bedtime	**Bedtime**	Milk
Ice cream	Eggnog	Custard
Milk	Junket	

TABLE 18–6. Full Liquid Diet

Basic foods to include daily		
Milk	1 qt	As beverage, cocoa, with cereal, in soups; dry skim milk may be added
Eggs	2–3	Soft custard, eggnog
Vegetables	2–4 tbsp	Strained, with meat, in cream soup, strained juice
Fruit	1 pt	Strained juice
Cereals	2 servings	Gruel
Fats	As tolerated	Cream; butter in soups, cereals
Desserts	2 or 3 servings	Custard, junket, gelatin, ice cream, sherbet
Soups	1 or 2 servings	Clear broth, beef juice, cream soup
Miscellaneous	As desired	Tea, coffee, gingerale, sugar

Sample meal plan

Breakfast	**Lunch or Supper**	**Dinner**
Fruit juice, strained	Beef broth with strained vegetables	Strained cream soup
Gruel with butter, milk	Eggnog	Custard
Coffee, cream, sugar	Sherbet, hot beverage	Milk, hot beverage

Between-meal snacks
Fruit juices, milk drinks, allowed desserts, etc.

TABLE 18–7. Soft Diet

Total Food for the Day	Sample Meal Plan	Your Diet
Milk and cheese 2 serv. Milk, cocoa, frappés, eggnogs; cottage cheese, any melted cheese sauce	**Breakfast** Fruit juice Hot cereal with milk Egg Toast with butter Coffee with cream and sugar	**Breakfast** Grapefruit juice Oatmeal with milk and sugar Poached egg on buttered toast Coffee with cream and sugar
Eggs 1 serv. Soft-cooked, poached, scrambled, creamed, omelet		
Meat 2 serv. Minced veal, lamb, beef, liver, fowl; chopped fish	**Lunch** Broiled meat patty Potato Vegetable Fruit dessert Tea or coffee	**Lunch** Lamb pattie with gravy Mashed potato with butter Tender asparagus Tapioca pudding with pineapple Coffee with cream and sugar
Vegetables 2 serv. Cooked and finely chopped; choose from carrots, asparagus tips, beets, peas, squash, beans, spinach; potatoes may be baked, mashed, boiled, creamed		
Fruit 2 serv. Any cooked fruits, finely chopped; raw banana	**Dinner** Strained cream soup Chopped fish Rice with sauce Vegetable Dessert Milk	**Dinner** Cream of mushroom soup Baked haddock with cheese sauce Rice with tomato gravy Mashed squash with butter Coconut custard Milk
Bread and Cereals 4 serv. Refined, enriched; also noodles, macaroni, etc.		
Dessert as desired Plain cakes, custard, gelatin, simple puddings, ice cream, sherbet	**Extras** Milk drink Fruit or vegetable juice	**Extras** Eggnog Orange juice with vanilla ice cream
Beverages as desired Carbonated beverages, tea, coffee		

TABLE 18–8. Additional Sample Menus for Soft Diet

Breakfast	Breakfast	Breakfast
Orange juice	Prune juice	Grapefruit juice
Farina with milk	Oatmeal with milk	Farina with milk
Soft-cooked egg	Poached egg	Scrambled egg
Toast with butter	Toast with butter	Bran muffin with butter
Coffee with cream and sugar	Coffee with cream and sugar	Coffee with cream and sugar
Lunch or Supper	**Lunch or supper**	**Lunch or supper**
Broiled hamburger	Tomato juice	Asparagus tips on toast
Mashed potato	Ground turkey on toast,	with cheese sauce
Strained carrots	gravy, cranberry jelly	Butterscotch pudding
Canned pears	Applesauce	with whipped cream
Tea or coffee	Milk	Tea or coffee
Dinner	**Dinner**	**Dinner**
Strained cream soup	Minced roast beef, gravy	Vegetable soup
Flaked haddock	Tender asparagus	Lamb pattie, gravy
Baked potato	Rice with gravy or butter	Mashed potato
Mashed squash	Tapioca pudding	Mashed turnip
Custard	Tea or coffee	Milk
Milk		Tea or coffee
Tea or coffee		

manage," should be avoided. It is best to supply a specific list of foods and beverages that the patient likes and that will provide nutrients for support.

If the surgery was done under local anesthesia, strongly advise the patient to drink nothing but cold beverages until the anesthesia has completely worn off. Other liquids or soft foods such as those listed in Tables 18–4 to 18–8, may be taken as tolerated. The personalized diet prescription should take into consideration the food likes and dislikes of the patient and should be in a suitable modified form. Liquid and soft diets can be made varied and appetizing as well as adequate in quality and quantity. The proprietary nutritional supplements already mentioned (Sustacal, Ensure, and so forth), may also be suggested. The extra time, effort, and thought expended in writing the diet prescription will be appreciated by the patient. These supportive measures can help to make the patient more comfortable and can hasten recovery from the surgery.

SUMMARY: PERIODONTAL SURGERY

Patients undergoing periodontal surgery require special attention to their nutrient needs and to methods for adequate feeding.

As a rule, the stresses of infection and surgery increase the requirements for calories, proteins, vitamins, minerals, and water to as much as double the usual needs. Malnutrition cannot be condoned; diets made up of liquids and soft foods can be adequate, appetizing, and varied by liquifying foods in a blender and then using proprietary supplements, as listed in Table 18–3.

The well-being of the periodontal surgery patient will be considerably enhanced, and recovery and convalescence will be speeded if the patient's nutritional needs during this stressful period are met.

REFERENCES

1. Jakush, J. Diet, nutrition and oral health; a rational approach for the dental practice. J. Am. Dent. Assoc. 109:20, 1984.
2. Alfano, M. C. Controversies, perspectives and clinical implications of nutrition in periodontal disease. Dent. Clin. North Am. 20:519, 1976.
3. Vogel, R. I.; Alvares, O. F. Nutrition and periodontal disease. In Pollack, R. L.; Kravitz, E., eds. Nutrition in Oral Health and Disease, pp. 136–150. Philadelphia, Lea & Febiger, 1985.
4. Navia, J. M. Research advances and needs in nutrition in oral health and disease. In Pollack, R. L.; Kravitz, E., eds. Nutrition in Oral Health and Disease, pp. 426–467. Philadelphia, Lea & Febiger, 1985.
5. Navia, J. M. Nutrition in oral health and disease. In Stallard, R. E., ed. A Textbook of Preventive Dentistry, 2nd ed., pp. 118–119. Philadelphia, W.B. Saunders Co., 1982.
6. Socransky, S. S. Relationship of bacteria to the etiology of periodontal disease. J. Dent. Res. 49:203, 1970.
7. Nisengard, R. J. The role of immunology in periodontal disease. J. Periodontol. 48:505, 1977.
8. Alfano, M. C. Effect of acute ascorbic acid deficiency on DNA content and permeability of guinea pig oral mucosal epithelium. Arch. Oral Biol. 23:929, 1978.
9. Vogel, R. I.; Deasy, M. J. The effect of folic acid on experimentally produced gingivitis. J. Prevent. Dent. 5:30, 1978.
10. Russell, A. L. International nutrition surveys: a summary of preliminary dental findings. J. Dent. Res. 42:233, 1963.
11. Mallek, H. An investigation of the role of ascorbic acid and iron in the etiology of gingivitis in humans. Ph.D. dissertation. Massachusetts Institute of Technology, 1978.
12. Poires, W. J.; Strain, W. H.; Rob, C. G. Zinc deficiency in delayed healing and chronic disease. Geol. Soc. Am. Mem. 123:73, 1971.
13. Krook, L. L., et al. Reversibility of nutritional osteoporosis: physico-chemical data on bones from an experimental study in dogs. J. Nutr. 101:233, 1971.
14. Scrimshaw, N. S.; Suskind, M. Interactions of nutrition and infection. Dent. Clin. North Am. 20:461, 1976.
15. O'Rourke, J. T. The relation of the physical character of the diet to the health of the periodontal tissues. Am. J. Orthod. Oral Surg. 33:687, 1947.
16. Sreebny, L. M. Effect of physical consistency of food on the crevicular complex and the salivary glands. Int. Dent. J. 22:394, 1972.

19

Effects of Diet and Nutrition on the Health of the Elderly, Especially Dental-Oral Health and Nutrient-Drug Interactions

DIETARY AND NUTRITIONAL NEEDS OF THE ELDERLY

Since the turn of the century, the increase in the number of elderly (persons aged 65 and older) in the United States has been ninefold. In 1986, they represented 12% of the population of the United States.[1] The fastest growing segment of this group includes persons over the age of 75.[2] Life expectancy has increased from the age of 45 in 1900 to the age of 72 for men and 77 for women in the 1980s. This shift is due in part to improved dietary practices and better overall health.[3]

Factors that influence food selection and eating habits of the elderly adversely are low income, loneliness, and poor cooking facilities. Lack of knowledge about and interest in desirable food choices also contributes to the poor nutritional status of the elderly. Dental and medical infirmities that interfere with chewing, digestion, or metabolism can also contribute to a poor nutritional status. Certain nutritionally related maladies—e.g., diabetes, obesity, cardiovascular disease, osteoporosis, and cancer—require special dietary regimens that may necessitate the combined guidance and supervision of a team of specialists in medicine, dentistry, dietetics, sociology, and psychology. In addition to the basic goal of providing the elderly person with an adequate, well-balanced diet, nutritionists incorporate into meal and menu planning the types of foods and their preparation that are acceptable, affordable, and manageable by the elderly.*

---

*In a study of 691 Massachusetts free-living elderly persons conducted by the U.S. Department of Agriculture's Human Nutrition Research Center on Aging (HNRC) at Tufts University, it was found that loss of teeth, low income, and education were better predictors of inadequate nutrition than demographic factors such as living alone or being homebound. We investigated a subset (206) of the HNRC study population and found that as teeth are lost, the nutritional quality of the diet declines. The biggest decline comes at the point at which an entire arch of teeth has been lost and then replaced by a complete denture.[3a, 3b] Risk factors for root caries are actively being researched. In our study we found that individuals who consumed a high-starch diet had a 50% higher root caries rate than those who did not.

Recommended Dietary Allowances (RDA)

Recommended dietary allowances for the elderly currently are based on extrapolations from the nutrient and calorie needs of adults up to the age of 50. RDA includes two age groupings for energy allowance—persons aged 51 to 75 and those aged 76 or older.[4] But the RDA for vitamins and minerals includes only one age grouping—those aged 51 and older. Data are not yet available for a more detailed breakdown.

Protein Requirements

The RDA for protein for persons aged 51 and over is 0.8 g protein/kg body weight per day. However, because of the general decline in energy intake as age increases, the recommendation is that the elderly should satisfy 12% or more of their energy intake with protein-rich foods.[4]

Mineral Requirements

According to the 1980 edition of Recommended Dietary Allowances, 800 mg/day of *calcium* for adults 51 years of age and older is advisable.[4] Based on newer knowledge, it is recommended especially that postmenopausal women have a calcium intake of 1000 to 1500 mg/day in order for them to enjoy the benefits of good skeletal strength.[5] The intake of 1000 to 1500 mg/day is thought to be more desirable for preventing osteoporosis, currently a major cause of hip and other bone fractures in American women 65 years of age and older.[6]

Osteoporosis is a metabolic bone disease that is believed to result from combined deficiencies of dietary calcium and an estrogen that are the major causes of (1) decreased bone mass, (2) spontaneous bone fractures, and (3) subsequent disabilities.[7] About 25% of American women 65 years of age and older suffer from osteoporosis. It occurs but rarely in men in the same age range. The nutritional factors that contribute to osteoporosis are

1. Insufficient intake of calcium-rich foods
2. Increased urinary excretion of calcium
3. Decreased blood level of 1,25-dihydroxycholecalciferol (vitamin D)

Vitamin D is essential for the regulation and promotion of the intestinal absorption of calcium and phosphorus (see Chap. 9). These three nutrients should be available simultaneously in adequate amounts in order to ensure the mineralization of the osteoid tissue. Although the requirement of the elderly for vitamin D is not precisely known, it is probably greater than that for young adults.[8] Bone demineralization is hastened and increased by such non-nutritional factors as (1) inadequate amount of physical exercise, e.g., walking, jogging, bicycling, swimming, and so forth; (2) immobilization of an extremity after an accident beyond the necessary period for healing; and (3) an estrogen deficiency.

The low dietary intake of calcium-rich foods—hard cheeses, milk, and dark green leafy vegetables (the darker the green, the more the calcium), such as mustard and turnip greens, collards, and kale—has been shown to be one of the several factors that can contribute significantly to a greater than usual loss of the alveolar bony ridge in edentulous patients aged 50 or older who elect to have immediate full upper or lower dentures or both. The rapid shrinkage of alveolar bone creates a void between the denture and the ridge that contributes to an unstable prosthesis and loss of some masticatory function and efficiency. This last loss can limit food choices to liquid and soft foods that do not provide the chewing stimulus for the bone mineralization necessary for maintaining alveolar ridge height.

It is advisable for a dentist who plans to insert a full upper or lower denture or both to prescribe a diet rich in calcium plus supplemental calcium carbonate tablets to be taken daily for 4 weeks or more before the removal of the remaining teeth and the insertion of the dentures. Presurgical calcium build-up may slow the rate of loss of alveolar ridge height, possibly contributing significantly to stabilizing the prosthesis and making the patient more comfortable and tolerant of it.[9]

In addition to calcium and vitamin D deficiencies, other nutrient inadequacies may occur in older patients. For example, although iron requirements for the elderly are low because menstruation and growth phases have ceased, exact iron requirement for this group has not yet been established. Only after factors influencing iron utilization are better understood can requirements be established.[10]

Zinc utilization declines with advancing age because intestinal absorption decreases after the age of 65 years. Thus it is conceivable that some of the clinical findings of decreased taste acuity, mental lethargy, and slow wound healing may be the results of a zinc deficiency.[11]

Vitamin Requirements

Elderly persons usually ingest foods rich in *vitamin A* sparingly; thus the intake is substantially below the RDA for vitamin A.[12] In spite of this, hypervitaminosis A may be more of a problem than a vitamin A deficiency because of an increase in vitamin A absorption and excessive use of multivitamin tablet supplements by the elderly.

The elderly are frequently deficient in *vitamin D* because of the lack of sun exposure and an inability to synthesize vitamin D in skin and convert it in the kidney.[13]

Vitamin E deficiency in the elderly does not seem to be a problem. Therefore the use of megavitamin E preparations is not indicated. Total plasma vitamin E levels increase with age.[14]

Vitamin C intake generally declines with age.[15] An inverse correlation between age and ascorbate levels in whole blood, plasma, and leukocytes has been reported.[16]

Vitamin B complex deficiencies are seen mainly in alcoholics because they do not eat enough bread or cereals. Enrichment of bread and flour products with vitamin B complex (thiamin, riboflavin, and niacin) by the baker or cereal manufacturer is mandatory.[17]

Folacin intake is adequate for most elderly persons in spite of the fact that it generally falls below the RDA of 500 µg, which may be high according to Rosenberg et al.[18]

Vitamin B₆ (pyridoxine) deficiency ranges from 50% to 90% of the elderly affected, which may be an important cause of the increased prevalence of the carpal tunnel syndrome (an inflamed tendon attached to the wrist bone) in the elderly.[19]

NUTRITIONALLY RELATED ORAL PROBLEMS IN ELDERLY PATIENTS

One of the major functions of nutritional fitness is to prevent or slow down the onset of those degenerative and disease conditions associated with aging that occur in the mouth, such as loss of taste, xerostomia (dry mouth), burning and sore tongue, oral mucous membrane disease, temporomandibular joint discomfort, periodontal disease, and osteoporosis of the alveolar bone.

Alterations in Gustation and Olfaction

Gustation (taste perception) is mediated through the papillae, taste buds, and free nerve endings that are found primarily in the tongue but also over the hard and soft palates and in the pharynx. In general, the number of these structures appears to decrease with age.

Four modalities of taste are perceived by the tongue—salt, sweet, sour, and bitter. The tongue is more sensitive to salt and sweet, whereas the palate with its complex network of receptors is more sensitive to sour and bitter.

Olfaction is the act of perceiving odors; the odors of food contribute to its palatability. The olfactory sense, or sense of smell, is the special chemical sense that is activated by stimulation of the olfactory receptors situated in the upper part of the nasal cavity. In contrast with gustation, olfaction can be stimulated by extremely low chemical concentrations.

In the process of aging, taste perception diminishes—the perception for salt at any early age and for sweet a little later—in part as a result of hyperkeratinization of the epithelium that may occlude the taste bud ducts. Vitamin A inadequacy may be associated with such epithelial hyperkeratinization. On the other hand, the receptors for bitter taste in the circumvallate papillae of the tongue seem to survive the aging process. If there are no systemic contraindications, increased use of condiments such as pepper usually provides more flavor to food. Certainly the palatability of food will be improved if its aroma is pleasant and if it has the proper texture and temperature.

There is a need to expand studies on the chemical senses in aging and to determine if alterations in taste and smell in elderly individuals can be correlated with neuroanatomical or physiological findings. In addition, the contribution of oral hygiene practices, of food habits, and of cultural, social, and individual variables must be considered in studies dealing with taste and smell in the elderly in the future. Oral hygiene practices should be checked because the presence of unpleasant tastes (dysgeusia) may be due to the discharge of crevicular fluid from the gingiva when chewing.[20]

Xerostomia (Dry Mouth)

Xerostomia is a condition commonly found in the elderly. It is not a direct consequence of the aging process but may result from one or more factors affecting salivary secretion. Emotions (especially fear or anxiety), neuroses, organic brain disorders, and drug therapy all can cause xerostomia. Many drugs are known to produce dry mouth as a side effect. Some of the commonly prescribed groups of drugs that produce xerostomia are antihypertensives, anticonvulsants, antidepressants, tranquilizers, and anti-Parkinson drugs. In addition, salivary gland function may be diminished by obstruction of the duct with a salivary stone, therapeutic radiation for head and neck cancer, infection such as mumps, Sjögren's syndrome (an autoimmune disorder), lupus erythematosus, biliary cirrhosis, polymyositis or dermatomyositis, or sarcoid and autoimmune hemolytic anemia.

Since saliva lubricates the oral mucosa, the lack of saliva creates a dry and often painful mucosa. Without significant salivary flow, food debris will remain in the mouth, where it is fermented by dental plaque bacteria to organic acids that initiate the dental caries process. A major function of saliva, which contains calcium phosphates, is to buffer the acids and to remineralize the eroded enamel surface.

In addition, the lack of saliva can affect the nutritional status in a number of ways:

1. It hinders the chewing of food because it prevents the formation of a bolus.

2. It makes the mouth sore and chewing painful.

3. It makes swallowing difficult due to the loss of saliva's lubricating effect.

4. It can cause changes in taste perception that decrease adequate food intake.

Since 1979 a comprehensive oral health management program for patients with xerostomia has been instituted at Tufts University School of Dental Medicine. Most of the oral complications associated with xerostomia and hypo-mineralization can be successfully prevented or at least markedly reduced in severity.

The caries-preventive aspect of the system is based on previous correlated ultrastructural and chemical studies on sound, exposed dentin, and carious dental tissues.[21] It was concluded from this research that there are inherent cariostatic mechanisms within the oral cavity.

The oral health management program includes intensive fluoride treatment over a 1-month period to raise the fluoride concentration of both the enamel and the exposed dentinal surfaces to levels that protect against caries. Supersaturated calcium phosphate mouth rinses are also utilized to augment the physiological maintenance system and provide new nucleation sites for mineral growth. In order to stimulate salivary secretion, the patients are supplied with inert chewing gum. Patients are instructed in proper home care oral hygiene and are given nutrition counseling.

Painful, Burning Tongue

A painful, burning tongue is often encountered in nutritional anemias associated with deficiencies of vitamin B_{12}, folic acid, or iron.

Vitamin B$_{12}$ deficiency (pernicious anemia), seen with increased frequency in older people, particularly in women, is characterized by a triad of symptoms: generalized weakness; a sore, painful tongue; and numbness or tingling of the extremities. In some cases, the tongue symptoms are the first sign of pernicious anemia. The tongue is generally described as dark red, rather than the normal pink, either in its entirety or in patches scattered over the dorsum (upper surface) and lateral borders. Characteristically, there is gradual atrophy of the papillae that results in a smooth, or bald, tongue. On occasion the oral mucosa exhibits a pale yellowish tinge similar to that noted on the skin. Not uncommonly in anemic patients, the oral mucosa becomes sensitive and intolerant to dentures.

Achlorhydria (absence of hydrochloric acid in stomach secretions), sensory disturbances, difficulty in walking, incoordination, and loss of vibratory sensations are other characteristic features of pernicious anemia. The major treatment of pernicious anemia consists of intramuscular administration of vitamin B$_{12}$.

Folic acid deficiency, like vitamin B$_{12}$ deficiency, causes a megaloblastic anemia. It occurs in poorly nourished people, especially those with malabsorption disorders, and is characterized clinically by glossodynia, glossitis (pain or inflammation of the tongue), stomatitis (inflammation of the mouth), diarrhea, and general weakness. It differs from vitamin B$_{12}$ deficiency in that the patient shows no central nervous system involvement, a normal Schilling test, presence of hydrochloric acid in the gastric juices, and low folate levels in serum and white blood cells.

Treatment is to supplement the diet with 5 to 15 mg of folacin tablets daily until reticulocytes in the blood increase; this improvement is maintained with doses of 2 to 5 mg daily. The best food sources of folic acid are yeast, liver, fresh green vegetables, and fruits. (B$_{12}$ deficiency should be ruled out as a cause of megaloblastic anemia prior to folate treatment.)

Elderly patients who live on a tea-and-toast diet are prime candidates for iron deficiency anemia; an adequately nourished older man or postmenopausal woman would probably not have this problem unless there is hemorrhage.

The oral manifestations of iron deficiency anemia are glossitis (inflamed tongue) and fissures at the corners of the mouth. The papillae of the tongue are atrophied, giving the tongue a smooth, shiny red appearance. Nutritional management consists of ingesting iron-rich or enriched foods, such as liver, eggs, and cereals, as well as iron supplements (1 g of ferrous sulfate in four divided doses daily).

Oral Mucous Membrane Problems

The mucous membranes of the lips, the buccal and palatal tissues, and the floor of the mouth change with age. The patient's chief complaints are a burning sensation, pain, and dryness of the mouth, as well as cracks in the lips. Chewing and swallowing become difficult, and taste is altered. The epithelial membrane is thin, friable, and easily injured. It heals slowly because of impaired circulation. If the salivary deficiency is pronounced, the oral mucosa may be dry, atrophic, and sometimes inflamed, but more often it is pale and translucent.

Aging produces change in the blood vessels, particularly atherosclerotic changes. Varicosities (unnatural swollen veins) are often noted on the underside of the tongue and in the floor of the mouth, and are related to varicosities found elsewhere. Lipid accumulation in the walls of the medium-sized sublingual arteries is a result of high intake of lipids, especially saturated fats and cholesterol.

The palatal mucosa is often hyperkeratotic and thickened in the elderly patient. The glandular tissue is apparently replaced by connective tissue, and the epithelial mass increases.

Cheilosis, inflammation of the lips caused by vitamin B complex deficiency, is manifested by vertical fissuring of the lips. A redness along the line of closure of the lips as a result of superficial denudation (deprivation of a surface of its epithelial covering) and increased inflammation can be seen. Lesions at the angles of the mouth start out pale in color, then become macerated (degenerative, discolored, and softened) and as a result of secondary infection, form yellow encrusted fissures.

Therapeutic doses of vitamin B complex and vitamin C (for example, Theragran, Cebefortis, Allbee with C, or a generic type) as well as a balanced, varied, adequate diet are the nutritional means for managing these problems. Of course, social, emotional, and economic factors, which influence food selection and general interest in diet, have to be managed in order to achieve any lasting, beneficial health effects.

Temporomandibular Joint Pain

As a result of masticating very firm foods over many years or as a result of bruxism (teeth grinding), attrition (wearing down) of the incisal and occlusal surfaces takes place. The resulting teeth have shortened anatomical crowns, exposed dentin, and wide, flattened chewing surfaces. This type of tooth wear can produce overclosure of the jaws and affect the relations of the mandibular condyle to the glenoid fossa. With age, the glenoid fossa can become shallower and the head of the condyle, flatter. Thus it is possible for the meniscus, or articular disc between the condyle and fossa, to be perforated or damaged by this change in temporomandibular relationships, causing pain and limitation of range of movement of the jaws.

Another common cause of overclosure, or loss of vertical dimension, is partial or complete edentulism without prosthetic replacement. This can produce a narrow and depressed (sunken) lip line because of a loss of adequate support and muscle tone. The circumoral skin becomes wrinkled, producing a "purse-string" appearance so characteristic of the elderly.

It is also possible that degenerative changes, such as osteoarthritis (seen in other joints of the body), can affect the temporomandibular joint and can also produce the articular disc changes that create the clicking of the jaw and discomfort in the ear. There may even be limitation to opening of the mouth, which may permit only a small-sized bolus of food.

For temporary prevention of overclosure, an acrylic night guard can be used. Once the proper and comfortable intermaxillary vertical dimension is ascertained, fixed bridgework or a partial denture should be constructed. The patient should be advised to select foods of medium to soft consistency in order to prevent excessive occlusal wear of the intact dentition.

Alveolar Osteoporosis

The physiological lability of alveolar bone is maintained by a sensitive balance between bone formation and bone resorption, which is regulated by local and systemic influences. The alveolar bone participates in the maintenance of body calcium balance. Calcium is constantly being deposited and withdrawn from the alveolar bone to provide for the needs of other tissues and to maintain the calcium level of the blood. The calcium in the cancellous trabeculae (spongy bone) is more readily available than that from compact bone. Conversely, easily mobilizable calcium is deposited in the trabecular rather than the cortical portions of bone.

Because alveolar bone acts as a reservoir of mineral ions to maintain more vital functions, it is susceptible to osteoporosis. With aging, bone becomes less dense. Because of this alveolar susceptibility to osteoporosis, some investigators have suggested that internal alveolar resorption may result from dietary calcium deficiency or phosphorus excess, or a combination of both. In fact, increased alveolar bone density has been noted in patients who have been given daily calcium supplements of 1 g/day for a year. However, this did not prove, as was suggested, that there was a direct cause-and-effect relationship between calcium deficiency and initiation of periodontal disease, because osteoporosis of the alveolar bone and periodontal disease are not the same.

Alveolar bone undergoes constant remodeling in response to occlusal (closure) forces. Osteoclasts and osteoblasts redistribute bone substance to meet new functional demands most efficiently. Bone is removed where it is no longer needed and added where new needs arise. When occlusal forces are reduced, bone is resorbed, bone height is diminished, and the number and thickness of the trabeculae are reduced. This is termed bone disuse, or nonfunctional atrophy.

In the elderly, there tends to be a relative increase in bone disease and resorption compared with deposition. With the loss of teeth, the alveolar process no longer serves its primary function of tooth support and therefore is resorbed. So much bone is lost in this way that the mandibular and maxillary ridges sometimes approach flatness. This loss in vertical height of bone and the changing of the angle of the mandible is manifested as a loss in face height in older people.

Wical and Swoope investigated the relationship between the dietary combination of calcium and phosphorus and the resorption of alveolar bone in edentulous patients.[22] They compared the diets of subjects who had minimal bone resorption with subjects who had severe alveolar bone loss. The results indicated a direct cause-and-effect relationship between low calcium intake or calcium-phosphorus imbalance and severe ridge resorption.

In a later study, Wical and Brusse reported that the ingestion of calcium and vitamin D dietary supplements reduced postextraction alveolar bone resorption by 36%.[23] They administered 750 to 1000 mg of calcium and 375 to 400 IU of vitamin D daily to patients who had a low calcium or a high phosphorus intake or both. This dietary supplementation, they believed, helped increase the resistance of the alveolar bone to both mechanical and nutritional biochemical stresses.

DIET, NUTRITION, AND DRUG INTERACTIONS

The elderly account for 40% of acute hospital bed days and 15% of psychiatric disturbances. They have a 20% chance of being admitted to nursing care facilities. Four per cent of persons aged 65 to 74 years and 20% of those 75 years or older have organic brain impairment.

On an average, the elderly take 13 prescriptions per year, three times as much as the population under age 65. Of the ambulatory 85% and of institutionalized almost 95% receive drugs; 25% of all the elderly are dependent on prescription drugs for activities of daily living.

The most common medications are analgesics and cardiovascular and psychotropic medications, especially those with sedative and hypnotic effects.

More than 50% of elderly patients in skilled nursing care facilities are given psychotropic medications (those that affect mental activity). Persons who take these medications also use more prescription drugs of other kinds and tend to consult physicians about medications more often than older persons who do not take them. With age there is an altered sensitivity to psychotropic medications that can lead to central nervous system toxicity if the medication level is not adjusted. The body's ability to absorb, bind, metabolize, and accept drugs changes with age. It is generally recommended to start with half the normal adult dose and slowly increase it to a therapeutic level. With the numerous medications given the elderly, care should be taken to avoid adverse drug interactions and drug-nutrient interactions. Medications can interact if one changes the metabolism of others through enzyme induction, by altering binding to plasma proteins and tissue receptor sites, by interfering with the transportation of drug to receptor sites, and by delaying or enhancing excretion. These interactions are dose-dependent and vary from individual to individual (see Table 19–2).

There are three sites at which medications and food may interact.

1. *Absorption site.* Drugs may interfere with or enhance absorption.

2. *Interference with metabolic pathways,* i.e., any induced changes in distribution, transport, and utilization of nutrients and the capacity of the kidneys to retain or eliminate drugs and nutrients.

3. *Excretion site.* Drugs may alter kidney capacity to retain or excrete certain nutrients.

A number of drugs affect (1) the body's use of nutrients, (2) appetite and food intake (Table 19–1), or (3) nutrient absorption or metabolism or both (Table 19–2). Also, requirements of persons who receive certain drugs over long periods are different from those who have not taken these drugs before. The purpose of this section is to inform the clinician how to minimize drug-induced malnutrition in geriatric patients.

Effects of Drugs on Appetite, Taste, and Food Intake

When phenothiazine tranquilizers or benzodiazepines (Librium, Valium) are given in high dosages to elderly patients, food intake diminishes.[24] On the other hand, patients who want a drug prescription to increase appetite and food intake

TABLE 19–1. Drugs That Exert an Effect on Taste and Appetite

Reduce Taste	Alter Taste Perception	Cause Metallic Taste	Cause Bitter Taste	Decrease Appetite	Stimulate Appetite
Azathioprine	Captopril	Allopurinol	Carbamazepine	Anticonvulsants	Antihistamines
Baclofen	Griseofulvin	Ethambutol	Phenylbutazone	Antineoplastic agents	Benzodiazepine
Carbamazepine	Lithium carbonate	Gold compounds		Carbonic anhydrase inhibitors	Hypoglycemic agents
Chlormezanone				Digitalis glycosides	Phenothiazine tranquilizers
Clofibrate				Estrogens	Steroids
Lincomycin				Flurazepam	Tricyclic antidepressants
Methimazole				Indomethacin	
Penicillamine				Lithium salts	
Phenylbutazone				Metronidazole	
Sulfasalazine				Monoamine oxidase inhibitors	
				Procainamide	
				Tetracyclines	
				Thiazide diuretics	
				Tolazemide	

Adapted from Scavone, J. M. Drug-food and drug-nutrient interactions. Natl. Assoc. Retail Druggists J., vol. 108, pp. 69–73, 1986.

TABLE 19–2. Effects of Drugs on Nutrients

Drug	Nutrient Affected	Effect
Phenytoin	Folate	Destroys folate
	Vitamin D	Inhibits synthesis of 1,25-dihydroxycholecalciferol
	Pyridoxine	Inhibits enzyme to decrease cellular level
Isoniazid (antituberculosis)	Vitamin D, pyridoxine, calcium	Long-term use leads to high urinary loss
Cimetidine	Vitamin D	Impairs metabolism to kidney
	Calcium	Decreases calcium absorption
Antacids	Folate, iron	Inhibit absorption
Fiber	Calcium	Increases fecal loss of calcium complex with free carboxyl groups of polysaccharides
Phytates	Calcium, zinc	Interfere with absorption
Oxalates	Calcium, zinc	Interfere with absorption
Protein	Calcium	Increases loss in urine
Phosphorus	Calcium	Unfavorable calcium to phosphorus ratio leads to bone loss
Antacids	Phosphorus, calcium	Precipitates phosphorus
Aluminum		Leads to bone loss
Magnesium		Increases fecal loss of calcium
Glucocorticoids	Calcium	Calciurea, osteoporosis
Furosemide	Calcium, sodium	Loss by kidney
Alcohol	Folate, thiamin, riboflavin, niacin, pyridoxine, retinol, magnesium, zinc	Displaces food (void of nutrients; leads to nutritional deficiencies)
Cholestyramine	Folate, fat, and fat-soluble vitamins	Binding in gastrointestinal tract
Tetracycline	Iron, calcium	Formation of insoluble complexes; long-term use leads to excessive loss in urine, skeletal demineralization
Neomycin	Fat malabsorption decreases fat-soluble vitamins	Induces morphological change in mucosal cells in intestine
Amphetamines	Decreased food intake	Anorectic
Mazindol		
Chlorpromazine	Increased food intake	Orectic
Diazepam		Hypotension, respiratory depression
Diuretics	Potassium (loss)	EKG change
Laxatives and mineral oil	Fat-soluble vitamins, essential (fatty acids)	Solubilizes these nutrients, decreasing their absorption
Oral contraceptives	Folate	Block absorption, inhibit brush border enzymes

Table continued on following page

TABLE 19–2. Effects of Drugs on Nutrients *Continued*

Drug	Nutrient Affected	Effect
Vitamin C in high doses	Selenium, copper	Inhibits intestinal absorption
Zinc in high doses	Copper	Inhibits absorption
Mycomycin	All nutrients	Malabsorption syndrome, cytotoxic to intestinal mucosa
Coumarin	Vitamin K	Inhibits metabolism
Caffeine	Iron, calcium	Decreases absorption

are given amitriptyline (Elavil) and gain a significant amount of weight. Patients taking Elavil seem to have a craving for sweets.[25] In persons who take antidepressant drugs (e.g., combination of tricyclics and monoamine oxidase inhibitors), weight gain results in a high percentage of cases.[26]

Over-the-counter weight-reducing drugs that may contain bulking agents such as methylcellulose and mild stimulants such as phenylpropanolamine (an ephedrinelike drug) do not have a significant effect on food intake or obesity.

Cancer chemotherapeutic drugs can induce nausea and vomiting and thus loss of appetite.

When phenothiazine tranquilizers are given to elderly patients so that their level of consciousness is depressed, food intake may also be reduced. It is important to appreciate the fact that a patient whose diet marginally includes the required nutrients may develop a nutritional, especially a vitamin, deficiency when given appetite-reducing drugs.[27]

Drugs and Nutrient Absorption

Drugs that cause malabsorption are (1) mineral oil, a laxative that solubilizes the fat-soluble vitamins A, D, K, and beta-carotene; (2) antacids that increase the pH of the lumen of the intestine and thus decrease the absorption of folacin; (3) colchicine and neomycin, which cause intestinal mucosal damage and the subsequent loss of fat, nitrogen, lactose, sodium, potassium, calcium, iron, and vitamin B_{12}; and (4) dilantin, which can cause mucosal damage and accelerate the metabolism of vitamin D with a resulting loss of calcium.[28]

Problems of Food Intake, Digestion, and Utilization

A major problem of many elderly persons is a limited physiological capability to digest and absorb foods. This begins with an inability to chew food thoroughly because of an inadequate or poorly functioning dentition. In addition, their appetite is diminished and their appreciation of flavorful tastes is lacking, which will diminish their food intake.

Sometimes an elderly patient will eat too much too rapidly and suffer gastric distress. Epigastric distress and flatulence are not uncommon after eating such foods as broccoli, Brussels sprouts, cabbage, cucumbers, onions, radishes, melons, peas, and beans. The efficiency of the digestion, absorption, and utilization of nutrients is probably impaired in the elderly because of diminished amounts of digestive enzymes and atrophy of the alimentary mucosa.

Older people may be subject to constipation as a result of the diminished tone of their intestinal muscles. To compensate for this natural physiological infirmity, foods high in fiber content, such as raw fruits and raw vegetables, should be recommended. If roughage is not allowed because of ulcer problems, the intake of six to eight cups of water per day and cooked prunes or figs or their juices or bran cereals may be recommended.

SOCIAL AND PSYCHOLOGICAL FACTORS THAT CONTRIBUTE TO MALNUTRITION IN THE ELDERLY

Social Factors

Social problems such as loneliness and apathy are important causes of malnutrition. There are five million older persons in the United States who live alone and prepare meals for themselves. A woman living alone may regard cooking as drudgery rather than the joy it used to be when she was preparing meals for her family. Some men have no food preparation skills at all. For the older person, eating with other people is an important way to socialize. Eating alone not only takes away the incentive for eating a well-balanced, varied, adequate diet but it also creates a negative attitude about food and stifles interest in eating. The importance of sociability is clearly demonstrated in care facilities and homes for the aged, where people take their meals in common dining rooms that provide congenial companionship, stimulating conversation, and pleasant surroundings. These contribute to good eating habits, high morale, and good health.

Psychological Factors

An older patient may develop loss of appetite, cravings for particular foods, nausea at the sight of food, indigestion, or an insatiable appetite as a result of anxiety or some other abnormal emotional states.

Elderly people, especially those in their 60s or 70s, sometimes suffer from overeating. Overeating reflects the boredom of an old person whose days often contain so little of interest or value that eating becomes the most important satisfaction and the reason for living. It has also been theorized that some senior citizens overeat because a sense of satiety, or fullness, acts as a sedative; it makes them drowsy and renders them less acutely aware of the unpleasantness of their situation.

It is not uncommon to find rigidity in food habits among the elderly. Food prejudices can be an adaptive technique designed to avoid anxiety. Security is achieved by maintaining rigid attitudes and rituals in which food acceptances play a part. In addition, elderly patients who have followed certain patterns for many years are not generally receptive to new ideas. Many of them have developed relatively inflexible ideas as to which foods are good or bad for them. Attempts to wean these individuals from food prejudices must be cautious in view of the listed factors and these patients' diminished capacities for dealing with anxiety.

MODIFYING FOOD SELECTION AND FOOD HABITS

The problem of selecting a properly nutritious diet for an elderly person is not simple, because one or more of the following environmental factors may influence food selection and eating habits:

- *Deficient dentition.* One cannot eat and chew normally without teeth or with teeth that are painful and in need of treatment. In Table 19–3 are a list of desirable foods and ways to modify them so that they will be easier to eat.
- *Low income.* Lack of money to buy healthful foods is a major cause of malnutrition in the elderly. Practical information on low-cost foods is available. Some cities provide a Dial-A-Dietitian service. This information can also be secured by writing to the Consumer Information Center, Public Documents Distribution Center Dept. A-7, Pueblo, Colorado 81001.
- *Ingrained food patterns.* Food likes and dislikes are often founded on years of more or less satisfactory personal experience and in many instances are almost unalterable.
- *Excessive introspection.* This may amount to preoccupation with one's health in general or with functioning of the gastrointestinal tract in particular.
- *Loss of independence.* The sense of not belonging and of having no job responsibility quickly eradicates the desire to reach any reasonable objective, such as keeping adequately nourished.

Several modifications in food preparation and service can be used to lift the spirits of the gerodontic patient. The sense of taste that is lost when the roof of the mouth is covered by dentures can be partially compensated by using herbs

TABLE 19–3. Modifying the Form of Desirable Foods That Otherwise May be Difficult to Chew

Foods Causing Difficulty	Modification
Steaks and chops	Tender fish; hamburger; meatloaf; chopped meat or fish in casseroles, and meat spreads
Celery stalks	Chopped celery in gelatin or in egg and tuna salad
Raw carrots and peppers	Cut into smaller pieces; incorporate in gelatin, in tuna or egg salad, or in omelets
Corn on the cob	Creamed corn, canned kernel corn
Baked or fried potatoes	Mashed potatoes, spaghetti, noodles, macaroni, and cooked cereal
Sandwiches	Trim crusts of fresh bread; use soft fillings
Apples, raw	Baked apple, applesauce
Lettuce, salads	Chop finely
Fruits, raw	Juices; cooked and canned fruits

and condiments and serving foods that are tolerably hot, thus making the patient more aware of the food aromas. Also, use of onions, chives, parsley, and other herbs can heighten food flavors for denture wearers. For maximum taste sensation, the use of sharply contrasting flavors in combinations (such as sweet and sour) has proved beneficial.

Besides the physiological, psychological, and social factors mentioned, food patterns are influenced by cultural and educational factors, and by the availability of foods. It is thus understandable that changing the food habits of elderly persons is not an easy task. It is easy to say that it cannot be done. Nevertheless, through persistent and rational nutrition education, food habits can be modified. We do not suggest drastic changes, but if the environmental factors are improved and with expression of concern for the patient, significant progress can be made in realistically and constructively modifying food habits.

FOOD RECOMMENDED FOR THE ELDERLY

The Five Food Groups

Since foods and mixtures of foods are more easily understood by the laity than nutrients, they have been used as a guide for teaching good eating habits. All the nutrients necessary for optimal health in the desirable amounts can be obtained by eating a variety of foods in adequate amounts from the Five Food Groups (Chap. 14). These are

1. Four servings of vegetables and fruits, subdivided into three categories:
   a. Two servings of good sources of vitamin C, such as citrus fruits, salad greens, and raw cabbage
   b. One serving of a good source of provitamin A, such as deep green and yellow vegetables or fruits
   c. One serving of potatoes and other vegetables and fruits
2. Four servings of enriched bread, cereals, and flour products
3. Two servings of milk and milk-based foods, such as cheese (but not butter)
4. Two servings of meats, fish, poultry, eggs, dried beans and peas, and nuts
5. Additional miscellaneous foods, including fats and oils, sugar and alcohol; the only serving recommendation is for about 2 to 4 tablespoons of polyunsaturated fats, which supply essential fatty acids.

The recommended minimum number of servings of the first four food groups provides about 1200 calories, which probably is not completely adequate calorically. With the addition of butter, margarine, oils, or one or two added servings from any of the food groups, the desirable 1400 to 2200 calorie range for females and the 2200 to 2800 calorie range for males aged 51 to 75 years can readily be obtained. For those in the 76 years and older group, the energy needs are 1200 to 2000 calories for females and 1650 to 2450 calories for males.

VEGETABLE-FRUIT GROUP

This group is important for its contribution of vitamins A and C and fiber, although individual foods in this group vary widely in how much of these they provide. The dark green and deep yellow vegetables are good sources of vitamin

A, and raw fruits and vegetables can provide significant amounts of fiber to the diet.

Although fruits and vegetables (especially those high in vitamin C) are extremely important in maintaining tissue health, they are often lacking or minimal in the diet of elderly persons. One reason is that fresh fruits and vegetables are often quite expensive. However, frozen citrus concentrates (juices) are quite economical, as are canned or frozen fruits, juices, and vegetables. Fresh fruits and vegetables are always cheaper in season. And although the fancy canned and frozen brands of vegetables, with added mushrooms or onions, may be more eye-appealing and attractive, they are no more nutritious than the less expensive brands.

For desserts, adding varieties of fruits and juices to plain gelatin helps to vary the fruit intake in the diet and is less expensive than prepared, flavored gelatin desserts.

BREAD-CEREAL GROUP

Whole-grain or enriched flour products are important sources of B vitamins and iron.

It is wise to make sure that all patients are using whole-grain or enriched bread products; otherwise, little but calories is gained and many essential nutrients will be missing.

Commercially baked bread is usually cheaper than bakery bread and rolls. Day-old baked products are usually the best buys. Sugar-coated cereals are usually more expensive than the unsugared varieties and also add unwanted calories.

MILK-CHEESE GROUP

Milk and Cheddar-type cheeses are the least expensive and best sources of calcium, vitamin D, and riboflavin in the American diet. Milk and cheese are also good sources of high-quality protein. Cottage cheese is equivalent to lean meat in protein, as is Cheddar cheese. These cheeses can be combined with macaroni, potatoes, and bread to make nutritious dishes that are relatively inexpensive, or they can be added to salads or used with fruit and crackers for dessert.

Milk costs can be cut by one-third by the use of dried skim milk. Purchasing dried milk powder in large quantities is also economical. Evaporated milk may be used for coffee and tea; it is less expensive than cream.

MEAT POULTRY, FISH, AND BEANS GROUP

These foods are valued for the protein, phosphorus, vitamins B_6 and B_{12}, and other vitamins and minerals they provide.

Cheaper cuts of meat are just as nourishing as the more expensive steaks. Beef brisket, pot roast, stew meat, and chuck roast can be cooked slowly in a little water to tenderize them. Lower-cost cuts of meat that are not all gristle, bone, and fat can also be ground or chopped. As a contributor of quality protein, lean hamburger provides the same essential amino acids as, for example, lamb chops. It is also wise to purchase beef, lamb, or pork liver instead of the more expensive calves' liver. Chicken, turkey, and fish (fresh, frozen, or canned) are often cheaper than meats.

Dried peas, beans, and nuts are actually the cheapest sources of iron and proteins, but the protein is not as high in quality as that found in meat, fish, and poultry. Nevertheless, these legumes make valuable contributions to the diet and may be used in casseroles with meat, fish, and poultry.

Eggs are also a source of high-quality protein. The food value of Grade A and Grade B eggs is exactly the same, and brown eggs are equally as nutritious as white but are usually more expensive.

Fats, Sugar, and Alcohol Group

Margarine is less expensive than butter and has approximately the same food value. Margarine made with polyunsaturated fats, such as corn oil or safflower oil, will also minimize the risk of formation of cholesterol. Sugar is a food additive that has no nutrient density and is used primarily for flavor and calories.

Since the Food Groups in the amounts recommended provide about 1200 calories, they may not meet the caloric requirements of the patient. By eating more servings from the food groups or by the *judicious, moderate* use of such additional foods as butter, margarine, oils, and sugars, calorie needs can be met. These additional foods should neither be ignored nor overemphasized because, as already pointed out, they can easily contribute to increased weight and other systemic problems associated with obesity. Alcohol can enhance weight gain or in excess can replace nutritious foods leading to deficiencies.

It is important to realize that foods specific to any ethnic group are just as much a part of the Food Groups as are our familiar American foods. Table 19–4 shows some of the ethnic variations of the Food Groups.

Meal Plans

As the digestive process slows down with age, meal size and spacing may be adjusted. Large, heavy meals tend to decrease efficient absorption and use of nutrients. It may be better to spread food intake more evenly throughout the day and to avoid the three traditional meals. For some persons, large meals at the end of the day may disturb the sleep. Others believe that a snack at bedtime helps them to sleep better. Many persons enjoy a snack between meals. This is to be encouraged, but elderly patients should be taught what foods constitute healthful snacks.

The following daily meal plan may be optimal for senior citizens, but it is not necessarily practical at the very beginning of diet modification:

BREAKFAST

Fruit or fruit juice
Egg (limit to two per week if need to lower cholesterol
     or saturated fat), whole-grain cereal, or both
Whole wheat or enriched toast
Enriched margarine or butter
Hot beverage

TABLE 19–4. Some Ethnic, Cultural, and Regional Variations on the 5–Food Groups Guide

Nationality	Milk	Meat	Fruits-Vegetables	Breads-Cereals	Sweets	Fats	Special Customs
Greek and Middle East	Yogurt, goat's milk, goat's cheese, and thick sour milk	Lamb, birds, mussels, frogs, squid, anchovies, lentils, almonds, pistachios, and chickpeas	Grape leaves, eggplant, okra, cabbage, peppers, turnips, and dried fruits	Cracked wheat, bulgar, flat bread, dark bread, whole wheat and cornmeal breads	Honey, bakalava, and sweet pastries	Olive oil, lard, and lamb fat	Nuts, pumpkin seeds, olives and fruits, bread at every meal, spices and garlic, pickled and salted foods, caraway, sesame and poppy seeds
Jewish	Cream cheese and sour cream	Lox (smoked salmon), chicken livers, pickled and smoked meats	Borscht (beet soup), kugel (potato-noodle pudding dish), and cooked dried fruits	Kasha (groats), challah, matzoth, bagels, bulgar, potato flour, and barley	Sweet pastries often made with fruits and poppy or sesame seeds, and strudels	Chicken fat	Dietary laws forbid certain foods and govern certain food combinations

Puerto Rican	Native White cheese	Dry salted cod, pork, sausage, and tripe	Viandas (starchy root), sweet potato, green and ripe bananas, tapioca, avacado, breadfruit, and many fruit juices	Gruel and oatmeal	Rice pudding, special fruit gum dessert	Salt pork, lard	Peppers, oregano, anise, olives, raisins, and starchy roots
Japanese		Seafood	Seaweed, pickled fruits, bamboo shoots, bean sprouts, dried mushrooms, pickles, lotus root, and white radishes	Rice			Soy sauces and green teas
United States (Southern Section)		Black-eyed peas, hog jowls, and ham hocks	Collard greens, mustard greens, beet greens, and okra	Hot breads, corn bread, and hominy grits	Molasses	Salt pork, fatback	

LUNCH OR SUPPER

Main dish (macaroni and cheese, fish, poultry, meat, cottage cheese) or creamed soup
Vegetables (cooked or in salad)
Whole-wheat or enriched bread
Butter or enriched margarine
Fruit or simple dessert

MIDAFTERNOON OR BEDTIME SNACK

Milk and crackers or fruit juice

Foods that furnish practically no nutrients but many calories, such as rich sauces, gravies, pies, frosted cakes, sweet puddings, sugar, candies, and fried and fatty foods should be eliminated.

For those elderly patients who complain about a sensitive digestive system, a practical suggestion is to eat something warm or cooked at each meal and also to eat four or five light meals instead of two or three heavy ones. If one eats a large meal at noon rather than at night, distress due to indigestion at bedtime will be less likely.

PRACTICAL PROCEDURE FOR NUTRITIONAL GUIDANCE OF THE ELDERLY

For giving the preceding information the following step-by-step office procedure is recommended.

Step 1. Determine What the Patient Is Presently Eating. This is best done by having the patient keep a 3- to 5-day food diary. Simply asking the patient what he or she ate at or between meals during the last 24-hour period may not elicit an accurate account of the patient's typical diet.

Step 2. Determine Some of the Reasons for Food Selection. It is important to understand the reasons that motivate the patient to eat only tea and toast, for example. Is it loneliness? Economic problems? Lack of interest? Digestive problems?

Step 3. Evaluate the Adequacy of the Diet. Review each day of the food diary and determine if the amounts and kinds of foods actually eaten are more, the same, or less than recommended. A simple evaluation sheet that blocks off the Food Groups into days, such as the one shown in Figure 19–1, might be useful. Credit each average serving of a food in the proper block.

Step 4. Write a Diet Prescription. On the basis of information acquired from the diet evaluation sheet and from the personal and medical history, the dentist should be able to prescribe an acceptable personalized diet that is balanced, varied, and adequate for the dental-oral health problem. This is done by simply substituting at first (for example, fat-free milk instead of coffee) rather than by increasing or decreasing the total food intake. In other words, emphasize qualitative rather than quantitative improvements. After some initial changes have been accepted, the patient may be more amenable to further improvements.

Method for Assessing Adequacy of a Diet, Especially for Patients Aged 60 or Older

FOOD GROUP	PORTION SIZE CONSIDERED ONE SERVING	DAY 1	DAY 2	DAY 3	AVER-AGE	INTAKE RECOM-MENDED	ACTUAL	DIFFER-ENCE
Vegetable and Fruit	*Vitamin C Rich* 4–6 oz citrus juice ½ grapefruit, cantaloupe 1 medium orange					1–2		
	Vitamin A Rich ½ c carrots, broccoli, spinach, corn and other deep green and yellow types					1		
	Other ½ c potatoes, peas, string beans 1 medium apple					1		
Bread and Cereal	1 slice bread 1 oz (¾ c) dry cereal ½–¾ c cooked cereal, pasta					2–3		
Milk and Cheese	1 c (8 oz) milk, yogurt 1½ oz cheddar, processed cheese 1–1½ c cottage cheese					2		
Meat, Poultry Fish and Beans	2–3 oz cooked lean meat, fish, poultry 2 eggs 4 tbsp peanut butter 1 c cooked dried peas, beans or lentils					2		

°For each serving of food eaten, place a check mark in the appropriate block.

FIGURE 19–1.

Table 19–3 contains suggestions for modifying some desirable foods for patients who can manage only soft foods. Eating less food at mealtimes can be easily accomplished by omitting desserts and using them as between-meal snacks instead.

An alternative procedure for assessment of nutritional status and management of a geriatric dental patient is shown in Figure 19–2.

DIETARY SUGGESTIONS FOR DENTURE WEARERS

Food Preferences

Hartsook made a study of food preferences, dietary adequacy, and sense of taste in a group of 46 patients whose ages ranged from 37 to 78 years and who wore either full or partial dentures.[29] She found that the adequacy of these patients' diets did not differ markedly from that of similar age groups in the

Name: _____ M, S, W, Age: _____

Address: _____ Home Phone: _____

Occupation: _____ Business Phone: _____

Complaints

GENERAL	+	−	ORAL			+	−	OTHER
Loss of weight			Thirst					
Loss of appetite			Bleeding gums					
Apathy			Loose teeth					
Tiredness			Sore lips					
Nervousness			Burning tongue					
Gastrointestinal			Breath odor					
problems			Toothache					
			Denture sore spots					
			Dental cavities					
			Loss of taste and smell					
			Mucous membrane lesions					

PRESENT ILLNESS

Medical History

PERSONAL	+	−	FAMILY	+	−	MEDICATIONS	+	−
Allergy			Diabetes			Antihistamines		
Atherosclerosis			Coronary heart			Atropine		
Diabetes			disease			Belladonna		
Hyperthyroidism			Hypertension			Banthine		
Liver disease			Osteoporosis			Sleeping pills		
Gallbladder disease			Cancer			Others		
Osteoporosis			Arthritis					
Hypertension								
Vision and/or hearing								
impaired								
Tumors								

Personal and Social History

DAILY ROUTINE:	+	−		+	−
Lives alone			Literacy		
Withdrawn			Television & radio		
Confined to house			Physical handicap		
Inadequate income					

FIGURE 19–2. Case history outline for assessment and management of nutritional status in a geriatric dental patient.

Illustration continued on opposite page

Diet History

Appetite: Good _____ Fair _____ Poor _____
Person responsible for food preparation _____
Eat with family or alone? _____
Is there a craving for sweets? _____
Bedtime snacks _____
Fluorides in communal water supply? _____
Do you chew your food thoroughly? _____
Do you have any difficulty biting into raw fruit, corn on the cob, sandwiches,
    and so forth?
_____
Do you prefer soft to firm foods (e.g., cooked to raw vegetables or ground to
    chewy meat)?
_____
Is eating a pleasurable, satisfying experience? _____
Prepare own meals? _____
Precooked meals or TV dinners? _____
Read food labels, newspaper, and articles about nutrition? _____
Watch food preparation programs on TV? _____

Diet Evaluation

INADEQUACIES IN DIET	Desirable Servings	Actual Servings
Fruit and vegetables	4	_____
Bread and cereal	4	_____
Meat, fish, chicken, and legumes	2	_____
Milk and milk products	2	_____

EATING HABITS
No. of meals per day _____
No. of between-meal snacks _____
Types of snacks: Sugar-sweetened _____ Fruits and vegetables _____

General Clinical Observations

Dry skin
Edema
Skeletal

Oral Clinical Observations

Angular stomatitis _____
Glossitis _____
Pallor of the oral mucosa _____
Plaque score _____
Periodontal pocket score _____
Gingival bleeding index _____
Total number of teeth _____
Number of carious teeth _____
Carious surfaces: Cervical _____ Occlusal _____ Proximal _____

FIGURE 19–2 Continued

Illustration continued on following page

Diagnosis

Oral findings: _____

Primary causes: _____

Caused by (educational, social, psychological, or systemic factors): _____

Management

DIET PRESCRIPTION

1. Quality of diet: _____

   _____

2. Balance of meals: _____

   _____

3. Elimination of plaque-forming sweets: _____

   _____

4. Suggested meal plan:
   Breakfast:

   Lunch:

   Dinner:

   Extras:

FIGURE 19–2 Continued

general population; that the subjects aged 70 or more had the least adequate diets; and that the highest percentage of patients with a satisfactory dietary pattern appeared in the group aged 50 to 60.

She also found that all subjects, regardless of whether they wore full or partial dentures, preferred beef. Raw vegetables were best eaten in chopped form in salads. Fresh fruits, except for apples, were eaten whole. Apples were peeled, quartered, and cored before eating. Berry seeds had a tendency to be annoying because they slipped under dentures, causing some discomfort. Toasted or plain bread could be eaten equally well, with no problem. However, nuts and candy, particularly caramels and chewing gum, seemed to be difficult for the denture wearers to manage.

Helping New Denture Wearers Learn to Chew

The ability to manage the physical consistency of food can be made easier for a new denture wearer if an analysis of the jaw movements involved in mastication is made. The process of eating actually involves three steps: biting, or incising; chewing, or pulverizing; and, finally, swallowing.

Incising food involves a grasping and tearing action by the incisor teeth requiring opening the mouth wide, an action that can cause dislodgement of the denture by the pulling action of overtensed muscle. When the leverage force of the incising action is exerted in the anterior segment of the mouth, the only equal and opposite force to prevent dislodging the denture is the seal created by the postdam compressive force of the denture on the soft palate. The counter-dislodgement forces in the incising action are not as effective as, for example, the balancing forces of the occlusal surfaces of the bicuspid and molars used in the chewing process. This makes the first step, the incising action, the most difficult of all three masticating actions.

The chewing and pulverizing of the bolus of the food by the molars and bicuspids are less difficult than incising, but still, the coordination of the many muscles of mastication that produce the hinge and sliding movement of the mandible during eating requires some experience. With patience and persistence, these movements can be mastered as long as there are no sore spots or cuspal interferences created by the dentures.

Actually, the easiest and least complex step in the eating process is that of swallowing. Deglutition, with the exception of initially propelling the bolus back to the pharynx, is an involuntary action.

Therefore although the logical sequence of eating food is biting, chewing, and swallowing, it is much easier for the new denture patient to master this complex of masticatory movements in the reverse order, namely, swallowing first, chewing second, and biting last. Consequently, food of a consistency that will require only swallowing, such as liquids, should be prescribed for the first day or two after insertion of the denture. The use of soft foods is advocated for the next few days, and a firm or regular diet can be eaten by the end of the week. Regardless of its consistency, the diet can be made varied, balanced, and adequate, as will be shown in the following dietary suggestions.

Diet for the First Day After Denture Insertion[30]

On the first postinsertion day, a new denture wearer can choose from the following foods, which are essentially liquids and are arranged according to the four basic food groups:

- Vegetable-fruit group: juices
- Bread-cereal group: gruels cooked in either milk or water
- Milk group: fluid milk may be taken in any form
- Meat group: for the first day or so eggs will be the first food choice; they may be taken in eggnogs; pureed meats, meat broths, or soups may also be eaten

A sample menu using the liquid foods should include a glass of milk at least once a day and tea, coffee, or caffeine-free coffee, as desired:

Breakfast: Orange juice, strained oatmeal gruel with milk
Lunch: Cream of tomato soup, junket
Dinner: Strained cream of chicken soup, vanilla ice cream
Between meals: Eggnog, ginger ale with ice cream; cocoa or other milk drink, or even the new low-calorie nutritionally complete mixtures.

Diet for the Second and Third Days After Denture Insertion

For the second and third postinsertion days, the denture patient can use soft foods that require a minimum of chewing:

- Vegetable-fruit group: in addition to fruit and vegetable juices, tender cooked fruits and vegetables (skins and seeds must be removed), such as tender asparagus tips, cooked carrots, tender green beans, cooked or canned peaches, pears, and apricots
- Bread-cereal group: cooked cereals such as Cream of Wheat or Wheatena; milk toast and softened bread; boiled rice, spaghetti, macaroni, or noodles
- Milk group: fluid milk, cottage cheese
- Meat group: chopped beef, ground liver, tender chicken or fish in a cream sauce or even children's junior food preparations; eggs may be scrambled or soft cooked; dried peas may be used in a thick, strained soup

These foods from the daily food guide can readily be arranged into three balanced and adequate meals if the following simple steps are followed:

1. Bread or some breadstuff or cereal at each meal and some meals with both cereal and bread

2. Milk as a beverage or in foods at two of the meals

3. At least one serving from the vegetable-fruit group at each meal, citrus fruit usually at breakfast; the three or more other servings could be divided between noon and evening meals

4. One of the servings from the meat group at the evening meal and the other at the noon meal or breakfast or divided between two meals

5. A serving from either the milk or the meat group is needed at each of the three meals or a serving from both

A sample menu using soft foods would include butter or margarine with the meals, a glass of milk at least once a day, tea or coffee as desired:

Breakfast: Prune juice, soft-cooked egg, toast
Lunch: Cream of asparagus soup, cottage cheese and peaches, bread, and gingerbread
Dinner: Meat loaf with tomato sauce, creamed potatoes, green peas, bread, tapioca pudding

Diet for the Fourth Day and Later

By the fourth day, or as soon as all the sore spots have healed, in addition to the soft diet, firmer foods can be eaten. In most instances, these foods should be cut into small pieces before eating.

A sample menu using firm foods would include butter or margarine with the meals, a glass of milk at least once a day, and tea or coffee as desired.

Breakfast: Orange juice, scrambled eggs (hot cereal replaces eggs for a low-cholesterol diet), toast
Lunch: Swiss steak, mashed potatoes, broccoli, bread, chocolate pudding
Dinner: Welsh rarebit, carrot-apple salad, ice cream

In general, it has been found that raw vegetables and sandwiches are the foods least preferred by denture wearers.[31] In fact, raw vegetables require more force during mastication to prepare them for swallowing than most other foods.[32]

Therefore if the denture patient is able to manage sandwiches and salads, the ultimate in denture success and patient achievement will have been realized.

SUMMARY

Providing for the food, diet, and nutritional needs of elderly patients should be considered an indispensable part of total dental care and supportive management. It is the responsibility of the dentist to provide the patient with this nutritional information for achieving optimal oral health, because what helps prevent oral disease will be equally useful in preventing general illness.

If the clinician bears in mind that the calorie needs for an older patient are less but that all other nutrient requirements are as high in old age as they were in youth, the geriatric patient will be well cared for. Certainly, special environmental, physiological, and psychological problems also need to be considered.

The best possible general advice is that the patient's daily diet should include vegetables and fruits; bread and cereals; milk and cheese; and poultry, fish, and legumes plus significant amounts of water (4 to 8 glasses per day). We suggest that there be more emphasis on high-quality protein foods and a generous selection of vegetables and fruits and that there be somewhat less emphasis on fats and sugars, in order to avoid an excess of calories. For the geriatric wearer of new dentures, each diet prescription should be based on an analysis and evaluation of the person's food habits and reasons for them and the actual food intake. Furthermore, the physical nature of the diet should be consistent with the patient's experience and ability to swallow, chew, and bite with the dental prosthesis, and with other medical problems, such as diabetes diets, low cholesterol diets, and so on.

REFERENCES

1. Blumberg, J.B. Nutrient requirements for the healthy elderly. Contemp. Nutr., 11(6):1–2, 1986.
2. Butler, R.N.; McGuire, E.A.H. Foreword to symposium on evidence relating selected vitamins and minerals to health and disease in the elderly population in the United States. Am. J. Clin. Nutr. 36(Suppl.):977, 1982.
3. Young, E.F. Nutrition, aging and the aged. Med. Clin. North Am. 67:295, 1983.
3a. McGandy, R.B.; Russell, R.M.; Hartz, S.C., et al. Nutritional status survey of healthy noninstitutionalized elderly: energy and nutrient intakes from three day diet records and nutrient supplements. Nutr. Res. (in press).
3b. Papas, A.; Heffernen, J.H. Nutrition and preventive needs of the elderly. American Dental Association Clinical Geriatric Dentistry 1986 Symposium. Chicago, Sept. 1986.
4. Committee on Dietary Allowances, Food and Nutrition Board, National Academy of Sciences-National Research Council. Recommended Dietary Allowances, 9th rev. ed. Washington, D.C., National Academy Press, 1980.
5. National Institute of Arthritis, Diabetes and Digestive and Kidney Diseases. Osteoporosis, Cause, Treatment, Prevention. NIH Publication no. 83-2226. Washington, D.C., GPO, April 1983.
6. Nutrition and the elderly. Dairy Council Digest 54(4): July-August 1983.
7. Heaney, R.P.; Gallagher, J.C.; Johnston, C.C., et al. Calcium nutrition and bone health in the elderly. Am. J. Clin. Nutr. 36(Suppl.):986, 1982.
8. Parfitt, A.M.; Gallagher, J.C.; Heaney, R.P., et al. Vitamin D and bone health in the elderly. Am. J. Clin. Nutr. 36(Suppl.):1014, 1982.
9. Rogoff, G.S.; Galburt, R.B.; Nizel, A.E. Role of dietary calcium and vitamin D in alveolar bone health. In Rubin, R.P.; Weiss, G.B.; Putney, J.W., eds. Calcium in Biological Systems. pp. 591–595. New York, Plenum Publishing Corp., 1985.

10. Lynch, S.R.; Finch, C.A., et al. Iron status of elderly Americans. Am. J. Clin. Nutr. 36(Suppl.):1032, 1982.
11. Sandstead, H.A., et al. Zinc nutriture in the elderly in relation to taste acuity, immune response, and wound healing. Am. J. Clin Nutr. 36(Suppl.):1046, 1982.
12. Bowman, B.B.; Rosenberg, I.H. Assessment of the nutritional status of the elderly. Am. J. Clin. Nutr. 36(Suppl.):1142, 1982.
13. Newton, H.M.V., et al. The relations between vitamin D_2 and D_3 in the diet and plasma 25,OH-D_2 and 25,OH-D_3 in elderly women in Great Britain. Am. J. Clin. Nutr. 41:760, 1985.
14. Vatassery, G.T., et al. Changes in vitamin E concentrations in human plasma and platelets with age. J. Am. Col. Nutr. 4:369, 1983.
15. Yearick, E. S., et al. Nutritional status of the elderly: dietary and biochemical findings. J. Gerontol. 5:663, 1980.
16. Loh, H.S. The relationship between dietary ascorbic acid intake and buffy coat and plasma ascorbic acid concentrations at different ages. Int. J. Vitam. Nutr. Res. 42:80, 1972.
17. Ibes, F.L.; Blass, J.P.; Brin, M., et al. Folate nutrition in the elderly. Am. J. Clin. Nutr. 36(Suppl.):1060, 1982.
18. Rosenberg, I.H.; Bowman, B.B.; Cooper, B.A., et al. Folate nutrition in the elderly. J. Am. Clin. Nutr. 36(Suppl.):1000, 1982.
19. Guilland, J.C., et al. Evaluation of the pyridoxine intake and pyridoxine status among aged institutionalized people. Int. J. Vitam. Nutr. Res. 54:185, 1984.
20. Alfano, M.C. The origin of gingival fluid. J. Theor. Biol. 47:127, 1974.
21. Johansen, E.; Olsen, T. Topical fluorides in the prevention and arrest of dental caries. In Johansen E.; Taves, D.R., eds. Continuing Evaluation of the Use of Fluorides. Boulder, Col., Westview Press, 1979.
22. Wical, K.E.; Swoope, C.C. Studies of residual ridge resorption. Part II, The relationship of dietary calcium and phosphorus to residual ridge resorption. J. Prosthet. Dent. 32:13, 1974.
23. Wical, K. E.; Brusse, P. Effects of calcium and vitamin D supplement on alveolar ridge resorption in immediate denture patients. J. Prosthet. Dent. 41:4, 1979.
24. Dickerson, J.W.T.; Walker, R. Nutrition, age and drug metabolism. Proc. Nutr. Soc. 33:191, 1974.
25. Arenillas, L. Amitriptyline and body weight. Lancet 1:432, 1964.
26. Gander, D.R.; Lord, M.B. Treatment of depressive illnesses with combined antidepressants. Lancet 2:107, 1965.
27. Roe, D.A. Drugs, diet and nutrition. Am. Pharm. 18(10):62, 1978.
28. Roe, D.A. Nutrient and drug interactions. Nutr. Rev. 42:141, 1984.
29. Hartsook, E.I. Food selection, dietary adequacy and related dental problems of patients with dental prostheses. J. Prosthet. Dent. 32:32, 1974.
30. Nizel, A.E. Role of nutrition in the oral health of the aging patient. In Winkler, S., et al. Essentials of Complete Denture Prosthodontics, pp. 480–492. Philadelphia, W.B. Saunders Co., 1979.
31. Yurkstas, A.; Emerson, H. Dietary selections of persons with natural and artificial teeth. J. Prosthet. Dent. 14:695, 1964.
32. Yurkstas, A.; Curby, W.A. Force analysis of prosthetic appliances during function. J. Prosthet. Dent. 3:83, 1953.

20

How to Deliver and Market a Preventive Dentistry Service, Including Nutritional Counseling

WHAT IS PREVENTIVE DENTISTRY? WHY PRACTICE IT?

In the 1980s, physicians and dentists are expected not only to cure patients but also to keep them well. Thus health professionals should provide their patients with an effective preventive program.

Glickman aptly described the dental profession's responsibility: "The idea of preventing disease is not new; the idea that teeth should be cleaned is not new. What is new is the realization that to fulfill the franchise it holds for the oral health of the public, dentistry must shift the emphasis from the repair of disease-damaged tissues to the prevention of disease—and that the time to do it is now."[1]

Preventive dentistry deals with the *causes* (both direct and indirect) of such common problems as dental caries and periodontal disease. Direct causes are those factors that affect the chemistry and structure of the tooth, its supporting structures, and its oral environment. Indirect causes are the environmental, systemic, psychological, and social factors influencing the patient's attitudes, oral hygiene practices, food choices, and eating habits. No one will deny that it is the dentist's professional responsibility to deal with the causes as well as the effects of dental-oral diseases. Patients not only expect this service but in fact demand it. Further, to ignore the practice of preventive dentistry may be unprofessional or even unethical. Some dentists have been accused and sued for malpractice for not recognizing the existence of or for not dealing with the causes of a condition such as periodontal disease.

Some practitioners claim properly that they are practicing preventive dentistry by extending the margins of the cavity preparations into self-cleansing areas when restoring their patients' carious teeth. They are indeed practicing *secondary prevention* by *controlling* and thus delaying the progress of recurrent caries. But is it not more rewarding to ensure the health of the natural dentition by practicing *primary prevention*, which deals with *inhibiting* the potential causes of dental caries (e.g., poor plaque control or poor food selection, or both)?

Is Providing a Primary Preventive Dentistry Service Against the Interests of the General Dental Practitioner?

Superficially, it might appear that a dentist's income will suffer if he or she promotes primary preventive dentistry services. The fact is that the opposite occurs. The income increases. How?

1. Practitioners who deliver the proper combination of preventive dentistry services will establish a reputation in the community of being *thorough, caring*, and *willing* to explain and to advise patients on the daily home care procedures that can help preserve their natural teeth in most instances for a lifetime. Word-of-mouth advertising by satisfied and appreciative patients will result in the referral of more new patients, the mainstay of any dental practice.

2. Practitioners will be able to use the time of their dental hygienists more effectively. An increase in preventive dentistry services rendered by dental hygienists will of course generate more income. These auxiliaries can be employed full time, because they are trained to take dental x-rays, thoroughly chart the mouth, and provide a comprehensive preventive dentistry service, which includes plaque control instruction, scaling and prophylaxis, application of topical fluorides, application of fissure sealants, and nutrition counseling when indicated.

3. Patients appreciate the continued use of their natural teeth, which is made possible as a result of such an all-inclusive preventive dentistry program. However, if the primary preventive services are ineffective, saving the natural teeth by secondary disease control measures, namely, restorations, will be much appreciated even when they involve such services as endodontics, periodontics, and the fabrication of crowns. These latter necessary services, which require much time and skill, must be paid for by the patients, but these procedures are seen as worthwhile because the patients will have preserved their natural teeth.

In short, a practice will flourish when it identifies preventive services as an essential component of an all-inclusive dental health care service.

WHAT ARE THE WEAKNESSES IN THE PRACTICE OF PREVENTIVE DENTISTRY? HOW CAN THEY BE ELIMINATED?

The two major weaknesses in some of the present practices of preventive dentistry are (1) a less-than-effective, limited preventive service deals with only a *few* causes, rather than a comprehensive service dealing with *all* the known causes; and (2) preventive dental services are not delivered in an *orderly, organized, objective,* and *thorough fashion* consisting of a history, examination, diagnosis, and management procedures.

Comprehensive Versus Limited Preventive Services

Before the 1940s, preventive dentistry consisted of (1) a dental hygiene service, i.e., scaling and oral prophylaxis twice a year in order to inhibit under usual circumstances the development of periodontal disease and (2) a dental examination for caries and defective restorations.

From the late 1940s, as a result of the discovery of the caries-inhibitory properties of fluoride, professionally applied topical fluorides have been accepted as another essential preventive office procedure.

However, there are at least five more chairside and counseling services that can significantly contribute to making preventive services comprehensive and useful:

1. A complete dental hygiene home care counseling service that includes plaque control instruction and the prescription of fluoride oral rinses when indicated

2. Personalized dietary or nutrition counseling plus the prescription of fluoride supplements when indicated

3. Application of fissure sealants in deep pits and fissures of posterior teeth

4. Fabrication of mouth guards to prevent possible tooth fractures when engaged in contact sports

5. Fabrication of space maintainers to prevent malocclusion and tooth arrangement irregularities after the removal of a permanent tooth in an adolescent

Why then the limitation to only two preventive dentistry services? Reasons for this incomplete, inadequate approach include lack of knowledge or experience in the following areas:

- Preventive evaluation and diagnosis
- Performance and delivery of effective counseling that will motivate patients to carry out home care dental regimens for optimal oral health
- Delivery of a preventive service that can be monitored
- Requests for adequate fees for preventive services
- Requests for inclusion of the additional five preventive services as part of the ordinary preventive dental insurance package

Preventive Dentistry: Evangelism or Pragmatic Chairside and Counseling Services?

About 10 years ago there was a movement to give preventive dentistry its rightful place in general dental practice. Although the philosophy was readily adopted by the profession, a delivery method was lacking. A transition from theory to practice was needed but was not happening. No wonder the preventive dentistry bubble burst. On the other hand, we would like to suggest that there is a pragmatic office procedure, that there is a method for visualizing and measuring in quantitative terms the clinical effects of preventive dentistry services, and that there is a practice-management aspect that is remunerative.

We believe that the time is now to convince ourselves, our patients, and insurance carriers that preventive dentistry is not a theoretical, esoteric service but rather is an essential one that is objective and that can be monitored.[2]

We have found the following to be a realistic, visit-by-visit, step-by-step office procedure for delivering a substantive, comprehensive, preventive dentistry service that can be both profitable and inwardly rewarding.

OFFICE PROCEDURE FOR DELIVERY OF A COMPREHENSIVE AND OBJECTIVE PREVENTIVE SERVICE

A bare minimum of two visits is essential for the delivery of an adequate preventive service. There may be instances when three, four, or even five visits may be necessary to accomplish all the indicated services and for the patients to be able to care for themselves adequately.

Visit 1

PROCEDURES

- Do a case history and examination to arrive at a diagnosis
- Establish the appropriate preventive management program
- Educate the patient about the causes and effects of dental caries and periodontal disease
- Instruct the patient on a home care oral hygiene program
- When indicated, instruct the patient on how to keep a 5-day food diary.

STEP 1: IDENTIFYING DATA ON CASE RECORD (Fig. 20–1)

The name, address, age, nationality, occupation, and so forth are ascertained in order to establish whether there is a correlation between the dental condition and these identifying data. For example, a propensity toward periodontal disease is found in Far Eastern population groups.

STEP 2. PREVENTIVE HISTORY (Fig. 20–1)

A preventive history is primarily concerned with establishing the patient's oral hygiene habits and the environmental (social, psychological, economic) factors that may influence behavior and habits. These last may have a bearing on the dental health status.

We ask all patients to demonstrate their usual oral hygiene home care procedures to establish how effectively they execute them.

Also, we are interested in knowing their vocation, avocation, and daily routine, which can influence food choices and eating habits.

STEP 3. PREVENTIVE EXAMINATION (Fig. 20–1)

We record the Caries Score, the Gingival Index, Plaque Score, and Dental Health Diet Score. The numerical values for each of these conditions provides an objective measurement rather than a qualitative description of some of the clinical conditions that are associated with dental caries and periodontal disease.

Dental Caries Score. The dental caries score is important because it can express in a single set of figures the number of decayed and filled tooth surfaces (DFS) at a certain time. This can serve as the baseline from which future caries increments can be calculated. Thus a condition of rampant caries, usual and customary caries experience, or caries resistance can be established.

Name: __Robert Myers__ Age: _16_ Sex: _M_ Nationality: _U.S. Citizen_

Occupation: __Student__ Height: _6'3"_ Actual Weight: _175_ Desired Weight: _180_

Preventive History

PAST AND PRESENT HISTORY

Fluoride intake: (Water supply, lozenges, topicals, rinses, dentrifice for how long?)
MDC water supply fluoridated in 1978; no fluoride lozenges or rinse;
topical fluoride tmt. once at age 10

Oral hygiene habits: (Brush, floss, how often, time spent)?
Brushes teeth before breakfast, for a few seconds;
no definite method. Never uses floss.

FAMILY DENTAL HISTORY

(Caries, periodontal disease, edentulism in parents and siblings?)
Father: full dentures at age 42; lost teeth owing to caries.
Mother: lost 4 teeth owing to periodontitis; remaining teeth sound due
to extensive tmt. Sister (age 18) has good dental health.

SOCIAL HISTORY

(Habits, daily routine: include activity [sedentary, athletic, etc.], interests, hobbies, etc.)
Robert attends high school and is a member of the varsity basketball
team. During summer vacation he helps out in family business (small
grocery store). After school he does homework, rides his bicycle, or
practices basketball. Evenings are spent watching T.V. or listening to stereo.

HOME AND FAMILY SITUATION

(Live alone or with friends or with family? Who buys food and prepares meals? With whom
do you eat?)
Lives with parents and sister. Mother shops and prepares evening
meal. Family members make their own breakfast and lunch,
or buy them.

STRESSES

(At work, at home, etc.)
Robert's major stress is related to schoolwork: he wants to obtain
athletic scholarship for college & must keep grades high, while devoting
time to basketball.

Richard Roe, D.M.D.
Signature

Preventive Examination

CARIES SCORE

$$\frac{DFS}{All\ S} = \frac{number\ of\ decayed\ and\ filled\ surfaces\ present}{total\ number\ of\ tooth\ surfaces\ at\ risk} = {}^{15}/_{120}$$

(No. of ant. teeth × 4 + no. of post. teeth × 5)

ORAL HYGIENE STATUS Poor

Plaque control skills (thoroughness, dexterity?) Excellent dexterity, but lacks
thoroughness and a definite method of brushing.

	First Visit	Subsequent Visit	Case Completion
Gingival Index	10/24	8/24	4/24
Plaque Score	52%	78%	85%

FIGURE 20–1. Preventive dentistry record.

There are two acceptable methods for measuring the Caries Score. The first is by adding the number of decayed, missing, and filled tooth surfaces symbolized as DMFS. The second method, which omits the missing (M) surfaces, is more precise, because the number of teeth at risk varies considerably during the childhood years when the dentition is changing from deciduous to permanent. This method also eliminates the possibility that the cause of the missing tooth is other than caries. The formula is DFS/S (total number of decayed and filled surfaces divided by total number of surfaces at risk.)

Gingival Index (Fig. 20–2). The Gingival Index interprets quantitatively the relative degree of gingival inflammation or bleeding tendency. The degree of gingival redness, puffiness, and tendency to bleed around six teeth is ascertained. These teeth are representative of all the dentition from an anatomical and location standpoint.[3]

#9: the maxillary left central incisor
#12: the maxillary left first bicuspid
#3: the maxillary right first molar
#25: the mandibular right central incisor
#28: the mandibular right first bicuspid
#19: the mandibular left first molar

If any of these teeth are missing, their adjoining counterparts are used.

The degree of inflammation (0 to 3) of the gingiva on the mesial, distal, buccal, and lingual surfaces of the six representative teeth (a total of 24 surfaces at risk) is determined.[4]

0 = normal gingival appearance
1 = mildly inflamed gingiva
2 = moderately inflamed gingiva that bleed on probing
3 = severely inflamed gingiva with spontaneous bleeding

The grade degree of inflammation around each of these surfaces is added and divided by 24 (the total number of surfaces at risk). Therefore, the best gingival health index is 0/24 and the worst, as much as 72/24.

The Plaque-Free Score (Fig. 20–3). The Plaque-Free Score is determined from an examination of the presence of disclosed plaque on four surfaces—facial,

	Example				**Date**				**Date**				**Date**			
	M	B	D	L	M	B	D	L	M	B	D	L	M	B	D	L
UL central incisor	1	1	1	1												
UL 1st bicuspid	0	2	0	2												
UR 1st molar	0	0	0	0												
LR central incisor	3	3	3	3												
LR 1st bicuspid	0	0	0	0												
LL 1st molar	0	2	0	2												

FIGURE 20–2. *Chart for recording Gingival Index and Plaque-Free Score. Gingival Index, according to Löe and Silness. Key: 0 = normal, pink, and stippled; 1 = slight marginal redness; 2 = moderate inflammation (bleeding on probing); 3 = severe inflammation (spontaneous bleeding). Index = Total score/Total surfaces. In the example, Index = 24/24 = 1. (Modified from Löe, H.; Silness, J. Periodontal disease in pregnancy. I. Prevalence and severity. Acta Odontol. Scand. 21:533–551, 1963.)*

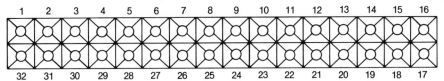

FIGURE 20–3. Tufts plaque-free index. A minimum of 80% of surfaces must be plaque-free before clinical periodontal services are rendered.

$$\frac{Total\ no.\ of\ surfaces\ with\ plaque}{Total\ no.\ of\ surfaces\ at\ risk} = plaque\ index$$

lingual, mesial, and distal. Presence of plaque is designated by shading in the appropriate surfaces. The acceptable minimal goal is 85% plaque-free.

Dental Health Diet Scores. Scores have been devised for dental caries and periodontal disease (Fig. 17–5). They are found by evaluating the points for the frequency of eating sugar-sweetened foods or other undesirable foods and the points for eating an adequate, balanced, and varied diet of protective foods, especially those rich in the nutrients necessary for good dental and periodontal health (Figs. 17–4 and 17–5). If the diet score is 64 or below, the patient needs detailed personalized nutritional counseling based upon a 5-day food diary.

STEP 4. PREVENTIVE DIAGNOSIS (Fig. 20–4)

The essential parts of the preventive diagnosis are the direct and indirect causes for the current condition or the anticipated state if existing oral hygiene and nutrition habits are continued.

The indirect factors are most important, because they deal with the patient's behavior. Without determining and understanding the contributing stimuli that influence a patient's daily activities and habits, an improvement in the patient's behavior is impossible.

STEP 5. PREVENTIVE MANAGEMENT REGIMEN

Scores and clinical conditions that indicate a specific preventive service are in Figure 20–4, a preventive diagnosis chart. Detailed techniques for performing each of these preventive services, i.e., plaque control counseling,[5] diet counseling for caries prevention and caries control (Chap. 17), prescribing fluoride,[6] applying topical fluorides[7], applying fissure sealants,[8] and making mouth guards and space maintainers,[9] are described elsewhere.[10]

STEP 6. TEACHING ABOUT THE CAUSES AND EFFECTS OF DENTAL CARIES AND PERIODONTAL DISEASE

Teaching aids such as ivorene tooth models depicting dental caries or periodontal disease and booklets with photographs and charts of the oral structures in health and disease such as the "Chairside Instructor" (from the American Dental Association) are recommended. For us, one of the best teaching aids has been sketching diagrams of the tooth, supporting structures, and the

Dietary Status:
1. Food allergies, food likes and dislikes, and eating habits

2. Dental health diet score

3. Dietary deficiencies or excesses

Preventive Diagnosis:
Oral diagnosis (caries rate? gingivitis? other?)

Primary causes

Results from (educational, social, psychological, or systemic factors)

Preventive Management (Circle the Relevant Phrase):
1. No preventive services indicated

2. Following preventive services indicated; signify by the word "needed"

3. Following preventive services not indicated; signify by the words "not needed"

	Treatment Plan
PVPH Plaque Control Counseling	
PVNT Nutrition Counseling	
PVOR Fluoride Oral Rinse	
PVTF Topical Fluoride	
PVMG Mouthguard	
PVFS Fissure Sealants	

Instructor's Signature

Home Care Instructions and Prescriptions:
1. Plaque control instruction (suggested methods for improvement):

2. Types of toothbrush, interdental cleansing device, oral rinse, dentrifice prescribed:

3. Dietary modification prescribed:

Patient Attitude and Knowledge (pretest vs. post-test results):

FIGURE 20–4. Preventive Diagnosis Chart.

factors that contribute to each of the steps in the dental caries or periodontal disease processes or both. This method holds the patients' interest and they seem to learn more than with any other educational tool.

It is important that simple, nontechnical language be used. The gingival location for plaque accumulation, the gingival crevice, is best understood if it is referred to as the "cuff" of the gum tissue around the tooth. Also, the use of analogies to an everyday experience can make some points clearer to the patient.

STEP 7. PLAQUE CONTROL COUNSELING

Demonstrate the use of disclosing solution and the appropriate techniques with the toothbrush, floss, or interdental cleansing devices (rubber tips, perioaids, stimudents) for removing the plaque without injury to the tooth and especially to the gingival tissues. Have the patient repeat these techniques and demonstrate dexterity and proficiency. Correct errors and concentrate on improving problem areas.

STEP 8. KEEPING A 5-DAY FOOD DIARY

If the Dental Health Diet Score is 56 or less, the patient needs dietary or nutritional counseling and should be given a 5-day food diary to complete. It is important to instruct patients about keeping an accurate and complete food diary. This is best done by reviewing the patient's previous 24-hour food intake and recording type of food, its preparation, amount, and the time when each meal or between-meal snack was eaten. The sequence of eating foods should also be kept accurately. Special attention is paid to including the snacks, chewing gum, candies, cookies, soft drinks, and other extras eaten during a day. For the step-by-step procedures for making a dietary (for the caries patient) or nutritional (for the periodontal patient) diagnosis and management see Chap. 17 and 18, respectively.

Visit 2 (5 to 7 Days Later)

PROCEDURES

- Record Gingival Index and Plaque Score; compare with those of Visit 1
- Review plaque control procedures if Plaque Score is below 80% plaque-free
- Perform scaling and oral prophylaxis
- Apply topical fluorides, if indicated
- Give dietary or nutritional counseling if indicated

Visit 3 (or 4) (1 or More Weeks Later)

PROCEDURES

- Record Gingival Index and Plaque Score and compare with those of Visit 2
- Review plaque control procedure if Plaque Score is below 80% plaque-free
- Recheck dietary changes and behavioral changes
- Apply sealants or fabricate mouthguards (for tooth protection in contact sports) or space maintainers to prevent malocclusion
- Assess patient's oral health knowledge and attitude about the value of preventive services

SUGGESTED FEES FOR PREVENTIVE DENTISTRY SERVICES

In the past, dentists have not charged for professional services that did not necessitate "wet finger" technical procedures with results that were objective. Fortunately, most practicing dentists today consider subjective services such as diagnosis and treatment planning based on clinical and radiographic findings worth a fee.

The counseling services dealing with plaque control and dietary (for caries) and nutritional (for periodontal problems) guidance are similar to oral diagnosis in that they are judgmental and advisory rather than technical or mechanical. Similarly, they should be compensated on the basis of amount of time spent in counseling and motivating the patient to be diligent about home care preventive procedures.

An equitable fee for counseling can be easily determined by deciding what a dental hygienist should gross for the office in an 8-hour day. Since hygienists usually are responsible for providing most preventive services, one can use their expected gross intake per day as a baseline figure for any portion of that time that is spent in counseling. For example, the customary fee for a scaling and oral prophylaxis performed by a dental hygienist currently varies from approximately $25.00 to $35.00 per hour. Thus if two or more visits are required for plaque control instruction or diet counseling, the total suggested fee is calculated on the customary hourly rate. A preventive dentistry service should include a prophylaxis, scaling, oral health education, and plaque control instructions, and nutrition counseling if needed. Additional visits for reinforcement, if necessary, will require an additional fee.

Keep in mind that the initial reaction to any fee may be unsettling. But as when periodontal and endodontic fees were first established, based on the significant benefits to the patient, the special knowledge and training required for the performance of the service, and the time spent, the suggested preventive fees seem reasonable.

SUMMARY

Preventive dentistry services must be considered an integral part of any total patient care service. Based on current knowledge, a comprehensive preventive dentistry service constitutes much more than the limited services that have been practiced. Only by including additional services, particularly plaque control counseling and nutritional guidance can the major causes of the common dental problems—dental caries and periodontal disease—be dealt with adequately.

The important point is that judgments and advice based on substantive findings (expressed numerically) are as much a part of the practice of dentistry as amalgam or gold restorations. Therefore an equitable fee based on the time spent for these preventive services should be charged.

Finally, the American Dental Association has recognized these preventive services as bonafide ones and has given them a code number. Therefore these services should be charged to insured and uninsured patients alike. The preventive services and fees should be itemized on insurance claim forms so that the third-party payers can develop a utilization and a customary fee profile for preventive dentistry services. This should help insurance companies sell a broader dental benefit coverage to prospective customers and should also assist prompt reimbursement for the comprehensive preventive dentistry services being provided by the dentist and dental hygienist.

In conclusion, the Council on Dental Health of the American Dental Association makes this statement regarding preventive dentistry:

The Council has long supported the concept of preventive dentistry and in 1971 adopted the following policy:[11]

The importance of effective preventive oral health practices in the dental office is recognized and the implementation of such programs in the care and treatment of every dental patient is encouraged. A wide range of procedures can be incorporated into a preventive dental program. Recommended procedures include

• Complete medical history and clinical diagnosis, including hard and soft tissue examination and occlusal evaluation

• Examination for oral manifestations of systemic disease

• Oral prophylaxis with periodic recall, as indicated

• Prescription of supplemental dietary fluoride in fluoride-deficient areas

• Nutritional analysis and dietary counseling with regard to oral health and what promotes good dental health

• Laboratory tests to determine caries activity and susceptibility, as indicated

• Oral biopsy and cytology, as indicated

• An effective plaque control program to include individual oral hygiene instruction, toothbrushing technique, flossing technique, use of disclosing tablets or solutions, as indicated

• Procedures to prevent or intercept malocclusion including habit control, use of space maintainers, prevention of premature loss of teeth

• Construction of mouth protectors for use in contact sports

• Patient education involving discussion of good health and the cause of dental disease, and the distribution of health education literature and preservation of audio-visual materials. . . .

REFERENCES

1. Glickman, I. Chairside preventive dentistry. Dent. Clin. North Am. 16:607, 1972.
2. Nizel, A. E. How to deliver a comprehensive preventive dentistry service that dental insurance carriers can underwrite. J. Am. Dent. Assoc. 92:911, 1976.
3. Ramfjord, S. P. The periodontal index (PDI). J. Periodontol. 38:602, 1967.
4. Löe, H.; Silness, J. Periodontal disease in pregnancy. I. Prevalence and severity. Acta Odont. Scand. 21:533, 1963.
5. Less, W. Mechanics of teaching plaque control. Dent. Clin. North Am. 16:647, 1972.
6. Council on Dental Therapeutics. Prescribing fluoride supplements. In Accepted Dental Therapeutics, 37th ed., pp. 293–294. Chicago, American Dental Association, 1977.
7. Katz, S.; McDonald, J. L.; Stookey, G. K. Preventive Dentistry in Action, pp. 167–188. Upper Montclair, N.J., D.C.P. Publishing, 1972.
8. Buonocore, M. G. Adhesives for pit and fissure caries control. Dent. Clin. North Am. 16:693, 1972.
9. Burstone, C. J. Preventive orthodontics. In Bernier, J. L.; Muhler, J.C., eds. Improving Dental Practice Through Preventive Measures, 3rd ed., pp. 204–224. St. Louis, Mo., C.V. Mosby Co., 1975.
10. Palmer, C.; Rounds, M. Clinical Preventive Dentistry, Student Manual. Boston, Mass., Tufts University School of Dental Medicine, 1988.
11. Council on Dental Health, American Dental Association. In Transactions 1971, p. 53. 112th Annual Session, Proceedings of Conference on Preventive Dentistry, Atlantic City, N.J., Oct. 10–14, 1971.

Appendix 1

Table of Nutritive Values of Foods

Appendix 1 is a compilation of information from two sources, U.S. and Canadian: a shortened version of a table that appears on pages 10–61 in the Home and Garden Bulletin Number 72, authored by Susan E. Gebhardt and Ruth H. Matthews, published in 1960, plus items from "Nutrient Value of Some Common Foods," revised in 1987, published by the authority of the Minister of National Health and Welfare, Health Services and Promotion Branch in cooperation with Health Protection Branch, Canada. The Canadian material is reproduced with permission of the Minister of Supply and Services Canada. The unabridged version of the Home and Garden Bulletin table was revised in 1981 and was published by the Human Nutrition Information Service of the U.S. Department of Agriculture.

We are including only the nutritive values of foods that can help promote dental-oral health. These foods are dairy products; eggs; fish and shellfish; fruits and fruit juices; grain products; legumes, nuts, and seeds; meat and meat products; poultry and poultry products; mixed dishes including some fast foods; and finally vegetables and vegetable products. Also included are food sources of vitamins B_6, B_{12}, D, and E, and of folacin, iodine, magnesium, and zinc.

Please note: Tr in the table indicates that a nutrient is present in trace amounts. A superscript 1 in the Food Energy column means that the value is given in kilocalories.

Item No.	Foods, Approximate Measures, Units, and Weight (Weight of Edible Portion Only)	Grams	Water (%)	Food Energy (cal)	Protein (g)	Fat (g)	Saturated (g)	Mono-unsaturated (g)	Poly-unsaturated (g)
	Dairy Products								
	Butter. See Fats and Oils (items 128–130)								
	Cheese								
	Natural								
30	Blue	1 oz	28	42	100	6	8	5.3	2.2	0.2
	Brick	45	41	167[1]	10	13	8		Tr
31	Camembert (3 wedges per 4-oz container)	1 wedge	38	52	115	8	9	5.8	2.7	0.3
	Cheddar								
32	Cut pieces	1 oz	28	37	115	7	9	6.0	2.7	0.3
33		1 in³	17	37	70	4	6	3.6	1.6	0.2
34	Shredded	1 c	113	37	455	28	37	23.8	10.6	1.1
	Cottage (curd not pressed down)								
	Creamed (cottage cheese, 4% fat)								
35	Large curd	1 c	225	79	235	28	10	6.4	2.9	0.3
36	Small curd	1 c	210	79	215	26	9	6.0	2.7	0.3
37	With fruit	1 c	226	72	280	22	8	4.9	2.2	0.2
38	Lowfat (2%)	1 c	226	79	205	31	4	2.8	1.2	0.1
39	Uncreamed (cottage cheese dry curd, less than ½% fat)	1 c	145	80	125	25	1	0.4	0.2	Tr
40	Cream	1 oz	28	54	100	2	10	6.2	2.8	0.4
41	Feta	1 oz	28	55	75	4	6	4.2	1.3	0.2
	Gouda	45	41	164[1]	11	13	8		Tr
	Gruyere	45	33	186[1]	13	15	9		Tr
	Mozzarella, made with								
42	Whole milk	1 oz	28	54	80	6	6	3.7	1.9	0.2
43	Part skim milk (low moisture)	1 oz	28	49	80	8	5	3.1	1.4	0.1
44	Muenster	1 oz	28	42	105	7	9	5.4	2.5	0.2
	Parmesan, grated								
45	Cup, not pressed down	1 c	100	18	455	42	302	19.1	8.7	0.7
46	Tablespoon	1 tbsp	5	18	25	2	2	1.0	0.4	Tr
47	Ounce	1 oz	28	18	130	12	9	5.4	2.5	0.2
48	Provolone	1 oz	28	41	100	7	8	4.8	2.1	0.2
	Ricotta, made with								
49	Whole milk	1 c	246	72	430	28	32	20.4	8.9	0.9
50	Part skim milk	1 c	246	74	340	28	19	12.1	5.7	0.6
51	Swiss	1 oz	28	37	105	8	8	5.0	2.1	0.3
	Pasteurized process cheese								
52	American	1 oz	28	39	105	6	9	5.6	2.5	0.3
53	Swiss	1 oz	28	42	95	7	7	4.5	2.0	0.2
54	Pasteurized process cheese food, American	1 oz	28	43	95	6	7	4.4	2.0	0.2
55	Pasteurized process cheese spread, American	1 oz	28	48	80	5	6	3.8	1.8	0.2
	Cream, sweet								
56	Half-and-half (cream and milk)	1 c	242	81	315	7	28	17.3	8.0	1.0
57		1 tbsp	15	81	20	Tr	2	1.1	0.5	0.1
58	Light, coffee, or table	1 c	240	74	470	6	46	28.8	13.4	1.7
59		1 tbsp	15	74	30	Tr	3	1.8	0.8	0.1

| | | | | | | | Nutrients in Indicated Quantity | | | | | | |

Cholesterol (mg)	Carbohydrate (g)	Calcium (mg)	Phosphorus (mg)	Iron (mg)	Potassium (mg)	Sodium (mg)	Vitamin A Value		Thiamin (mg)	Riboflavin (mg)	Niacin (mg)	Ascorbic Acid (mg)	Item No.
							IU	RE					
21	1	150	110	0.1	73	396	200	65	0.01	0.11	0.3	0	30
42	1	303		0.2	61	252	136		Tr	0.16	2.5	0	
27	Tr	147	132	0.1	71	320	350	96	0.01	0.19	0.2	0	31
30	Tr	204	145	0.2	28	176	300	86	0.01	0.11	Tr	0	32
18	Tr	123	87	0.1	17	105	180	52	Tr	0.06	Tr	0	33
119	1	815	579	0.8	111	701	1,200	342	0.03	0.42	0.1	0	34
34	6	135	297	0.3	190	911	370	108	0.05	0.37	0.3	Tr	35
31	6	126	277	0.3	177	850	340	101	0.04	0.34	0.3	Tr	36
25	30	108	236	0.2	151	915	280	81	0.04	0.29	0.2	Tr	37
19	8	155	340	0.4	217	918	160	45	0.05	0.42	0.3	Tr	38
10	3	46	151	0.3	47	19	40	12	0.04	0.21	0.2	0	39
31	1	23	30	0.3	34	84	400	124	Tr	0.06	Tr	0	40
25	1	140	96	0.2	18	316	130	36	0.04	0.24	0.3	0	41
52	1	321		0.1	55	376		80	0.01	0.15	2.7	0	
50	Tr	455		Tr	36	151		135	0.03	0.13	3.2	0	
22	1	147	105	0.1	19	106	220	68	Tr	0.07	Tr	0	42
15	1	207	149	0.1	27	150	180	54	0.01	0.10	Tr	0	43
27	Tr	203	133	0.1	38	178	320	90	Tr	0.09	Tr	0	44
79	4	1,376	807	1.0	107	1,861	700	173	0.05	0.39	0.3	0	45
4	Tr	69	40	Tr	5	93	40	9	Tr	0.02	Tr	0	46
22	1	390	229	0.3	30	528	200	49	0.01	0.11	0.1	0	47
20	1	214	141	0.1	39	248	230	75	0.01	0.09	Tr	0	48
124	7	509	389	0.9	257	207	1,210	330	0.03	0.48	0.3	0	49
76	13	669	449	1.1	307	307	1,060	278	0.05	0.46	0.2	0	50
26	1	272	171	Tr	31	74	240	72	0.01	0.10	Tr	0	51
27	Tr	174	211	0.1	46	406	340	82	0.01	0.10	Tr	0	52
24	1	219	216	0.2	61	388	230	65	Tr	0.08	Tr	0	53
18	2	163	130	0.2	79	337	260	62	0.01	0.13	Tr	0	54
16	2	159	202	0.1	69	381	220	54	0.01	0.12	Tr	0	55
89	10	254	230	0.2	314	98	1,050	259	0.08	0.36	0.2	2	56
6	1	16	14	Tr	19	6	70	16	0.01	0.02	Tr	Tr	57
159	9	231	192	0.1	292	95	1,730	437	0.08	0.36	0.1	2	58
10	1	14	12	Tr	18	6	100	27	Tr	0.02	Tr	Tr	59

Table continued on following page

Item No.	Foods, Approximate Measures, Units, and Weight (Weight of Edible Portion Only)		Grams	Water (%)	Food Energy (cal)	Pro-tein (g)	Fat (g)	Saturated (g)	Mono-unsaturated (g)	Poly-unsaturated (g)
								Fatty Acids		
	Whipping, unwhipped (volume about double when whipped)									
60	Light	1 c	239	64	700	5	74	46.2	21.7	2.1
61		1 tbsp	15	64	45	Tr	5	2.9	1.4	0.1
62	Heavy	1 c	238	58	820	5	88	54.8	25.4	3.3
63		1 tbsp	15	58	50	Tr	6	3.5	1.6	0.2
64	Whipped topping (pressurized)	1 c	60	61	155	2	13	8.3	3.9	0.5
65		1 tbsp	3	61	10	Tr	1	0.4	0.2	Tr
66	Cream, sour	1 c	230	71	495	7	48	30.0	13.9	1.8
67		1 tbsp	12	71	25	Tr	3	1.6	0.7	0.1
	Cream products, imitation (made with vegetable fat)									
	Sweet									
	Whipped topping									
72	Powdered, made with whole milk	1 c	80	67	150	3	10	8.5	0.7	0.2
73		1 tbsp	4	67	10	Tr	Tr	0.4	Tr	Tr
74	Pressurized	1 c	70	60	185	1	16	13.2	1.3	0.2
75		1 tbsp	4	60	10	Tr	1	0.8	0.1	Tr
76	Sour dressing (filled cream type product, nonbutterfat)	1 c	235	75	415	8	39	31.2	4.6	1.1
77		1 tbsp	12	75	20	Tr	2	1.6	0.2	0.1
	Ice cream. See Milk desserts, frozen (items 106–111)									
	Ice milk. See Milk desserts, frozen (items 112–114)									
	Milk									
	Fluid									
78	Whole (3.3% fat)	1 c	244	88	150	8	8	5.1	2.4	0.3
	Lowfat (2%)									
79	No milk solids added	1 c	244	89	120	8	5	2.9	1.4	0.2
80	Milk solids added, label claim less than 10 g of protein per cup	1 c	245	89	125	9	5	2.9	1.4	0.2
	Lowfat (1%)									
81	No milk solids added	1 c	244	90	100	8	3	1.6	0.7	0.1
82	Milk solids added, label claim less than 10 g of protein per cup	1 c	245	90	105	9	2	1.5	0.7	0.1
	Nonfat (skim)									
	No milk solids added	1 c	245	91	85	8	Tr	0.3	0.1	Tr
84	Milk solids added, label claim less than 10 g of protein per cup	1 c	245	90	90	9	1	0.4	0.2	Tr
85	Buttermilk	1 c	245	90	100	8	2	1.3	0.6	0.1
	Goat, whole	250 ml	258	87	178[1]	9	11	7		Tr

Nutrients in Indicated Quantity

Cholesterol (mg)	Carbohydrate (g)	Calcium (mg)	Phosphorus (mg)	Iron (mg)	Potassium (mg)	Sodium (mg)	Vitamin A Value		Thiamin (mg)	Riboflavin (mg)	Niacin (mg)	Ascorbic Acid (mg)	Item No.
							IU	RE					
265	7	166	146	0.1	231	82	2,690	705	0.06	0.30	0.1	1	60
17	Tr	10	9	Tr	15	5	170	44	Tr	0.02	Tr	Tr	61
326	7	154	149	0.1	179	89	3,500	1,002	0.05	0.26	0.1	1	62
21	Tr	10	9	Tr	11	6	220	63	Tr	0.02	Tr	Tr	63
46	7	61	54	Tr	88	78	550	124	0.02	0.04	Tr	0	64
2	Tr	3	3	Tr	4	4	30	6	Tr	Tr	Tr	0	65
102	10	268	195	0.1	331	123	1,820	448	0.08	0.34	0.2	2	66
5	1	14	10	Tr	17′	6	90	23	Tr	0.02	Tr	Tr	67
8	13	72	69	Tr	121	53	290*	39*	0.02	0.09	Tr	1	72
Tr	1	4	3	Tr	6	3	10*	2*	Tr	Tr	Tr	Tr	73
0	11	4	13	Tr	13	43	330*	33*	0.00	0.00	0.0	0	74
0	1	Tr	1	Tr	1	2	20*	2*	0.00	0.00	0.0	0	75
13	11	266	205	0.1	380	113	20	5	0.09	0.38	0.2	2	76
1	1	14	10	Tr	19	6	Tr	Tr	Tr	0.02	Tr	Tr	77
33	11	291	228	0.1	370	120	310	76	0.09	0.40	0.2	2	78
18	12	297	232	0.1	377	122	500	139	0.10	0.40	0.2	2	79
18	12	313	245	0.1	397	128	500	140	0.10	0.42	0.2	2	80
10	12	300	235	0.1	381	123	500	144	0.10	0.41	0.2	2	81
10	12	313	245	0.1	397	128	500	145	0.10	0.42	0.2	2	82
4	12	302	247	0.1	406	126	500	149	0.09	0.34	0.2	2	83
5	12	316	255	0.1	418	130	500	149	0.10	0.43	0.2	2	84
9	12	285	219	0.1	371	257	80	20	0.08	0.38	0.1	2	85
29	11	344		0.1	527	128		144	0.12	0.36	2.6	3	

Table continued on following page

*Vitamin A value is largely from beta-carotene used for coloring.

Item No.	Foods, Approximate Measures, Units, and Weight (Weight of Edible Portion Only)		Grams	Water (%)	Food Energy (cal)	Protein (g)	Fat (g)	Fatty Acids		
								Saturated (g)	Monounsaturated (g)	Polyunsaturated (g)
	Human whole, mature	250 ml	260	88	181[1]	3	11	5		1
	Soybean, fluid	250 ml	258	92	85[1]	9	4	0		0
	Canned, evaporated									
87	Whole milk	1 c	252	74	340	17	19	11.6	5.9	0.6
	Lowfat (2%) undiluted	250 ml	268	78	246[1]	20	5	3	Tr	21
88	Skim milk	1 c	255	79	200	19	1	0.3	0.2	Tr
	Dried									
89	Buttermilk	1 c	120	3	465	41	7	4.3	2.0	0.3
	Nonfat, instant:									
90	Envelope, 3.2 oz net wt*	1 envelope	91	4	325	32	1	0.4	0.2	Tr
91	Cup	1 c	68	4	245	24	Tr	0.3	0.1	Tr
	Whole milk	15 ml	8	2	40[1]	2	2	1		Tr
	Milk beverages									
	Cocoa and chocolate-flavored beverages									
95	Powder containing nonfat dry milk	1 oz	28	1	100	3	1	0.6	0.3	Tr
96	Prepared (6 oz water plus 1 oz powder)	1 serving	206	86	100	3	1	0.6	0.3	Tr
97	Powder without nonfat dry milk	¾ oz	21	1	75	1	1	0.3	0.2	Tr
98	Prepared (8 oz whole milk plus ¾ oz powder)	1 serving	265	81	225	9	9	5.4	2.5	0.3
99	Eggnog (commercial)	1 c	254	74	340	10	19	11.3	5.7	0.9
	Malted milk									
	Chocolate									
100	Powder	¾ oz	21	2	85	1	1	0.5	0.3	0.1
100	Prepared (8 oz whole milk plus ¾ oz powder)	1 serving	265	81	235	9	9	5.5	2.7	0.4
	Natural									
102	Powder	¾ oz	21	3	85	3	2	0.9	0.5	0.3
103	Prepared (8 oz whole milk plus ¾ oz powder)	1 serving	265	81	235	11	10	6.0	2.9	0.6
	Shakes, thick									
104	Chocolate	10-oz container	283	72	335	9	8	4.8	2.2	0.3
105	Vanilla	10-oz container	283	74	315	11	9	5.3	2.5	0.3
	Milk desserts, frozen									
	Ice cream, vanilla									
	Regular (about 11% fat)									
106	Hardened	½ gal	1,064	61	2,155	38	115	71.3	33.1	4.3
107		1 c	33	61	270	5	14	8.9	4.1	0.5
108		3 fl oz	50	61	100	2	5	3.4	1.6	0.2
109	Soft serve (frozen custard)	1c	173	60	375	7	23	13.5	6.7	1.0
110	Rich (about 15% fat), hardened	½ gal	1,188	59	2,805	33	190	118.3	54.9	7.1
111		1 c	148	59	350	4	24	14.7	6.8	0.9

*Yields 1 qt of fluid milk when reconstituted according to package directions.

Nutrients in Indicated Quantity

Cholesterol (mg)	Carbohydrate (g)	Calcium (mg)	Phosphorus (mg)	Iron (mg)	Potassium (mg)	Sodium (mg)	Vitamin A Value IU	Vitamin A Value RE	Thiamin (mg)	Riboflavin (mg)	Niacin (mg)	Ascorbic Acid (mg)	Item No.
36	18	84		Tr	133	44		166	0.04	0.09	1.2	13	
0	6	54		2.1	506	0		10	0.21	0.08	2.1	0	
74	25	657	510	0.5	764	267	610	136	0.12	0.80	0.5	5	87
21	30	738		0.6	851	296		314	0.12	0.84	5.1	44	
9	29	738	497	0.7	845	293	1,000	298	0.11	0.79	0.4	3	88
83	59	1,421	1,119	0.4	1,910	621	260	65	0.47	1.89	1.1	7	89
17	47	1,120	896	0.3	1,552	499	2,160*	646*	0.38	1.59	0.8	5	90
12	35	837	670	0.2	1,160	373	1,610*	483*	0.28	1.19	0.6	4	91
8	3	73		Tr	106	30		22	0.02	0.10	0.5	Tr	
1	22	90	88	0.3	223	139	Tr	Tr	0.03	0.17	0.2	Tr	95
1	22	90	88	0.3	223	139	Tr	Tr	0.03	0.17	0.2	Tr	96
0	19	7	26	0.7	136	56	Tr	Tr	Tr	0.03	0.1	Tr	97
33	30	298	254	0.9	508	176	310	76	0.10	0.43	0.3	3	98
149	34	330	278	0.5	420	138	890	203	0.09	0.48	0.3	4	99
1	18	13	37	0.4	130	49	20	5	0.04	0.04	0.4	0	100
34	29	304	265	0.5	500	168	330	80	0.14	0.43	0.7	2	101
4	15	56	79	0.2	159	96	70	17	0.11	0.14	1.1	0	102
37	27	347	307	0.3	529	215	380	93	0.20	0.54	1.3	2	103
30	60	374	357	0.9	634	314	240	59	0.13	0.63	0.4	0	104
33	50	413	326	0.3	517	270	320	79	0.08	0.55	0.4	0	105
476	254	1,406	1,075	1.0	2,052	929	4,340	1,064	0.42	2.63	1.1	6	106
59	32	176	134	0.1	257	116	540	133	0.05	0.33	0.1	1	107
22	12	66	51	Tr	96	44	200	50	0.02	0.12	0.1	Tr	108
153	38	236	199	0.4	338	153	790	199	0.08	0.45	0.2	1	109
703	256	1,213	927	0.8	1,771	868	7,200	1,758	0.36	2.27	0.9	5	110
88	32	151	115	0.1	221	108	900	219	0.04	0.28	0.1	1	111

Table continued on following page

*With added vitamin A.

Item No.	Foods, Approximate Measures, Units, and Weight (Weight of Edible Portion Only)		Grams	Water (%)	Food Energy (cal)	Pro-tein (g)	Fat (g)	Fatty Acids		
								Satu-rated (g)	Mono-unsatu-rated (g)	Poly-unsatu-rated (g)
	Ice milk, vanilla									
112	Hardened (about 4% fat)	½ gal	1,048	69	1,470	41	45	2.81	13.0	1.7
113		1 c	131	69	185	5	6	3.5	1.6	0.2
114	Soft serve (about 3% fat)	1 c	175	70	225	8	5	2.9	1.3	0.2
	Pudding									
	Canned, chocolate	125 ml	132	68	191[1]	3	10	9		Tr
	Canned, vanilla	125 ml	132	69	205[1]	2	9	9		Tr
	Cornstarch, cooked	125 ml	137	70	170[1]	5	4	2		Tr
	Cornstarch, instant with whole milk	125 ml	137	69	171[1]	4	3	2		Tr
	Custard, baked	125 ml	140	77	161[1]	8	8	4		Tr
	Mix, low calorie, pre-pared with skim milk	125 ml	137	78	137[1]	4	3	Tr		Tr
	Tapioca (minute)	125 ml	87	72	117[1]	4	4	2		Tr
115	Sherbet (about 2% fat)	½ gal	1,542	66	2,160	17	31	19.0	8.8	1.1
		1 c	193	66	270	2	4	2.4	1.1	0.1
	Yogurt									
	With added milk solids									
	Made with lowfat milk									
117	Fruit-flavored*	8-oz con-tainer	227	74	230	10	2	1.6	0.7	0.1
118	Plain	8-oz con-tainer	227	85	145	12	4	2.3	1.0	0.1
119	Made with nonfat milk	8-oz con-tainer	227	85	125	13	Tr	0.3	0.1	Tr
	Without added milk solids									
120	Made with whole milk	8-oz con-tainer	227	88	140	8	7	4.8	2.0	0.2
	Frozen, fruit, 6.3% fat		125	—	148[1]	4	5	—		—
	Eggs									
	Eggs, large (24 oz per dozen)									
	Raw									
121	Whole, without shell	1 egg	50	75	80	6	6	1.7	2.2	0.7
122	White	1 white	33	88	15	3	Tr	0.0	0.0	0.0
123	Yolk	1 yolk	17	49	65	3	6	1.7	2.2	0.7
	Cooked									
124	Fried in butter	1 egg	46	68	95	6	7	2.7	2.7	0.8
125	Hard-cooked, shell re-moved	1 egg	50	75	80	6	6	1.7	2.2	0.7
126	Poached	1 egg	50	74	80	6	6	1.7	2.2	0.7
127	Scrambled (milk added) in butter; also omelet	1 egg	64	73	110	7	8	3.2	2.9	0.8
	Substitute, frozen (yolk replaced)	60 ml	61	73	97[1]	7	7	1		4

*Carbohydrate content varies widely because of amount of sugar added and amount and solids content of added flavoring. Consult the label if more precise values for carbohydrate and calories are needed.

Nutrients in Indicated Quantity

Cholesterol (mg)	Carbohydrate (g)	Calcium (mg)	Phosphorus (mg)	Iron (mg)	Potassium (mg)	Sodium (mg)	Vitamin A Value		Thiamin (mg)	Riboflavin (mg)	Niacin (mg)	Ascorbic Acid (mg)	Item No.
							IU	RE					
146	232	1,409	1,035	1.5	2,117	836	1,710	419	0.61	2.78	0.9	6	112
18	29	176	129	0.2	265	105	210	52	0.08	0.35	0.1	1	113
13	38	274	202	0.3	412	163	175	44	0.12	0.54	0.2	1	114
Tr	28	69		1.1	236	265		29	0.04	0.16	1.1	Tr	
Tr	31	73		0.2	144	284		Tr	0.03	0.11	0.9	Tr	
16	31	140		0.4	186	177		53	0.03	0.21	1.0	Tr	
15	33	197		0.7	177	170		53	0.04	0.21	0.9	1	
147	16	157		0.6	204	111		147	0.06	0.27	1.5	Tr	
2	27	197		0.7	194	190		21	0.04	0.21	0.1	Tr	
84	15	91		0.3	117	136		76	0.04	0.16	0.9	Tr	
113	469	827	594	2.5	1,585	706	1,480	308	0.26	0.71	1.0	31	115
14	59	103	74	0.3	198	88	190	39	0.03	0.09	0.1	4	116
10	43	345	271	0.2	442	133	100	25	0.08	0.40	0.2	1	117
14	16	415	326	0.2	531	159	150	36	0.10	0.49	0.3	2	118
4	17	452	355	0.2	579	174	20	5	0.11	0.53	0.3	2	119
29	11	274	215	0.1	351	105	280	68	0.07	0.32	0.2	1	120
—	23	145		—	199	63		—	0.03	0.27	0.2	4	
274	1	28	90	1.0	65	69	260	78	0.04	0.15	Tr	0	121
0	Tr	4	4	Tr	45	50	0	0	Tr	0.09	Tr	0	122
272	Tr	26	86	0.9	15	8	310	94	0.04	0.07	Tr	0	123
278	1	29	91	1.1	66	162	320	94	0.04	0.14	Tr	0	124
274	1	28	90	1.0	65	69	260	78	0.04	0.14	Tr	0	125
273	1	28	90	1.0	65	146	260	78	0.03	0.13	Tr	0	126
282	2	54	109	1.0	97	176	350	102	0.04	0.18	Tr	Tr	127
1	2	44		1.2	130	122		82	0.07	0.24	18	Tr	

Table continued on following page

| | | | | | | | | Fatty Acids | | |
| | | | | | | | | Satu- | Mono- unsatu- | Poly- unsatu- |
Item No.	Foods, Approximate Measures, Units, and Weight (Weight of Edible Portion Only)		Grams	Water (%)	Food Energy (cal)	Pro- tein (g)	Fat (g)	rated (g)	rated (g)	rated (g)
	Fats and Oils									
	Butter (4 sticks per lb)									
128	Stick	½ c	113	16	810	1	92	57.1	26.4	3.4
129	Tablespoon (⅛ stick)	1 tbsp	14	16	100	Tr	11	7.1	3.3	0.4
130	Pat (1 in square, ⅓ in high; 90 per lb)	1 pat	5	16	35	Tr	4	2.5	1.2	0.2
131	Fats, cooking (vegetable shortenings)	1 c	205	0	1,810	0	205	51.3	91.2	53.5
132		1 tbsp	13	0	115	0	13	3.3	5.8	3.4
133	Lard	1 c	205	0	1,850	0	205	80.4	92.5	23.0
134		1 tbsp	13	0	115	0	13	5.1	5.9	1.5
	Margarine									
135	Imitation (about 40% fat), soft	8-oz con- tainer	227	58	785	1	88	17.5	35.6	31.3
136		1 tbsp	14	58	50	Tr	5	1.1	2.2	1.9
	Regular (about 80% fat) Hard (4 sticks per lb)									
137	Stick	½ cup	113	16	810	1	91	17.9	40.5	28.7
138	Tablespoon (⅛ stick)	1 tbsp	14	16	100	Tr	11	2.2	5.0	3.6
139	Pat (1 in square, ⅓ in high; 90 per lb)	1 pat	5	16	35	Tr	4	0.8	1.8	1.3
140	Soft	8-oz con- tainer	227	16	1,625	2	183	31.3	64.7	78.5
141		1 tbsp	14	16	100	Tr	11	1.9	4.0	4.8
	Spread (about 60% fat) Hard (4 sticks per lb)									
142	Stick	½ c	113	37	610	1	69	15.9	29.4	20.5
143	Tablespoon (⅛ stick)	1 tbsp	14	37	75	Tr	9	2.0	3.6	2.5
144	Pat (1 in square, ⅓ in high; 90 per lb)	1 pat	5	37	25	Tr	3	0.7	1.3	0.9
145	Soft	8-oz con- tainer	227	37	1,225	1	138	29.1	71.5	31.3
146		1 tbsp	14	37	75	Tr	9	1.8	4.4	1.9
	Oils, salad and cooking									
	Canola (rapeseed, colza)	250 ml	230	0	2,033[1]	0	230	17	77	0
	Canola (rapeseed, colza)	15 ml	14	0	24[1]	0	14	1	5	0
147	Corn	1 c	218	0	1,925	0	218	27.7	52.8	128.0
148		1 tbsp	14	0	125	0	14	1.8	3.4	8.2
149	Olive	1 c	216	0	1,910	0	216	29.2	159.2	18.1
150		1 tbsp	14	0	125	0	14	1.9	10.3	1.2
151	Peanut	1 c	216	0	1,910	0	216	36.5	99.8	69.1
152		1 tbsp	14	0	125	0	14	2.4	6.5	4.5
153	Safflower	1 c	218	0	1,925	0	218	19.8	26.4	162.4
154		1 tbsp	14	0	125	0	14	1.3	1.7	10.4
155	Soybean oil, hydrogen- ated (partially hard- ened)	1 c	218	0	1,925	0	218	32.5	93.7	82.0
156		1 tbsp	14	0	125	0	14	2.1	6.0	5.3

Nutrients in Indicated Quantity

Cholesterol (mg)	Carbohydrate (g)	Calcium (mg)	Phosphorus (mg)	Iron (mg)	Potassium (mg)	Sodium (mg)	Vitamin A Value		Thiamin (mg)	Riboflavin (mg)	Niacin (mg)	Ascorbic Acid (mg)	Item No.
							IU	RE					
247	Tr	27	26	0.2	29	933*	3,460†	852†	0.01	0.04	Tr	0	128
31	Tr	3	3	Tr	4	116	430†	106†	Tr	Tr	Tr	0	129
11	Tr	1	1	Tr	1	41*	150†	38†	Tr	Tr	Tr	0	130
0	0	0	0	0.0	0	0	0	0	0.00	0.00	0.0	0	131
0	0	0	0	0.0	0	0	0	0	0.00	0.00	0.0	0	132
195	0	0	0	0.0	0	0	0	0	0.00	0.00	0.0	0	133
12	0	0	0	0.0	0	0	0	0	0.00	0.00	0.0	0	134
0	1	40	31	0.0	57	2,178‡	7,510§	2,254§	0.01	0.05	Tr	Tr	135
0	Tr	2	2	0.0	4	134‡	460§	139§	Tr	Tr	Tr	Tr	136
0	1	34	26	0.1	48	1,066‡	3,740§	1,122§	0.01	0.04	Tr	Tr	137
0	Tr	4	3	Tr	6	132‡	460§	139§	Tr	0.01	Tr	Tr	138
0	Tr	1	1	Tr	2	47‡	170§	50§	Tr	Tr	Tr	Tr	139
0	1	60	46	0.0	86	2,449‡	7,510§	2,254§	0.02	0.07	Tr	Tr	140
0	Tr	4	3	0.0	5	151‡	460§	139§	Tr	Tr	Tr	Tr	141
0	0	24	18	0.0	34	1,123‡	3,740§	1,122§	0.01	0.03	Tr	Tr	142
0	0	3	2	0.0	4	139‡	460§	139§	Tr	Tr	Tr	Tr	143
0	0	1	1	0.0	1	50‡	170§	50§	Tr	Tr	Tr	Tr	144
0	0	47	37	0.0	68	2,256‡	7,510§	2,254§	0.02	0.06	Tr	Tr	145
0	0	3	2	0.0	4	139‡	460§	139§	Tr	Tr	Tr	Tr	146
0	0	0	0	0.0	0	0	0	0	0.00	0.00	0.0	0	
0	0	0	0	0.0	0	0	0	0	0.00	0.00	0.0	0	
0	0	0	0	0.0	0	0	0	0	0.00	0.00	0.0	0	147
0	0	0	0	0.0	0	0	0	0	0.00	0.00	0.0	0	148
0	0	0	0	0.0	0	0	0	0	0.00	0.00	0.0	0	149
0	0	0	0	0.0	0	0	0	0	0.00	0.00	0.0	0	150
0	0	0	0	0.0	0	0	0	0	0.00	0.00	0.0	0	151
0	0	0	0	0.0	0	0	0	0	0.00	0.00	0.0	0	152
0	0	0	0	0.0	0	0	0	0	0.00	0.00	0.0	0	153
0	0	0	0	0.0	0	0	0	0	0.00	0.00	0.0	0	154
0	0	0	0	0.0	0	0	0	0	0.00	0.00	0.0	0	155
0	0	0	0	0.0	0	0	0	0	0.00	0.00	0.0	0	156

Table continued on following page

*For salted butter; unsalted butter contains 12 mg sodium per stick, 2 mg per tbsp, or 1 mg per pat.
†Values for vitamin A are year-round average.
‡For salted margarine.
§Based on average vitamin A content of fortified margarine. Federal specifications for fortified margarine require a minimum of 15,000 IU per pound.

								Fatty Acids		
Item No.	Foods, Approximate Measures, Units, and Weight (Weight of Edible Portion Only)		Grams	Water (%)	Food Energy (cal)	Pro-tein (g)	Fat (g)	Satu-rated (g)	Mono-unsatu-rated (g)	Poly-unsatu-rated (g)
157	Soybean-cottonseed oil blend, hydrogenated	1 c	218	0	1,925	0	218	39.2	64.3	104.9
158		1 tbsp	14	0	125	0	14	2.5	4.1	6.7
159	Sunflower	1 c	218	0	1,925	0	218	22.5	42.5	143.2
160		1 tbsp	14	0	125	0	14	1.4	2.7	9.2
	Salad dressings									
	Commercial									
161	Blue cheese	1 tbsp	15	32	75	1	8	1.5	1.8	4.2
	French									
162	Regular	1 tbsp	16	35	85	Tr	9	1.4	4.0	3.5
163	Low calorie	1 tbsp	16	75	25	Tr	2	0.2	0.3	1.0
	Italian									
164	Regular	1 tbsp	15	34	80	Tr	9	1.3	3.7	3.2
165	Low calorie	1 tbsp	15	86	5	Tr	Tr	Tr	Tr	Tr
	Mayonnaise									
166	Regular	1 tbsp	14	15	100	Tr	11	1.7	3.2	5.8
167	Imitation	1 tbsp	15	63	35	Tr	3	0.5	0.7	1.6
168	Mayonnaise type	1 tbsp	15	40	60	Tr	5	0.7	1.4	2.7
169	Tartar sauce	1 tbsp	14	34	75	Tr	8	1.2	2.6	3.9
	Thousand island									
170	Regular	1 tbsp	16	46	60	Tr	6	1.0	1.3	3.2
171	Low calorie	1 tbsp	15	69	25	Tr	2	0.2	0.4	0.9
	Prepared from home recipe									
172	Cooked type*	1 tbsp	16	69	25	1	2	0.5	0.6	0.3
173	Vinegar and oil	1 tbsp	16	47	70	0	8	1.5	2.4	3.9
	Fish and Shellfish									
	Anchovy	3 fillets	12	59	21[1]	2	1	Tr	Tr	7
	Bluefish, baked or broiled, 12 × 7 × 1 cm	1 piece	92	68	146[1]	24	5	Tr	Tr	64
	Clams									
174	Raw, meat only	3 oz	85	82	65	11	1	0.3	0.3	0.3
175	Canned, drained solids	3 oz	85	77	85	13	2	0.5	0.5	0.4
	Cod, fresh, broiled, 10 × 4 × 2 cm	1 piece	88	65	150[1]	25	5	Tr	Tr	71
176	Crabmeat, canned	1 c	135	77	135	23	3	0.5	0.8	1.4
177	Fish sticks, frozen, reheated (stick, 4 × 1 × ½ in)	1 fish stick	28	52	70	6	3	0.8	1.4	0.8
	Flounder or sole, baked, with lemon juice									
178	With butter	3 oz	85	73	120	16	6	3.2	1.5	0.5
179	With margarine	3 oz	85	73	120	16	6	1.2	2.3	1.9
180	Without added fat	3 oz	85	78	80	17	1	0.3	0.2	0.4
181	Haddock, breaded, fried†	3 oz	85	61	175	17	9	2.4	3.9	2.4
182	Halibut, broiled, with butter and lemon juice	3 oz	85	67	140	20	6	3.3	1.6	0.7
183	Herring, pickled	3 oz	85	59	190	17	13	4.3	4.6	3.1
	Lobster, canned	150 ml	92	77	87[1]	17	1	0	0	78
	Mackerel, canned, solids and liquid	150 ml	95	66	174[1]	18	11	3	—	89
184	Ocean perch, breaded, fried†	1 fillet	85	59	185	16	11	2.6	4.6	2.8

*Fatty acid values apply to products made with regular margarine.
†Dipped in egg, milk, and breadcrumbs; fried in vegetable shortening.

Nutrients in Indicated Quantity

Cholesterol (mg)	Carbohydrate (g)	Calcium (mg)	Phosphorus (mg)	Iron (mg)	Potassium (mg)	Sodium (mg)	Vitamin A Value		Thiamin (mg)	Riboflavin (mg)	Niacin (mg)	Ascorbic Acid (mg)	Item No.
							IU	RE					
0	0	0	0	0.0	0	0	0	0	0.00	0.00	0.0	0	157
0	0	0	0	0.0	0	0	0	0	0.00	0.00	0.0	0	158
0	0	0	0	0.0	0	0	0	0	0.00	0.00	0.0	0	159
0	0	0	0	0.0	0	0	0	0	0.00	0.00	0.0	0	160
3	1	12	11	Tr	6	164	30	10	Tr	0.02	Tr	Tr	161
0	1	2	1	Tr	2	188	Tr	Tr	Tr	Tr	Tr	Tr	162
0	2	6	5	Tr	3	306	Tr	Tr	Tr	Tr	Tr	Tr	163
0	1	1	1	Tr	5	162	30	3	Tr	Tr	Tr	Tr	164
0	2	1	1	Tr	4	136	Tr	Tr	Tr	Tr	Tr	Tr	165
8	Tr	3	4	0.1	5	80	40	12	0.00	0.00	Tr	0	166
4	2	Tr	Tr	0.0	2	75	0	0	0.00	0.00	0.0	0	167
4	4	2	4	Tr	1	107	30	13	Tr	Tr	Tr	0	168
4	1	3	4	0.1	11	182	30	9	Tr	Tr	0.0	Tr	169
4	2	2	3	0.1	18	112	50	15	Tr	Tr	Tr	0	170
2	2	2	3	0.1	17	150	50	14	Tr	Tr	Tr	0	171
9	2	13	14	0.1	19	117	70	20	0.01	0.02	Tr	Tr	172
0	Tr	0	0	0.0	1	Tr	0	0	0.00	0.00	0.0	0	173
7	Tr	20		0.3	71	99	8		Tr	0.02	1.1	0	
64	0	27		0.6	386	96	14		0.10	0.09	6.2	0	
43	2	59	138	2.6	154	102	90	26	0.09	0.15	1.1	9	174
54	2	47	116	3.5	119	102	90	26	0.01	0.09	0.9	3	175
71	0	27		0.9	358	97	48		0.07	0.10	7.2	0	
135	1	61	246	1.1	149	1,350	50	14	0.11	0.11	2.6	0	176
26	4	11	58	0.3	94	53	20	5	0.03	0.05	0.6	0	177
68	Tr	13	187	0.3	272	145	210	54	0.05	0.08	1.6	1	178
55	Tr	14	187	0.3	273	151	230	69	0.05	0.08	1.6	1	179
59	Tr	13	197	0.3	286	101	30	10	0.05	0.08	1.7	1	180
75	7	34	183	1.0	270	123	70	20	0.06	0.10	2.9	0	181
62	Tr	14	206	0.7	441	103	610	174	0.06	0.07	7.7	1	182
85	0	29	128	0.9	85	850	110	33	0.04	0.18	2.8	0	183
78	Tr	60		0.7	166	193	0		0.09	0.06	4.5	0	
89	0	176		2.0	399	70	123		0.06	0.20	8.9	0	
66	7	31	191	1.2	241	138	70	20	0.10	0.11	2.0	0	184

Table continued on following page

Item No.	Foods, Approximate Measures, Units, and Weight (Weight of Edible Portion Only)		Grams	Water (%)	Food Energy (cal)	Pro-tein (g)	Fat (g)	Satu-rated (g)	Mono-unsatu-rated (g)	Poly-unsatu-rated (g)
									Fatty Acids	
	Oysters									
185	Raw, meat only (13–19 medium Selects)	1 c	240	85	160	20	4	1.4	0.5	1.4
186	Breaded, fried*	1 oyster	45	65	90	5	5	1.4	2.1	1.4
	Salmon									
187	Canned (pink), solids and liquid	3 oz	85	71	120	17	5	0.9	1.5	2.1
188	Baked (red)	3 oz	85	67	140	21	5	1.2	2.4	1.4
189	Smoked	3 oz	85	59	150	18	8	2.6	3.9	0.7
190	Sardines, Atlantic, canned in oil, drained solids	3 oz	85	62	175	20	9	2.1	3.7	2.9
191	Scallops, breaded, frozen, reheated	6 scallops	90	59	195	15	10	2.5	4.1	2.5
	Steamed	7 scallops	90	73	101[1]	21	1	0	0	48
	Shrimp									
192	Canned, drained solids	3 oz	85	70	100	21	1	0.2	0.2	0.4
193	French fried (7 medium)†	3 oz	85	55	200	16	10	2.5	4.1	2.6
194	Trout, broiled, with butter and lemon juice	3 oz	85	63	175	21	9	4.1	2.9	1.6
	Tuna, canned, drained solids									
195	Oil pack, chunk light	3 oz	85	61	165	24	7	1.4	1.9	3.1
196	Water pack, solid white	3 oz	85	63	135	30	1	0.3	0.2	0.3
197	Tuna salad‡	1 c	205	63	375	33	19	3.3	4.9	9.2
	Whitefish, baked stuffed, 12 × 7 × 1 cm	1 piece	92	63	198[1]	14	13	4	—	40
	Fruits and Fruit Juices									
	Apples									
	Raw									
	Unpeeled, without cores									
198	2¾-in diam. (about 3 per lb with cores)	1 apple	138	84	80	Tr	Tr	0.1	Tr	0.1
199	3¼-in diam. (about 2 per lb with cores)	1 apple	212	84	125	Tr	1	0.1	Tr	0.2
200	Peeled, sliced	1 c	110	84	65	Tr	Tr	0.1	Tr	0.1
201	Dried, sulfured	10 rings	64	32	155	1	Tr	Tr	Tr	0.1
202	Apple juice, bottled or canned§	1 c	248	88	115	Tr	Tr	Tr	Tr	0.1
204	Applesauce, canned, unsweetened	1 c	244	88	105	Tr	Tr	Tr	Tr	Tr
	Apricots									
205	Raw, without pits (about 3 12 per lb with pits)	apricots	106	86	50	1	Tr	Tr	0.2	0.1
	Canned (fruit and liquid)									
208	Juice pack	1 c	248	87	120	2	Tr	Tr	Tr	Tr
209		3 halves	84	87	40	1	Tr	Tr	Tr	Tr

*Dipped in egg, milk, and breadcrumbs; fried in vegetable shortening.
†Dipped in egg, breadcrumbs, and flour; fried in vegetable shortening.
‡Made with drained chunk light tuna, celery, onion, pickle relish, and mayonnaise-type salad dressing.
§Also applies to pasteurized apple cider.

| | | | | | | | Nutrients in Indicated Quantity | | | | | | |

Cholesterol (mg)	Carbohydrate (g)	Calcium (mg)	Phosphorus (mg)	Iron (mg)	Potassium (mg)	Sodium (mg)	Vitamin A Value IU	Vitamin A Value RE	Thiamin (mg)	Riboflavin (mg)	Niacin (mg)	Ascorbic Acid (mg)	Item No.
120	8	226	343	15.6	290	175	740	223	0.34	0.43	6.0	24	185
35	5	49	73	3.0	64	70	150	44	0.07	0.10	1.3	4	186
34	0	167*	243	0.7	307	443	60	18	0.03	0.15	6.8	0	187
60	0	26	269	0.5	305	55	290	87	0.18	0.14	5.5	0	188
51	0	12	208	0.8	327	1,700	260	77	0.17	0.17	6.8	0	189
85	0	371*	424	2.6	349	425	190	56	0.03	0.17	4.6	0	190
70	10	39	203	2.0	369	298	70	21	0.11	0.11	1.6	0	191
48	3	104		2.7	428	239	27		0.09	0.05	5.0	0	
128	1	98	224	1.4	1	1,955	50	15	0.01	0.03	1.5	0	192
168	11	61	154	2.0	189	384	90	26	0.06	0.09	2.8	0	193
71	Tr	26	259	1.0	297	122	230	60	0.07	0.07	2.3	1	194
55	0	7	199	1.6	298	303	70	20	0.04	0.09	10.1	0	195
48	0	17	202	0.6	255	468	110	32	0.03	0.10	13.4	0	196
80	19	31	281	2.5	531	877	230	53	0.06	0.14	13.3	6	197
40	5	33		0.5	268	179	552		0.10	0.10	4.7	0	
0	21	10	10	0.2	159	Tr	70	7	0.02	0.02	0.1	8	198
0	32	15	15	0.4	244	Tr	110	11	0.04	0.03	0.2	12	199
0	16	4	8	0.1	124	Tr	50	5	0.02	0.01	0.1	4	200
0	42	9	24	0.9	288	56†	0	0	0.00	0.10	0.6	2	201
0	29	17	17	0.9	295	7	Tr	Tr	0.05	0.04	0.2	2‡	202
0	28	7	17	0.3	183	5	70	7	0.03	0.06	0.5	3	204
0	12	15	20	0.6	314	1	2,770	277	0.03	0.04	0.6	11	205
0	31	30	50	0.7	409	10	4,190	419	0.04	0.05	0.9	12	208
0	10	10	17	0.3	139	3	1,420	142	0.02	0.02	0.3	4	209

Table continued on following page

*If bones are discarded, value for calcium will be greatly reduced.
†Sodium bisulfite used to preserve color; unsulfited product would contain less sodium.
‡Without added ascorbic acid. For value with added ascorbic acid, refer to label.

Item No.	Foods, Approximate Measures, Units, and Weight (Weight of Edible Portion Only)		Grams	Water (%)	Food Energy (cal)	Pro-tein (g)	Fat (g)	Fatty Acids		
								Satu-rated (g)	Mono-unsatu-rated (g)	Poly-unsatu-rated (g)
	Dried									
210	Uncooked (28 large or 37 medium halves per cup)	1 c	130	31	310	5	1	Tr	0.3	0.1
211	Cooked, unsweetened, fruit and liquid	1 c	250	76	210	3	Tr	Tr	0.2	0.1
212	Apricot, nectar, canned	1 c	251	85	140	1	Tr	Tr	0.1	Tr
	Avocados, raw, whole, without skin and seed									
213	California (about 2 per lb with skin and seed)	1 avocado	173	73	305	4	30	4.5	19.4	3.5
214	Florida (about 1 per lb with skin and seed)	1 avocado	304	80	340	5	27	5.3	14.8	4.5
	Bananas, raw, without peel									
215	Whole (about 2½ per lb with peel)	1 banana	114	74	105	1	1	0.2	Tr	0.1
216	Sliced	1 c	150	74	140	2	1	0.3	0.1	0.1
217	Blackberries, raw	1 c	144	86	75	1	1	0.2	0.1	0.1
218	Blueberries, raw	1 c	145	85	80	1	1	Tr	0.1	0.3
	Cantaloupe. See Melons (item 251)									
	Cherries									
221	Sour, red, pitted, canned, water pack	1 c	244	90	90	2	Tr	0.1	0.1	0.1
222	Sweet, raw, without pits and stems	10 cherries	68	81	50	1	1	0.1	0.2	0.2
	Cranberries, whole, raw	250 ml	100	87	49[1]	Tr	Tr	0	—	0
	Cranberry juice, cocktail, bottled	250 ml	267	85	155[1]	Tr	Tr	0	—	0
	Dates									
225	Whole, without pits	10 dates	83	23	230	2	Tr	0.1	0.1	Tr
226	Chopped	1 c	178	23	490	4	1	0.3	0.2	Tr
	Fruit cocktail, canned, fruit and liquid									
229	Juice pack	1 c	248	87	115	1	Tr	Tr	Tr	Tr
	Water pack	250ml	259	91	83[1]	1	Tr	Tr	Tr	0
	Fruit-flavored drinks									
	Canned or bottled, vitamin C added	250 ml	264	88	127[1]	0	0	0	0	0
	Crystals, water and vitamin C added	250 ml	284	88	117[1]	0	0	0	0	0
	Grapefruit									
230	Raw, without peel, membrane and seeds (3¾-in diam., 1 lb 1 oz, whole, with refuse)	½ grape-fruit	120	91	40	1	Tr	Tr	Tr	Tr
	Grapefruit juice									
232	Raw	1 c	247	90	95	1	Tr	Tr	Tr	0.1
233	Canned, unsweetened	1 c	247	90	95	1	Tr	Tr	Tr	0.1
	Frozen concentrate, unsweetened									
235	Undiluted	6 fl oz can	207	62	300	4	1	0.1	0.1	0.2
236	Diluted with 3 parts water by volume	1 c	247	89	100	1	Tr	Tr	Tr	0.1

| | | | | | | | Nutrients in Indicated Quantity | | | | | | |

| Cho-les-terol (mg) | Carbo-hydrate (g) | Cal-cium (mg) | Phos-phorus (mg) | Iron (mg) | Potas-sium (mg) | Sodium (mg) | Vitamin A Value | | Thia-min (mg) | Ribo-flavin (mg) | Nia-cin (mg) | Ascor-bic Acid (mg) | Item No. |
							IU	RE					
0	80	59	152	6.1	1,791	13	9.410	941	0.01	0.20	3.9	3	210
0	55	40	103	4.2	1,222	8	5,910	591	0.02	0.08	2.4	4	211
0	36	18	23	1.0	286	8	3,300	330	0.02	0.04	0.7	2*	212
0	12	19	73	2.0	1,097	21	1,060	106	0.19	0.21	3.3	14	213
0	27	33	119	1.6	1,484	15	1,860	186	0.33	0.37	5.8	24	214
0	27	7	23	0.4	451	1	90	9	0.05	0.11	0.6	10	215
0	35	9	30	0.5	594	2	120	12	0.07	0.15	0.8	14	216
0	18	46	30	0.8	282	Tr	240	24	0.04	0.06	0.6	30	217
0	20	9	15	0.2	129	9	150	15	0.07	0.07	0.5	19	218
0	22	27	24	3.3	239	17	1,840	184	0.04	0.10	0.4	5	221
0	11	10	13	0.3	152	Tr	150	15	0.03	0.04	0.3	5	222
0	13	7		0.2	71	1		5	0.03	0.02	0.2	14	
0	40	8		0.4	64	11		0	0.01	0.04	0.1	60	
0	61	27	33	1.0	541	2	40	4	0.07	0.08	1.8	0	225
0	131	57	71	2.0	1,161	5	90	9	0.16	0.18	3.9	0	226
0	29	20	35	0.5	236	10	760	76	0.03	0.04	1.0	7	229
0	22	13		0.6	243	10		65	0.04	0.03	1.1	5	
0	32	18		0.6	42	37		4	0.03	0.03	Tr	61	
0	31	78		0.1	1	19		0	0	0	0	60	
0	10	14	10	0.1	167	Tr	10†	1†	0.04	0.02	0.3	41	230
0	23	22	37	0.5	400	2	20	2	0.10	0.05	0.5	94	232
0	22	17	27	0.5	378	2	20	2	0.10	0.05	0.6	72	233
0	72	56	101	1.0	1,002	6	60	6	0.30	0.16	1.6	248	235
0	24	20	35	0.3	336	2	20	2	0.10	0.05	0.5	83	236

Table continued on following page

*Without added ascorbic acid. For value with added ascorbic acid, refer to label.
†For white grapefruit; pink grapefruit have about 310 IU or 31 RE.

Item No.	Foods, Approximate Measures, Units, and Weight (Weight of Edible Portion Only)		Grams	Water (%)	Food Energy (cal)	Pro-tein (g)	Fat (g)	Fatty Acids		
								Satu-rated (g)	Mono-unsatu-rated (g)	Poly-unsatu-rated (g)
	Grapes, Canadian type (slip skin), raw	10 grapes	24	81	15[1]	Tr	Tr	Tr	Tr	Tr
	Grapes, European type (adherent skin), raw									
237	Thompson Seedless	10 grapes	50	81	35	Tr	Tr	0.1	Tr	0.1
238	Tokay and Emperor, seedless types	10 grapes	57	81	40	Tr	Tr	0.1	Tr	0.1
242	Kiwifruit, raw, without skin (about 5 per lb with skin)	1 kiwi-fruit	76	83	45	1	Tr	Tr	0.1	0.1
243	Lemons, raw, without peel and seeds (about 4 per lb with peel and seeds)	1 lemon	58	89	15	1	Tr	Tr	Tr	0.1
	Lemon juice									
244	Raw	1 c	244	91	60	1	Tr	Tr	Tr	Tr
245	Canned or bottled, un-sweetened	1 c	244	92	50	1	1	0.1	Tr	0.2
246		1 tbsp	15	92	5	Tr	Tr	Tr	Tr	Tr
247	Frozen, single-strength, unsweetened	6 fl oz can	244	92	55	1	1	0.1	Tr	0.2
	Lime juice									
248	Raw	1 c	246	90	65	1	Tr	Tr	Tr	0.1
249	Canned, unsweetened	1 c	246	93	50	1	1	0.1	0.1	0.2
250	Mangos, raw, without skin and seed (about 1½ per lb with skin and seed)	1 mango	207	82	135	1	1	0.1	0.2	0.1
	Melons, raw, without rind and cavity contents									
251	Cantaloupe, orange-fleshed (5-in diam., 2⅓ lb, whole, with rind and cavity contents)	½ melon	267	90	95	2	1	0.1	0.1	0.3
252	Honeydew (6½-in diam., 5¼ lb, whole, with rind and cavity contents)	⅒ melon	129	90	45	1	Tr	Tr	Tr	0.1
253	Nectarines, raw, without pits (about 3 per lb with pits)	1 nec-tarine	136	86	65	1	1	0.1	0.2	0.3
	Oranges, raw									
254	Whole, without peel and seeds (2⅝-in diam., about 2½ per lb, with peel and seeds)	1 orange	131	87	60	1	Tr	Tr	Tr	Tr
255	Sections without mem-branes	1 c	180	87	85	2	Tr	Tr	Tr	Tr
	Orange juice									
256	Raw, all varieties	1 c	248	88	110	2	Tr	0.1	0.1	0.1
257	Canned, unsweetened	1 c	249	89	105	1	Tr	Tr	0.1	0.1
258	Chilled	1 c	249	88	110	2	1	0.1	0.1	0.2
	Frozen concentrate									
259	Undiluted	6 fl oz can	213	58	340	5	Tr	0.1	0.1	0.1
260	Diluted with 3 parts water by volume	1 c	249	88	110	2	Tr	Tr	Tr	Tr

Nutrients in Indicated Quantity

Cholesterol (mg)	Carbohydrate (g)	Calcium (mg)	Phosphorus (mg)	Iron (mg)	Potassium (mg)	Sodium (mg)	Vitamin A Value		Thiamin (mg)	Riboflavin (mg)	Niacin (mg)	Ascorbic Acid (mg)	Item No.
							IU	RE					
0	4	3		Tr	46	Tr		2	0.02	0.01	Tr	Tr	
0	9	6	7	0.1	93	1	40	4	0.05	0.03	0.2	5	237
0	10	6	7	0.1	105	1	40	4	0.05	0.03	0.2	6	238
0	11	20	30	0.3	252	4	130	13	0.02	0.04	0.4	74	242
0	5	15	9	0.3	80	1	20	2	0.02	0.01	0.1	31	243
0	21	17	15	0.1	303	2	50	5	0.07	0.02	0.2	112	244
0	16	27	22	0.3	249	51*	40	4	0.10	0.02	0.5	61	245
0	1	2	1	Tr	15	3*	Tr	Tr	0.01	Tr	Tr	4	246
0	16	20	20	0.3	217	2	30	3	0.14	0.03	0.3	77	247
0	22	22	17	0.1	268	2	20	2	0.05	0.02	0.2	72	248
0	16	30	25	0.6	185	39*	40	4	0.08	0.01	0.4	16	249
0	35	21	23	0.3	323	4	8,060	806	0.12	0.12	1.2	57	250
0	22	29	45	0.6	825	24	8,610	861	0.10	0.06	1.5	113	251
0	12	8	13	0.1	350	13	50	5	0.10	0.02	0.8	32	252
0	16	7	22	0.2	288	Tr	1,000	100	0.02	0.06	1.3	7	253
0	15	52	18	0.1	237	Tr	270	27	0.11	0.05	0.4	70	254
0	21	72	25	0.2	326	Tr	370	37	0.16	0.07	0.5	96	255
0	26	27	42	0.5	496	2	500	50	0.22	0.07	1.0	124	256
0	25	20	35	1.1	436	5	440	44	0.15	0.07	0.8	86	257
0	25	25	27	0.4	473	2	190	19	0.28	0.05	0.7	82	258
0	81	68	121	0.7	1,436	6	590	59	0.60	0.14	1.5	294	259
0	27	22	40	0.2	473	2	190	19	0.20	0.04	0.5	97	260

Table continued on following page

*Sodium benzoate and sodium bisulfite added as preservatives.

Item No.	Foods, Approximate Measures, Units, and Weight (Weight of Edible Portion Only)		Grams	Water (%)	Food Energy (cal)	Pro-tein (g)	Fat (g)	Fatty Acids		
								Satu-rated (g)	Mono-unsatu-rated (g)	Poly-unsatu-rated (g)
261	Orange and grapefruit juice, canned	1 c	247	89	105	1	Tr	Tr	Tr	Tr
262	Papayas, raw, ½-in cubes									
	Peaches									
	Raw	1 c	140	86	65	1	Tr	0.1	0.1	Tr
263	Whole, 2½-in diam., peeled, pitted (about 4 per lb with peels and pits)	1 peach	87	88	35	1	Tr	Tr	Tr	Tr
264	Sliced	1c	170	88	75	1	Tr	Tr	0.1	0.1
267	Canned, fruit and liquid, juice pack									
		1 c	248	87	110	2	Tr	Tr	Tr	Tr
268		1 half	77	87	35	Tr	Tr	Tr	Tr	Tr
	Canned halves or slices, water pack	250 ml	258	93	62[1]	1	Tr	Tr	Tr	0
	Peaches									
	Dried									
269	Uncooked	1 c	160	32	380	6	1	0.1	0.4	0.6
270	Cooked, unsweetened, fruit and liquid	1 c	258	78	200	3	1	0.1	0.2	0.3
271	Frozen, sliced, sweetened	10-oz con-tainer	284	75	265	2	Tr	Tr	0.1	0.2
272		1 c	250	75	235	2	Tr	Tr	0.1	0.2
	Pears									
	Raw, with skin, cored									
273	Bartlett, 2½-in diam. (about 2½ per lb with cores and stems)	1 pear	166	84	100	1	1	Tr	0.1	0.2
274	Bosc, 2½-in diam. (about 3 per lb with cores and stems)	1 pear	141	84	85	1	1	Tr	0.1	0.1
275	D'Anjou, 3-in diam. (about 2 per lb with cores and stems)	1 pear	200	84	120	1	1	Tr	0.2	0.2
278	Canned, fruit and liquid, juice pack	1 c	248	86	125	1	Tr	Tr	Tr	Tr
279		1 half	77	86	40	Tr	Tr	Tr	Tr	Tr
	Pineapple									
280	Raw, diced	1 c	155	87	75	1	1	Tr	0.1	0.2
	Canned, fruit and liquid									
	Juice pack									
283	Chunks or tidbits	1 c	250	84	150	1	Tr	Tr	Tr	0.1
284	Slices	1 slice	58	84	35	Tr	Tr	Tr	Tr	Tr
	Water pack, cubes	250 ml	260	91	83[1]	1	Tr	Tr		Tr
285	Pineapple juice, unsweet-ened, canned	1 c	250	86	140	1	Tr	Tr	Tr	0.1
	Plantains, without peel									
286	Raw	1 plan-tain	179	65	220	2	1	0.3	0.1	0.1
287	Cooked, boiled, sliced	1 c	154	67	180	1	Tr	0.1	Tr	0.1
	Plums, without pits									
	Raw									
288	2⅛-in diam. (about 6½ per lb with pits)	1 plum	66	85	35	1	Tr	Tr	0.3	0.1

Nutrients in Indicated Quantity

Cholesterol (mg)	Carbohydrate (g)	Calcium (mg)	Phosphorus (mg)	Iron (mg)	Potassium (mg)	Sodium (mg)	Vitamin A Value		Thiamin (mg)	Riboflavin (mg)	Niacin (mg)	Ascorbic Acid (mg)	Item No.
							IU	RE					
0	25	20	35	1.1	390	7	290	29	0.14	0.07	0.8	72	261
0	17	35	12	0.3	247	9	400	40	0.04	0.04	0.5	92	262
0	10	4	10	0.1	171	Tr	470	47	0.01	0.04	0.9	6	263
0	19	9	20	0.2	335	Tr	910	91	0.03	0.07	1.7	11	264
0	29	15	42	0.7	317	10	940	94	0.02	0.04	1.4	9	267
0	9	5	13	0.2	99	3	290	29	0.01	0.01	0.4	3	268
0	16	5		0.8	255	8	137		0.02	0.05	1.4	7	
0	98	45	190	6.5	1,594	11	3,460	346	Tr	0.34	7.0	8	269
0	51	23	98	3.4	826	5	510	51	0.01	0.05	3.9	10	270
0	68	9	31	1.1	369	17	810	81	0.04	0.10	1.9	268*	271
0	60	8	28	0.9	325	15	710	71	0.03	0.09	1.6	236*	272
0	25	18	18	0.4	208	Tr	30	3	0.03	0.07	0.2	7	273
0	21	16	16	0.4	176	Tr	30	3	0.03	0.06	0.1	6	274
0	30	22	22	0.5	250	Tr	40	4	0.04	0.08	0.2	8	275
0	32	22	30	0.7	238	10	10	1	0.03	0.03	0.5	4	278
0	10	7	9	0.2	74	3	Tr	Tr	0.01	0.01	0.2	1	279
0	19	11	11	0.6	175	2	40	4	0.14	0.06	0.7	24	280
0	39	35	15	0.7	305	3	100	10	0.24	0.05	0.7	24	283
0	9	8	3	0.2	71	1	20	2	0.06	0.01	0.2	6	284
0	22	39		1.0	330	3	5		0.24	0.07	1.0	20	
0	34	43	20	0.7	335	3	10	1	0.14	0.06	0.6	27	285
0	57	5	61	1.1	893	7	2,020	202	0.09	0.10	1.2	33	286
0	48	3	43	0.9	716	8	1,400	140	0.07	0.08	1.2	17	287
0	9	3	7	0.1	114	Tr	210	21	0.03	0.06	0.3	6	288

Table continued on following page

*With added ascorbic acid.

Item No.	Foods, Approximate Measures, Units, and Weight (Weight of Edible Portion Only)		Grams	Water (%)	Food Energy (cal)	Pro- tein (g)	Fat (g)	Satu- rated (g)	Fatty Acids Mono- unsatu- rated (g)	Poly- unsatu- rated (g)
289	1½-in diam. (about 15 per lb with pits)	1 plum	28	85	15	Tr	Tr	Tr	0.1	Tr
292	Canned, purple, fruit and liquid, juice pack	1 c	252	84	145	1	Tr	Tr	Tr	Tr
293		3 plums	95	84	55	Tr	Tr	Tr	Tr	Tr
	Prunes, dried									
294	Uncooked	4 extra large or 5 large prunes	49	32	115	1	Tr	Tr	0.2	0.1
295	Cooked, unsweetened, fruit and liquid	1 c	212	70	225	2	Tr	Tr	0.3	0.1
296	Prune juice, canned or bottled	1 c	256	81	180	2	Tr	Tr	0.1	Tr
	Raisins, seedless									
297	Cup, not pressed down	1 c	145	15	435	5	1	0.2	Tr	0.2
298	Packet, ½ oz (1½ tbsp)	1 packet	14	15	40	Tr	Tr	Tr	Tr	Tr
299	Raspberries, raw	1 c	123	87	60	1	1	Tr	0.1	0.4
	Rhubarb									
	Raw, diced	250 ml	129	94	27[1]	1	Tr			0
	Strawberries									
303	Raw, capped, whole	1 c	149	92	45	1	1	Tr	0.1	0.3
	Frozen, unsweetened	250 ml	157	90	55[1]	Tr	Tr	Tr		Tr
	Tangerines									
306	Raw, without peel and seeds (2⅜-in diam., about 4 per lb, with peel and seeds)	1 tanger- ine	84	88	35	1	Tr	Tr	Tr	Tr
307	Canned, light syrup, fruit and liquid	1 c	252	83	155	1	Tr	Tr	Tr	0.1
	Watermelon, raw, without rind and seeds									
309	Piece (4 by 8 in wedge with rind and seeds; 1/16 of 32⅔-lb melon, 10 by 16 in)	1 piece	482	92	155	3	2	0.3	0.2	1.0
310	Diced	1 c	160	92	50	1	1	0.1	0.1	0.3
	Grain Products									
311	Bagels, plain or water, en- riched, 3½-in diam.*	1 bagel	68	29	200	7	2	0.3	0.5	0.7
312	Barley, pearled, light, un- cooked	1 cup	200	11	700	16	2	0.3	0.2	0.9
	Biscuits, baking powder, 2- in diam. (enriched flour, vegetable short- ening)									
313	From home recipe	1 biscuit	28	28	100	2	5	1.2	2.0	1.3
314	From mix	1 biscuit	28	29	95	2	3	0.8	1.4	0.9
315	From refrigerated dough	1 biscuit	20	30	65	1	2	0.6	0.9	0.6
	Breadcrumbs, enriched									
316	Dry, grated Soft. See White bread (item 351)	1 c	100	7	390	13	5	1.5	1.6	1.0

*Egg bagels have 44 mg cholesterol and 22 IU or 7 RE vitamin A per bagel.

Nutrients in Indicated Quantity

Cho-les-terol (mg)	Carbo-hydrate (g)	Cal-cium (mg)	Phos-phorus (mg)	Iron (mg)	Potas-sium (mg)	Sodium (mg)	Vitamin A Value IU	RE	Thia-min (mg)	Ribo-flavin (mg)	Nia-cin (mg)	Ascor-bic Acid (mg)	Item No.
0	4	1	3	Tr	48	Tr	90	9	0.01	0.03	0.1	3	289
0	38	25	38	0.9	388	3	2,540	254	0.06	0.15	1.2	7	292
0	14	10	14	0.3	146	1	960	96	0.02	0.06	0.4	3	293
0	31	25	39	1.2	365	2	970	97	0.04	0.08	1.0	2	294
0	60	49	74	2.4	708	4	650	65	0.05	0.21	1.5	6	295
0	45	31	64	3.0	707	10	10	1	0.04	0.18	2.0	10	296
0	115	71	141	3.0	1.089	17	10	1	0.23	0.13	1.2	5	297
0	11	7	14	0.3	105	2	Tr	Tr	0.02	0.01	0.1	Tr	298
0	14	27	15	0.7	187	Tr	160	16	0.04	0.11	1.1	31	299
0	6	111		0.3	372	5	13		0.03	0.04	0.6	10	
0	10	21	28	0.6	247	1	40	4	0.03	0.10	0.3	84	303
0	14	25		1.2	232	3	6		0.04	0.06	0.9	65	
0	9	12	8	0.1	132	1	770	77	0.09	0.02	0.1	26	306
0	41	18	25	0.9	197	15	2,120	212	0.13	0.11	1.1	50	307
0	35	39	43	0.8	559	10	1,760	176	0.39	0.10	1.0	46	309
0	11	13	14	0.3	186	3	590	59	0.13	0.03	0.3	15	310
0	38	29	46	1.8	50	245	0	0	0.26	0.20	2.4	0	311
0	158	32	378	4.2	320	6	0	0	0.24	0.10	6.2	0	312
Tr	13	47	36	0.7	32	195	10	3	0.08	0.08	0.8	Tr	313
Tr	14	58	128	0.7	56	262	20	4	0.12	0.11	0.8	Tr	314
1	10	4	79	0.5	18	249	0	0	0.08	0.05	0.7	0	315
5	73	122	141	4.1	152	736	0	0	0.35	0.35	4.8	0	316

Table continued on following page

| | | | | | Food | Pro- | | | Fatty Acids | |
| | Foods, Approximate Measures, | | | Water | Energy | tein | Fat | Satu-rated | Mono-unsatu-rated | Poly-unsatu-rated |
Item No.	Units, and Weight (Weight of Edible Portion Only)		Grams	(%)	(cal)	(g)	(g)	(g)	(g)	(g)
	Breads									
317	Boston brown bread, canned, slice, 3¼ in by ½ in*	1 slice	45	45	95	2	1	0.3	0.1	0.1
	Cracked-wheat bread (¾ enriched wheat flour, ¼ cracked wheat flour)*									
318	Loaf, 1 lb	1 loaf	454	35	1,190	42	16	3.1	4.3	5.7
319	Slice (18 per loaf)	1 slice	25	35	65	2	1	0.2	0.2	0.3
320	Toasted	1 slice	21	26	65	2	1	0.2	0.2	0.3
	French or Vienna bread, enriched*									
321	Loaf, 1 lb	1 loaf	454	34	1,270	43	18	3.8	5.7	5.9
322	Slice French, 5 by 2½ by 1 in	1 slice	35	34	100	3	1	0.3	0.4	0.5
323	Vienna, 4¾ by 4 by ½ in	1 slice	25	34	70	2	1	0.2	0.3	0.3
	Italian bread, enriched									
324	Loaf, 1 lb	1 loaf	454	32	1,255	41	4	0.6	0.3	1.6
325	Slice, 4½ by 3¼ by ¾ in	1 slice	30	32	85	3	Tr	Tr	Tr	0.1
	Melba toast	1 piece	4	5	16[1]	Tr	Tr	—	—	—
	Mixed-grain bread, en-riched*									
326	Loaf, 1 lb	1 loaf	454	37	1,165	45	17	3.2	4.1	6.5
327	Slice (18 per loaf)	1 slice	25	37	65	2	1	0.2	0.2	0.4
328	Toasted	1 slice	23	27	65	2	1	0.2	0.2	0.4
	Oatmeal bread, enriched*									
329	Loaf, 1 lb	1 loaf	454	37	1,145	38	20	3.7	7.1	8.2
330	Slice (18 per loaf)	1 slice	25	37	65	2	1	0.2	0.4	0.5
331	Toasted	1 slice	23	30	65	2	1	0.2	0.4	0.5
332	Pita bread, enriched, white, 6½-in diam.	1 pita	60	31	165	6	1	0.1	0.1	0.4
	Pumpernickel (⅔ rye flour, ⅓ enriched wheat flour)*									
333	Loaf, 1 lb	1 loaf	454	37	1,160	42	16	2.6	3.6	6.4
334	Slice, 5 by 4 by ⅜ in	1 slice	32	37	80	3	1	0.2	0.3	0.5
335	Toasted	1 slice	29	28	80	3	1	0.2	0.3	0.5
	Raisin bread, enriched*									
336	Loaf, 1 lb	1 loaf	454	33	1,260	37	18	4.1	6.5	6.7
337	Slice (18 per loaf)	1 slice	25	33	65	2	1	0.2	0.3	0.4
338	Toasted	1 slice	21	24	65	2	1	0.2	0.3	0.4
	Rye bread, light (⅔ enriched wheat flour, ⅓ rye flour)*									
339	Loaf, 1 lb	1 loaf	454	37	1,190	38	17	3.3	5.2	5.5
340	Slice, 4¾ by 3¾ by ⁷⁄₁₆ in	1 slice	25	37	65	2	1	0.2	0.3	0.3
341	Toasted	1 slice	22	28	65	2	1	0.2	0.3	0.3
	Rye bread, dark, pumpernickel	1 slice	32	34	79[1]	3	Tr	Tr		Tr

*Made with vegetable shortening.

							Vitamin A Value					Ascor-	
Cho-les-terol (mg)	Carbo-hydrate (g)	Cal-cium (mg)	Phos-phorus (mg)	Iron (mg)	Potas-sium (mg)	Sodium (mg)	IU	RE	Thia-min (mg)	Ribo-flavin (mg)	Nia-cin (mg)	bic Acid (mg)	Item No.
3	21	41	72	0.9	131	113	0*	0*	0.06	0.04	0.7	0	317
0	227	295	581	12.1	608	1,966	Tr	Tr	1.73	1.73	15.3	Tr	318
0	12	16	32	0.7	34	106	Tr	Tr	0.10	0.09	0.8	Tr	319
0	12	16	32	0.7	34	106	Tr	Tr	0.07	0.09	0.8	Tr	320
0	230	499	386	14.0	409	2,633	Tr	Tr	2.09	1.59	18.2	Tr	321
0	18	39	30	1.1	32	203	Tr	Tr	0.16	0.12	1.4	Tr	322
0	13	28	21	0.8	23	145	Tr	Tr	0.12	0.09	1.0	Tr	323
0	256	77	350	12.7	336	2,656	0	0	1.80	1.10	15.0	0	324
0	17	5	23	0.8	22	176	0	0	0.12	0.07	1.0	0	325
—	3	5		0.1	6	29	0		Tr	0.01	0.1	0	
0	212	472	962	14.8	990	1,870	Tr	Tr	1.77	1.73	18.9	Tr	326
0	12	27	55	0.8	56	106	Tr	Tr	0.10	0.10	1.1	Tr	327
0	12	27	55	0.8	56	106	Tr	Tr	0.08	0.10	1.1	Tr	328
0	212	267	563	12.0	707	2,231	0	0	2.09	1.20	15.4	0	329
0	12	15	31	0.7	39	124	0	0	0.12	0.07	0.9	0	330
0	12	15	31	0.7	39	124	0	0	0.09	0.07	0.9	0	331
0	33	49	60	1.4	71	339	0	0	0.27	0.12	2.2	0	332
0	218	322	990	12.4	1,966	2,461	0	0	1.54	2.36	15.0	0	333
0	16	23	71	0.9	141	177	0	0	0.11	0.17	1.1	0	334
0	16	23	71	0.9	141	177	0	0	0.09	0.17	1.1	0	335
0	239	463	395	14.1	1,058	1,657	Tr	Tr	1.50	2.81	18.6	Tr	336
0	13	25	22	0.8	59	92	Tr	Tr	0.08	0.15	1.0	Tr	337
0	13	25	22	0.8	59	92	Tr	Tr	0.06	0.15	1.0	Tr	338
0	218	363	658	12.3	926	3,164	0	0	1.86	1.45	15.0	0	339
0	12	20	36	0.7	51	175	0	0	0.10	0.08	0.8	0	340
0	12	20	36	0.7	51	175	0	0	0.08	0.08	0.8	0	341
Tr	17	27		0.8	145	182		0	0.07	0.05	1.0	0	

Table continued on following page

*Made with white cornmeal. If made with yellow cornmeal, value is 32 IU or 3 RE.

| | | | | | | | | Fatty Acids | |
Item No.	Foods, Approximate Measures, Units, and Weight (Weight of Edible Portion Only)	Grams	Water (%)	Food Energy (cal)	Pro-tein (g)	Fat (g)	Satu-rated (g)	Mono-unsatu-rated (g)	Poly-unsatu-rated (g)
	Wheat bread, enriched*								
342	Loaf, 1 lb	1 loaf	454	37	1,160	43	19	3.9	7.3	4.5
343	Slice (18 per loaf)	1 slice	25	37	65	2	1	0.2	0.4	0.3
344	Toasted	1 slice	23	28	65	3	1	0.2	0.4	0.3
	White bread, enriched*								
345	Loaf, 1 lb	1 loaf	454	37	1,210	38	18	5.6	6.5	4.2
346	Slice (18 per loaf)	1 slice	25	37	65	2	1	0.3	0.4	0.2
347	Toasted	1 slice	22	28	65	2	1	0.3	0.4	0.2
348	Slice (22 per loaf)	1 slice	20	37	55	2	1	0.2	0.3	0.2
349	Toasted	1 slice	17	28	55	2	1	0.2	0.3	0.2
350	Cubes	1 c	30	37	80	2	1	0.4	0.4	0.3
351	Crumbs, soft	1 c	45	37	120	4	2	0.6	0.6	0.4
	Whole-wheat bread*								
352	Loaf, 1 lb	1 loaf	454	38	1,110	44	20	5.8	6.8	5.2
353	Slice (16 per loaf)	1 slice	28	38	70	3	1	0.4	0.4	0.3
354	Toasted	1 slice	25	29	70	3	1	0.4	0.4	0.3
	Bread stuffing (from enriched bread), prepared from mix								
355	Dry type	1 c	140	33	500	9	31	6.1	13.3	9.6
356	Moist type	1 c	203	61	420	9	26	5.3	11.3	8.0
	Breakfast cereals								
	Hot type, cooked								
	Corn (hominy) grits								
357	Regular and quick, enriched	1 c	242	85	145	3	Tr	Tr	0.1	0.2
358	Instant, plain	1 pkt	137	85	80	2	Tr	Tr	Tr	0.1
	Cream of Wheat								
359	Regular, quick, instant	1 c	244	86	140	4	Tr	0.1	Tr	0.2
360	Mix'n Eat, plain	1 pkt	142	82	100	3	Tr	Tr	Tr	0.1
361	Malt-O-Meal	1 c	240	88	120	4	Tr	Tr	Tr	0.1
	Oatmeal or rolled oats								
362	Regular, quick, instant, nonfortified	1 c	234	85	145	6	2	0.4	0.8	1.0
	Instant, fortified								
363	Plain	1 pkt	177	86	105	4	2	0.3	0.6	0.7
364	Flavored	1 pkt	164	76	160	5	2	0.3	0.7	0.8
	Red River	125 ml	125	—	82[1]	3	Tr	—		—
	Ready to eat								
365	All-Bran (about ⅓ c)	1 oz	28	3	70	4	1	0.1	0.1	0.3
	Bran flakes, whole wheat	200 ml	40	5	139[1]	4	Tr	—		—
	Bran, bran buds	125 ml	44	3	122[1]	5	Tr	—		—
	Bran, 100%	125 ml	35	3	90[1]	4	Tr	Tr		Tr
	Cheerios (about 1¼ c)	1 oz	28	5	110	4	2	0.3	0.6	0.7
	Corn bran	200 ml	30	2	118[1]	2	1	—		—

*Made with vegetable shortening.

Nutrients in Indicated Quantity

Cholesterol (mg)	Carbohydrate (g)	Calcium (mg)	Phosphorus (mg)	Iron (mg)	Potassium (mg)	Sodium (mg)	Vitamin A Value IU	Vitamin A Value RE	Thiamin (mg)	Riboflavin (mg)	Niacin (mg)	Ascorbic Acid (mg)	Item No.
0	213	572	835	15.8	627	2,447	Tr	Tr	2.09	1.45	20.5	Tr	342
0	12	32	47	0.9	35	138	Tr	Tr	0.12	0.08	1.2	Tr	343
0	12	32	47	0.9	35	138	Tr	Tr	0.10	0.08	1.2	Tr	344
0	222	572	490	12.9	508	2,334	Tr	Tr	2.13	1.41	17.0	Tr	345
0	12	32	27	0.7	28	129	Tr	Tr	0.12	0.08	0.9	Tr	346
0	12	32	27	0.7	28	129	Tr	Tr	0.09	0.08	0.9	Tr	347
0	10	25	21	0.6	22	101	Tr	Tr	0.09	0.06	0.7	Tr	348
0	10	25	21	0.6	22	101	Tr	Tr	0.07	0.06	0.7	Tr	349
0	15	38	32	0.9	34	154	Tr	Tr	0.14	0.09	1.1	Tr	350
0	22	57	49	1.3	50	231	Tr	Tr	0.21	0.14	1.7	Tr	351
0	206	327	1,180	15.5	799	2,887	Tr	Tr	1.59	0.95	17.4	Tr	352
0	13	20	74	1.0	50	180	Tr	Tr	0.10	0.06	1.1	Tr	353
0	13	20	74	1.0	50	180	Tr	Tr	0.08	0.06	1.1	Tr	354
0	50	92	136	2.2	126	1,254	910	273	0.17	0.20	2.5	0	355
67	40	81	134	2.0	118	1,023	850	256	0.10	0.18	1.6	0	356
0	31	0	29	1.5*	53	0†	0‡	0‡	0.24*	0.15*	2.0*	0	357
0	18	7	16	1.0*	29	343	0	0	0.18*	0.08*	1.3*	0	358
0	29	54§	43‖	10.9§	46	5‖,¶	0	0	0.24§	0.07§	1.5§	0	359
0	21	20§	20§	8.1§	38	241	1,250§	376§	0.43§	0.28§	5.0§	0	360
0	26	5	24§	9.6§	31	2**	0	0	0.48§	0.24§	5.8§	0	361
0	25	19	178	1.6	131	2††	40	4	0.26	0.05	0.3	0	362
0	18	163*	133	6.3*	99	285*	1,510*	453*	0.53*	0.28*	5.5*	0	363
0	31	168*	148	6.7*	137	254*	1,530*	460*	0.53*	0.38*	5.9*	Tr	364
0	16	—		0.4	—	7		0	0.04	Tr	1.1	0	
0	21	23	264	4.5§	350	320	1,250§	375§	0.37§	0.43§	5.0§	15§	365
0	32	1		5.3	175	291		4	80	0.4	2.7	0	
0	34	36		5.9	400	221		0	0.88	0.09	6.6	0	
0	29	27		4.7	431	—		0	0.70	0.13	8.9	10	
0	26	23		4.0	66	259		0	0.60	0.01	1.8	0	
0	20	48	134	4.5§	101	307	1,250§	375§	0.37*	0.43§	5.0§	15§	

Table continued on following page

*Nutrient added.

†Cooked without salt. If salt is added according to label recommendations, sodium content is 540 mg.

‡For white corn grits. Cooked yellow grits contain 145 IU or 14 RE.

§Value based on label declaration for added nutrients.

‖For regular and instant cereal. For quick cereal, phosphorus is 102 mg and sodium is 142 mg.

¶Cooked without salt. If salt is added according to label recommendations, sodium content is 390 mg.

**Cooked without salt. If salt is added according to label recommendations, sodium content is 324 mg.

††Cooked without salt. If salt is added according to label recommendations, sodium content is 374 mg.

Item No.	Foods, Approximate Measures, Units, and Weight (Weight of Edible Portion Only)		Grams	Water (%)	Food Energy (cal)	Pro-tein (g)	Fat (g)	Fatty Acids Satu-rated (g)	Mono-unsatu-rated (g)	Poly-unsatu-rated (g)
	Corn Flakes (about 1¼ c)									
368	Kellogg's	1 oz	28	3	110	2	Tr	Tr	Tr	Tr
369	Toasties	1 oz	28	3	110	2	Tr	Tr	Tr	Tr
	40% Bran Flakes									
370	Kellogg's (about ¾ c)	1 oz	28	3	90	4	1	0.1	0.1	0.3
371	Post (about ⅔ c)	1 oz	28	3	90	3	Tr	0.1	0.1	0.2
373	Golden Grahams (about ¾ c)	1 oz	28	2	110	2	1	0.7	0.1	0.2
	Granola, homemade	125 ml	64	3	312[1]	8	17	3		9
374	Grape-Nuts (about ¼ c)	1 oz	28	3	100	3	Tr	Tr	Tr	0.1
377	Nature Valley Granola (about ⅓ c)	1 oz	28	4	125	3	5	3.3	0.7	0.7
378	100% Natural Cereal (about ¼ c)	1 oz	28	2	135	3	6	4.1	1.2	0.5
379	Product 19 (about ¾ c)	1 oz	28	3	110	3	Tr	Tr	Tr	0.1
	Raisin Bran									
380	Kellogg's (about ¾ c)	1 oz	28	8	90	3	1	0.1	0.1	0.3
381	Post (about ½ c)	1 oz	28	9	85	3	1	0.1	0.1	0.3
	Rice Flakes	200 ml	27	5	103[1]	2	Tr	—		—
382	Rice Krispies (about 1 c)	1 oz	28	2	110	2	Tr	Tr	Tr	0.1
	Rice, puffed	250 ml	15	2	59[1]	Tr	Tr	—		—
383	Shredded Wheat (about ⅔ c)	1 oz	28	5	100	3	1	0.1	0.1	0.3
	Shreddies (whole wheat)	200 ml	44	5	169[1]	4	Tr	—		—
384	Special K (about 1⅓ c)	1 oz	28	2	110	6	Tr	Tr	Tr	Tr
388	Total (about 1 c)	1 oz	28	4	100	3	1	0.1	0.1	0.3
389	Trix (about 1 c)	1 oz	28	3	110	2	Tr	0.2	0.1	0.1
	Wheat, puffed	250 ml	13	2	50[1]	2	Tr	—		—
390	Wheaties (about 1 c)	1 oz	28	5	100	3	Tr	0.1	Tr	0.2
391	Buckwheat flour, light, sifted	1 c	98	12	340	6	1	0.2	0.4	0.4
392	Bulgur, uncooked	1 c	170	10	600	19	3	1.2	0.3	1.2
437	Corn chips	1-oz package	28	1	155	2	9	1.4	2.4	3.7
	Cornmeal									
438	Whole-ground, unbolted, dry form	1 c	122	12	435	11	5	0.5	1.1	2.5
439	Bolted (nearly whole-grain), dry form	1 c	122	12	440	11	4	0.5	0.9	2.2
	Degermed, enriched									
440	Dry form	1 c	138	12	500	11	2	0.2	0.4	0.9
441	Cooked	1 c	240	88	120	3	Tr	Tr	0.1	0.2
	Crackers*									
	Cheese									
442	Plain, 1-in square	10 crackers	10	4	50	1	3	0.9	1.2	0.3
443	Sandwich type (peanut butter)	1 sand-wich	8	3	40	1	2	0.4	0.8	0.3
444	Graham, plain, 2½-in square	2 crackers	14	5	60	1	1	0.4	0.6	0.4

Nutrients in Indicated Quantity

Cho-les-terol (mg)	Carbo-hydrate (g)	Cal-cium (mg)	Phos-phorus (mg)	Iron (mg)	Potas-sium (mg)	Sodium (mg)	Vitamin A Value		Thia-min (mg)	Ribo-flavin (mg)	Nia-cin (mg)	Ascor-bic Acid (mg)	Item No.
							IU	RE					
0	24	1	18	1.8*	26	351	1,250*	375*	0.37*	0.43*	5.0*	15*	368
0	24	1	12	0.7†	33	297	1,250*	375*	0.37*	0.43*	5.0*	0	369
0	22	14	139	8.1*	180	264	1,250*	375*	0.37*	0.43*	5.0*	0	370
0	22	12	179	4.5*	151	260	1,250*	375*	0.37*	0.43*	5.0*	0	371
Tr	24	17	41	4.5*	63	346	1,250*	375*	0.37*	0.43*	5.0*	15*	373
0	35	40		2.5	321	6		2	0.38	0.16	2.7	Tr	
0	23	11	71	1.2	95	197	1,250*	375*	0.37*	0.43*	5.0*	0	374
0	19	18	89	0.9	98	58	20	2	0.10	0.05	0.2	0	377
Tr	18	49	104	0.8	140	12	20	2	0.09	0.15	0.6	0	378
0	24	3	40	18.0*	44	325	5,000*	1,501*	1.50*	1.70*	20.0*	60*	379
0	21	10	105	3.5*	147	207	960*	288*	0.28*	0.34*	3.9*	0	380
0	21	13	119	4.5*	175	185	1,250*	375*	0.37*	0.43*	5.0*	0	381
0	24	8		3.6	—	—		0	0.54	0.02	1.6	0	
0	25	4	34	1.8*	29	340	1,250*	375*	0.37*	0.43*	5.0*	15*	382
0	14	1		Tr	17	1		0	Tr	0.01	0.5	0	
0	23	11	100	1.2	102	3	0	0	0.07	0.08	1.5	0	383
0	37	16		5.9	—	—		0	0.88	0.07	2.9	0	
Tr	21	8	55	4.5*	49	265	1,250*	375*	0.37*	0.43*	5.0*	15*	384
0	22	48	118	18.0*	106	352	5,000*	1,501*	1.50*	1.70*	20.0*	60*	388
0	25	6	19	4.5*	27	181	1,250*	375*	0.37*	0.43*	5.0*	15*	389
0	10	3		5	46	Tr		0	0.01	0.03	1.2	0	
0	23	43	98	4.5*	106	354	1,250*	375*	0.37*	0.43*	5.0*	15*	390
0	78	11	86	1.0	314	2	0	0	0.08	0.04	0.4	0	391
0	129	49	575	9.5	389	7	0	0	0.48	0.24	7.7	0	392
0	16	35	52	0.5	52	233	110	11	0.04	0.05	0.4	1	437
0	90	24	312	2.2	346	1	620	62	0.46	0.13	2.4	0	438
0	91	21	272	2.2	303	1	590	59	0.37	0.10	2.3	0	439
0	108	8	137	5.9	166	1	610	61	0.61	0.36	4.8	0	440
0	26	2	34	1.4	38	0	140	14	0.14	0.10	1.2	0	441
6	6	11	17	0.3	17	112	20	5	0.05	0.04	0.4	0	442
1	5	7	25	0.3	17	90	Tr	Tr	0.04	0.03	0.6	0	443
0	11	6	20	0.4	36	86	0	0	0.02	0.03	0.6	0	444

Table continued on following page

*Value based on label declaration for added nutrients.
†Nutrient added.

Item No.	Foods, Approximate Measures, Units, and Weight (Weight of Edible Portion Only)		Grams	Water (%)	Food Energy (cal)	Pro-tein (g)	Fat (g)	Satu-rated (g)	Mono-unsatu-rated (g)	Poly-unsatu-rated (g)
									Fatty Acids	
445	Melba toast, plain	1 piece	5	4	20	1	Tr	0.1	0.1	0.1
446	Rye wafers, whole-grain, 1⅛ by 3½ in	2 wafers	14	5	55	1	1	0.3	0.4	0.3
447	Saltines*	4 crackers	12	4	50	1	1	0.5	0.4	0.2
448	Snack-type, standard	1 round cracker	3	3	15	Tr	1	0.2	0.4	0.1
449	Wheat, thin	4 crackers	8	3	35	1	1	0.5	0.5	0.4
450	Whole-wheat wafers	2 crackers	8	4	35	1	2	0.5	0.6	0.4
451	Croissants, made with enriched flour, 4½ by 4 by 1¾ in	1 croissant	57	22	235	5	12	3.5	6.7	1.4
458	English muffins, plain, enriched	1 muffin	57	42	140	5	1	0.3	0.2	0.3
459	Toasted	1 muffin	50	29	140	5	1	0.3	0.2	0.3
	Flour									
	Carob	250 ml	148	11	266[1]	7	2	Tr		Tr
	Cornstarch	125 ml	68	12	246[1]	Tr	0	0		0
	Potato	250 ml	38	8	133[2]	3	Tr	Tr		Tr
	Rye, light	250 ml	100	11	357[1]	9	1	Tr		Tr
	Soybean, defatted	250 ml	106	8	346[2]	50	Tr	0		0
	Wheat. See Wheat flours (items 520–524)									
460	French toast, from home recipe	1 slice	65	53	155	6	7	1.6	2.0	1.6
	Macaroni, enriched, cooked (cut lengths, elbows, shells)									
461	Firm stage (hot)	1 c	130	64	190	7	1	0.1	0.1	0.3
	Tender stage									
462	Cold	1 c	105	72	115	4	Tr	0.1	0.1	0.2
463	Hot	1 c	140	72	155	5	1	0.1	0.1	0.2
	Muffins made with en-riched flour, 2½-in diam., 1½ in high									
	From home recipe									
464	Blueberry†	1 muffin	45	37	135	3	5	1.5	2.1	1.2
465	Bran‡	1 muffin	45	35	125	3	6	1.4	1.6	2.3
466	Corn (enriched, de-germed cornmeal and flour)†	1 muffin	45	33	145	3	5	1.5	2.2	1.4
	From commercial mix (egg and water added)									
467	Blueberry	1 muffin	45	33	140	3	5	1.4	2.0	1.2
468	Bran	1 muffin	45	28	140	3	4	1.3	1.6	1.0
469	Corn	1 muffin	45	30	145	3	6	1.7	2.3	1.4
470	Noodles (egg noodles), en-riched, cooked	1 c	160	70	200	7	2	0.5	0.6	0.6
471	Noodles, chow mein, canned	1 c	45	11	220	6	11	2.1	7.3	0.4

*Made with lard.
†Made with vegetable shortening.
‡Made with vegetable oil.

Nutrients in Indicated Quantity

Cho-les-terol (mg)	Carbo-hydrate (g)	Cal-cium (mg)	Phos-phorus (mg)	Iron (mg)	Potas-sium (mg)	Sodium (mg)	Vitamin A Value		Thia-min (mg)	Ribo-flavin (mg)	Nia-cin (mg)	Ascor-bic Acid (mg)	Item No.
							IU	RE					
0	4	6	10	0.1	11	44	0	0	0.01	0.01	0.1	0	445
0	10	7	44	0.5	65	115	0	0	0.06	0.03	0.5	0	446
4	9	3	12	0.5	17	165	0	0	0.06	0.05	0.6	0	447
0	2	3	6	0.1	4	30	Tr	Tr	0.01	0.01	0.1	0	448
0	5	3	15	0.3	17	69	Tr	Tr	0.04	0.03	0.4	0	449
0	5	3	22	0.2	31	59	0	0	0.02	0.03	0.4	0	450
13	27	20	64	2.1	68	452	50	13	0.17	0.13	1.3	0	451
0	27	96	67	1.7	331	378	0	0	0.26	0.19	2.2	0	458
0	27	96	67	1.7	331	378	0	0	0.23	0.19	2.2	0	459
0	119	521		6.0	1,348	25		Tr	0.07	0.07	2.4	0	
0	60	0		0	0	0		0	0	0	0	0	
0	30	13		6.5	603	13		0	0.16	0.05	2.1	7	
0	78	22		1.1	156	1		0	0.15	0.07	2.3	0	
0	40	281		11.8	1,929	1		4	1.16	0.36	11.9	0	
112	17	72	85	1.3	86	257	110	32	0.12	0.16	1.0	Tr	460
0	39	14	85	2.1	103	1	0	0	0.23	0.13	1.8	0	461
0	24	8	53	1.3	64	1	0	0	0.15	0.08	1.2	0	462
0	32	11	70	1.7	85	1	0	0	0.20	0.11	1.5	0	463
19	20	54	46	0.9	47	198	40	9	0.10	0.11	0.9	1	464
24	19	60	125	1.4	99	189	230	30	0.11	0.13	1.3	3	465
23	21	66	59	0.9	57	169	80	15	0.11	0.11	0.9	Tr	466
45	22	15	90	0.9	54	225	50	11	0.10	0.17	1.1	Tr	467
28	24	27	182	1.7	50	385	100	14	0.08	0.12	1.9	0	468
42	22	30	128	1.3	31	291	90	16	0.09	0.09	0.8	Tr	469
50	37	16	94	2.6	70	3	110	34	0.22	0.13	1.9	0	470
5	26	14	41	0.4	33	450	0	0	0.05	0.03	0.6	0	471

Table continued on following page

Item No.	Foods, Approximate Measures, Units, and Weight (Weight of Edible Portion Only)		Grams	Water (%)	Food Energy (cal)	Pro-tein (g)	Fat (g)	Satu-rated (g)	Mono-unsatu-rated (g)	Poly-unsatu-rated (g)
									Fatty Acids	
	Pancakes, 4-in diam.									
472	Buckwheat, from mix (with buckwheat and enriched flours), egg and milk added	1 pan-cake	27	58	55	2	2	0.9	0.9	0.5
	Plain									
473	From home recipe us-ing enriched flour	1 pan-cake	27	50	60	2	2	0.5	0.8	0.5
474	From mix (with en-riched flour), egg, milk, and oil added	1 pan-cake	27	54	60	2	2	0.5	0.9	0.5
	Piecrust, made with en-riched flour and vege-table shortening, baked									
475	From home recipe, 9-in diam.	1 pie shell	180	15	900	11	60	14.8	25.9	15.7
476	From mix, 9-in diam.	Piecrust for 2-crust pie	320	19	1,485	20	93	22.7	41.0	25.0
	Popcorn, popped									
497	Air-popped, unsalted	1 c	8	4	30	1	Tr	Tr	0.1	0.2
498	Popped in vegetable oil, salted	1 c	11	3	55	1	3	0.5	1.4	1.2
	Pretzels, made with en-riched flour									
500	Stick, 2¼ in long	10 pretz-els	3	3	10	Tr	Tr	Tr	Tr	Tr
501	Twisted, dutch, 2¾ by 2⅝ in	1 pretzels	16	3	65	2	1	0.1	0.2	0.2
502	Twisted, thin, 3¼ by 2¼ by ¼ in	10 pretz-els	60	3	240	6	2	0.4	0.8	0.6
	Rice									
503	Brown, cooked, served hot	1 c	195	70	230	5	1	0.3	0.3	0.4
	White enriched Commercial varieties, all types									
504	Raw	1 c	185	12	670	12	1	0.2	0.2	0.3
505	Cooked, served hot	1 c	205	73	225	4	Tr	0.1	0.1	0.1
506	Instant, ready-to-serve, hot	1 c	165	73	180	4	0	0.1	0.1	0.1
	Parboiled									
507	Raw	1 c	185	10	685	14	1	0.1	0.1	0.2
	Cooked, served hot	1 c	175	73	185	4	Tr	Tr	Tr	0.1
	Rolls, enriched Commercial									
509	Dinner, 2½-in diam., 2 in high	1 roll	28	32	85	2	2	0.5	0.8	0.6
510	Frankfurter and ham-burger (8 per 11½-oz pkg.)	1 roll	40	34	115	3	2	0.5	0.8	0.6
511	Hard, 3¾-in diam., 2 in high	1 roll	50	25	155	5	2	0.4	0.5	0.6
512	Hoagie or submarine, 11½ by 3 by 2½ in	1 roll	135	31	400	11	8	1.8	3.0	2.2

Nutrients in Indicated Quantity

Cho-les-terol (mg)	Carbo-hydrate (g)	Cal-cium (mg)	Phos-phorus (mg)	Iron (mg)	Potas-sium (mg)	Sodium (mg)	Vitamin A Value		Thia-min (mg)	Ribo-flavin (mg)	Nia-cin (mg)	Ascor-bic Acid (mg)	Item No.
							IU	RE					
20	6	59	91	0.4	66	125	60	17	0.04	0.05	0.2	Tr	472
16	9	27	38	0.5	33	115	30	10	0.06	0.07	0.5	Tr	473
16	8	36	71	0.7	43	160	30	7	0.09	0.12	0.8	Tr	474
0	79	25	90	4.5	90	1,100	0	0	0.54	0.40	5.0	0	475
0	141	131	272	9.3	179	2,602	0	0	1.06	0.80	9.9	0	476
0	6	1	22	0.2	20	Tr	10	1	0.03	0.01	0.2	0	497
0	6	3	31	0.3	19	86	20	2	0.01	0.02	0.1	0	498
0	2	1	3	0.1	3	48	0	0	0.01	0.01	0.1	0	500
0	13	4	15	0.3	16	258	0	0	0.05	0.04	0.7	0	501
0	48	16	55	1.2	61	966	0	0	0.19	0.15	2.6	0	502
0	50	23	142	1.0	137	0	0	0	0.18	0.04	2.7	0	503
0	149	44	174	5.4	170	9	0	0	0.81	0.06	6.5	0	504
0	50	21	57	1.8	57	0	0	0	0.23	0.02	2.1	0	505
0	40	5	31	1.3	0	0	0	0	0.21	0.02	1.7	0	506
0	150	111	370	5.4	278	17	0	0	0.81	0.07	6.5	0	507
0	41	33	100	1.4	75	0	0	0	0.19	0.02	2.1	0	508
Tr	14	33	44	0.8	36	155	Tr	Tr	0.14	0.09	1.1	Tr	509
Tr	20	54	44	1.2	56	241	Tr	Tr	0.20	0.13	1.6	Tr	510
Tr	30	24	46	1.4	49	313	0	0	0.20	0.12	1.7	0	511
Tr	72	100	115	3.8	128	683	0	0	0.54	0.33	4.5	0	512

Table continued on following page

| | | | | | | Fatty Acids | | |
Item No.	Foods, Approximate Measures, Units, and Weight (Weight of Edible Portion Only)		Grams	Water (%)	Food Energy (cal)	Pro-tein (g)	Fat (g)	Satu-rated (g)	Mono-unsatu-rated (g)	Poly-unsatu-rated (g)
	From home recipe									
513	Dinner, 2½-in diam., 2 in high	1 roll	35	26	120	3	3	0.8	1.2	0.9
	Spaghetti, enriched, cooked									
514	Firm stage, al dente, served hot	1 c	130	64	190	7	1	0.1	0.1	0.3
515	Tender stage, served hot	1 c	140	73	155	5	1	0.1	0.1	0.2
517	Tortillas, corn	1 tortilla	30	45	65	2	1	0.1	0.3	0.6
	Waffles, made with en-riched flour, 7-in diam.									
518	From home recipe	1 waffle	75	37	245	7	13	4.0	4.9	2.6
519	From mix, egg and milk added	1 waffle	75	42	205	7	8	2.7	2.9	1.5
	Wheat bran	15 ml	3	12	6[1]	Tr	Tr	Tr		Tr
	Wheat flours									
	All-purpose or family flour, enriched									
520	Sifted, spooned	1 c	115	12	420	12	1	0.2	0.1	0.5
521	Unsifted, spooned	1 c	125	12	455	13	1	0.2	0.1	0.5
522	Cake or pastry flour, en-riched, sifted, spooned	1 c	96	12	350	7	1	0.1	0.1	0.3
523	Self-rising, enriched un-sifted spooned	1 c	125	12	440	12	1	0.2	0.1	0.5
524	Whole-wheat, from hard wheats, stirred	1 c	120	12	400	16	2	0.3	0.3	1.1
	Wheat germ	15 ml	7	12	25[1]	2	Tr	Tr		Tr
Legumes, Nuts, and Seeds										
525	Almonds, shelled Slivered, packed	1 c	135	4	795	27	70	6.7	45.8	14.8
526	Whole	1 oz	28	4	165	6	15	1.4	9.6	3.1
	Beans, dry									
	Cooked, drained									
527	Black	1 c	171	66	225	15	1	0.1	0.1	0.5
	Common white	250 ml	195	69	230[1]	15	1	Tr		Tr
528	Great Northern	1 c	180	69	210	14	1	0.1	0.1	0.6
529	Lima	1 c	190	64	260	16	1	0.2	0.1	0.5
530	Pea (navy)	1 c	190	69	225	15	1	0.1	0.1	0.7
531	Pinto	1 c	180	65	265	15	1	0.1	0.1	0.5
	Red kidney	250 ml	195	69	230[1]	15	Tr	Tr		Tr
	Canned, solids and liquids									
	White with									
532	Frankfurters (sliced)	1 c	255	71	365	19	18	7.4	8.8	0.7
533	Pork and tomato sauce	1 c	255	71	310	16	7	2.4	2.7	0.7
534	Pork and sweet sauce	1 c	255	66	385	16	12	4.3	4.9	1.2
535	Red kidney	1 c	255	76	230	15	1	0.1	0.1	0.6
536	Black-eyed peas, dry, cooked (with residual cooking liquid)	1 c	250	80	190	13	1	0.2	Tr	0.3
537	Brazil nuts, shelled	1 oz	28	3	185	4	19	4.6	6.5	6.8
	Cashew nuts, salted									
539	Dry roasted	1 c	137	2	785	21	63	12.5	37.4	10.7
540		1 oz	28	2	165	4	13	2.6	7.7	2.2

Nutrients in Indicated Quantity

Cholesterol (mg)	Carbohydrate (g)	Calcium (mg)	Phosphorus (mg)	Iron (mg)	Potassium (mg)	Sodium (mg)	Vitamin A Value IU	RE	Thiamin (mg)	Riboflavin (mg)	Niacin (mg)	Ascorbic Acid (mg)	Item No.
12	20	16	36	1.1	41	98	30	8	0.12	0.12	1.2	0	513
0	39	14	85	2.0	103	1	0	0	0.23	0.13	1.8	0	514
0	32	11	70	1.7	85	1	0	0	0.20	0.11	1.5	0	515
0	13	42	55	0.6	43	1	80	8	0.05	0.03	0.4	0	517
102	26	154	135	1.5	129	445	140	39	0.18	0.24	1.5	Tr	518
59	27	179	257	1.2	146	515	170	49	0.14	0.23	0.9	Tr	519
0	2	4		0.4	34	Tr		0	0.02	0.01	0.7	0	
0	88	18	100	5.1	109	2	0	0	0.73	0.46	6.1	0	520
0	95	20	109	5.5	119	3	0	0	0.80	0.50	6.6	0	521
0	76	16	70	4.2	91	2	0	0	0.58	0.38	5.1	0	522
0	93	331	583	5.5	113	1,349	0	0	0.80	0.50	6.6	0	523
0	85	49	446	5.2	444	4	0	0	66	0.14	5.2	0	524
0	3	5		0.7	58	Tr		0	0.14	0.05	0.6	0	
0	28	359	702	4.9	988	15	0	0	0.28	1.05	4.5	1	525
0	6	75	147	1.0	208	3	0	0	0.06	0.22	1.0	Tr	526
0	41	47	239	2.9	608	1	Tr	Tr	0.43	0.05	0.9	0	527
0	41	98		5.3	811	14		0	0.27	0.14	4.1	0	
0	38	90	266	4.9	749	13	0	0	0.25	0.13	1.3	0	528
0	49	55	293	5.9	1,163	4	0	0	0.25	0.11	1.3	0	529
0	40	95	281	5.1	790	13	0	0	0.27	0.13	1.3	0	530
0	49	86	296	5.4	882	3	Tr	Tr	0.33	0.16	0.7	0	531
0	42	74		4.7	663	6		1	0.22	0.12	4.2	0	
30	32	94	303	4.8	668	1,374	330	33	0.18	0.15	3.3	Tr	532
10	48	138	235	4.6	536	1,181	330	33	0.20	0.08	1.5	5	533
10	54	161	291	5.9	536	969	330	33	0.15	0.10	1.3	5	534
0	42	74	278	4.6	673	968	10	1	0.13	0.10	1.5	0	535
0	35	43	238	3.3	573	20	30	3	0.40	0.10	1.0	0	536
0	4	50	170	1.0	170	1	Tr	Tr	0.28	0.03	0.5	Tr	537
0	45	62	671	8.2	774	877*	0	0	0.27	0.27	1.9	0	539
0	9	13	139	1.7	160	181*	0	0	0.06	0.06	0.4	0	540

Table continued on following page

*Cashews without salt contain 21 mg sodium/cup or mg/oz.

| | | | | | | | | Fatty Acids | |
| | | | | | | | Satu- | Mono-
unsatu- | Poly-
unsatu- |
Item No.	Foods, Approximate Measures, Units, and Weight (Weight of Edible Portion Only)		Grams	Water (%)	Food Energy (cal)	Pro- tein (g)	Fat (g)	rated (g)	rated (g)	rated (g)
541	Roasted in oil	1 c	130	4	750	21	63	12.4	36.9	10.6
542		1 oz	28	4	165	5	14	2.7	8.1	2.3
543	Chestnuts, European (Ital- ian), roasted, shelled	1 c	143	40	350	5	3	0.6	1.1	1.2
544	Chickpeas, cooked, drained	1 c	163	60	270	15	4	0.4	0.9	1.9
	Coconut Raw									
545	Piece, about 2 by 2 by ½ in	1 piece	45	47	160	1	15	13.4	0.6	0.2
546	Shredded or grated	1 c	80	47	285	3	27	23.8	1.1	0.3
548	Filberts (hazelnuts), chopped	1 c	115	5	725	15	72	5.3	56.5	6.9
549		1 oz	28	5	180	4	18	1.3	13.9	1.7
550	Lentils, dry, cooked	1 c	200	72	215	16	1	0.1	0.2	0.5
551	Macadamia nuts, roasted in oil, salted	1 c	134	2	960	10	103	15.4	80.9	1.8
552		1 oz	28	2	205	2	22	3.2	17.1	0.4
	Mixed nuts, with peanuts, salted									
553	Dry roasted	1 oz	28	2	170	5	15	2.0	8.9	3.1
554	Roasted in oil	1 oz	28	2	175	5	16	2.5	9.0	3.8
555	Peanuts, roasted in oil, salted	1 c	145	2	840	39	71	9.9	35.5	22.6
556		1 oz	28	2	165	8	14	1.9	6.9	4.4
557	Peanut butter	1 tbsp	16	1	95	5	8	1.4	4.0	2.5
	Salt added	15 ml	16	1	95[1]	5	8	1		2
558	Peas, split, dry, cooked	1 c	200	70	230	16	1	0.1	0.1	0.3
559	Pecans, halves	1 c	108	5	720	8	73	5.9	45.5	18.1
560		1 oz	28	5	190	2	19	1.5	12.0	4.7
561	Pine nuts (pinyons), shelled	1 oz	28	6	160	3	17	2.7	6.5	7.3
562	Pistachio nuts, dried, shelled	1 oz	28	4	165	6	14	1.7	9.3	2.1
	Dry roasted, salt added	125 ml	68	2	412[1]	10	36	5		5
563	Pumpkin and squash ker- nels, dry, hulled	1 oz	28	7	155	7	13	2.5	4.0	5.9
564	Refried beans, canned	1 c	290	72	295	18	3	0.4	0.6	1.4
565	Sesame seeds, dry, hulled	1 tbsp	8	5	45	2	4	0.6	1.7	1.9
566	Soybeans, dry, cooked, drained	1 c	180	71	235	20	10	1.3	1.9	5.3
	Soy products									
567	Miso	1 c	276	53	470	29	13	1.8	2.6	7.3
568	Tofu, piece 2½ by 2¾ by 1 in	1 piece	120	85	85	9	5	0.7	1.0	2.9
569	Sunflower seeds, dry, hulled	1 oz	28	5	160	6	14	1.5	2.7	9.3
570	Tahini	1 tbsp	15	3	90	3	8	1.1	3.0	3.5
	Walnuts									
571	Black, chopped	1 c	125	4	760	30	71	4.5	15.9	46.9
572		1 oz	28	4	170	7	16	1.0	3.6	10.6
573	English or Persian, pieces or chips	1 c	120	4	770	17	74	6.7	17.0	47.0
574		1 oz	28	4	180	4	18	1.6	4.0	11.1

Nutrients in Indicated Quantity

Cho-les-terol (mg)	Carbo-hydrate (g)	Cal-cium (mg)	Phos-phorus (mg)	Iron (mg)	Potas-sium (mg)	Sodium (mg)	Vitamin A Value		Thia-min (mg)	Ribo-flavin (mg)	Nia-cin (mg)	Ascor-bic Acid (mg)	Item No.
							IU	RE					
0	37	53	554	5.3	689	814*	0	0	0.55	0.23	2.3	0	541
0	8	12	121	1.2	150	177	0	0	0.12	0.05	0.5	0	542
0	76	41	153	1.3	847	3	30	3	0.35	0.25	1.9	37	543
0	45	80	273	4.9	475	11	Tr	Tr	0.18	0.09	0.9	0	544
0	7	6	51	1.1	160	9	0	0	0.03	0.01	0.2	1	545
0	12	11	90	1.9	285	16	0	0	0.05	0.02	0.4	3	546
0	18	216	359	3.8	512	3	80	8	0.58	0.13	1.3	1	548
0	4	53	88	0.9	126	1	20	2	0.14	0.03	0.3	Tr	549
0	38	50	238	4.2	498	26	40	4	0.14	0.12	1.2	0	550
0	17	60	268	2.4	441	348†	10	1	0.29	0.15	2.7	0	551
0	4	13	57	0.5	93	74†	Tr	Tr	0.06	0.03	0.6	0	552
0	7	20	123	1.0	169	190‡	Tr	Tr	0.06	0.06	1.3	0	553
0	6	31	131	0.9	165	185‡	10	1	0.14	0.06	1.4	Tr	554
0	27	125	734	2.8	1,019	626§	0	0	0.42	0.15	21.5	0	555
0	5	24	143	0.5	199	122§	0	0	0.08	0.03	4.2	0	556
0	3	5	60	0.3	110	75	0	0	0.02	0.02	2.2	0	557
0	3	5		0.3	110	75		0	0.02	0.02	3.1	0	
0	42	22	178	3.4	592	26	80	8	0.30	0.18	1.8	0	558
0	20	39	314	2.3	423	1	140	14	0.92	0.14	1.0	2	559
0	5	10	83	0.6	111	Tr	40	4	0.24	0.04	0.3	1	560
0	5	2	10	0.9	178	20	10	1	0.35	0.06	1.2	1	561
0	7	38	143	1.9	310	2	70	7	0.23	0.05	0.3	Tr	562
0	19	48		2.2	660	530		16	0.29	0.17	3.3	5	
0	5	12	333	4.2	229	5	110	11	0.06	0.09	0.5	Tr	563
0	51	141	245	5.1	1,141	1,228	0	0	0.14	0.16	1.4	17	564
0	1	11	62	0.6	33	3	10	1	0.06	0.01	0.4	0	565
0	19	131	322	4.9	972	4	50	5	0.38	0.16	1.1	0	566
0	65	188	853	4.7	922	8,142	110	11	0.17	0.28	0.8	0	567
0	3	108	151	2.3	50	8	0	0	0.07	0.04	0.1	0	568
0	5	33	200	1.9	195	1	10	1	0.65	0.07	1.3	Tr	569
0	3	21	119	0.7	69	5	10	1	0.24	0.02	0.8	1	570
0	15	73	580	3.8	655	1	370	37	0.27	0.14	0.9	Tr	571
0	3	16	132	0.9	149	Tr	80	8	0.06	0.03	0.2	Tr	572
0	22	113	380	2.9	602	12	150	15	0.46	0.18	1.3	4	573
0	5	27	90	0.7	142	3	40	4	0.11	0.04	0.3	1	574

Table continued on following page

*Cashews without salt contain 22 mg sodium/cup or 5 mg/oz.
†Macadamia nuts without salt contain 9 mg sodium/cup or 2 mg oz.
‡Mixed nuts without salt contain 3 mg sodium/oz.
§Peanuts without salt contain 22 mg sodium/cup or 4 mg/oz.

								Fatty Acids		
Item No.	Foods, Approximate Measures, Units, and Weight (Weight of Edible Portion Only)	Grams	Water (%)	Food Energy (cal)	Pro-tein (g)	Fat (g)	Satu-rated (g)	Mono-unsatu-rated (g)	Poly-unsatu-rated (g)
	Meat and Meat Products									
	Beef, cooked*									
	Corned, brisket, cooked	90	60	226[1]	16	17	6		Tr	
	Corned, hash with potatoes	232	67	420[1]	20	26	13		Tr	
250 ml										
	Cuts braised, simmered, or pot roasted									
	Relatively fat such as chuck blade									
575	Lean and fat, piece, 2½ by 2½ by ¾ in 3 oz	85	43	325	22	26	10.8	11.7	0.9
576	Lean only from item 575 2.2 oz	62	53	170	19	9	3.9	4.2	0.3
	Relatively lean, such as bottom round									
577	Lean and fat, piece, 4½ by 2¼ by ½ in 3 oz	85	54	220	25	13	4.8	5.7	0.5
578	Lean only from item 577 2.8 oz	78	57	175	25	8	2.7	3.4	0.3
	Ground beef, broiled, patty, 3 by ⅝ in									
579	Lean 3 oz	85	56	230	21	16	6.2	6.9	0.6
580	Regular 3 oz	85	54	245	20	18	6.9	7.7	0.7
	Ground beef, regular, pan-fried medium, 8-cm diam. × 1.5 cm 1 patty	88	52	269[1]	21	20	8		Tr	
	Ground beef, regular, pan-fried, well done, 8-cm diam. × 1.5 cm 1 patty	88	53	252[1]	24	17	7		Tr	
581	Heart, lean, braised 3 oz	85	65	150	24	5	1.2	0.8	1.6
582	Liver, fried, slice, 6½ by 2⅜ by ⅜ in† 3 oz	85	56	185	23	7	2.5	3.6	1.3
	Calves, fried, 8 × 6 × 0.6 cm 3 slices	95	51	248[1]	28	13	3		Tr	
	Roast, oven cooked, no liquid added									
	Relatively fat, such as rib									
583	Lean and fat, 2 pieces, 4⅛ by 2¼ by ¼ in 3 oz	85	46	315	19	26	10.8	11.4	0.9
584	Lean only from item 583 2.2 oz	61	57	150	17	9	3.6	3.7	0.3
	Relatively lean, such as eye of round									
585	Lean and fat, 2 pieces, 2½ by 2½ by ⅜ in 3 oz	85	57	205	23	12	4.9	5.4	0.5
586	Lean only from item 585 2.6 oz	75	63	135	22	5	1.9	2.1	0.2
	Roast, rump, roasted, 11 × 6 × 0.6 cm									
	Lean and fat 2 pieces	88	58	205[1]	26	10	5		Tr	
	Lean only 2 pieces	89	60	177[1]	27	7	3		Tr	

*Outer layer of fat was removed to within approximately ½ inch of the lean. Deposits of fat within the cut were not removed.
†Fried in vegetable shortening.

Nutrients in Indicated Quantity

Cholesterol (mg)	Carbohydrate (g)	Calcium (mg)	Phosphorus (mg)	Iron (mg)	Potassium (mg)	Sodium (mg)	Vitamin A Value		Thiamin (mg)	Riboflavin (mg)	Niacin (mg)	Ascorbic Acid (mg)	Item No.
							IU	RE					
88	Tr	7		1.7	131	1021		—	0.02	0.15	5.2	0	
77	25	30		4.6	464	1253		0	0.02	0.21	8.6	0	
87	0	11	163	2.5	163	53	Tr	Tr	0.06	0.19	2.0	0	575
66	0	8	146	2.3	163	44	Tr	Tr	0.05	0.17	1.7	0	576
81	0	5	217	2.8	248	43	Tr	Tr	0.06	0.21	3.3	0	577
75	0	4	212	2.7	240	40	Tr	Tr	0.06	0.20	3.0	0	578
74	0	9	134	1.8	256	65	Tr	Tr	0.04	0.18	4.4	0	579
76	0	9	144	2.1	248	70	Tr	Tr	0.03	0.16	4.9	0	580
63	0	10		2.2	264	74		—	0.03	0.18	9.5	0	
70	0	11		2.4	292	82		—	0.04	0.19	10.6	0	
164	0	5	213	6.4	198	54	Tr	Tr	0.12	1.31	3.4	5	581
410	7	9	392	5.3	309	90	30,690*	9,120*	0.18	3.52	12.3	23	582
416	4	12		13.5	430	112		9,320	0.23	3.96	20.8	35	
72	0	8	145	2.0	246	54	Tr	Tr	0.06	0.16	3.1	0	583
49	0	5	127	1.7	218	45	Tr	Tr	0.05	0.13	2.7	0	584
62	0	5	177	1.6	308	50	Tr	Tr	0.07	0.14	3.0	0	585
52	0	3	170	1.5	297	46	Tr	Tr	0.07	0.13	2.8	0	586
66	0	5		2.0	340	56		—	0.08	0.22	7.5	0	
66	0	5		2.1	360	60		—	0.09	0.24	8.1	0	

Table continued on following page

*Value varies widely.

Item No.	Foods, Approximate Measures, Units, and Weight (Weight of Edible Portion Only)	Grams	Water (%)	Food Energy (cal)	Protein (g)	Fat (g)	Saturated (g)	Monounsaturated (g)	Polyunsaturated (g)
	Steak								
	Sirloin, broiled								
587	Lean and fat, piece, 2½ by 2½ by ¾ in 3 oz	85	53	240	23	15	6.4	6.9	0.6
588	Lean only from item 587 2.5 oz	72	59	150	22	6	2.6	2.8	0.3
	Steak, inside (top) round, 11 × 6 × 1.2 cm								
	Lean and fat 1 piece	88	61	154[1]	26	5	2		Tr
	Lean only 1 piece	88	63	144[1]	26	3	1		Tr
	Stewing, simmered, lean only 250 ml	148	58	335[1]	49	14	5		Tr
	Sweetbreads (thymus), braised 1 slice	90	53	287[1]	20	22	—		—
	Tongue, simmered	90	56	255[1]	20	19	8		Tr
589	Beef, canned, corned 3 oz	85	59	185	22	10	4.2	4.9	0.4
590	Beef, dried, chipped 2.5 oz	72	48	145	24	4	1.8	2.0	0.2
	Creton 15 ml	13	60	59[1]	2	5	2		Tr
	Lamb, cooked								
	Chops, (3 per lb with bone)								
	Arm, braised								
591	Lean and fat 2.2 oz	63	44	220	20	15	6.9	6.0	0.9
592	Lean only from item 591 1.7 oz	48	49	135	17	7	2.9	2.6	0.4
	Loin, broiled								
593	Lean and fat 2.8 oz	80	54	235	22	16	7.3	6.4	1.0
594	Lean only from item 593 2.3 oz	64	61	140	19	6	2.6	2.4	0.4
	Leg, roasted								
595	Lean and fat, 2 pieces, 4⅛ by 2¼ by ¼ in 3 oz	85	59	205	22	13	5.6	4.9	0.8
596	Lean only from item 595 2.6 oz	73	64	140	20	6	2.4	2.2	0.4
	Rib, roasted								
597	Lean and fat, 3 pieces, 2½ by 2½ by ¼ in 3 oz	85	47	315	18	26	12.1	10.6	1.5
598	Lean only from 597 2 oz	57	60	130	15	7	3.2	3.0	0.5
	Liverwurst 15 ml	15	52	49[1]	2	4	2		Tr
	Pork, cured, cooked								
	Bacon								
599	Regular 3 medium slices	19	13	110	6	9	3.3	4.5	1.1
600	Canadian style 2 slices	46	62	85	11	4	1.3	1.9	0.4
	Ham, light cure, roasted								
601	Lean and fat, 2 pieces, 4⅛ by 2¼ by ¼ in 3 oz	85	58	205	18	14	5.1	6.7	1.5
602	Lean only from item 601 2.4 oz	68	66	105	17	4	1.3	1.7	0.4
603	Ham, canned, roasted, 2 pieces, 4⅛ by 2¼ by ¼ in 3 oz	85	67	140	18	7	2.4	3.5	0.8
	Luncheon meat								
604	Canned, spiced or unspiced, slice, 3 by 2 by ½ in 2 slices	42	52	140	5	13	4.5	6.0	1.5
605	Chopped ham (8 slices per 6-oz pkg) 2 slices	42	64	95	7	7	2.4	3.4	0.9

Nutrients in Indicated Quantity

Cho-les-terol (mg)	Carbo-hydrate (g)	Cal-cium (mg)	Phos-phorus (mg)	Iron (mg)	Potas-sium (mg)	Sodium (mg)	Vitamin A Value IU	RE	Thia-min (mg)	Ribo-flavin (mg)	Nia-cin (mg)	Ascor-bic Acid (mg)	Item No.
77	0	9	186	2.6	306	53	Tr	Tr	0.10	0.23	3.3	0	587
64	0	8	176	2.4	290	48	Tr	Tr	0.09	0.22	3.1	0	588
57	0	4		2.4	339	43		—	0.10	0.23	10.2	0	
57	0	5		2.5	352	45		—	0.10	0.24	10.5	0	
128	0	12		4.7	511	70		—	0.12	0.42	12.5	0	
265	0	—		1.3	390	104		0	—	—	—	27	
96	Tr	6		3.1	162	54		—	0.03	0.32	4.5	Tr	
80	0	17	90	3.7	51	802	Tr	Tr	0.02	0.20	2.9	0	589
46	0	14	287	2.3	142	3,053	Tr	Tr	0.05	0.23	2.7	0	590
11	Tr	2		0.3	25	37		Tr	0.05	0.02	0.8	Tr	
77	0	16	132	1.5	195	46	Tr	Tr	0.04	0.16	4.4	0	591
59	0	12	111	1.3	162	36	Tr	Tr	0.03	0.13	3.0	0	592
78	0	16	162	1.4	272	62	Tr	Tr	0.09	0.21	5.5	0	593
60	0	12	145	1.3	241	54	Tr	Tr	0.08	0.18	4.4	0	594
78	0	8	162	1.7	273	57	Tr	Tr	0.09	0.24	5.5	0	595
65	0	6	150	1.5	247	50	Tr	Tr	0.08	0.20	4.6	0	596
77	0	19	139	1.4	224	60	Tr	Tr	0.08	0.18	5.5	0	597
50	0	12	111	1.0	179	46	Tr	Tr	0.05	0.13	3.5	0	598
24	Tr	4		1.0	26	129		1,245	0.04	0.16	1.0	0	
16	Tr	2	64	0.3	92	303	0	0	0.13	0.05	1.4	6	599
27	1	5	136	0.4	179	711	0	0	0.38	0.09	3.2	10	600
53	0	6	182	0.7	243	1,009	0	0	0.51	0.19	3.8	0	601
37	0	5	154	0.6	215	902	0	0	0.46	0.17	3.4	0	602
35	Tr	6	188	0.9	298	908	0	0	0.82	0.21	4.3	19*	603
26	1	3	34	0.3	90	541	0	0	0.15	0.08	1.3	Tr	604
21	0	3	65	0.3	134	576	0	0	0.27	0.09	1.6	8*	605

Table continued on following page

*Contains added sodium ascorbate. If sodium ascorbate is not added, ascorbic acid content is negligible.

								Fatty Acids		
Item No.	Foods, Approximate Measures, Units, and Weight (Weight of Edible Portion Only)		Grams	Water (%)	Food Energy (cal)	Pro-tein (g)	Fat (g)	Satu-rated (g)	Mono-unsatu-rated (g)	Poly-unsatu-rated (g)
	Cooked ham (8 slices per 8-oz pkg)									
606	Regular	2 slices	57	65	105	10	6	1.9	2.8	0.7
607	Extra lean	2 slices	57	71	75	11	3	0.9	1.3	0.3
	Pork, fresh, cooked									
	Chop, loin (cut 3 per lb with bone)									
	Broiled									
608	Lean and fat	3.1 oz	87	50	275	24	19	7.0	8.8	2.2
609	Lean only from item 608	2.5 oz	72	57	165	23	8	2.6	3.4	0.9
	Pan fried									
610	Lean and fat	3.1 oz	89	45	335	21	27	9.8	12.5	3.1
611	Lean only from item 610	2.4 oz	67	54	180	19	11	3.7	4.8	1.3
	Ham (leg), roasted									
612	Lean and fat, piece, 2½ by 2½ by ¾ in	3 oz	85	53	250	21	18	6.4	8.1	2.0
613	Lean only from item 612	2.5 oz	72	60	160	20	8	2.7	3.6	1.0
	Liver, braised, 16 × 6 × 1 cm	1 slice	86	64	142[1]	22	4	1		Tr
	Rib, roasted									
614	Lean and fat, piece, 2½ by ¾ in	3 oz	85	51	270	21	20	7.2	9.2	2.3
615	Lean only from item 614	2.5 oz	71	57	175	20	10	3.4	4.4	1.2
	Shoulder cut, braised									
616	Lean and fat, 3 pieces, 2½ by 2½ by ¼ in	3 oz	85	47	295	23	22	7.9	10.0	2.4
617	Lean only from item 616	2.4 oz	67	54	165	22	8	2.8	3.7	1.0
	Spareribs, braised, lean and fat	2 medium	70	40	278[1]	20	21	8		2
	Sausages (See also Luncheon meats, items 604–607)									
	Blood sausage or pudding, 12 × 0.2 cm	1 slice	30	47	113[1]	4	10	4		1
618	Bologna, slice (8 per 8-oz pkg)	2 slices	57	54	180	7	16	6.1	7.6	1.4
	Beef and pork, 11 × 0.2 cm	1 slice	22	54	70[1]	3	6	2		Tr
	Turkey, 11 × 0.2 cm	1 slice	22	65	44[1]	3	3	1		Tr
619	Braunschweiger, slice (6 per 6-oz pkg)	2 slices	57	48	205	8	18	6.2	8.5	2.1
620	Brown and serve (10–11 per 8-oz pkg), browned	1 link	13	45	50	2	5	1.7	2.2	0.5
621	Frankfurter (10 per 1-lb pkg), cooked (reheated)	1 frank-furter	45	54	145	5	13	4.8	6.2	1.2
	Chicken, 12 per 450-g package	1 frank-furter	37	58	95[1]	5	7	2		1
	Turkey, 12 per 450-g package	1 frank-furter	37	63	84[1]	5	7	2		2
622	Pork link (16 per 1-lb pkg), cooked*	1 link	13	45	50	3	4	1.4	1.8	0.5

*One patty (8 per pound) or bulk sausage is equivalent to 2 links.

| | | | | | | | Nutrients in Indicated Quantity | | | | | | |

Cholesterol (mg)	Carbohydrate (g)	Calcium (mg)	Phosphorus (mg)	Iron (mg)	Potassium (mg)	Sodium (mg)	Vitamin A Value		Thiamin (mg)	Riboflavin (mg)	Niacin (mg)	Ascorbic Acid (mg)	Item No.
							IU	RE					
32	2	4	141	0.6	189	751	0	0	0.49	0.14	3.0	16*	606
27	1	4	124	0.4	200	815	0	0	0.53	0.13	2.8	15*	607
84	0	3	184	0.7	312	61	10	3	0.87	0.24	4.3	Tr	608
71	0	4	176	0.7	302	56	10	1	0.83	0.22	4.0	Tr	609
92	0	4	190	0.7	323	64	10	3	0.91	0.24	4.6	Tr	610
72	0	3	178	0.7	305	57	10	1	0.84	0.22	4.0	Tr	611
79	0	5	210	0.9	280	50	10	2	0.54	0.27	3.9	Tr	612
68	0	5	202	0.8	269	46	10	1	0.50	0.25	3.6	Tr	613
305	3	9		15.4	129	42		4,643	0.22	1.89	12.5	20	
69	0	9	190	0.8	313	37	10	3	0.50	0.24	4.2	Tr	614
56	0	8	182	0.7	300	33	10	2	0.45	0.22	3.8	Tr	615
93	0	6	162	1.4	286	75	10	3	0.46	0.26	4.4	Tr	616
76	0	5	151	1.3	271	68	10	1	0.40	0.24	4.0	Tr	617
85	0	33		1.3	224	65		2	0.29	0.27	8.4	0	
36	Tr	2		1.9	11	204		0	0.02	0.04	1.3	0	
31	2	7	52	0.9	103	581	0	0	0.10	0.08	1.5	12*	618
12	Tr	3		0.3	40	224		0	0.04	0.03	1.0	5	
22	Tr	18		0.3	44	193		0	0.01	0.04	1.2	0	
89	2	5	96	5.3	113	652	8,010	2,405	0.14	0.87	4.8	6*	619
9	Tr	1	14	0.1	25	105	0	0	0.05	0.02	0.4	0	620
23	1	5	39	0.5	75	504	0	0	0.09	0.05	1.2	12*	621
37	3	35		0.7	31	507		14	0.02	0.04	1.8	0	
40	Tr	39		0.7	66	528		0	0.02	0.07	2.2	0	
11	Tr	4	24	0.2	47	168	0	0	0.10	0.03	0.6	Tr	622

Table continued on following page

*Contains added sodium ascorbate. If sodium ascorbate is not added, ascorbic acid content is negligible.

Item No.	Foods, Approximate Measures, Units, and Weight (Weight of Edible Portion Only)		Grams	Water (%)	Food Energy (cal)	Pro-tein (g)	Fat (g)	Fatty Acids		
								Satu-rated (g)	Mono-unsatu-rated (g)	Poly-unsatu-rated (g)
	Salami									
623	Cooked type, slice (8 per 8-oz pkg)	2 slices	57	60	145	8	11	4.6	5.2	1.2
624	Dry type, slice (12 per 4-oz pkg)	2 slices	20	35	85	5	7	2.4	3.4	0.6
625	Sandwich spread (pork, beef)	1 tbsp	15	60	35	1	3	0.9	1.1	0.4
626	Vienna sausage (7 per 4-oz can)	1 sausage	16	60	45	2	4	1.5	2.0	0.3
	Veal, medium fat, cooked, bone removed									
627	Cutlet, 4⅛ by 2¼ by ½ in, braised or broiled	3 oz	85	60	185	23	9	4.1	4.1	0.6
628	Rib, 2 pieces 4⅛ by 2¼ by ¼ in, roasted	3 oz	85	55	230	23	14	6.0	6.0	1.0

Mixed Dishes, Wild Game, and Fast Foods

Item No.	Foods, Approximate Measures, Units, and Weight (Weight of Edible Portion Only)		Grams	Water (%)	Food Energy (cal)	Pro-tein (g)	Fat (g)	Satu-rated (g)	Mono-unsatu-rated (g)	Poly-unsatu-rated (g)
	Wild game									
	Bear, polar, flesh, simmered		90	61	163[1]	33	4	—		—
	Beaver, roasted		90	56	223	26	12	5		2
	Caribou, cooked		90	—	157	34	1	—		—
	Hare or rabbit, cooked		90	—	194	26	9	—		—
	Moose, cooked		90	—	158	31	3	—		—
	Muskrat or porcupine, roasted		90	67	138	24	4	2		Tr
	Ptarmigan (grouse), roasted, meat only		90	62	156	28	5	—		—
	Seal, cooked		90	60	165[1]	23	8	—		—
	Mixed dishes									
	Beans and frankfurters, canned	250 ml	269	71	387[1]	20	19	8		8
	Beans with tomato sauce and pork, canned	250 ml	269	71	328[1]	16	7	3		Tr
629	Beef and vegetable stew, from home recipe	1 c	245	82	220	16	11	4.4	4.5	0.5
630	Beef pot pie, from home recipe, baked, piece, ⅓ of 9-in diam. pie*	1 piece	210	55	515	21	30	7.9	12.9	7.4
631	Chicken à la king, cooked, from home recipe	1 c	245	68	470	27	34	12.9	13.4	6.2
632	Chicken and noodles, cooked, from home recipe	1 c	240	71	365	22	18	5.1	7.1	3.9
	Chicken chow mein									
633	Canned	1 c	250	89	95	7	Tr	0.1	0.1	0.8
634	From home recipe	1 c	250	78	255	31	10	4.1	4.9	3.5
635	Chicken pot pie, from home recipe, baked, piece, ⅓ of 9-in diam. pie*	1 piece	232	57	545	23	31	10.3	15.5	6.6
636	Chili con carne									
	With beans, canned	1 c	255	72	340	19	16	5.8	7.2	1.0
	Without beans, canned	250 ml	269	67	538[1]	28	40	19		0
637	Chop suey with beef and pork, from home recipe	1 c	250	75	300	26	17	4.3	7.4	4.2

*Crust made with vegetable shortening and enriched flour.

Nutrients in Indicated Quantity

Cho-les-terol (mg)	Carbo-hydrate (g)	Cal-cium (mg)	Phos-phorus (mg)	Iron (mg)	Potas-sium (mg)	Sodium (mg)	Vitamin A Value IU	RE	Thia-min (mg)	Ribo-flavin (mg)	Nia-cin (mg)	Ascor-bic Acid (mg)	Item No.
37	1	7	66	1.5	113	607	0	0	0.14	0.21	2.0	7*	623
16	1	2	28	0.3	76	372	0	0	0.12	0.06	1.0	5*	624
6	2	2	9	0.1	17	152	10	1	0.03	0.02	0.3	0	625
8	Tr	2	8	0.1	16	152	0	0	0.01	0.02	0.3	0	626
109	0	9	196	0.8	258	56	Tr	Tr	0.06	0.21	4.6	0	627
109	0	10	211	0.7	259	57	Tr	Tr	0.11	0.26	6.6	0	628
—	0	16		6.5	—	—		378	0.01	0.63	9.3	0	
90	0	19		1.4	331	37		0	0.07	0.34	15.0	0	
—	0	17		3.1	—	—		6	0.10	0.57	10.4	0	
—	0	19		1.4	—	—		0	0.05	0.06	15.3	0	
—	0	9		3.0	—	—		52	0.04	0.30	10.1	0	
90	0	19		1.4	331	37		27	0.14	0.19	14.7	0	
—	0	27		6.8	423	86		—	0.29	0.49	13.1	0	
—	0	23		18.6	147	80		—	0.14	0.54	—	Tr	
35	34	100		5.1	705	1,450		35	0.19	0.16	7.2	0	
11	51	145		4.8	565	1,245		35	0.22	0.08	4.6	5	
71	15	29	184	2.9	613	292	5,690	568	0.15	0.17	4.7	17	629
42	39	29	149	3.8	334	596	4,220	517	0.29	0.29	4.8	6	630
221	12	127	358	2.5	404	760	1,130	272	0.10	0.42	5.4	12	631
103	26	26	247	2.2	149	600	430	130	0.05	0.17	4.3	Tr	632
8	18	45	85	1.3	418	725	150	28	0.05	0.10	1.0	13	633
75	10	58	293	2.5	473	718	280	50	0.08	0.23	4.3	10	634
56	42	70	232	3.0	343	594	7,220	735	0.32	0.32	4.9	5	635
28	31	82	321	4.3	594	1,354	150	15	0.08	0.18	3.3	8	636
70	16	102		3.8	627	1,428		40	0.05	0.32	11.0	0	
68	13	60	248	4.8	425	1,053	600	60	0.28	0.38	5.0	33	637

Table continued on following page

*Contains added sodium ascorbate. If sodium ascorbate is not added, ascorbic acid content is negligible.

Item No.	Foods, Approximate Measures, Units, and Weight (Weight of Edible Portion Only)		Grams	Water (%)	Food Energy (cal)	Pro-tein (g)	Fat (g)	Fatty Acids		
								Satu-rated (g)	Mono-unsatu-rated (g)	Poly-unsatu-rated (g)
	Chow mein, chicken									
	Canned, without									
	noodles	250 ml	264	89	100[1]	7	Tr	0		0
	Home recipe, without									
	noodles	250 ml	264	78	269[1]	33	11	3		3
	Macaroni (enriched) and cheese									
638	Canned†	1 c	240	80	230	9	10	4.7	2.9	1.3
639	From home recipe‡	1 c	200	58	430	17	22	9.8	7.4	3.6
	Meat loaf, homemade, 10 × 8 × 1 cm	1 slice	73	64	117[1]	12	6	—		—
640	Quiche Lorraine, ⅛ of 8-in diam. quiche*	1 slice	176	47	600	13	48	23.2	17.8	4.1
	Spaghetti (enriched) in tomato sauce with cheese									
641	Canned	1 c	250	80	190	6	2	0.4	0.4	0.5
642	From home recipe	1 c	250	77	260	9	9	3.0	3.6	1.2
	Spaghetti (enriched) with meatballs and tomato sauce									
643	Canned	1 c	250	78	260	12	10	2.4	3.9	3.1
644	From home recipe	1 c	248	70	330	19	12	3.9	4.4	2.2
	Tourtière (pork pie), ⅙ of 23-cm diam.	1 sector	139	37	482[1]	21	30	8		5
	Fast food entrees:									
	Cheeseburger									
645	Regular	1 sand-wich	112	46	300	15	15	7.3	5.6	1.0
646	4-oz patty	1 sand-wich	194	46	525	30	31	15.1	12.2	1.4
	Chicken, fried. See Poultry and Poultry Products (items 656–659)									
647	Enchilada	1 enchi-lada	230	72	235	20	16	7.7	6.7	0.6
648	English muffin, egg, cheese, and bacon	1 sand-wich	138	49	360	18	18	8.0	8.0	0.7
	Fish sandwich									
649	Regular, with cheese	1 sand-wich	140	43	420	16	23	6.3	6.9	7.7
650	Large, without cheese	1 sand-wich	170	48	470	18	27	6.3	8.7	9.5
	Hamburger									
651	Regular	1 sand-wich	98	46	245	12	11	4.4	5.3	0.5
652	4-oz patty	1 sand-wich	174	50	445	25	21	7.1	11.7	0.6
653	Pizza, cheese ⅛ of 15-in diam. pizza*	1 slice	120	46	290	15	9	4.1	2.6	1.3
	Pizza, sausage, ⅛ of 35-cm diam. pizza	1 slice	65	43	183[1]	8	9	2		Tr
654	Roast beef sandwich	1 sand-wich	150	52	345	22	13	3.5	6.9	1.8
655	Taco	1 taco	81	55	195	9	11	4.1	5.5	0.8

*Crust made with vegetable shortening and enriched flour.
†Made with corn oil.
‡Made with margarine.

							Vitamin A Value					Ascor-	
Cho-les-terol (mg)	Carbo-hydrate (g)	Cal-cium (mg)	Phos-phorus (mg)	Iron (mg)	Potas-sium (mg)	Sodium (mg)	IU	RE	Thia-min (mg)	Ribo-flavin (mg)	Nia-cin (mg)	bic Acid (mg)	Item No.
8	19	48		1.3	441	766		16	0.05	0.11	2.3	13	
82	11	61		2.6	499	758		29	0.08	0.24	10.5	11	
24	26	199	182	1.0	139	730	260	72	0.12	0.24	1.0	Tr	638
44	40	362	322	1.8	240	1,086	860	232	0.20	0.40	1.8	1	639
67	3	28		1.7	273	477		—	0.05	0.14	8.1	1	
285	29	211	276	1.0	283	653	1,640	454	0.11	0.32	Tr	Tr	640
3	39	40	88	2.8	303	955	930	120	0.35	0.28	4.5	10	641
8	37	80	135	2.3	408	955	1,080	140	0.25	0.18	2.3	13	642
23	29	53	113	3.3	245	1,220	1,000	100	0.15	0.18	2.3	5	643
89	39	124	236	3.7	665	1,009	1,590	159	0.25	0.30	4.0	22	644
53	32	27		3.9	235	707		3	0.56	0.32	8.2	Tr	
44	28	135	174	2.3	219	672	340	65	0.26	0.24	3.7	1	645
104	40	236	320	4.5	407	1,224	670	128	0.33	0.48	7.4	3	646
19	24	322	662	11.0	2,180	4,451	2,720	352	0.18	0.26	Tr	Tr	647
213	31	197	290	3.1	201	832	650	160	0.46	0.50	3.7	1	648
56	39	132	223	1.8	274	667	160	25	0.32	0.26	3.3	2	649
91	41	61	246	2.2	375	621	110	15	0.35	0.23	3.5	1	650
32	28	56	107	2.2	202	463	80	14	0.23	0.24	3.8	1	651
71	38	75	225	4.8	404	763	160	28	0.38	0.38	7.8	1	652
56	39	220	216	1.6	230	699	750	106	0.34	0.29	4.2	2	653
19	18	122		0.9	127	434		109	0.05	0.12	2.4	6	
55	34	60	222	4.0	338	757	240	32	0.40	0.33	6.0	2	654
21	15	109	134	1.2	263	456	420	57	0.09	0.07	1.4	1	655

Table continued on following page

							Fatty Acids		
Item No.	Foods, Approximate Measures, Units, and Weight (Weight of Edible Portion Only)	Grams	Water (%)	Food Energy (cal)	Pro-tein (g)	Fat (g)	Satu-rated (g)	Mono-unsatu-rated (g)	Poly-unsatu-rated (g)
	Poultry and Poultry Products								
	Chicken								
	Fried, flesh, with skin*								
	Batter dipped								
656	Breast, ½ breast (5.6 oz with bones)	4.9 oz 140	52	365	35	18	4.9	7.6	4.3
657	Drumstick (3.4 oz with bones)	2.5 oz 72	53	195	16	11	3.0	4.6	2.7
	Flour coated								
658	Breast, ½ breast (4.2 oz with bones)	3.5 oz 98	57	220	31	9	2.4	3.4	1.9
659	Drumstick (2.6 oz with bones)	1.7 oz 49	57	120	13	7	1.8	2.7	1.6
	Roasted, flesh only								
660	Breast, ½ breast (4.2 oz with bones and skin)	3.0 oz 86	65	140	27	3	0.9	1.1	0.7
661	Drumstick, (2.9 oz with bones and skin)	1.6 oz 44	67	75	12	2	0.7	0.8	0.6
662	Stewed, flesh only, light and dark meat, chopped or diced	1 c 140	67	250	38	9	2.6	3.3	2.2
663	Chicken liver, cooked	1 liver 20	68	30	5	1	0.4	0.3	0.2
664	Duck, roasted, flesh only	½ duck 221	64	445	52	25	9.2	8.2	3.2
	Turkey, roasted, flesh only								
665	Dark meat, piece, 2½ by 1⅝ by ¼ in	4 pieces 85	63	160	24	6	2.1	1.4	1.8
666	Light meat, piece, 4 by 2 by ¼ in	2 pieces 85	66	135	25	3	0.9	0.5	0.7
	Light and dark meat								
667	Chopped or diced	1 c 140	65	240	41	7	2.3	1.4	2.0
668	Pieces (1 slice white meat, 4 by 2 by ¼ in and 2 slices dark meat, 2½ by 1⅝ by ¼ in)	3 pieces 85	65	145	25	4	1.4	0.9	1.2
	Poultry food products								
	Chicken								
669	Canned, boneless	5 oz 142	69	235	31	11	3.1	4.5	2.5
670	Frankfurter (10 per 1-lb pkg)	1 frank-furter 45	58	115	6	9	2.5	3.8	1.8
671	Roll, light (6 slices per 6-oz pkg)	2 slices 57	69	90	11	4	1.1	1.7	0.9
	Turkey								
672	Gravy and turkey, frozen	5-oz pack-age 142	85	95	8	4	1.2	1.4	0.7
673	Ham, cured turkey thigh meat (8 slices per 8-oz pkg)	2 slices 57	71	75	11	3	1.0	0.7	0.9
674	Loaf, breast meat (8 slices per 6-oz pkg)	2 slices 42	72	45	10	1	0.2	0.2	0.1
675	Patties, breaded, bat-tered, fried (2¼ oz)	patty 64	50	180	9	12	3.0	4.8	3.0
676	Roast, boneless, frozen, seasoned, light and dark meat, cooked	3 oz 85	68	130	18	5	1.6	1.0	1.4

*Fried in vegetable shortening.

							Vitamin A Value					Ascor-	
Cho-les-terol (mg)	Carbo-hydrate (g)	Cal-cium (mg)	Phos-phorus (mg)	Iron (mg)	Potas-sium (mg)	Sodium (mg)	IU	RE	Thia-min (mg)	Ribo-flavin (mg)	Nia-cin (mg)	bic Acid (mg)	Item No.

Nutrients in Indicated Quantity

119	13	28	259	1.8	281	385	90	28	0.16	0.20	14.7	0	656
62	6	12	106	1.0	134	194	60	19	0.08	0.15	3.7	0	657
87	2	16	228	1.2	254	74	50	15	0.08	0.13	13.5	0	658
44	1	6	86	0.7	112	44	40	12	0.04	0.11	3.0	0	659
73	0	13	196	0.9	220	64	20	5	0.06	0.10	11.8	0	660
41	0	5	81	0.6	108	42	30	8	0.03	0.10	2.7	0	661
116	0	20	210	1.6	252	98	70	21	0.07	0.23	8.6	0	662
126	Tr	3	62	1.7	28	10	3,270	983	0.03	0.35	0.9	3	663
197	0	27	449	6.0	557	144	170	51	0.57	1.04	11.3	0	664
72	0	27	173	2.0	246	67	0	0	0.05	0.21	3.1	0	665
59	0	16	186	1.1	259	54	0	0	0.05	0.11	5.8	0	666
106	0	35	298	2.5	417	98	0	0	0.09	0.25	7.6	0	667
65	0	21	181	1.5	253	60	0	0	0.05	0.15	4.6	0	668
88	0	20	158	2.2	196	714	170	48	0.02	0.18	9.0	3	669
45	3	43	48	0.9	38	616	60	17	0.03	0.05	1.4	0	670
28	1	24	89	0.6	129	331	50	14	0.04	0.07	3.0	0	671
26	7	20	115	1.3	87	787	60	18	0.03	0.18	2.6	0	672
32	Tr	6	108	1.6	184	565	0	0	0.03	0.14	2.0	0	673
17	0	3	97	0.2	118	608	0	0	0.02	0.05	3.5	0*	674
40	10	9	173	1.4	176	512	20	7	0.06	0.12	1.5	0	675
45	3	4	207	1.4	253	578	0	0	0.04	0.14	5.3	0	676

Table continued on following page

*If sodium ascorbate is added, product contains 11 mg ascorbic acid.

Item No.	Foods, Approximate Measures, Units, and Weight (Weight of Edible Portion Only)		Grams	Water (%)	Food Energy (cal)	Pro-tein (g)	Fat (g)	Satu-rated (g)	Mono-unsatu-rated (g)	Poly-unsatu-rated (g)
									Fatty Acids	
	Soups, Sauces, and Gravies									
	Soups									
	Canned, condensed									
	Prepared with equal volume of milk									
677	Clam chowder, New England	1 c	248	85	165	9	7	3.0	2.3	1.1
678	Cream of chicken	1 c	248	85	190	7	11	4.6	4.5	1.6
679	Cream of mushroom	1 c	248	85	205	6	14	5.1	3.0	4.6
680	Tomato	1 c	248	85	160	6	6	2.9	1.6	1.1
	Prepared with equal volume of water									
681	Bean with bacon	1 c	253	84	170	8	6	1.5	2.2	1.8
682	Beef broth, bouillon, consomme	1 c	240	98	15	3	1	0.3	0.2	Tr
683	Beef noodle	1 c	244	92	85	5	3	1.1	1.2	0.5
684	Chicken noodle	1 c	241	92	75	4	2	0.7	1.1	0.6
685	Chicken rice	1 c	241	94	60	4	2	0.5	0.9	0.4
686	Clam chowder, Manhattan	1 c	244	90	80	4	2	0.4	0.4	1.3
687	Cream of chicken	1 c	244	91	115	3	7	2.1	3.3	1.5
688	Cream of mushroom	1 c	244	90	130	2	9	2.4	1.7	4.2
689	Minestrone	1 c	241	91	80	4	3	0.6	0.7	1.1
690	Pea, green	1 c	250	83	165	9	3	1.4	1.0	0.4
691	Tomato	1 c	244	90	85	2	2	0.4	0.4	1.0
692	Vegetable beef	1 c	244	92	80	6	2	0.9	0.8	0.1
693	Vegetarian	1 c	241	92	70	2	2	0.3	0.8	0.7
	Dehydrated									
	Unprepared									
694	Bouillon	1 pkt	6	3	15	1	1	0.3	0.2	Tr
695	Onion	1 pkt	7	4	20	1	Tr	0.1	0.2	Tr
	Prepared with water									
696	Chicken noodle	1 pkt (6-fl-oz)	188	94	40	2	1	0.2	0.4	0.3
697	Onion	1 pkt (6-fl-oz)	184	96	20	1	Tr	0.1	0.2	0.1
698	Tomato vegetable	1 pkt (6-fl-oz)	189	94	40	1	1	0.3	0.2	0.1
	Sauces									
	From dry mix									
699	Cheese, prepared with milk	1 c	279	77	305	16	17	9.3	5.3	1.6
700	Hollandaise, prepared with water	1 c	259	84	240	5	20	11.6	5.9	0.9
701	White sauce, prepared with milk	1 c	264	81	240	10	13	6.4	4.7	1.7
	From home recipe									
702	White sauce, medium*	1 c	250	73	395	10	30	9.1	11.9	7.2
	Ready to serve									
703	Barbecue	1 tbsp	16	81	10	Tr	Tr	Tr	0.1	0.1
704	Soy	1 tbsp	18	68	10	2	0	0.0	0.0	0.0
	Gravies									
	Canned									
705	Beef	1 c	233	87	125	9	5	2.7	2.3	0.2
706	Chicken	1 c	238	85	190	5	14	3.4	6.1	3.6
707	Mushroom	1 c	238	89	120	3	6	1.0	2.8	2.4

*Made with enriched flour, margarine, and whole milk.

							Vitamin A Value					Ascor-	
Cho-les-terol (mg)	Carbo-hydrate (g)	Cal-cium (mg)	Phos-phorus (mg)	Iron (mg)	Potas-sium (mg)	Sodium (mg)	IU	RE	Thia-min (mg)	Ribo-flavin (mg)	Nia-cin (mg)	bic Acid (mg)	Item No.

Nutrients in Indicated Quantity

Cholesterol	Carbohydrate	Calcium	Phosphorus	Iron	Potassium	Sodium	IU	RE	Thiamin	Riboflavin	Niacin	Ascorbic	Item No.
22	17	186	156	1.5	300	992	160	40	0.07	0.24	1.0	3	677
27	15	181	151	0.7	273	1,047	710	94	0.07	0.26	0.9	1	678
20	15	179	156	0.6	270	1,076	150	37	0.08	0.28	0.9	2	679
17	22	159	149	1.8	449	932	850	109	0.13	0.25	1.5	68	680
3	23	81	132	2.0	402	951	890	89	0.09	0.03	0.6	2	681
Tr	Tr	14	31	0.4	130	782	0	0	Tr	0.05	1.9	0	682
5	9	15	46	1.1	100	952	630	63	0.07	0.06	1.1	Tr	683
7	9	17	36	0.8	55	1,106	710	71	0.05	0.06	1.4	Tr	684
7	7	17	22	0.7	101	815	660	66	0.02	0.02	1.1	Tr	685
2	12	34	59	1.9	261	1,808	920	92	0.06	0.05	1.3	3	686
10	9	34	37	0.6	88	986	560	56	0.03	0.06	0.8	Tr	687
2	9	46	49	0.5	100	1,032	0	0	0.05	0.09	0.7	1	688
2	11	34	55	0.9	313	911	2,340	234	0.05	0.04	0.9	1	689
0	27	28	125	2.0	988	200	20	0.11	0.07	1.2	2	690
0	17	12	34	1.8	264	871	690	69	0.09	0.05	1.4	66	691
5	10	17	41	1.1	173	956	1,890	189	0.04	0.05	1.0	2	692
0	12	22	34	1.1	210	822	3,010	301	0.05	0.05	0.9	1	693
1	1	4	19	0.1	27	1,019	Tr	Tr	Tr	0.01	0.3	0	694
Tr	4	10	23	0.1	47	627	Tr	Tr	0.02	0.04	0.4	Tr	695
2	6	24	24	0.4	23	957	50	5	0.05	0.04	0.7	Tr	696
0	4	9	22	0.1	48	635	Tr	Tr	0.02	0.04	0.4	Tr	697
0	8	6	23	0.5	78	856	140	14	0.04	0.03	0.6	5	698
53	23	569	438	0.3	552	1,565	390	117	0.15	0.56	0.3	2	699
52	14	124	127	0.9	124	1,564	730	220	0.05	0.18	0.1	Tr	700
34	21	425	256	0.3	444	797	310	92	0.08	0.45	0.5	3	701
32	24	292	238	0.9	381	888	1,190	340	0.15	0.43	0.8	2	702
0	2	3	3	0.1	28	130	140	14	Tr	Tr	0.1	1	703
0	2	3	38	0.5	64	1,029	0	0	0.01	0.02	0.6	0	704
7	11	14	70	1.6	189	117	0	0	0.07	0.08	1.5	0	705
5	13	48	69	1.1	259	1,373	880	264	0.04	0.10	1.1	0	706
0	13	17	36	1.6	252	1,357	0	0	0.08	0.15	1.6	0	707

Table continued on following page

Item No.	Foods, Approximate Measures, Units, and Weight (Weight of Edible Portion Only)		Grams	Water (%)	Food Energy (cal)	Pro-tein (g)	Fat (g)	Fatty Acids		
								Satu-rated (g)	Mono-unsatu-rated (g)	Poly-unsatu-rated (g)
	From dry mix									
708	Brown	1 c	261	91	80	3	2	0.9	0.8	0.1
709	Chicken	1 c	260	91	85	3	2	0.5	0.9	0.4
	Vegetables and Vegetable Products									
750	Alfalfa seeds, sprouted, raw	1 c	33	91	10	1	Tr	Tr	Tr	0.1
751	Artichokes, globe or French, cooked, drained	1 arti-choke	120	87	55	3	Tr	Tr	Tr	0.1
	Asparagus, green Cooked, drained From raw									
752	Cuts and tips	1 c	180	92	45	5	1	0.1	Tr	0.2
753	Spears, ½ in diam. at base	4 spears	60	92	15	2	Tr	Tr	Tr	0.1
	From frozen									
754	Cuts and tips	1 c	180	91	50	5	1	0.2	Tr	0.3
755	Spears, ½ in. diam. at base	4 spears	60	91	15	2	Tr	0.1	Tr	0.1
756	Canned, spears, ½ in diam. at base	4 spears	80	95	10	1	Tr	Tr	Tr	0.1
757	Bamboo shoots, canned, drained	1 c	131	94	25	2	1	0.1	Tr	0.2
	Beans Green, yellow, or Italian Canned, drained	250 ml	144	93	29[1]	2	Tr	Tr		Tr
	Frozen, boiled, drained	250 ml	144	92	37[1]	2	Tr	Tr		Tr
	Lima, immature seeds, frozen, cooked, drained									
758	Thick-seeded types (Fordhooks)	1 c	170	74	170	10	1	0.1	Tr	0.3
759	Thin-seeded types (baby limas)	1 c	180	72	190	12	1	0.1	Tr	0.3
	Snap Cooked, drained									
760	From raw (cut and French style)	1 c	125	89	45	2	Tr	0.1	Tr	0.2
761	From frozen (cut)	1 c	135	92	35	2	Tr	Tr	Tr	0.1
762	Canned, drained solids (cut)	1 c	135	93	25	2	Tr	Tr	Tr	0.1
	Beans, mature. See Beans, dry (items 527–535) and Black-eyed peas, dry (item 536)									
	Bean sprouts (mung)									
763	Raw	1 c	104	90	30	3	Tr	Tr	Tr	0.1
764	Cooked, drained	1 c	124	93	25	3	Tr	Tr	Tr	Tr
	Stir-fried	250 ml	131	84	66[1]	6	Tr	Tr		Tr
	Beets Cooked, drained									
765	Diced or sliced	1 c	170	91	55	2	Tr	Tr	Tr	Tr
766	Whole beets, 2-in-diam.	2 beets	100	91	30	1	Tr	Tr	Tr	Tr

Nutrients in Indicated Quantity

Cho-les-terol (mg)	Carbo-hydrate (g)	Cal-cium (mg)	Phos-phorus (mg)	Iron (mg)	Potas-sium (mg)	Sodium (mg)	Vitamin A Value		Thia-min (mg)	Ribo-flavin (mg)	Nia-cin (mg)	Ascor-bic Acid (mg)	Item No.
							IU	RE					
2	14	66	47	0.2	61	1,147	0	0	0.04	0.09	0.9	0	708
3	14	39	47	0.3	62	1,134	0	0	0.05	0.15	0.8	3	709
0	1	11	23	0.3	26	2	50	5	0.03	0.04	0.2	3	750
0	12	47	72	1.6	316	79	170	17	0.07	0.06	0.7	9	751
0	8	43	110	1.2	558	7	1,490	149	0.18	0.22	1.9	49	752
0	3	14	37	0.4	186	2	500	50	0.06	0.07	0.6	16	753
0	9	41	99	1.2	392	7	1,470	147	0.12	0.19	1.9	44	754
0	3	14	33	0.4	131	2	490	49	0.04	0.06	0.6	15	755
0	2	11	30	0.5	122	278‖	380	38	0.04	0.07	0.7	13	756
0	4	10	33	0.4	105	9	10	1	0.03	0.03	0.2	1	757
0	6	37		1.3	157	361		50	0.02	0.08	0.6	7	
0	9	65		1.2	161	19		76	0.07	0.11	0.9	12	
0	32	37	107	2.3	694	90	320	32	0.13	0.10	1.8	22	758
0	35	50	202	3.5	740	52	300	30	0.13	0.10	1.4	10	759
0	10	58	49	1.6	374	4	830*	83*	0.09	0.12	0.8	12	760
0	8	61	32	1.1	151	18	710†	71†	0.06	0.10	0.6	11	761
0	6	35	26	1.2	147	339‡	470§	47§	0.02	0.08	0.3	6	762
0	6	14	56	0.9	155	6	20	2	0.09	0.13	0.8	14	763
0	5	15	35	0.8	125	12	20	2	0.06	0.13	1.0	14	764
0	14	17		2.5	287	12		4	0.18	0.24	2.8	21	
0	11	19	53	1.1	530	83	20	2	0.05	0.02	0.5	9	765
0	7	11	31	0.6	312	49	10	1	0.03	0.01	0.3	6	766

Table continued on following page

*For green varieties; yellow varieties contain 101 IU or 10 RE.
†For green varieties; yellow varieties contain 151 IU or 15 RE.
‡For regular pack; special dietary pack contains 3 mg sodium.
§For green varieties; yellow varieties contain 142 IU or 14 RE.
‖For regular pack; special dietary pack contains 3 mg sodium.

| | | | | | | | | Fatty Acids | | |
Item No.	Foods, Approximate Measures, Units, and Weight (Weight of Edible Portion Only)		Grams	Water (%)	Food Energy (cal)	Pro- tein (g)	Fat (g)	Satu- rated (g)	Mono- unsatu- rated (g)	Poly- unsatu- rated (g)
767	Canned, drained solids, diced or sliced	1 c	170	91	55	2	Tr	Tr	Tr	0.1
768	Beet greens, leaves and stems, cooked, drained	1 c	144	89	40	4	Tr	Tr	0.1	0.1
	Black-eyed peas, immature seeds, cooked and drained									
769	From raw	1 c	165	72	180	13	1	0.3	0.1	0.6
770	From frozen	1 c	170	66	225	14	1	0.3	0.1	0.5
	Broccoli									
771	Raw	1 spear	151	91	40	4	1	0.1	Tr	0.3
	Cooked, drained									
	From raw									
772	Spear, medium	1 spear	180	90	50	5	1	0.1	Tr	0.2
773	Spears, cut into ½-in pieces	1 c	155	90	45	5	Tr	0.1	Tr	0.2
	From frozen									
774	Piece, 4½ to 5 in long	1 piece	30	91	10	1	Tr	Tr	Tr	Tr
775	Chopped	1 c	185	91	50	6	Tr	Tr	Tr	0.1
	Brussels sprouts, cooked, drained									
776	From raw, 7–8 sprouts, 1¼ to 1½-in diam.	1 c	155	87	60	4	1	0.2	0.1	0.4
777	From frozen	1 c	155	87	65	6	1	0.1	Tr	0.3
	Cabbage, common varieties									
778	Raw, coarsely shredded or sliced	1 c	70	93	15	1	Tr	Tr	Tr	0.1
779	Cooked, drained	1 c	150	94	30	1	Tr	Tr	Tr	0.2
	Cabbage, Chinese									
780	Pak-choi, cooked, drained	1 c	170	96	20	3	Tr	Tr	Tr	0.1
781	Pe-tsai, raw, 1-in pieces	1 c	76	94	10	1	Tr	Tr	Tr	0.1
782	Cabbage, red, raw, coarsely shredded or sliced	1 c	70	92	20	1	Tr	Tr	Tr	0.1
783	Cabbage, savoy, raw, coarsely shredded or sliced	1 c	70	91	20	1	Tr	Tr	Tr	Tr
	Carrots									
	Raw, without crowns and tips, scraped									
784	Whole, 7½ by 1⅛ in, or strips, 2½ to 3 in long	1 carrot or 18 strips	72	88	30	1	Tr	Tr	Tr	0.1
785	Grated	1 c	110	88	45	1	Tr	Tr	Tr	0.1
	Cooked, sliced, drained									
786	From raw	1 c	156	87	70	2	Tr	0.1	Tr	0.1
787	From frozen	1 c	146	90	55	2	Tr	Tr	Tr	0.1
788	Canned, sliced, drained solids	1 c	146	93	35	1	Tr	0.1	Tr	0.1
	Cauliflower									
789	Raw, (flowerets)	1 c	100	92	25	2	Tr	Tr	Tr	0.1
	Cooked, drained									
790	From raw (flowerets)	1 c	125	93	30	2	Tr	Tr	Tr	0.1
791	From frozen (flowerets)	1 c	180	94	35	3	Tr	0.1	Tr	0.2

							Vitamin A Value				Ascor-	
Cho-les-terol (mg)	Carbo-hydrate (g)	Cal-cium (mg)	Phos-phorus (mg)	Iron (mg)	Potas-sium (mg)	Sodium (mg)	IU	RE	Thia-min (mg)	Ribo-flavin (mg)	Nia-cin (mg)	bic Acid (mg)	Item No.
0	12	26	29	3.1	252	466*	20	2	0.02	0.07	0.3	7	767
0	8	164	59	2.7	1,309	347	7,340	734	0.17	0.42	0.7	36	768
0	30	46	196	2.4	693	7	1,050	105	0.11	0.18	1.8	3	769
0	40	39	207	3.6	638	9	130	13	0.44	0.11	1.2	4	770
0	8	72	100	1.3	491	41	2,330	233	0.10	0.18	1.0	141	771
0	10	205	86	2.1	293	20	2,540	254	0.15	0.37	1.4	113	772
0	9	177	74	1.8	253	17	2,180	218	0.13	0.32	1.2	97	773
0	2	15	17	0.2	54	7	570	57	0.02	0.02	0.1	12	774
0	10	94	102	1.1	333	44	3,500	350	0.10	0.15	0.8	74	775
0	13	56	87	1.9	491	33	1,110	111	0.17	0.12	0.9	96	776
0	13	37	84	1.1	504	36	910	91	0.16	0.18	0.8	71	777
0	4	33	16	0.4	172	13	90	9	0.04	0.02	0.2	33	778
0	7	50	38	0.6	308	29	130	13	0.09	0.08	0.3	36	779
0	3	158	49	1.8	631	58	4,370	437	0.05	0.11	0.7	44	780
0	2	59	22	0.2	181	7	910	91	0.03	0.04	0.3	21	781
0	4	36	29	0.3	144	8	30	3	0.04	0.02	0.2	40	782
0	4	25	29	0.3	161	20	700	70	0.05	0.02	0.2	22	783
0	7	19	32	0.4	233	25	20,250	2,025	0.07	0.04	0.7	7	784
0	11	30	48	0.6	355	39	30,940	3,094	0.11	0.06	1.0	10	785
0	16	48	47	1.0	354	103	38,300	3,830	0.05	0.09	0.8	4	786
0	12	41	38	0.7	231	86	25,850	2,585	0.04	0.05	0.6	4	787
0	8	37	35	0.9	261	352†	20,110	2,011	0.03	0.04	0.8	4	788
0	5	29	46	0.6	355	15	20	2	0.08	0.06	0.6	72	789
0	6	34	44	0.5	404	8	20	2	0.08	0.07	0.7	69	790
0	7	31	43	0.7	250	32	40	4	0.07	0.10	0.6	56	791

Table continued on following page

*For regular pack; special dietary pack contains 78 mg sodium.
†For regular pack; special dietary pack contains 61 mg sodium.

Item No.	Foods, Approximate Measures, Units, and Weight (Weight of Edible Portion Only)		Grams	Water (%)	Food Energy (cal)	Pro-tein (g)	Fat (g)	Fatty Acids		
								Satu-rated (g)	Mono-unsatu-rated (g)	Poly-unsatu-rated (g)
	Celery, pascal type, raw									
792	Stalk, large outer, 8 by 1½ in (at root end)	1 stalk	40	95	5	Tr	Tr	Tr	Tr	Tr
	Pieces, boiled drained	250 ml	158	95	24[1]	Tr	Tr	Tr		Tr
793	Pieces, diced	1 c	120	95	20	1	Tr	Tr	Tr	0.1
	Chard, swiss, boiled, drained	250 ml	185	93	37[1]	3	Tr	0		0
	Coleslaw (cabbage salad)	250 ml	127	82	88[1]	2	3	Tr		2
	Collards, cooked, drained									
794	From raw (leaves without stems)	1 c	190	96	25	2	Tr	0.1	Tr	0.2
795	From frozen (chopped)	1 c	170	88	60	5	1	0.1	0.1	0.4
	Corn, sweet									
	Cooked, drained									
796	From raw, ear 5 by 1¾ in	1 ear	77	70	85	3	1	0.2	0.3	0.5
	From frozen									
797	Ear, trimmed to about 3½ in long	1 ear	63	73	60	2	Tr	0.1	0.1	0.2
798	Kernels	1 c	165	76	135	5	Tr	Tr	Tr	0.1
	Canned									
799	Cream style	1 c	256	79	185	4	1	0.2	0.3	0.5
800	Whole kernel, vacuum pack	1 c	210	77	165	5	1	0.2	0.3	0.5
	Cowpeas. See Black-eyed peas, immature (items 769, 770), mature (item 536)									
801	Cucumber, with peel, slices, ⅛ in thick (large, 2⅛-in diam.; small, 1¾-in diam.)	6 large or 8 small slices	28	96	5	Tr	Tr	Tr	Tr	Tr
802	Dandelion greens, cooked, drained	1 c	105	90	35	2	1	0.1	Tr	0.3
803	Eggplant, cooked, steamed	1 c	96	92	25	1	Tr	Tr	Tr	0.1
804	Endive, curly (including escarole), raw, small pieces	1 c	50	94	10	1	Tr	Tr	Tr	Tr
	Fiddlehead greens, frozen cooked	250 ml	150	93	30[1]	4	Tr	—		—
805	Jerusalem artichoke, raw, sliced	1 c	150	78	115	3	Tr	0.0	Tr	Tr
	Kale, cooked, drained									
806	From raw, chopped	1 c	130	91	40	2	1	0.1	Tr	0.3
807	From frozen, chopped	1 c	130	91	40	4	1	0.1	Tr	0.3
808	Kohlrabi, thickened bulb-like stems, cooked, drained, diced	1 c	165	90	50	3	Tr	Tr	Tr	0.1
	Lettuce, raw									
	Butterhead, as Boston types									
809	Head, 5-in diam	1 head	163	96	20	2	Tr	Tr	Tr	0.2
810	Leaves	1 outer or 2 inner leaves	15	96	Tr	Tr	Tr	Tr	Tr	Tr

Nutrients in Indicated Quantity

Cholesterol (mg)	Carbohydrate (g)	Calcium (mg)	Phosphorus (mg)	Iron (mg)	Potassium (mg)	Sodium (mg)	Vitamin A Value IU	RE	Thiamin (mg)	Riboflavin (mg)	Niacin (mg)	Ascorbic Acid (mg)	Item No.
0	1	14	10	0.2	114	35	50	5	0.01	0.01	0.1	3	792
0	6	57		0.2	559	101		17	0.04	0.05	0.6	7	
0	4	43	31	0.6	341	106	150	15	0.04	0.04	0.4	8	793
0	8	107		4.2	1016	331		581	0.06	0.16	1.2	33	
10	2	57		0.7	230	29		104	0.08	0.08	0.7	42	
0	5	148	19	0.8	177	36	4,220	422	0.03	0.08	0.4	19	794
0	12	357	46	1.9	427	85	10,170	1,017	0.08	0.20	1.1	45	795
0	19	2	79	0.5	192	13	170*	17*	0.17	0.06	1.2	5	796
0	14	2	47	0.4	158	3	130*	13*	0.11	0.04	1.0	3	797
0	34	3	78	0.5	229	8	410*	41*	0.11	0.12	2.1	4	798
0	46	8	131	1.0	343	730†	250*	25*	0.06	0.14	2.5	12	799
0	41	11	134	0.9	391	571‡	510*	51*	0.09	0.15	2.5	17	800
0	1	4	5	0.1	42	1	10	1	0.01	0.01	0.1	1	801
0	7	147	44	1.9	244	46	12,290	1,229	0.14	0.18	0.5	19	802
0	6	6	21	0.3	238	3	60	6	0.07	0.02	0.6	1	803
0	2	26	14	0.4	157	11	1,030	103	0.04	0.04	0.2	3	804
0	5	8		1.2	332	2		—	0	0.38	—	14	
0	26	21	117	5.1	644	6	30	3	0.30	0.09	2.0	6	805
0	7	94	36	1.2	296	30	9,620	962	0.07	0.09	0.7	53	806
0	7	179	36	1.2	417	20	8,260	826	0.06	0.15	0.9	33	807
0	11	41	74	0.7	561	35	60	6	0.07	0.03	0.6	89	808
0	4	52	38	0.5	419	8	1,580	158	0.10	0.10	0.5	13	809
0	Tr	5	3	Tr	39	1	150	15	0.01	0.01	Tr	1	810

Table continued on following page

*For yellow varieties; white varieties contain only a trace of vitamin A.
†For regular pack; special dietary pack cotnains 8 mg sodium.
‡For regular pack; special dietary pack contains 6 mg sodium.

Item No.	Foods, Approximate Measures, Units, and Weight (Weight of Edible Portion Only)		Grams	Water (%)	Food Energy (cal)	Protein (g)	Fat (g)	Fatty Acids		
								Saturated (g)	Mono-unsaturated (g)	Poly-unsaturated (g)
	Crisphead, as iceberg									
811	Head, 6-in diam	1 head	539	96	70	5	1	0.1	Tr	0.5
812	Wedge, ¼ of head	1 wedge	135	96	20	1	Tr	Tr	Tr	0.1
813	Pieces, chopped or shredded	1 c	55	96	5	1	Tr	Tr	Tr	0.1
814	Looseleaf (bunching varieties including romaine or cos), chopped or shredded pieces	1 c	56	94	10	1	Tr	Tr	Tr	0.1
	Mushrooms									
815	Raw, sliced or chopped	1 c	70	92	20	1	Tr	Tr	Tr	0.1
816	Cooked, drained	1 c	156	91	40	3	1	0.1	Tr	0.3
817	Canned, drained solids	1 c	156	91	35	3	Tr	0.1	Tr	0.2
818	Mustard greens, without stems and midribs, cooked, drained	1 c	140	94	20	3	Tr	Tr	0.2	0.1
819	Okra pods, 3 by ⅝ in, cooked	8 pods	85	90	25	2	Tr	Tr	Tr	Tr
	Onions									
	Raw									
820	Chopped	1 c	160	91	55	2	Tr	0.1	0.1	0.2
821	Sliced	1 c	115	91	40	1	Tr	0.1	Tr	0.1
822	Cooked (whole or sliced), drained	1 c	210	92	60	2	Tr	0.1	Tr	0.1
	Frozen, chopped, boiled, drained	250 ml	222	92	62[1]	2	Tr	Tr		Tr
823	Onions, spring, raw, bulb (⅜-in diam.) and white portion of top	6 onions	30	92	10	1	Tr	Tr	Tr	Tr
824	Onion rings, breaded, pan-fried, frozen, prepared	2 rings	20	29	80	1	5	1.7	2.2	1.0
	Parsley									
825	Raw	10 sprigs	10	88	5	Tr	Tr	Tr	Tr	Tr
826	Freeze-dried	1 tbsp	0.4	2	Tr	Tr	Tr	Tr	Tr	Tr
827	Parsnips, cooked (diced or 2-in lengths), drained	1 c	156	78	125	2	Tr	0.1	0.2	0.1
828	Peas, edible pod									
	Cooked, drained	1 c	160	89	65	5	Tr	0.1	Tr	0.2
	Raw	250 ml	153	89	64[1]	4	Tr	Tr		Tr
	Peas, green									
	Boiled, drained	250 ml	169	78	142[1]	9	Tr	Tr		Tr
829	Canned, drained solids	1 c	170	82	115	8	1	0.1	0.1	0.3
830	Frozen, cooked, drained	1 c	160	80	125	8	Tr	0.1	Tr	0.2
	Peppers									
831	Hot chili, raw	1 pepper	45	88	20	1	Tr	Tr	Tr	Tr
	Sweet (about 5 per lb, whole), stem and seeds removed									
832	Raw	1 pepper	74	93	20	1	Tr	Tr	Tr	0.2
833	Cooked, drained	1 pepper	73	95	15	Tr	Tr	Tr	Tr	0.1

Nutrients in Indicated Quantity

Cho-les-terol (mg)	Carbo-hydrate (g)	Cal-cium (mg)	Phos-phorus (mg)	Iron (mg)	Potas-sium (mg)	Sodium (mg)	Vitamin A Value		Thia-min (mg)	Ribo-flavin (mg)	Nia-cin (mg)	Ascor-bic Acid (mg)	Item No.
							IU	RE					
0	11	102	108	2.7	852	49	1,780	178	0.25	0.16	1.0	21	811
0	3	26	27	0.7	213	12	450	45	0.06	0.04	0.3	5	812
0	1	10	11	0.3	87	5	180	18	0.03	0.02	0.1	2	813
0	2	38	14	0.8	148	5	1,060	106	0.03	0.04	0.2	10	814
0	3	4	73	0.9	259	3	0	0	0.07	0.31	2.9	2	815
0	8	9	136	2.7	555	3	0	0	0.11	0.47	7.0	6	816
0	8	17	103	1.2	201	663	0	0	0.13	0.03	2.5	0	817
0	3	104	57	1.0	283	22	4,240	424	0.06	0.09	0.6	35	818
0	6	54	48	0.4	274	4	490	49	0.11	0.05	0.7	14	819
0	12	40	46	0.6	248	3	0	0	0.10	0.02	0.2	13	820
0	8	29	33	0.4	178	2	0	0	0.07	0.01	0.1	10	821
0	13	57	48	0.4	319	17	0	0	0.09	0.02	0.2	12	822
0	15	36		0.7	240	27		7	0.05	0.06	0.7	6	
0	2	18	10	0.6	77	1	1,500	150	0.02	0.04	0.1	14	823
0	8	6	16	0.3	26	75	50	5	0.06	0.03	0.7	Tr	824
0	1	13	4	0.6	54	4	520	52	0.01	0.01	0.1	9	825
0	Tr	1	2	0.2	25	2	250	25	Tr	0.01	Tr	1	826
0	30	58	108	0.9	573	16	0	0	0.13	0.08	1.1	20	827
0	11	67	88	3.2	384	6	210	21	0.20	0.12	0.9	77	828
0	12	66		3.2	306	6		21	0.23	0.12	1.6	92	
0	26	46		2.6	458	5		101	0.44	0.25	4.5	24	
0	21	34	114	1.6	294	372*	1,310	131	0.21	0.13	1.2	16	829
0	23	38	144	2.5	269	139	1,070	107	0.45	0.16	2.4	16	830
0	4	8	21	0.5	153	3	4,840†	484†	0.04	0.04	0.4	109	831
0	4	4	16	0.9	144	2	390‡	39‡	0.06	0.04	0.4	95§	832
0	3	3	11	0.6	94	1	280‖	28‖	0.04	0.03	0.3	81¶	833

Table continued on following page

*For regular pack; special pack contains 3 mg sodium.
†For red peppers; green peppers contain 350 IU or 35 RE.
‡For green peppers; red peppers contain 4,220 IU or 422 RE.
§For green peppers; red peppers contain 141 mg ascorbic acid.
‖For green peppers; red peppers contain 2,740 IU or 274 RE.
¶For green peppers; red peppers contain 121 mg ascorbic acid.

Item No.	Foods, Approximate Measures, Units, and Weight (Weight of Edible Portion Only)		Grams	Water (%)	Food Energy (cal)	Pro- tein (g)	Fat (g)	Satu- rated (g)	Mono- unsatu- rated (g)	Poly- unsatu- rated (g)
								Fatty Acids		
	Potatoes, cooked									
	Baked (about 2 per lb, raw)									
834	With skin	1 potato	202	71	220	5	Tr	0.1	Tr	0.1
835	Flesh only	1 potato	156	75	145	3	Tr	Tr	Tr	0.1
	Boiled (about 3 per lb, raw)									
836	Peeled after boiling	1 potato	136	77	120	3	Tr	Tr	Tr	0.1
837	Peeled before boiling	1 potato	135	77	115	2	Tr	Tr	Tr	0.1
	French fried, strip, 2 to 3½ in long, frozen									
838	Oven heated	10 strips	50	53	110	2	4	2.1	1.8	0.3
839	Fried in vegetable oil	10 strips	50	38	160	2	8	2.5	1.6	3.8
	Microwaved, flesh and skin, 12 cm long	1	206	72	216[1]	5	Tr	Tr		Tr
	Potato products, prepared									
	Au gratin									
840	From dry mix	1 c	245	79	230	6	10	6.3	2.9	0.3
841	From home recipe	1 c	245	74	325	12	19	11.6	5.3	0.7
842	Hashed brown, from fro- zen	1 c	156	56	340	5	18	7.0	8.0	2.1
	Hashed brown, home pre- pared	250 ml	165	75	252[1]	4	23	9		3
	Mashed									
	From home recipe									
843	Milk added	1 c	210	78	160	4	1	0.7	0.3	0.1
844	Milk and margarine added	1 c	210	76	225	4	9	2.2	3.7	2.5
845	From dehydrated flakes (without milk), water, milk, butter, and salt added	1 c	210	76	235	4	12	7.2	3.3	0.5
846	Potato salad, made with mayonnaise	1 c	250	76	360	7	21	3.6	6.2	9.3
	Scalloped									
847	From dry mix	1 c	245	79	230	5	11	6.5	3.0	0.5
848	From home recipe	1 c	245	81	210	7	9	5.5	2.5	0.4
849	Potato chips	10 chips	20	3	105	1	7	1.8	1.2	3.6
	Pumpkin									
850	Cooked from raw, mashed	1 c	245	94	50	2	Tr	0.1	Tr	Tr
851	Canned	1 c	245	90	85	3	1	0.4	0.1	Tr
852	Radishes, raw, stem ends, rootlets cut off	4 radishes	18	95	5	Tr	Tr	Tr	Tr	Tr
853	Sauerkraut, canned, solids and liquid	1 c	236	93	45	2	Tr	0.1	Tr	0.1
	Seaweed									
854	Kelp, raw	1 oz	28	82	10	Tr	Tr	0.1	Tr	Tr
855	Spirulina, dried	1 oz	28	5	80	16	2	0.8	0.2	0.6
	Southern peas. See Black- eyed peas, immature (items 769, 770), mature (item 536)									
	Spinach									
856	Raw, chopped	1 c	55	92	10	2	Tr	Tr	Tr	0.1

Nutrients in Indicated Quantity

Cholesterol (mg)	Carbohydrate (g)	Calcium (mg)	Phosphorus (mg)	Iron (mg)	Potassium (mg)	Sodium (mg)	Vitamin A Value		Thiamin (mg)	Riboflavin (mg)	Niacin (mg)	Ascorbic Acid (mg)	Item No.
							IU	RE					
0	51	20	115	2.7	844	16	0	0	0.22	0.07	3.3	26	834
0	34	8	78	0.5	610	8	0	0	0.16	0.03	2.2	20	835
0	27	7	60	0.4	515	5	0	0	0.14	0.03	2.0	18	836
0	27	11	54	0.4	443	7	0	0	0.13	0.03	1.8	10	837
0	17	5	43	0.7	229	16	0	0	0.06	0.02	1.2	5	838
0	20	10	47	0.4	366	108	0	0	0.09	0.01	1.6	5	839
0	50	23		2.6	921	16		0	0.25	0.07	4.8	31	
12	31	203	233	0.8	537	1,076	520	76	0.05	0.20	2.3	8	840
56	28	292	277	1.6	970	1,061	650	93	0.16	0.28	2.4	24	841
0	44	23	112	2.4	680	53	0	0	0.17	0.03	3.8	10	842
0	12	13		1.3	530	40		0	0.12	0.03	4.2	9	
4	37	55	101	0.6	628	636	40	12	0.18	0.08	2.3	14	843
4	35	55	97	0.5	607	620	360	42	0.18	0.08	2.3	13	844
29	32	103	118	0.5	489	697	380	44	0.23	0.11	1.4	20	845
170	28	48	130	1.6	635	1,323	520	83	0.19	0.15	2.2	25	846
27	31	88	137	0.9	497	835	360	51	0.05	0.14	2.5	8	847
29	26	140	154	1.4	926	821	330	47	0.17	0.23	2.6	26	848
0	10	5	31	0.2	260	94	0	0	0.03	Tr	0.8	8	849
0	12	37	74	1.4	564	2	2,650	265	0.08	0.19	1.0	12	850
0	20	64	86	3.4	505	12	54,040	5,404	0.06	0.13	0.9	10	851
0	1	4	3	0.1	42	4	Tr	Tr	Tr	0.01	0.1	4	852
0	10	71	47	3.5	401	1,560	40	4	0.05	0.05	0.3	35	853
0	3	48	12	0.8	25	66	30	3	0.01	0.04	0.1	(*)	854
0	7	34	33	8.1	386	297	160	16	0.67	1.04	3.6	3	855
0	2	54	27	1.5	307	43	3,690	369	0.04	0.10	0.4	15	856

Table continued on following page

*Value not determined.

Item No.	Foods, Approximate Measures, Units, and Weight (Weight of Edible Portion Only)		Grams	Water (%)	Food Energy (cal)	Pro-tein (g)	Fat (g)	Fatty Acids		
								Satu-rated (g)	Mono-unsatu-rated (g)	Poly-unsatu-rated (g)
	Cooked, drained									
857	From raw	1 c	180	91	40	5	Tr	0.1	Tr	0.2
858	From frozen (leaf)	1 c	190	90	55	6	Tr	0.1	Tr	0.2
859	Canned, drained solids	1 c	214	92	50	6	1	0.2	Tr	0.4
860	Spinach souffle	1 c	136	74	220	11	18	7.1	6.8	3.1
	Squash, cooked									
861	Summer (all varieties), sliced, drained	1 c	180	94	35	2	1	0.1	Tr	0.2
862	Winter (all varieties), baked, cubes)	1 c	205	89	80	2	1	0.3	0.1	0.5
	Winter, butternut, frozen, boiled	250 ml	254	88	99[1]	3	Tr	Tr		Tr
	Winter, hubbard, boiled, mashed	250 ml	249	91	75[1]	4	Tr	Tr		Tr
	Sunchoke. See Jerusalem artichoke (item 805)									
	Sweet potatoes									
	Cooked (raw, 5 by 2 in; about 2½ per lb)									
863	Baked in skin, peeled	1 potato	114	73	115	2	Tr	Tr	Tr	0.1
864	Boiled, without skin	1 potato	151	73	160	2	Tr	0.1	Tr	0.2
	Canned									
866	Solid pack (mashed)	1 c	255	74	260	5	1	0.1	Tr	0.2
867	Vacuum pack, piece 2¾ by 1 in	1 piece	40	76	35	1	Tr	Tr	Tr	Tr
	Tomatoes									
868	Raw, 2⅗-in diam (3 per 12-oz pkg.)	1 tomato	123	94	25	1	Tr	Tr	Tr	0.1
869	Canned, solids and liquid	1 c	240	94	50	2	1	0.1	0.1	0.2
	Canned, stewed	250 ml	269	91	70[1]	3	Tr	Tr		Tr
870	Tomato juice, canned	1 c	244	94	40	2	Tr	Tr	Tr	0.1
	Tomato products, canned									
871	Paste	1 c	262	74	220	10	2	0.3	0.4	0.9
872	Puree	1 c	250	87	105	4	Tr	Tr	Tr	0.1
873	Sauce	1 c	245	89	75	3	Tr	0.1	0.1	0.2
874	Turnips, Cooked, diced	1 c	156	94	30	1	Tr	Tr	Tr	0.1
	Raw, cubed	250 ml	137	92	37[1]	1	Tr	Tr		Tr
	Turnip greens, cooked, drained									
875	From raw (leaves and stems)	1 c	144	93	30	2	Tr	0.1	Tr	0.1
876	From frozen (chopped)	1 c	164	90	50	5	1	0.2	Tr	0.3
877	Vegetable juice cocktail, canned	1 c	242	94	45	2	Tr	Tr	Tr	0.1
	Vegetables, mixed									
878	Canned, drained solids	1 c	163	87	75	4	Tr	0.1	Tr	0.2
879	Frozen, cooked, drained	1 c	182	83	105	5	Tr	0.1	Tr	0.1
880	Water chestnuts, canned	1 c	140	86	70	1	Tr	Tr	Tr	Tr

							Vitamin A Value					Ascor-	
Cho-les-terol (mg)	Carbo-hydrate (g)	Cal-cium (mg)	Phos-phorus (mg)	Iron (mg)	Potas-sium (mg)	Sodium (mg)	IU	RE	Thia-min (mg)	Ribo-flavin (mg)	Nia-cin (mg)	bic Acid (mg)	Item No.
0	7	245	101	6.4	839	126	14,740	1,474	0.17	0.42	0.9	18	857
0	10	277	91	2.9	566	163	14,790	1,479	0.11	0.32	0.8	23	858
0	7	272	94	4.9	740	683*	18,780	1,878	0.03	0.30	0.8	31	859
184	3	230	231	1.3	201	763	3,460	675	0.09	0.30	0.5	3	860
0	8	49	70	0.6	346	2	520	52	0.08	0.07	0.9	10	861
0	18	29	41	0.7	896	2	7,290	729	0.17	0.05	1.4	20	862
0	26	48		1.5	338	5		848	0.13	0.10	1.9	9	
0	16	25		0.7	533	12		998	0.11	0.07	1.7	16	
0	28	32	63	0.5	397	11	24,880	2,488	0.08	0.14	0.7	28	863
0	37	32	41	0.8	278	20	25,750	2,575	0.08	0.21	1.0	26	864
0	59	77	133	3.4	536	191	38,570	3,857	0.07	0.23	2.4	13	866
0	8	9	20	0.4	125	21	3,190	319	0.01	0.02	0.3	11	867
0	5	9	28	0.6	255	10	1,390	139	0.07	0.06	0.7	22	868
0	10	62	46	1.5	530	391†	1,450	145	0.11	0.07	1.8	36	869
0	17	89		2.0	643	683		148	0.12	0.09	2.2	36	
0	10	22	46	1.4	537	881‡	1,360	136	0.11	0.08	1.6	45	870
0	49	92	207	7.8	2,442	170§	6,470	647	0.41	0.50	8.4	111	871
0	25	38	100	2.3	1,050	50‖	3,400	340	0.18	0.14	4.3	88	872
0	18	34	78	1.9	909	1,482¶	2,400	240	0.16	0.14	2.8	32	873
0	8	34	30	0.3	211	78	0	0	0.04	0.04	0.5	18	874
0	9	41		0.4	262	92		0	0.06	0.04	0.8	29	
0	6	197	42	1.2	292	42	7,920	792	0.06	0.10	0.6	39	875
0	8	249	56	3.2	367	25	13,080	1,308	0.09	0.12	0.8	36	876
0	11	27	41	1.0	467	883	2,830	283	0.10	0.07	1.8	67	877
0	15	44	68	1.7	474	243	18,990	1,899	0.08	0.08	0.9	8	878
0	24	46	93	1.5	308	64	7,780	778	0.13	0.22	1.5	6	879
0	17	6	27	1.2	165	11	10	1	0.02	0.03	0.5	2	880

Table continued on following page

*With added salt; if none is added, sodium content is 58 mg.
†For regular pack; special dietary pack contains 31 mg sodium.
‡With added salt; if none is added, sodium content is 24 mg.
§With no added salt; if salt is added, sodium content is 2,070 mg.
‖With no added salt; if salt is added, sodium content is 998 mg.
¶With salt added.

Item No.	Foods, Approximate Measures, Units, and Weight (Weight of Edible Portion Only)	Grams	Water (%)	Food Energy (cal)	Pro-tein (g)	Fat (g)	Fatty Acids		
							Satu-rated (g)	Mono-unsatu-rated (g)	Poly-unsatu-rated (g)
	Miscellaneous Items								
	Baking powders for home use								
	Sodium aluminum sulfate								
881	With monocalcium phosphate monohydrate	1 tsp	3	2	5	Tr	0	0.0	0.0	0.0
882	With monocalcium phosphate monohydrate, calcium sulfate	1 tsp	2.9	1	5	Tr	0	0.0	0.0	0.0
883	Straight phosphate	1 tsp	3.8	2	5	Tr	0	0.0	0.0	0.0
884	Low sodium	1 tsp	4.3	1	5	Tr	0	0.0	0.0	0.0
	Bouillon cubes	1 cube	6	3	10	1	Tr	Tr		Tr
885	Catsup	1 c	273	69	290	5	1	0.2	0.2	0.4
886		1 tbsp	15	69	15	Tr	Tr	Tr	Tr	Tr
887	Celery seed	1 tsp	2	6	10	Tr	1	Tr	0.3	0.1
888	Chili powder	1 tsp	2.6	8	10	Tr	Tr	0.1	0.1	0.2
889	Chocolate, bitter or baking	1 oz	28	2	145	3	15	9.0	4.9	0.5
890	Cinnamon	1 tsp	2.3	10	5	Tr	Tr	Tr	Tr	Tr
	Coffee	250 ml	254	100	5[1]	Tr	0	0		0
891	Curry powder	1 tsp	2	10	5	Tr	Tr	(*)	(*)	(*)
892	Garlic powder	1 tsp	2.8	6	10	Tr	Tr	Tr	Tr	Tr
893	Gelatin, dry	1 envelope	7	13	25	6	Tr	Tr	Tr	Tr
	Dietetic, prepared with water	125 ml	127	99	10[1]	3	Tr	0		Tr
894	Mustard, prepared, yellow	1 tsp or individual packet	5	80	5	Tr	Tr	Tr	0.2	Tr
	Olives, canned									
895	Green	4 medium or 3 extra large	13	78	15	Tr	2	0.2	1.2	0.1
896	Ripe, Mission, pitted	3 small or 2 large	9	73	15	Tr	2	0.3	1.3	0.2
897	Onion powder	1 tsp	2.1	5	5	Tr	Tr	Tr	Tr	Tr
898	Oregano	1 tsp	1.5	7	5	Tr	Tr	Tr	Tr	0.1
899	Paprika	1 tsp	2.1	10	5	Tr	Tr	Tr	Tr	0.2
900	Pepper, black	1 tsp	2.1	11	5	Tr	Tr	Tr	Tr	Tr
	Pickles, cucumber									
901	Dill, medium, whole, 3¾ in long, 1¼-in diam.	1 pickle	65	93	5	Tr	Tr	Tr	Tr	0.1
902	Fresh-pack, slices 1½-in diam., ¼ in thick	2 slices	15	79	10	Tr	Tr	Tr	Tr	Tr
903	Sweet, gherkin, small, whole, about 2½ in long, ¾-in diam.	1 pickle	15	61	20	Tr	Tr	Tr	Tr	Tr
	Popcorn. See Grain Products (items 497–499)									
	Postum, made with water	250 ml	252	—	17	Tr	0	0		0
904	Relish, finely chopped, sweet	1 tbsp	15	63	20	Tr	Tr	Tr	Tr	Tr
905	Salt	1 tsp	5.5	0	0	0	0	0.0	0.0	0.0
	Shake and bake, dry	15 ml	6	5	24	Tr	Tr	Tr		Tr

*Value not determined.

Nutrients in Indicated Quantity

Cho-les-terol (mg)	Carbo-hydrate (g)	Cal-cium (mg)	Phos-phorus (mg)	Iron (mg)	Potas-sium (mg)	Sodium (mg)	Vitamin A Value		Thia-min (mg)	Ribo-flavin (mg)	Nia-cin (mg)	Ascor-bic Acid (mg)	Item No.
							IU	RE					
0	1	58	87	0.0	5	329	0	0	0.00	0.00	0.0	0	881
0	1	183	45	0.0	4	290	0	0	0.00	0.00	0.0	0	882
0	1	239	359	0.0	6	312	0	0	0.00	0.00	0.0	0	883
0	1	207	314	0.0	891	Tr	0	0	0.00	0.00	0.0	0	884
Tr	Tr	4		0.1	24	1440		Tr	0.01	0.01	0.4	0	
0	69	60	137	2.2	991	2,845	3,820	382	0.25	0.19	4.4	41	885
0	4	3	8	0.1	54	156	210	21	0.01	0.01	0.2	2	886
0	1	35	11	0.9	28	3	Tr	Tr	0.01	0.01	0.1	Tr	887
0	1	7	8	0.4	50	26	910	91	0.01	0.02	0.2	2	888
0	8	22	109	1.9	235	1	10	1	0.01	0.07	0.4	0	889
0	2	28	1	0.9	12	1	10	1	Tr	Tr	Tr	1	890
0	1	5		1.0	137	5	0	0	0	0	0.6	0	
0	1	10	7	0.6	31	1	20	2	0.01	0.01	0.1	Tr	891
0	2	2	12	0.1	31	1	0	0	0.01	Tr	Tr	Tr	892
0	0	1	0	0.0	2	6	0	0	0.00	0.00	0.0	0	893
0	Tr	0		0	47	9		0	0	0	0	0	
0	Tr	4	4	0.1	7	63	0	0	Tr	0.01	Tr	Tr	894
0	Tr	8	2	0.2	7	312	40	4	Tr	Tr	Tr	0	895
0	Tr	10	2	0.2	2	68	10	1	Tr	Tr	Tr	0	896
0	2	8	7	0.1	20	1	Tr	Tr	0.01	Tr	Tr	Tr	897
0	1	24	3	0.7	25	Tr	100	10	0.01	Tr	0.1	1	898
0	1	4	7	0.5	49	1	1,270	127	0.01	0.04	0.3	1	899
0	1	9	4	0.6	26	1	Tr	Tr	Tr	0.01	Tr	0	900
0	1	17	14	0.7	130	928	70	7	Tr	0.01	Tr	4	901
0	3	5	4	0.3	30	101	20	2	Tr	Tr	Tr	1	902
0	5	2	2	0.2	30	107	10	1	Tr	Tr	Tr	1	903
0	4	7		0.7	131	7		—	0.05	0	—	0	
0	5	3	2	0.1	30	107	20	2	Tr	Tr	0.0	1	904
0	0	14	3	Tr	Tr	2,132	0	0	0.00	0.00	0.0	0	905
0	4	4		0.2	12	210		0	0.01	0	0.2	0	

Table continued on following page

Item No.	Foods, Approximate Measures, Units, and Weight (Weight of Edible Portion Only)		Grams	Water (%)	Food Energy (cal)	Pro-tein (g)	Fat (g)	Fatty Acids		
								Satu-rated (g)	Mono-unsatu-rated (g)	Poly-unsatu-rated (g)
	Soft drinks, club soda (soda water)	280 ml	280	100	0	0	0	0		0
	Soft drinks, cola type beverage with aspartame	280 ml	280	100	3	Tr	0	0		0
	Soft drinks, tonic water	280 ml	289	91	98	0	0	0		0
	Tea, beverage	250 ml	254	100	3	0	0	0		0
	Tea, beverage, made from sweetened instant powder	250 ml	277	91	94	Tr	Tr	Tr		Tr
906	Vinegar, cider	1 tbsp	15	94	Tr	Tr	0	0.0	0.0	0.0
	Vinegar, white	15 ml	15	95	2	0	0	0		0
	Yeast									
907	Baker's, dry, active	1 pkg	7	5	20	3	Tr	Tr	0.1	Tr
908	Brewer's dry	1 tbsp	8	5	25	3	Tr	Tr	Tr	0.0

Cho-les-terol (mg)	Carbo-hydrate (g)	Cal-cium (mg)	Phos-phorus (mg)	Iron (mg)	Potas-sium (mg)	Sodium (mg)	Vitamin A Value IU	Vitamin A Value RE	Thia-min (mg)	Ribo-flavin (mg)	Nia-cin (mg)	Ascor-bic Acid (mg)	Item No.
							Nutrients in Indicated Quantity						
0	0	14		0	6	59		0	0	0	0	0	
0	Tr	11		0.1	0	17		0	0	0	0	0	
0	25	3		0	0	12		0	0	0	0	0	
0	Tr	0		Tr	94	8		0	0	0.04	0	0	
0	24	6		Tr	52	Tr		0	0	0.04	0.2	0	
0	1	1	1	0.1	15	Tr	0	0	0.00	0.00	0.0	0	906
0	Tr	0		0	2	Tr		0	0	0	0	0	
0	3	3	90	1.1	140	4	Tr	Tr	0.16	0.38	2.6	Tr	907
0	3	17*	140	1.4	152	10	Tr	Tr	1.25	0.34	3.0	Tr	908

*Value may vary from 6 to 60 mg.

Food Sources of Additional Nutrients

Vitamins

Vitamin B₆	Vitamin B₁₂*	Vitamin D
Bananas	Cheese	Egg yolk
Fish (most)	Fish	Liver
Liver and kidney	Liver and kidney	Saltwater fish
Meat	Meat	Vitamin D milk
Poultry	Milk	
Potatoes and sweet potatoes	Shellfish	
Whole-grain cereals	Whole egg and egg yolk	
Yeast		

Vitamin E	Folacin
Margarine	Dark green vegetables
Nuts	Dry beans and peas
Peanuts and peanut butter	Liver
Vegetable oils	Wheat germ
Whole-grain cereals	Yeast

Minerals

Iodine	Magnesium	Zinc
Iodized salt	Bananas	Cocoa
Seafood	Cocoa	Dry beans and peas
	Dark green vegetables (most)	Meat
	Dry beans and peas	Poultry
	Milk	Shellfish
	Nuts	Whole-grain cereals
	Whole-grain cereals	

*Present in foods of animal origin only.

Appendix 2

Food and Nutrition Board, National Academy of Sciences–National Research Council Recommended Daily Dietary Allowances,* Revised 1980

	Age (Years)	Weight kg	Weight lb	Height cm	Height in	Protein (g)	Fat-Soluble Vitamins Vita-min A (µg RE)†	Fat-Soluble Vitamins Vita-min D (µg)‡	Fat-Soluble Vitamins Vita-min E (mg α-TE)§	Water-Soluble Vitamins Vita-min C (mg)	Water-Soluble Vitamins Thia-min (mg)
Infants	0.0–0.5	6	13	60	24	kg × 2.2	420	10	3	35	0.3
	0.5–1.0	9	20	71	28	kg × 2.0	400	10	4	35	0.5
Children	1–3	13	29	90	35	23	400	10	5	45	0.7
	4–6	20	44	112	44	30	500	10	6	45	0.9
	7–10	28	62	132	52	34	700	10	7	45	1.2
Males	11–14	45	99	157	62	45	1000	10	8	50	1.4
	15–18	66	145	176	69	56	1000	10	10	60	1.4
	19–22	70	154	177	70	56	1000	7.5	10	60	1.5
	23–50	70	154	178	70	56	1000	5	10	60	1.4
	51+	70	154	178	70	56	1000	5	10	60	1.2
Females	11–14	46	101	157	62	46	800	10	8	50	1.1
	15–18	55	120	163	64	46	800	10	8	60	1.1
	19–22	55	120	163	64	44	800	7.5	8	60	1.1
	23–50	55	120	163	64	44	800	5	8	60	1.0
	51+	55	120	163	64	44	800	5	8	60	1.0
Pregnant						+30	+200	+5	+2	+20	+0.4
Lactating						+20	+400	+5	+3	+40	+0.5

*The allowances are intended to provide for individual variations among most normal persons as they live in the United States under usual environmental stresses. Diets should be based on a variety of common foods to provide other nutrients for which human requirements have been less well defined. See text for detailed discussion of allowances and of nutrients not tabulated. Note: The Recommended Daily Dietary Allowances (RDA) should not be confused with the U.S. Recommended Daily Allowances (USRDA). The RDA are amounts of nutrients recommended by the Food and Nutrition Board of the National Research Council and are considered adequate for maintenance of good nutrition in healthy persons in the United States. The allowances are revised from time to time in accordance with newer knowledge of nutritional needs.

The USRDA are the amounts of protein, vitamins, and minerals established by the Food and Drug Administration as standards for nutrition labeling. These allowances were derived from the RDA set by the Food and Nutrition Board. The USRDA for most nutrients approximates the highest RDA of the sex-age categories in this table, excluding the allowances for pregnant and lactating females. Therefore, a diet that furnishes the USRDA for a nutrient will furnish the RDA for most people and more than the RDA for many. USRDA are protein, 45 g (eggs, fish, meat, milk, poultry), 65 g (other foods); vitamin A, 5000 IU; thiamin, 1.5 mg; riboflavin, 1.7 mg; niacin, 20 mg; ascorbic acid, 60 mg; calcium, 1 g; phosphorus, 1 g; iron, 18 mg. For additional information on USRDA, see the Federal Register, vol. 38, no. 49 (March 14, 1973), pp. 6959–6960, and Agriculture Information Bulletin 382. "Nutrition Labeling—Tools for Its Use."
†Retinol equivalents: 1 RE = 1 µg retinol or 6 µg beta-carotene. See text for calculation of vitamin A activity of diets as REs.
‡As cholecalciferol; 10 µg cholecalciferol = 400 IU of vitamin D.
§Alpha-tocopherol equivalents; 1 mg d-alpha-tocopherol = 1 α-TE. See text for variation in allowances and calculation of vitamin E activity of the diet as alpha-tocopherol equivalents.

Food and Nutrition Board, National Academy of Sciences–National Research Council Recommended Daily Dietary Allowances, Revised 1980 *Continued*

Water-Soluble Vitamins					Minerals					
Ribo-flavin (mg)	Niacin (mg NE)‖	Vita-min B_6 (mg)	Fola-cin¶ (μg)	Vita-min B_{12} (μg)	Cal-cium (mg)	Phos-pho-rus (mg)	Mag-nesium (mg)	Iron (mg)	Zinc (mg)	Io-dine (μg)
0.4	6	0.3	30	0.5**	360	240	50	10	3	40
0.6	8	0.6	45	1.5	540	360	70	15	5	50
0.8	9	0.9	100	2.0	800	800	150	15	10	70
1.0	11	1.3	200	2.5	800	800	200	10	10	90
1.4	16	1.6	300	3.0	800	800	250	10	10	120
1.6	18	1.8	400	3.0	1200	1200	350	18	15	150
1.7	18	2.0	400	3.0	1200	1200	400	18	15	150
1.7	19	2.2	400	3.0	800	800	350	10	15	150
1.6	18	2.2	400	3.0	800	800	350	10	15	150
1.4	16	2.2	400	3.0	800	800	350	10	15	150
1.3	15	1.8	400	3.0	1200	1200	300	18	15	150
1.3	14	2.0	400	3.0	1200	1200	300	18	15	150
1.3	14	2.0	400	3.0	800	800	300	18	15	150
1.2	13	2.0	400	3.0	800	800	300	18	15	150
1.2	13	2.0	400	3.0	800	800	300	10	15	150
+0.3	+2	+0.6	+400	+1.0	+400	+400	+150	††	+5	+25
+0.5	+5	+0.5	+100	+1.0	+400	+400	+150	††	+10	+50

‖1 NE (niacin equivalent) is equal to 1 mg of niacin or 60 mg of dietary tryptophan.

¶The folacin allowances refer to dietary sources as determined by *Lactobacillus casei* assay after treatment with enzymes (conjugases) to make polyglutamyl forms of the vitamin available to the test organism.

**The recommended dietary allowance for vitamin B_{12} in infants is based on average concentration of the vitamin in human milk. The allowances after weaning are based on energy intake (as recommended by the American Academy of Pediatrics) and consideration of other factors, such as intestinal absorption; see text.

††The increased requirement during pregnancy cannot be met by the iron content of habitual American diets nor by the existing iron stores of many women; therefore the use of 30–60 mg of supplemental iron is recommended. Iron needs during lactation are not substantially different from those of nonpregnant women, but continued supplementation of the mother for 2–3 mo after parturition is advisable to replenish stores depleted by pregnancy.

Appendix 3

Estimated Safe and Adequate Daily Dietary Intakes of Selected Vitamins and Minerals*

	Age (Years)	Vitamins		
		Vitamin K (μg)	Biotin (μg)	Pantothenic Acid (mg)
Infants	0–0.05	12	35	2
	0.5–1	10–20	50	3
Children	1–3	15–30	65	3
and	4–6	20–40	85	3–4
adolescents	7–10	30–60	120	4–5
	11+	50–100	100–200	4–7
Adults		70–140	100–200	4–7

	Age (Years)	Trace Elements†					
		Copper (mg)	Manganese (mg)	Fluoride (mg)	Chromium (mg)	Selenium (mg)	Molybdenum (mg)
Infants	0–0.5	0.5–0.7	0.5–0.7	0.1–0.5	0.01–0.04	0.01–0.04	0.03–0.06
	0.5–1	0.7–1.0	0.7–1.0	0.2–1.0	0.02–0.06	0.02–0.06	0.04–0.08
Children	1–3	1.0–1.5	1.0–1.5	0.5–1.5	0.02–0.08	0.02–0.08	0.05–0.1
and	4–6	1.5–2.0	1.5–2.0	1.0–2.5	0.03–0.12	0.03–0.12	0.06–0.15
adolescents	7–10	2.0–2.5	2.0–3.0	1.5–2.5	0.05–0.2	0.05–0.2	0.10–0.3
	11+	2.0–3.0	2.5–5.0	1.5–2.5	0.05–0.2	0.05–0.2	0.15–0.5
Adults		2.0–3.0	2.5–5.0	1.5–4.0	0.05–0.2	0.05–0.2	0.15–0.5

	Age (Years)	Electrolytes		
		Sodium (mg)	Potassium (mg)	Chloride (mg)
Infants	0–0.5	115–350	350–925	275–700
	0.5–1	250–750	425–1275	400–1200
Children	1–3	325–975	550–1650	500–1500
and	4–6	450–1350	775–2325	700–2100
adolescents	7–10	600–1800	1000–3000	925–2775
	11+	900–2700	1525–4575	1400–4200
Adults		1100–3300	1875–5625	1700–5100

*Because there is less information on which to base allowances, these figures are not given in the main table of RDA and are provided here in the form of ranges of recommended intakes.

†Since the toxic levels for many trace elements may be only several times usual intakes, the upper levels for the trace elements given in this table should not be habitually exceeded.

Appendix 4

Foods and Mixed Dishes Classified According to Food Group and Amounts Commonly Considered as One Serving

Foods and Mixed Dishes	Amount Commonly Considered as One Serving	Food Group
Apple	1 med. 3–4 oz	Veg.-fruit
Apple juice	½ c	Veg.-fruit
Apricots	3–4 oz, 2–3 med.	Veg.-fruit
Asparagus	½ c (4 oz)	Veg.-fruit
Avocado	½ c (4 oz)	Veg.-fruit
Bacon	2 slices	Fat
Bananas	1 med.	Veg.-fruit
Beans (dry)	½ c, cooked	Meat
Beans (fresh) green or wax	½ c, cooked (4 oz)	Veg.-fruit
Beef	2–3 oz, cooked hamburger	Meat
Beet greens	½ c (4 oz)	Veg.-fruit
Beets	½ c (4 oz)	Veg.-fruit
Berries	½ c (4 oz)	Veg.-fruit
Biscuits (baking powder)	1 med., 2 in diameter	Bread-cereal
Blanc mange	½ c	Milk (½)
		Sugar, 3 tsp
Bread, corn	1 piece, 2 in square	Bread-cereal
Bread, all varieties	1 slice (1 oz)	Bread-cereal
Broccoli	½ c (4 oz)	Veg.-fruit
Brussels sprouts	½ c (4 oz)	Veg.-fruit
Butter	1 tsp	Fat
Buttermilk	1 c	Milk
Cabbage	½ c (4 oz)	Veg.-fruit
Cantaloupe	¼ med. melon	Veg.-fruit
Carrots	½ c (4 oz)	Veg.-fruit
Cauliflower	½ c (4 oz)	Veg.-fruit
Cereals, cooked (oatmeal, corn meal, Cream of Wheat, etc.)	½ c (1 oz)	Bread-cereal
Cereals, ready-to-eat, flaked or puffed	¾–1 c (1 oz)	Bread-cereal
Celery	½ c (4 oz)	Veg.-fruit
Chard	½ c (4 oz)	Veg.-fruit
Cheese, Cheddar, American, Swiss	1 oz	Milk
Cheese, cream	2 tbsp	Fat
Cheese, soft type, cottage	½ c	Milk (⅓)
Cheese bits	½ c (10–20 crackers)	Bread-cereal
Cherries	3–4 oz, 15 large	Veg.-fruit
Chicken	½ breast or 1 leg and thigh (4 oz)	Meat
Chickory	½ c (4 oz)	Veg.-fruit
Clams	3–4 oz, cooked (½) c	Meat
Cocoa, made with milk	1 c	Milk

Table continued on following page

Foods and Mixed Dishes	Amount Commonly Considered as One Serving	Food Group
Collards	½ c (4 oz)	Veg.-fruit
Corn	½ c (4 oz)	Veg.-fruit
	1 ear, 5 in	
Crackers, round, thin	6 crackers	Bread-cereal
Saltines	3 crackers	Bread-cereal
Graham	3 crackers	Bread-cereal
Oyster	24 crackers	Bread-cereal
Cress	½ c (4 oz)	Veg.-fruit
Cucumbers	½ c (4 oz)	Veg.-fruit
Custard pudding	½ c	Milk (½)
		Sugar, 3 tsp
Dandelion greens	½ c (4 oz)	Veg.-fruit
Duck	2–3 oz, cooked	Meat
Egg, in any form	2	Meat
Eggplant	½ c (4 oz)	Veg.-fruit
English muffins	1 muffin	Bread-cereal
Escarole	½ c (4 oz)	Veg.-fruit
Figs, fresh	3 small	Veg.-fruit
Fish: cod, haddock, bass, mackerel, flounder, halibut	3–4 oz, cooked	Meat
Fish chowder	1⅓ c	Meat (½)
		Milk
		Veg.-fruit (½)
Grapefruit	½ med.	Veg.-fruit
Grapes	3–4 oz, 22 Tokay; 60 green, seedless	Veg.-fruit
Greens, all kinds, cooked	½ c	Veg.-fruit
Grits	½ c (1 oz)	Bread-cereal
Guava	3 oz	Veg.-fruit
Heart	2–3 oz, cooked	Meat
Honeydew melon	¼ melon; ½ c diced	Veg.-fruit
Ice cream	½ c	Milk (¼)
Kale	½ c (4 oz)	Veg.-fruit
Kidney	2–3 oz, cooked	Meat
Lamb	2 rib chops, ½ in thick	Meat
Lentils, dried	½ c, cooked	Meat
Lettuce	½ c (4 oz)	Veg.-fruit
Liver	2–3 oz, cooked	Meat
Lobster	2–3 oz, cooked	Meat
Macaroni	½ c	Bread-cereal
Macaroni and cheese	1 c (8 oz)	Bread-cereal
		Milk
Mango	3–4 oz	Veg.-fruit
Margarine	1 tsp	Fat
Mayonnaise	1 tbsp	Fat
Meat, lean: beef, lamb, pork veal	3–4 oz	Meat
Meat loaf	3–4 oz	Meat
		Bread-cereal (¼)
Meat stew	1 c (8 oz)	Veg.-fruit
Milk, (fresh, diluted, evaporated, reconstructed, or dried)	½ c	Milk
Muffins	1 med.	Bread-cereal
Mushrooms	½ c	Veg.-fruit
Nectarines	1 med.	Veg.-fruit
Noodles	½ c	Bread-cereal
Nuts	2 tbsp, ½ oz	Meat (¼)

Foods and Mixed Dishes	Amount Commonly Considered as One Serving	Food Group
Okra	½ c (4 oz)	Veg.-fruit
Olives	10–12	Fat
Onions	½ c (4 oz)	Veg.-fruit
Oranges	1 med., 3–4 oz	Veg.-fruit
Oysters	6–8 med.	Meat
Pancakes	1, 4-in pancake	Bread-cereal
Papaya	3–4 oz (½ c)	Veg.-fruit
Parsnips	½ c (4 oz)	Veg.-fruit
Peaches	1 med., 3–4 oz	Veg.-fruit
Peanut butter	2 tbsp	Meat (½)
Pears	1 med., 3–4 oz	Veg.-Fruit
Peas, dried	½ c, cooked	Meat
Peas, fresh or canned	½ c, cooked	Veg.-fruit
Peppers	½ c (4 oz)	Veg.-fruit
Pies, cream: 1 crust (custard, squash)	⅙ of a pie	Bread-cereal (½) Milk (½) Sugar, 2 tbsp
Pies, fruit: 2 crusts (apple, berry, peach, cherry, etc.)	⅙ of a pie	Bread-cereal Veg.-fruit Sugar, 2 tbsp
Pies, lemon meringue: 1 crust	⅙ of a pie	Bread-cereal (½) Sugar, 3 tbsp
Pineapple	3–4 oz, ½ c diced	Veg.-fruit
Plums	½ c (1 med.)	Veg.-fruit
Popcorn	¾–1 c	Bread-cereal
Pork	1 chop, 1 in thick	Meat
Popovers	1 popover	Bread-cereal
Potato chips	8–10 pieces	Bread-cereal
Potatoes	1 med., 3–4 oz	Veg.-fruit
Pretzel sticks	½ c (10–20 crackers)	Bread-cereal
Prunes	4 med.	Veg.-fruit
Rabbit	2–3 oz, cooked	Meat
Radishes	½ c (4 oz)	Veg.-fruit
Rice	½ c	Bread-cereal
Rolls, plain	1 roll, medium, Parker House or Cloverleaf	Bread-cereal
Rutabaga	½ c (4 oz)	Veg.-fruit
Ry-Krisp	4 crackers	Bread-cereal
Salmon	2–3 oz, cooked	Meat
Sandwiches	2 slices bread	Bread-cereal (2)
	Filling:	
	2 oz meat, fish, chicken, egg, or peanut butter	Meat (½)
	1 slice cheese	Milk
	lettuce, tomato	Veg.-fruit
Sardines	2–3 oz	Meat
Sauerkraut	½ c	Veg.-fruit
Sausage (bologna, frankfurters, liverwurst, etc.)	2–3 oz, 3 slices 1 large or 2 small frankfurters	Meat
Shredded wheat	¾–1 c, 1 oz	Bread-cereal
Shrimp	2–3 oz, cooked	Meat
Soup, clear, chicken or beef bouillon	1 c	Meat (½)

Table continued on following page

Foods and Mixed Dishes	Amount Commonly Considered as One Serving	Food Group
Soup, cream of tomato, asparagus, corn	1 c	Milk (½)
Soup, noodle, rice, or barley	1 c	Bread-cereal (½)
Soup, vegetable	1 c	Veg.-fruit
Spaghetti	½ c	Bread-cereal
Spaghetti (Italian style) with meat sauce	1 c spaghetti ½ c meat sauce	Bread-cereal (2) Meat (½)
Spinach	½ c (4 oz)	Veg.-fruit
Squash	½ c (4 oz)	Veg.-fruit
Strawberries	3–4 oz, 1 c	Veg.-fruit
Swordfish	2–3 oz, cooked	Meat
Tangerines	3–4 oz, 1 med.	Veg.-fruit
Tapioca pudding	½ c	Milk (½) Sugar, 3 tsp
Tomatoes	1 med., 3–4 oz	Veg.-fruit
Tortillas	1 med.	Bread-cereal
Tuna	2–3 oz, cooked	Meat
Turkey	2–3 oz, cooked	Meat
Turnip greens	½ c (4 oz)	Veg.-fruit
Turnips	½ c (4 oz)	Veg.-fruit
Veal	2–3 oz, cooked	Meat
Venison	2–3 oz, cooked	Meat
Waffles	½ med.	Bread-cereal
Watermelon	1/16 of a melon, ½ c diced	Veg.-fruit
White sauce, for creamed chicken, meat, fish, or vegetables	½ c	Milk (½)
Yams	1 med.	Veg.-fruit
Yogurt	1 c	Milk

Index

Page numbers in *italic* type indicate illustrations; page numbers followed by *t* refer to tables.